Manual of Neuroanesthesia

Manual of Neuroanesthesia
The Essentials

Edited By
Hemanshu Prabhakar
Charu Mahajan
Indu Kapoor

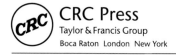

CRC Press
Taylor & Francis Group
Boca Raton London New York

CRC Press is an imprint of the
Taylor & Francis Group, an **informa** business

CRC Press
Taylor & Francis Group
6000 Broken Sound Parkway NW, Suite 300
Boca Raton, FL 33487-2742

© 2017 by Taylor & Francis Group, LLC
CRC Press is an imprint of Taylor & Francis Group, an Informa business

No claim to original U.S. Government works

Printed and bound in India by Replika Press Pvt. Ltd.

Printed on acid-free paper

International Standard Book Number-13: 978-1-4987-7170-2 (Hardback)

Visit the Taylor & Francis Web site at
http://www.taylorandfrancis.com

and the CRC Press Web site at
http://www.crcpress.com

Dedication

To our parents, teachers, and families, our "Pillars of Strength" – Pallavi Prabhakar, Atul Sharma, and Deepak Kapoor, and ones who make our world complete, Anavi, Namyah, Amyra, Nyra, and Ansh

Table of Contents

Foreword

It is a pleasure to contribute the foreword to *Manual of Neuroanesthesia: The Essentials*, an excellent book, brilliantly conceived and edited for rapid reference by the "occasional neuroanesthetist." Most of the currently available books on neuroanesthesia have been written primarily for "dedicated neuroanesthetists"; they can be quite overwhelming for residents, trainees, or private practitioners in general anesthesia practice, who have not been formally trained in neuroanesthesia but often need to manage patients with primary or concomitant neurosurgical/neurological disorders. This book addresses this gap. It has concise yet comprehensive "hands-on" information about the anesthetic management of these patients; Parts VII and XI are highly recommended. Additional chapters on basic principles of neuroanesthesia, neuroradiology, neurology, and critical care skillfully supplement this practical information and also make it a useful resource book for novice neuroanesthetists. Contributors to this book span the globe and are experts in their areas of clinical coverage. The language is simple and lucid; the chapters are short and easy to read. This book certainly occupies a niche among books on neuroanesthesia.

Monica S. Tandon

Preface

Manual of Neuroanesthesia: The Essentials covers all important aspects of neuroanesthesia and provides an overview of the subject.

This book is mainly targeted to "occasional neuroanesthesiologists," anesthesiologists who have not received any formal training in "neuroanesthesia" but occasionally provide anesthesia for patients related to various disciplines in neurosciences. This book gives basic details of neuroanesthesia and how management of different neurosurgical cases may differ. Simple issues such as neurological examination of patients and understanding CT and MRI scans along with anesthetic management are discussed in simple language, which would make this book a ready reckoner.

This book will also be useful for any medical practitioner associated with neurosurgical and allied branches such as neurology and neuroradiology. It will provide a quick and easy guide to understanding neuroanesthesia. It also provides insight into all possible aspects of anesthetic management of neurosurgical and commonly encountered neurological patients. It includes chapters related to allied specialities such as critical care, neurology, and neuroradiology.

The authors have done an excellent job writing chapters in the simplest manner for the targeted audience. In view of keeping the interest of readers, the authors have provided information on the discussed topic in the form of figures, elaborate tables, and boxes. We hope that this will engage them and help them to form their own differential diagnosis and plan a suitable anesthetic protocol for each situation. We also hope that patients will benefit from our readers' knowledge gained from this book. The editors are grateful to all the contributors who have made this work possible in a wonderful way.

Indu Kapoor
Charu Mahajan
Hemanshu Prabhakar

Editors

Hemanshu Prabhakar is a Professor in the Department of Neuroanaesthesiology and Critical Care at the All India Institute of Medical Sciences (AIIMS), New Delhi, India. He received his training in neuroanesthesia and completed his PhD at the same institute. He is a recipient of the AIIMS Excellence Award for notable contribution in academics and has more than 200 publications in national and international journals. Dr. Prabhakar is a reviewer for various national and international journals. He is also a review author for the Cochrane Collaboration and has a special interest in the evidence-based practice of neuroanesthesia. Dr. Prabhakar is a member of various national and international neuroanesthesia societies and is past secretary of the Indian Society of Neuroanesthesia and Critical Care. He has been an invited faculty for various national and international conferences. He is on the editorial board of the Indian Journal of Palliative Care and is the executive editor of the *Journal of Neuroanaesthesiology and Critical Care.*

Charu Mahajan is an Assistant Professor in the Department of Neuroanaesthesiology and Critical Care at the All India Institute of Medical Sciences (AIIMS), New Delhi, India. After completing her MD in anaesthesia, she did her DM neuroanaesthesia course at AIIMS and later joined the faculty in the parent department. She has over 60 publications in recognized national and international journals. She is a review author for the Cochrane Collaboration, and has authored chapters in various national and international books. She has received numerous awards for scientific paper presentations. Dr. Mahaja is a member of national and international societies and is a reviewer for various journals.

Indu Kapoor is an Assistant Professor in Neuroanesthesiology and Critical Care at the All India Institute of Medical Sciences (AIIMS), New Delhi, India. She received her training in neuroanesthesia at the same institute. She is the recipient of Dr. T N Jha Memorial Award awarded by the Indian Society of Anaesthesiologists (ISA) on the state and national level at Delhi and Chennai 2009. She has received the Smt. Chandra and Sh. Narayan Wadhwani Memorial Award for Best Outgoing Postgraduate in Anesthesia in University College of Medical Sciences, Delhi, in 2010. She has over 30 publications in national and international journals. She is a reviewer for national journals and is also a review author for the Cochrane Collaboration. Dr. Kapoor has special interest in the evidence-based practice of neuroanesthesia and is a member of various national societies. She is an invited faculty for various national conferences and has contributed chapters to various national and international books.

Contributors

Farzana Afroze
Albany Medical Center
Albany, New York

Alaa Abd-Elsayed
Department of Anesthesiology
University of Wisconsin School of Medicine
    and Public Health
Madison, Wisconsin

Zulfiqar Ali
SKIMS
Srinagar, Jammu and Kashmir, India

John Andrzejowski
Royal Hallamshire Hospital and
Sheffield Teaching Hospitals
    NHS Trust
Sheffield, UK

Salman Al Jerdi
University of Iowa
Burlington, Vermont

Marc-Alain Babi
Duke University
Durham, North Carolina

Sujoy Banik
Medanta - The Medicity
Gurugram, India

Hemant Bhagat
Postgraduate Institute of Medical Education
    and Research
Chandigarh, India

Prasanna U. Bidkar
JIPMER
Pondicherry, India

Rebecca Campbell
St Georges Healthcare Trust
London, UK

Nicole Collins
University of Wisconsin School of Medicine
    and Public Health
Madison, Wisconsin

Andrew Davidson
Royal Hallamshire Hospital
Sheffield, UK

S. Leve Joseph Devarajan
AIIMS
New Delhi, India

Judith Dinsmore
St Georges Healthcare Trust
London, UK

Jake Drinkwater
Royal Hallamshire Hospital
Sheffield, UK

Radhika Dua
SMS Medical College
Jaipur, India

Melissa Ehlers
Albany Medical Center
Albany, New York

Peter Farling
Royal Victoria Hospital
Belfast, Ireland, UK

Elizabeth A. M. Frost
Mount Sinai Medical Center, New York
New York, New York

Ravi K. Grandhi
College of Medicine, University of Cincinnati
Cincinnati, Ohio

Vinod K. Grover
Postgraduate Institute of Medical Education
    and Research
Chandigarh, India

Nidhi Gupta
Indraprastha Apollo Hospitals
New Delhi, India

Matthew J. Hammer
Northwestern University
Chicago, Illinois

Laura B. Hemmer
Northwestern University
Chicago, Illinois

Bhavna Hooda
Base Hospital
New Delhi, India

Michael L James
Duke University
Durham, North Carolina

Kiran Jangra
Postgraduate Institute of Medical Education
    and Research
Chandigarh, India

Stefan Jankowski
Royal Hallamshire Hospital
Sheffield, UK

Kavitha Jayaram
Nizam's Institute of Medical Sciences
Hyderabad, India

Majid Jehangir
SKIMS
Srinagar, Jammu and Kashmir, India

Sonia Kapil
Postgraduate Institute of Medical Education
    and Research
Chandigarh, India

Ankur Luthra
Postgraduate Institute of Medical Education
    and Research
Chandigarh, India

Katie Megaw
Royal Victoria Hospital
Belfast, Ireland, UK

Narmadha Lakshmi K.
JIPMER
Pondicherry, India

Samuel Y. Lee
Cleveland Clinic
USA

Helena Oechsner
Albany Medical Center
Albany, New York

Hemanshu Prabhakar
AIIMS
New Delhi, India

M. V. S. Satya Prakash
JIPMER
Pondicherry, India

Shobha Purohit
SMS Medical College
Jaipur, India

Yasir N. Shah
SKIMS
Srinagar, India

Altan Sahin
Hacettepe University School of Medicine
Turkey

Shaheen Shaikh
UMass Memorial Hospital
Worcester, Massachusetts

Gyaninder P. Singh
AIIMS
New Delhi, India

Vasudha Singhal
Medanta—The Medicity
Gurugram, India

Srilata Moningi
Nizam's Institute of Medical Sciences
Hyderabad, India

Swagata Tripathy
AIIMS, Bhubaneswar
India

Jamie Uejima
Northwestern University
Chicago, Illinois

Filiz Uzumcugil
Hacettepe University School of Medicine
Turkey

Ryan J. Vealey
Northwestern University
Chicago, Illinois

Sally H. Vitali
Boston Children's Hospital
Boston, Massachusetts

Basic principles of neuroanesthesia

Anatomical considerations

GYANINDER P SINGH

Introduction

The nervous system in humans can be divided into two main parts, the *central nervous system* and the *peripheral nervous system*. The brain and spinal cord form the main divisions of the central nervous system (CNS). The cranial and spinal nerves along with their ganglia comprise the peripheral nervous system (Table 1.1). The organization of nervous system is shown in the flow chart.

Central nervous system

Brain

The skull houses the brain and is composed of 28 bones that are mostly paired, but those situated in the midline are unpaired. Internally, the skull cavity is divided into the anterior, middle, and posterior cranial fossa. Vessels and nerves pass in and out of the skull through various foramina (Table 1.2).

The CNS develops from a hollow cylindrical tube called the *neural tube*. During embryogenesis, the developing brain (i.e., anterior part of the neural tube) is seen to be divided into five continuous parts (*telencephalon, diencephalon, mesencephalon, metencephalon,* and *myelencephalon*)

from anterior to posterior. As the developing brain enlarges, some regions overgrow the other areas. Thus, some areas get submerged (hidden from the surface) as the brain grows and folds over itself.[1] The cavity of the neural tube is retained as *ventricles* in the brain and *central canal* in the spinal cord, which forms a continuous channel filled with cerebrospinal fluid (CSF) (Figure 1.1).

Gross anatomy of the brain

The brain is enclosed in a bony cranial cavity and is surrounded by three layers of meninges: the outer *dura mater*, the middle *arachnoid mater*, and the innermost *pia mater*. The brain is divided into the forebrain, midbrain, and hindbrain[2] (Figure 1.2).

Forebrain

This is divided into the diencephalon (central part) and the telencephalon or *cerebrum*. Hidden from the surface of the brain, the diencephalon consists of a dorsal *thalamus* and a ventral *hypothalamus*, and the *subthalamus* and *epithalamus* as its other divisions. The thalamus is an important station for all sensory systems except the olfactory pathway. The subthalamus consists of the cranial part of *red nucleus* and the *substantia nigra*. The epithalamus consists of the *habenular nuclei* and the *pineal gland*. The habenular nucleus is the center for integration of the olfactory,

Organization of nervous system

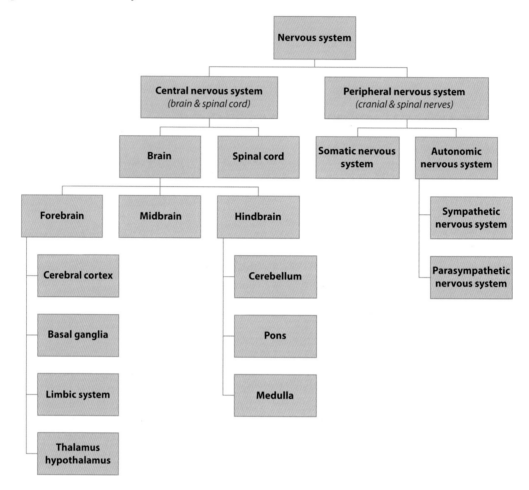

Table 1.1 Division of Nervous System and Cavities of the Brain and Spinal Cord

Central nervous system

	Cavities
a. Brain	
Forebrain (or prosencephalon)	
Telencephalon	Right and left lateral ventricles
Cerebral cortex, basal ganglia, limbic system	
Diencephalon	Third ventricle
Thalamus, hypothalamus	
Midbrain (or mesencephalon)	Cerebral aqueduct
Hindbrain (or rhombencephalon)	Fourth ventricle
Metencephalon	
Pons	
Cerebellum	
Myelencephalon	
Medulla oblongata	

(Continued)

b. Spinal cord   Central canal
   Cervical segments
   Thoracic segments
   Lumbar segments
   Coccygeal segments
Peripheral nervous system
a. Cranial nerves and their ganglia (12 pairs)
   12 cranial (I–XII) nerves
b. Spinal nerves and their ganglia (31 pairs)
   08 cervical
   12 thoracic
   05 lumbar
   05 sacral
   01 coccygeal

Table 1.2 Foramina of Skull and Structure Passing through Them

Cranial fossae (bones forming)	Foramina	Structures passing
Anterior cranial fossa	Cribriform plate of ethmoid	Olfactory nerve filaments
		Anterior ethmoidal nerves and vessels
(frontal, ethmoid,	Foramen cecum	Emissary vein
sphenoid: body	Anterior ethmoidal canal	Anterior ethmoidal nerve and vessels
and lesser wing)	Posterior ethmoidal canal	Posterior ethmoidal nerves and vessels
Middle cranial fossa	Optic canal	Optic nerve surrounded by meninges
(parietal, temporal,	Superior orbital fissure	Ophthalmic artery nerves: oculomotor, trochlear, abducent, lacrimal, frontal, nasociliary nerve, filaments from internal carotid artery, sympathetic plexus
sphenoid: body and greater wing)		Vessels: orbital branch of middle meningeal artery, recurrent branch of ophthalmic artery, superior ophthalmic vein, inferior ophthalmic vein
	Foramen rotundum	Maxillary nerve
	Foramen ovale	Mandibular nerve
		Accessory meningeal artery
		Lesser petrosal nerve
		Emissary vein
	Foramen spinosum	Meningeal branch of mandibular nerve
		Middle meningeal vessels
	Foramen lacerum	Internal carotid artery
		Greater petrosal nerve
		Deep petrosal nerve
		Nerve of pterygoid canal
		Meningeal branch of ascending pharyngeal artery
		Emissary vein
	Petrosal or innominate foramen (occasionally present)	Lesser petrosal nerve (if not through foramen ovale)

(Continued)

Table 1.2 Foramina of Skull and Structure Passing through Them *(Continued)*

Cranial fossae (*bones forming*)	Foramina	Structures passing
	Hiatus for greater petrosal nerve	Greater petrosal nerve
		Petrosal branch of middle meningeal artery
	Hiatus for lesser petrosal nerve	Lesser petrosal nerve
Posterior cranial fossa	Internal acoustic meatus	Facial nerve
		Vestibulocochlear nerve
(*occipital, temporal: petrous part*)	Jugular foramen	Labyrinthine artery
		Glossopharyngeal nerve
		Vagus nerve
		Accessory nerve Inferior petrosal sinus
		Internal jugular vein
		Meningeal branch of occipital artery
	Hypoglossal canal	Hypoglossal nerve and it srecurrent meningeal branch
		Meningeal branch of ascending pharyngeal artery
		Emissary vein
	Condylar canal	Meningeal branch of occipital artery
		Emissary vein
	Mastoid foramen	Meningeal branch of occipital artery
		Emissary vein
	Foramen magnum	Apical ligament of dens
		Tentorial membrane
		Medulla oblongata and meninges
		Lower end of cerebellar tonsils
		Spinal part of accessory nerve
		Meningeal branches of upper cervical nerves
		Vertebral arteries
		Anterior spinal artery
		Posterior spinal arteries

visceral, and somatic afferent pathways. The pineal gland does not contain nerve cells but adrenergic sympathetic fibers derived from the superior cervical sympathetic ganglia. The hypothalamus controls and integrates the functions of the autonomic nervous system and the endocrine system and plays a vital role in maintaining body homeostasis.[2]

The cerebrum forms the largest part of the brain and is grossly divided into four lobes: frontal, parietal, temporal, and occipital by the midline *interhemispheric fissure*, the *central sulcus*, and the lateral *Sylvian fissures* (Figure 1.3). It consists of two hemispheres connected by *corpus callosum* which is a mass of white matter. The hemispheres contain numerous *sulci (fissures)* and *gyri (folds)*. The cavity present in cerebral hemispheres is the *lateral ventricle*, which communicates with the third ventricle

through the *interventricular foramen (foramen of Monro)*. The two hemispheres are separated by the *longitudinal fissure* into which projects the *falx cerebri*. Within the hemispheres is a large mass of gray matter, the *basal ganglia*. The corona radiata is a collection of nerve fibers that pass to and from the cerebral cortex to the brain stem. *The internal capsule* is a part of the corona radiata that converges to pass between the basal ganglia.[2]

Midbrain

This connects the forebrain to the hindbrain and measures about 2 cm. It contains the cavity known as the *cerebral aqueduct (aqueduct of Sylvius)*. The aqueduct connects the third and fourth ventricles.

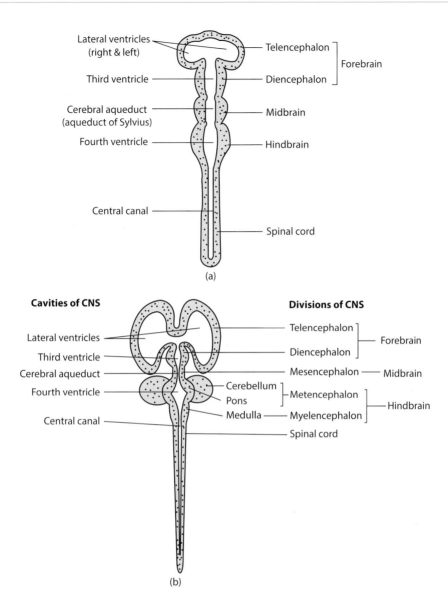

Figure 1.1 Longitudinal section of the brain and spinal cord showing cavities of different parts of the central nervous system (CNS). (a) Neural tube with various bulging or vesicles. (b) Vesicles of the brain forming different parts of the brain and spinal cord with their respective cavities.

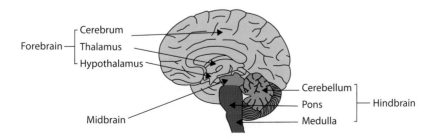

Figure 1.2 Division of the brain into forebrain, midbrain, and hindbrain.

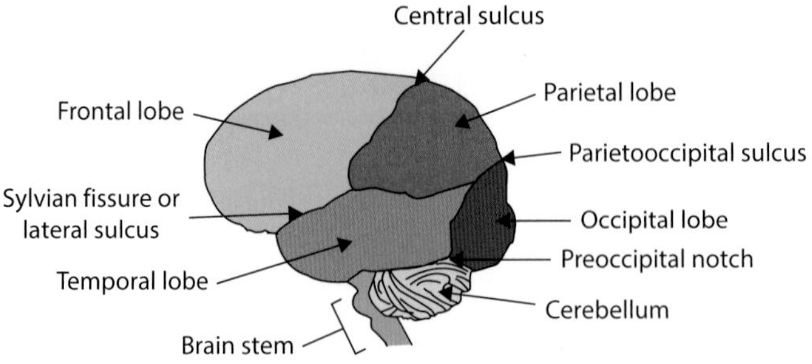

Figure 1.3 Lobes of the cerebrum (frontal, parietal, temporal, and occipital lobes) and the sulci dividing these lobes.

Hindbrain

This comprises the *medulla oblongata, pons,* and *cerebellum*. Both the medulla oblongata and the pons contain various nuclei and ascending and descending nerve tracts. Lying within the posterior fossa, the two cerebellar hemispheres are united by a *vermis* and connected to the midbrain, pons, and medulla oblongata through the *superior, middle,* and *inferior cerebellar peduncles*. The cerebellum unconsciously controls the smooth contraction of voluntary muscles and coordinates their actions, together with the relaxation of their antagonists.[3] The cavity of the hindbrain is called the *fourth ventricle.*

Brain stem

This comprises the medulla oblongata, pons, and midbrain and connects the spinal cord with the forebrain. The brainstem occupies the posterior cranial fossa and has important vital centers such as respiratory, cardiovascular, and center for consciousness. It also contains the nuclei for cranial nerves III through XII. It serves as a conduit for the ascending and the descending tracts connecting the spinal cord to the higher centers in the forebrain.

Arterial supply of the brain

The brain is supplied by the right and left internal carotid arteries (branches of common carotid artery) and the right and left vertebral arteries (branches of subclavian artery). The four arteries lie in the subarachnoid space in the cranial cavity.[2]

The *internal carotid artery* perforates the base of skull through the carotid canal and enters the cranial cavity through the foramen lacerum. It then runs through the cavernous sinus (S-shaped course) and perforates the dura mater and arachnoid mater to lie in the subarachnoid space and reach the lateral cerebral sulcus (Sylvian sulcus) where it ends by dividing into *anterior* and *middle cerebral arteries.*

The *vertebral artery* ascends through the foramen transversarium of the upper six cervical vertebrae and enters the skull through the foramen magnum. It pierces the dura mater and arachnoid mater to enter the subarachnoid space. The right and left vertebral arteries join at the lower border of the pons to form the *basilar artery*, which ascends on the ventral surface of the pons and divides into the *right* and *left posterior cerebral artery* at the upper border of the pons. The internal carotid and the vertebrobasilar systems anastomose in the interpeduncular fossa at the base of the brain forming the *circle of Willis* or *circulus arteriosus*[2] (Figure 1.4).

Arterial supply of the cerebral cortex

The cerebral cortex is supplied by the anterior, middle, and posterior cerebral arteries (Figure 1.5). The anterior, middle, and posterior cerebral arteries give rise to cortical and central branches. The cortical branches supply the cortex while the central or perforating branches penetrate deep into the substance of the cerebral hemisphere to supply deeper structures (such as the internal capsule, thalamus, hypothalamus, caudate nucleus, putamen, and globus pallidus). The cortical arteries give rise to branches that run perpendicularly into the substance of cerebral cortex. These are terminal or end arteries and do not anastomose with neighboring arteries. Blockage of these branches leads to necrosis of brain tissue supplied by that branch.[4]

Arterial supply of the brain stem

The *medulla* is supplied by the branches of vertebral arteries, namely anterior and posterior spinal arteries, posterior inferior cerebellar artery, and direct branches to medulla.

Arteries and their branches supplying the brain

Artery	Branches
Internal carotid arteries	Ophthalmic artery
	Posterior communicating artery
	Anterior choroidal artery
	Anterior cerebral artery
	Middle cerebral artery
Vertebral artery	Posterior inferior cerebellar artery
	Medullar arteries
	Posterior spinal artery
	Anterior spinal artery
	Meningeal artery
Basilar artery	Posterior cerebral artery
	Superior cerebellar artery
	Pontine arteries
	Labyrinthine arteries
	Anterior inferior cerebellar artery

Arteries contributing to the formation of the circle of Willis

- Anterior communicating artery
- Right and left anterior cerebral arteries
- Right and left internal carotid arteries
- Right and left posterior communicating arteries
- Right and left posterior cerebral arteries

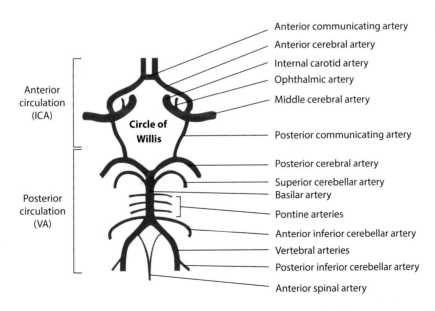

Figure 1.4 Arteries supplying the brain (note the formation of Circle of Willis). ICA, internal carotid artery; VA, vertebral artery.

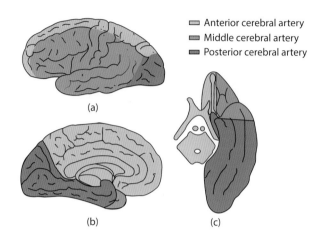

Anterior cerebral artery
Middle cerebral artery
Posterior cerebral artery

(a)

(b)   (c)

Figure 1.5 Arteries supplying the cerebral hemispheres: (a) superolateral surface, (b) medial surface, and (c) inferior surface.

The *pons* is supplied by the branches of the basilar artery, namely the anterior inferior cerebellar and superior cerebellar arteries and the pontine arteries.

The *midbrain* is mainly supplied by the branches of the basilar artery, namely the posterior cerebral arteries, superior cerebellar arteries, and direct branches from the basilar artery. It also receives branches from posterior communicating arteries.

Arterial supply of the cerebellum

The cerebellum is supplied by superior cerebellar and anterior inferior cerebellar arteries (branches of the basilar artery) and posterior inferior cerebellar arteries (branch of the vertebral artery).

Venous drainage of the brain

Veins draining the cerebral hemisphere consist of superficial and deep veins. Superficial veins drain the cerebral cortex and end in the neighboring venous sinuses, which are *superior cerebral veins, inferior cerebral veins*, and *superficial middle cerebral veins*. Deep veins drain the deeper structures (such as the thalamus, hypothalamus, caudate nucleus, putamen, internal capsule, corpus callosum, and choroid plexus) and join to form two *internal cerebral veins* and two *basal veins*. These veins drain into the *great cerebral vein* (*great vein of Galen*) that ends in the straight sinus. The cerebellum is drained by the *superior* and *inferior cerebellar veins* into the straight sinus and other neighboring venous sinuses.[1] The veins from the brain stem drain into the adjoining venous sinuses and inferiorly the veins from the medulla are continuous with the veins of the spinal cord.

All the veins draining the brain ultimately open into the various dural sinuses (i.e., superior sagittal, inferior sagittal, straight, cavernous, sphenoparietal, petrosal, occipital, transverse, and sigmoid sinuses). Blood from all these sinuses reaches the sigmoid sinus that ultimately drains into the internal jugular vein (Figure 1.6).

Nerve supply to the brain

The brain receives sensory stimuli and sends motor impulses to different parts of the body but is devoid of any sensation. However, the dura mater covering the brain and spinal cord possesses numerous sensory endings that are sensitive to stretching. The branches from the trigeminal, vagus, and the first three cervical spinal nerves and the branches from the cervical sympathetic trunk supply the dura covering the brain. Stimulation of the sensory endings in the dura produces referred pain to an area of skin supplied by these nerves, for example, from the supratentorial region, pain is referred to the skin of the head and face supplied by the trigeminal nerve and from the infratentorial region to the back of the neck and scalp (distribution of C2,C3).

The sympathetic fibers pass along the arteries forming the plexus over these vessels. These are postganglionic sympathetic fibers and stimulation of these causes vasoconstriction of the arteries supplying the brain.[5]

Spinal cord

The spinal cord is enclosed within a vertebral column that consists of 33 vertebrae: 7 cervical,

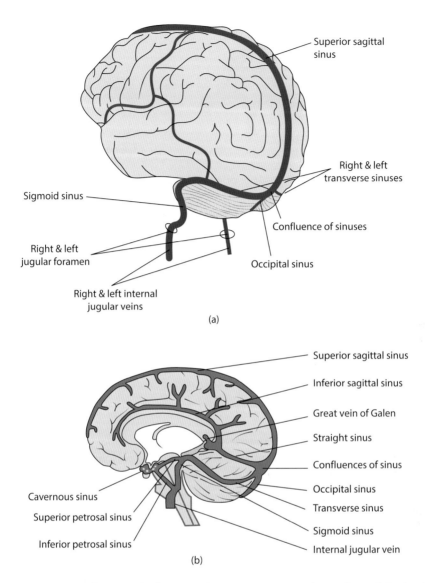

Figure 1.6 Venous sinuses draining the brain. (a) Venous sinuses on the surface of the brain. (b) Venous sinuses seen after removing the cerebral hemisphere on one side.

12 thoracic, 5 lumbar, 5 sacral, and 5 coccygeal vertebrae. A series of pairs of lateral intervertebral foramina transmits the spinal nerves and their associated vessels between adjacent vertebrae. The vertebral column has primary thoracic and pelvic curvatures that are convex dorsally. The secondary curvatures are the cervical and the lumbar lordoses (convex forward).[5] A typical vertebra has a ventral body, a dorsal vertebral arch, and a vertebral foramen. On each side of the arch are the pedicle and the lamina. The transverse processes arise from the junction of the pedicle and the lamina. The spinous process or vertebral spine projects

dorsally and caudally from the junction of the laminae (Figure 1.7). The *first cervical* or *atlas vertebra* is typically ring shaped and contains a transverse foramen that transmits the vertebral artery. The *second cervical* or *axis vertebra* is typically identified by the presence of the *odontoid process* or *dens*, projecting upward from the body. The *seventh cervical vertebra* or *vertebra prominence* has a prominent spinous process and is easily felt at the lower end of nuchal furrow. All thoracic vertebrae display lateral costal facets for articulation with the head and tubercle of the ribs. Lumbar vertebrae are large and do not contain costal facets and

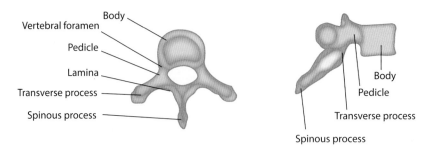

Figure 1.7 Parts of a typical vertebra: (a) superior view and (b) lateral view.

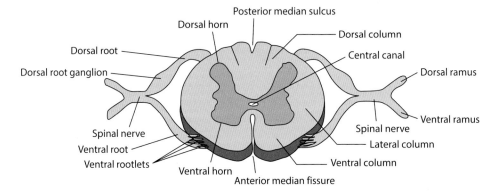

Figure 1.8 Transverse section of the spinal cord.

the intervertebral foramina. The five sacral vertebrae fuse to form the sacrum that is triangular in shape and articulates with the coccyx below. The coccyx is a small rudimentary bone that often fuses with the sacrum in later decades of life.

Gross anatomy of the spinal cord

The spinal cord begins as a continuation of the medulla oblongata at the foramen magnum and terminates at the level of the lower border of the first lumbar vertebra in adults. In children, it extends to the upper border of the third vertebra. In the cervical and lumbar regions, the cord is expanded into fusiform shape and is known as the *cervical* and *lumbar enlargement*, respectively. The lower end of the cord tapers to form *conus medullaris*. The dura and arachnoid mater along with the subarachnoid space containing CSF extend beyond the lower end of the cord up to the second sacral vertebra. The pia mater extends below the conus medullaris to form the *filum terminale* that ends by attaching to the first coccyx vertebra.[6] Thirty-one pairs of spinal nerves are attached to the spinal cord by the anterior or ventral (*motor*) roots and posterior or dorsal (*sensory*) roots. Each posterior root has a

ganglion (*dorsal root ganglion*) that contains cells giving rise to peripheral and central nerve fibers. Internally, the spinal cord has a core of gray matter surrounded by white matter. The butterfly-shaped gray matter has dorsal and ventral projections or *horns* (Figure 1.8). In the center of the spinal gray matter lies the vestigial ventricular system, the *central canal*.[6]

In general, the ascending sensory fibers are related to the general senses (touch, pain, pressure, vibration, heat, and proprioception). These fibers consist of third-order neurons extending from the peripheral receptor to the contralateral cerebral cortex. Primary fibers for pain, temperature, coarse touch, and pressure are carried via the *spinothalamic tract* in the spinal cord.[7] The *lateral spinothalamic tracts* are responsible for carrying pain and temperature sensations while the pressure and coarse touch sensations are carried by the *anterior spinothalamic tract*. Fibers for vibration, proprioception, and fine touch constitute the *dorsal* or *posterior white columns* (*fasciculus gracilis* and *fasciculus cuneatus*) of the spinal cord. The muscle joint sense is carried by the *anterior* and *posterior spinocerebellar tracts*. The ascending sensory tracts reach the thalamus and their third-order neurons, passing through the internal capsule, reach the cerebral cortex, where they terminate in the *postcentral gyrus* of the parietal lobe (*primary somatosensory cortex*). The *descending motor fibers* originate from the widespread areas of the cerebral cortex. Fibers terminating in the brain stem are termed *corticobulbar fibers* and they control the activity of the brain stem neurons. The *corticospinal fibers* descend into the spinal cord. Throughout the midbrain, pons, and medulla oblongata, groups of scattered nerve cells and fibers exist and are collectively known as *reticular formation*. The reticular formation controls the voluntary movement, the reflex activity, and also the autonomic activity.[7]

Arterial supply of the spinal cord

The spinal cord is supplied by three longitudinal arteries that run along its entire length. These are the *anterior spinal artery* and the two *posterior spinal arteries* (branches of vertebral arteries). Blood from the vertebral arteries reaches only up to the cervical segments of the cord. Lower down, the anterior and posterior spinal arteries are reinforced by the multiple small arteries, the *radicular arteries*. These radicular arteries arise from the spinal branches of the arteries outside the vertebral column (namely vertebral, ascending cervical, deep cervical, intercostal, lumbar, and sacral arteries), which reach the spinal cord through the intervertebral foramen along with the nerve roots.

One of the anterior radicular branches is often very large and is called the *arteria radicularis magna* (*artery of Adamkiewicz*).[2,8] Its position is variable but usually arises at the lower thoracic or upper lumbar vertebral level and may be responsible for supplying blood to the lower two-thirds of the spinal cord.[8]

The anterior spinal artery supplies the anterior two-thirds and the posterior spinal arteries supplies the posterior one-third of the spinal cord (Figure 1.9). The branches from the anterior and posterior spinal arteries anastomose to form the arterial plexus in the pia mater covering the spinal cord called the *arterial vasocorona* that sends branches into the substance of the cord.

Venous drainage of the spinal cord

Veins draining the spinal cord are arranged in six longitudinal channels, which are the *anteromedian* and *posteromedian channels* in the midline, and the *anterolateral* and *posterolateral channels* on each side. These channels are interconnected forming venous plexus. Blood from these channels is drained by *radicular veins* into another plexus of veins lying outside the dura mater (*epidural venous plexus*), which in turn drains into various segmental veins outside the vertebral column.

Nerve supply of the spinal cord

Similar to the brain, the spinal cord in itself is devoid of sensations. The dura mater covering the spinal cord possesses numerous sensory endings

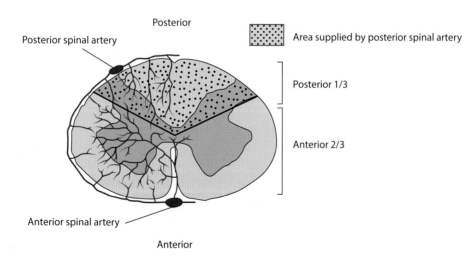

Figure 1.9 Transverse section of the spinal cord showing the area supplied by the anterior and posterior spinal arteries.

that are sensitive to stretching. *Meningeal branches from each spinal nerve* innervate the dura along the length of the spinal cord. Pain from the dura mater is referred to the area of skin supplied by that spinal nerve. Sympathetic fibers reach the dura along the blood vessels and are vasoconstrictor in function.

Peripheral nervous system

Cranial nerves

Twelve pairs of cranial nerves arise directly from the brain (Figure 1.10). The cranial nerves are labeled with Roman numerals I to XII. Some of the cranial nerves are either entirely sensory or entirely motor while others are mixed. The cranial nerves have central sensory and/or motor nuclei within the brain and their peripheral nerve fibers leave the cranium by passing through various foramina in the skull (Table 1.3).[9] All are distributed in the head and neck except the X cranial nerve that supplies the structures in the thorax and in the abdomen as well.

Spinal nerves

Thirty-one pairs of spinal nerves originate from the spinal cord. They are all mixed nerves, and they provide a two-way communication system between the spinal cord and parts of the arms, legs, neck, and trunk of the body. Although spinal nerves do not have individual names, they are grouped according to the level at which they arise from spinal cord, and each nerve is numbered in sequence. Hence, there are 8 pairs of *cervical nerves* (C1–C8), 12 pairs of *thoracic nerves* (T1–T12), 5 pairs of *lumbar nerves* (L1–L5), 5 pairs of *sacral nerves* (S1–S5), and 1 pair of coccygeal nerves (Co1). The nerves coming from the upper part of the spinal cord pass outward nearly horizontally, while those from the lower regions descend at sharp angles. This is the consequence of growth difference between the spinal cord and the vertebral column. In early life, the spinal cord extends the entire length of the vertebral column, but with age, the column grows faster than the cord. As a result, the adult spinal cord ends at the level between the first and second lumbar vertebrae, so the lumbar, sacral, and coccygeal nerves descend to their exits beyond the end of the cord.[9] Roots of the lumbar and sacral nerves below the level of termination of the spinal cord form a bundle of nerves descending vertically, which resembles the tail of a horse and is called the *cauda equine.*

Each spinal nerve is connected to the spinal cord by anterior (ventral) and posterior (dorsal) roots (Figure 1.10). The anterior root consists of efferent (motor) nerve fibers while the posterior root consists of afferent (sensory) nerve fibers. The posterior root contains a ganglion known as the *posterior* or *dorsal root ganglion*, which contains the cell body

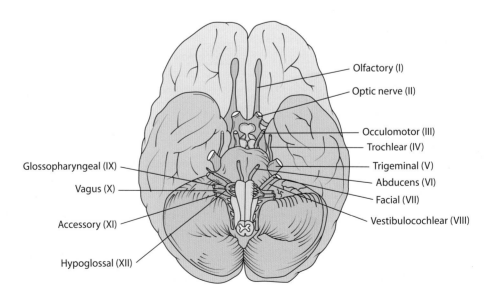

Figure 1.10 Origin of cranial nerves from the brain.

Table 1.3 Cranial Nerves

Cranial nerve	Name	Foramen	Structure supplied
I	Olfactory nerve	Cribriform plate of ethmoid	Nose (olfactory mucosa)
II	Optic nerve	Optic canal	Eyeball (rods and cones of retina)
III	Oculomotor nerve	Superior orbital fissure	Muscles of eyeball movement (superior rectus, medial rectus, inferior rectus, inferior oblique) Sphincter pupillae
IV	Trochlear nerve	Superior orbital fissure	Superior oblique
V	Trigeminal nerve	V1: superior orbital fissure V2: foramen rotundum V3: foramen ovale	Face (sensory) Muscles of mastication, tensor tympani, tensor palati
VI	Abducens nerve	Superior orbital fissure	Lateral rectus
VII	Facial nerve	Internal acoustic meatus	Posterior external ear canal, anterior 2/3 tongue (taste), facial muscles, salivary glands, lacrimal glands
VIII	Vestibulocochlear or auditory nerve	Internal acoustic meatus	Cochlea and vestibule of inner ear
IX	Glossopharyngeal nerve	Jugular foramen	Posterior 1/3 tongue (sensory), posterior 1/3 tongue (taste), middle ear, carotid body/sinus, stylopharyngeus, parotid gland
X	Vagus nerve	Jugular foramen	External ear, aortic arch/body, epiglottis, soft palate, pharynx, larynx, lungs, heart, gut except large intestine
XI	Accessory nerve	Jugular foramen	Trapezius sternocleidomastoid
XII	Hypoglossal nerve	Hypoglossal canal	Muscles of tongue

of the sensory neurons. The two nerve roots unite to form the spinal nerve. The spinal nerve divides into a large *anterior (ventral) ramus* and a small *posterior (dorsal) ramus* (Figure 1.11). The posterior ramus passes posteriorly to supply the skin and muscles of the back. The anterior ramus continues anteriorly and further divides into the anterior and lateral cutaneous branches to supply the muscles and skin over the anterior and lateral wall of the body (thorax and abdomen) and the muscles and skin of the limbs (cervical, lumbar, and sacral spinal nerves). The thoracic and upper 2 or 3 lumbar spinal nerves also give rise to branches to the paravertebral sympathetic trunk called white and gray rami communicantes.[2,9]

Autonomic nervous system

The autonomic nervous system controls the involuntary activities of various organs in the body and innervate structures such as the heart, blood vessels, smooth muscles, and glands. It is divided into sympathetic and parasympathetic nervous systems. Both the sympathetic and parasympathetic nervous systems have afferent and efferent nerve fibers that are distributed through the cranial and peripheral nerves.[2,3]

Sympathetic nervous system

Sympathetic nerve fibers (efferent) emerge from the first thoracic (T1) to second lumbar (L2) segment of the spinal cord (thoracolumbar outflow).

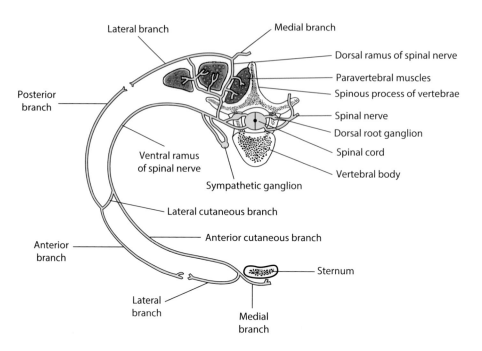

Figure 1.11 Spinal nerve and its branches.

This part of the spinal cord (T1-L2) possesses a *lateral horn* in addition to anterior and posterior horns present in the other part of the spinal cord. The cell body of the *sympathetic connector neuron* is located in the lateral horn of the spinal cord (Figure 1.12).[3] The myelinated axons of these cells pass through the anterior nerve root of the spinal nerve. From the spinal nerve, these fibers pass via the *white rami communicantes* to reach the paravertebral ganglion of the sympathetic trunk on either side of the vertebral column. These are the *preganglionic fibers*. Sympathetic trunks (or sympathetic chains) are elongated chains of sympathetic nerve fibers running along each side of the vertebral column (paravertebral) with a number of sympathetic ganglia along its length. The number of ganglia is variable.[8] Generally, there are 3 ganglia in the cervical region (superior, middle, and inferior cervical ganglia), 11–12 ganglia in the thoracic region, 4–5 ganglia in the lumbar region, and 4–5 ganglia in the sacral region. The two trunks end by joining caudally to form a single ganglion called the *ganglion impar*.[8] The inferior cervical and first thoracic ganglion are often fused to form the *stellate ganglion*.[2] Once the preganglionic fibers reach the ganglion of the sympathetic trunk, these fibers may take one of the following

courses (Figure 1.12).[2,8] (1) These fibers may synapse with another cell (postganglionic neuron) in the ganglion. The postganglionic nerve fibers (nonmyelinated) reach the spinal nerve via gray rami communicantes and are distributed via the branches of spinal nerves. (2) Some preganglionic fibers may travel up or down via the sympathetic trunk to reach another ganglion higher or lower in the sympathetic chain before synapsing with the postganglionic neurons. The postganglionic nerve fibers than pass through the gray rami communicantes to reach the spinal nerve and are distributed along with the nerve and its branches. (3) A few preganglionic fibers may leave the ganglion of sympathetic trunk without synapsing via the visceral branches of sympathetic trunk, such as cardiac, pulmonary, and splanchnic nerves, to reach the autonomic nerve plexuses (cardiac, pulmonary, celiac, mesenteric, and renal nerve plexuses). The preganglionic fibers synapse with the postganglionic fibers in these plexuses and the postganglionic fibers supply the blood vessels, smooth muscles, and glands of the visceral organs.[2,3]

The afferent sympathetic nerve fibers (myelinated) accompany the efferent fibers. Afferent fibers from the visceral organs travel to the spinal cord via the sympathetic ganglion. They reach the spinal

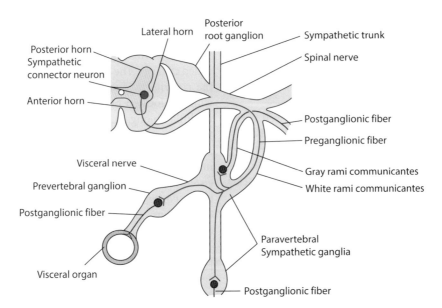

Figure 1.12 Arrangement of efferent sympathetic nerve fibers.

nerve via the white rami communicantes without synapsing in the ganglion. The cell body of these fibers lies in the posterior (dorsal) root ganglion of the spinal nerve. The afferent fibers are the peripheral processes of the neurons located in the posterior root ganglion. The central process of these neurons enters the spinal cord through the posterior root of spinal nerve. Here they may synapse with the sympathetic connector neuron to form the reflex arc or may ascend along the spinal cord to higher autonomic centers located in the brain (limbic system, thalamus, hypothalamus, and prefrontal cortex).[8]

Parasympathetic nervous system

Parasympathetic efferent fibers emerge from the brain and sacral segment of the spinal cord along with the cranial and sacral spinal nerves (craniosacral outflow). In the brain, the parasympathetic neurons are located in the brain stem and form part of nuclei of origin of cranial nerves III, VII, IX, and X.[2,3] The axons of these neurons pass through the corresponding cranial nerves to terminate in the peripheral parasympathetic ganglia. These axons constitute the preganglionic parasympathetic fibers. The parasympathetic ganglia associated with cranial nerve III is *ciliary ganglion*, VII is *submandibular ganglion*, and IX are *pterygopalatine* and *otic ganglia*. The preganglionic parasympathetic fibers in the vagus (X) cranial

nerve terminate in the autonomic nerve plexuses in the thorax and abdomen (cardiac, pulmonary, celiac, mesenteric, and renal plexuses).[8] These peripheral ganglia are located close to the viscera innervated. The postganglionic fibers from these ganglion are short, nonmyelinated, and supply various glands, eye, and thoracic and abdominal viscera. In the sacral region, the parasympathetic connector neurons are located in the gray matter of second, third, and fourth sacral segment of the spinal cord. The parasympathetic efferent fibers (myelinated) emerge from these sacral segments through the anterior roots of corresponding sacral spinal nerves. These preganglionic parasympathetic fibers than leave the spinal nerves to form the *pelvic splanchnic nerves* that terminate in the ganglia of *pelvic autonomic plexuses*. Here, the preganglionic fibers synapse with the postganglionic parasympathetic neurons and the postganglionic fibers (nonmyelinated) innervate the pelvic viscera and part of the large intestine.[8]

The afferent parasympathetic nerve fibers (myelinated) accompany the efferent fibers. They travel from the viscera along the cranial or spinal nerves to their cell bodies located in either the sensory ganglion of the cranial nerves or the posterior root ganglion of the sacral spinal nerve. The central axon from the cell bodies enters the CNS (brain or spinal cord) and either synapses with the connector neuron to form the reflex arc or ascends to higher centers of the autonomic nervous system (limbic system, thalamus, hypothalamus, and prefrontal cortex).[3,8]

Cerebrospinal fluid

The CSF fills the subarachnoid space as well as the ventricles of the brain and central canal of the spinal cord. It is formed by the choroid plexuses in the lateral, third and fourth ventricles of the brain.[1,2,10] The CSF formed in each of the lateral ventricles flows through the *foramen of Monro* (interventricular foramen) into the third ventricle and then through the *cerebral aqueduct* (aqueduct of Sylvius) to the fourth ventricle. From the fourth ventricle, it passes to the subarachnoid space through the three openings in the roof of the fourth ventricle (two lateral openings called the foramen of *Luschka* and a median opening called the foramen of *Magendie*) and into the central canal of the spinal cord. The CSF flows through the subarachnoid space around the brain and spinal cord and drains into the superior sagittal sinus through arachnoid granulations (*arachnoid villi*) (Figure 1.13).[2,10] The subarachnoid space closely follows the contours of the brain, but in certain regions the arachnoid mater diverges away to form large spaces filled with the CSF, called cisterns. The largest of these cisterns is called the *cisterna magna* or *cerebellomedullary cistern*, which is located between the cerebellum and the medulla oblongata. The CSF from the fourth ventricle passes into this cistern through the foramen of Luschka and foramen of Magendie.[1] Other major cisterns present are the *superior cistern* or *cisterna ambiens* between the cerebellum and midbrain, *pontine cistern or prepontine cistern* in front of the pons, and *interpeduncular cistern* between cerebral peduncles.

References

1. Hiatt JL, Gartner LP, editors. *Textbook of Head and Neck Anatomy*, 3rd ed. Philadelphia, PA: Lippincott Williams and Wilkins; 2001.
2. Snell RS, editor. *Clinical Anatomy for Medical Students*, 5th ed. Boston, MA: Little Brown and Company; 1995.

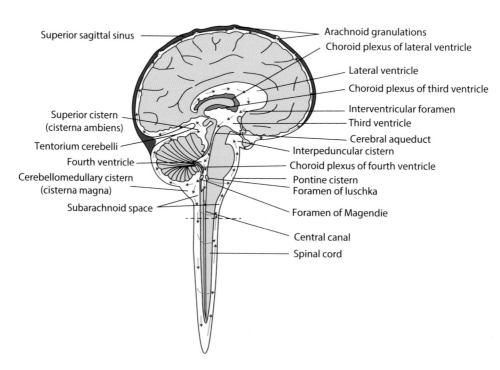

Figure 1.13 **Path of cerebrospinal fluid flow.**

3. Young PA, Young PH, Tolbert DL, editors. *Basic Clinical Neurosciences*, 2nd ed. Philadelphia, PA: Lippincott Williams and Wilkins; 2008.

4. Snell RS, editor. *Clinical Anatomy by Regions*, 9th ed. Philadelphia, PA: Lippincott Williams and Wilkins; 2012.

5. Standring S, Crossman AR, Fitzgerald MJT, editors. *The Anatomical Basis of Clinical Practice*, 39th ed. Philadelphia, PA: Elsevier Churchill Livingstone; 2005.

6. Romanes GJ. The central nervous system. In: Romanes GJ, editor. *Cunningham's Textbook of Anatomy*, 12th ed. Oxford, UK: Oxford University Press; 1981, pp. 609–738.

7. Sinnatamby CS, editor. *Last's Anatomy Regional and Applied*, 12th ed. Philadelphia, PA: Elsevier Churchill Livingstone; 2011.

8. Singh I. *Textbook of Anatomy*, 5th ed. New Delhi, IN: Jaypee Brothers Medical Publishers; 2011.

9. Romanes GJ. The peripheral nervous system. In: Romanes GJ, editor. *Cunningham's Textbook of Anatomy*, 12th ed. Oxford, UK: Oxford University Press; 1981, pp. 739–827.

10. Moore KI, Dalley AF, Agur AMR, editors. *Moore Clinical Oriented Anatomy*, 7th ed. Philadelphia, PA: Lippincott Williams and Wilkins; 2014.

2

Intracranial pressure

VASUDHA SINGHAL

Introduction

The concept of intracranial pressure (ICP) being a function of the volume and compliance of each component of the intracranial compartment was proposed by Monroe–Kellie doctrine in the nineteenth century. The brain, blood, and cerebrospinal fluid (CSF) exist in a state of volume equilibrium inside the semirigid skull box such that a change in the volume of one component is compensated by the change in the volume of the other; otherwise an increase in the ICP will ensue. Once the capacitance in the skull is exhausted, there is a sharp increase in the ICP resulting in intracranial hypertension (Figure 2.1), which may lead to severe neurological damage and even death. Prompt recognition of raised ICP and initiation of therapy targeted at reducing the ICP is therefore of paramount importance to prevent brain damage.

Pathophysiology of ICP

The main purpose of monitoring the ICP is to monitor the cerebral perfusion pressure (CPP), which is the pressure differential across the arteriovenous bed in the brain.[1,2]

CPP = MAP (Mean Arterial blood Pressure) – ICP

Furthermore, the cerebral blood flow (CBF) is determined by the following relation:

$$CBF = \frac{CPP}{CVR}$$

where CVR is the cerebrovascular resistance.

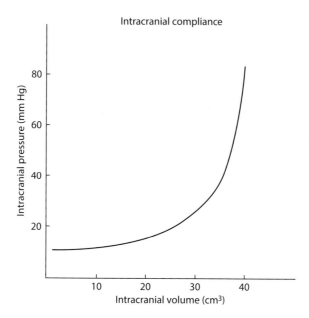

Figure 2.1 Intracranial compliance curve. An increase in the intracranial volume (up to 30 cm³) is well compensated by the capacitance of the cranial system. Further increases in volume result in sustained elevations in the intracranial pressure, causing brain herniation and death.

A constant CBF is maintained over a wide range of CPP in the face of physiological and pathological swings in MAP via constriction and dilatation of the microvascular networks. This buffer system, called autoregulation, is effective between an MAP of 60 and 150 mmHg.

To keep things simple, it can be said that the cranial biomechanical state is a function of the total CBF, intracranial compliance, and ICP. This changes with normal activities (e.g., change in body posture), aging, and head trauma and diseases (e.g., stroke, intracranial hemorrhage, hydrocephalus, Chiari malformations).

Normal ICP

ICP >15–20 mmHg: pathological, which warrants treatment.

Adults and older children	10–15 mmHg
Young children	3–7 mmHg
Full term infants	1.5–6 mmHg

ICP >40 mmHg: severe, uncontrolled hypertension, which could lead to catastrophic brain herniation and eventually death.[3,4]

Uses of ICP monitoring

- Helps to determine the CPP.
- Confirms or excludes intracranial hypertension—forms the basis of all intervention to lower ICP.
- Helps to assess whether therapy for decreasing ICP is effective.
- Suggests avoiding potentially dangerous treatment; if the ICP is not elevated.
- Can be therapeutic if intraventricular catheter is in place.
- Is useful in sedated and paralyzed patients in which conventional neurological assessment may not be possible.

Dynamics of ICP

The ICP and its waveforms provide information about intracranial dynamics and brain compliance, including the CPP, regulation of CBF and volume, absorption capacity of CSF, compensatory reserve of the brain, and content of vasogenic events. These parameters aid in the prediction of prognosis and survival following head injury and optimization of *CPP-guided therapy*.

ICP waveforms

A normal ICP trace is pulsatile, and reflects cardiac and respiratory cycles.[5,6]

The respiratory wave (2–10 mmHg) reflects changes in the intrathoracic pressure with respiration—it diminishes and eventually disappears with increase in ICP.

The pulse component of the normal ICP waveform (1–4 mmHg) generally consists of three peaks, which correlate with the arterial pressure waveform occurring with each cardiac cycle (Figure 2.2). These are as follows:

- P1 (*percussion wave*): This correlates with the arterial pulse transmitted through the choroid plexus into the CSF.
- P2 (*tidal wave*): This represents cerebral compliance and is a *reflection* of the arterial pulse wave bouncing off the springy brain parenchyma.
- P3 (*dicrotic wave*): This correlates with the closure of the aortic valve, which makes the trough prior to P3 the equivalent of the dicrotic notch.

> Visual inspection of waveforms can provide information about decreased intracranial compliance and altered intracranial dynamics, including:
>
> - Increased waveform amplitude
> - Elevated P2
> - Rounding of waveform
> - Appearance of plateau waves
>
> These all signify that intervention to decrease ICP is warranted.

When the ICP is increased and the intracranial compliance is decreased, pathological waves appear (Figure 2.3).[7]

- *Lundberg* A waves, or plateau waves: These are characteristic of conditions that lead to a markedly reduced intracranial compliance. They
  - Have an amplitude of 50–100 mmHg.
  - Occur for a duration of 5–10 minutes.

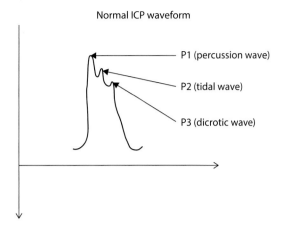

Normal ICP waveform

P1 (percussion wave)
P2 (tidal wave)
P3 (dicrotic wave)

Figure 2.2 Normal intracranial pressure waveform.

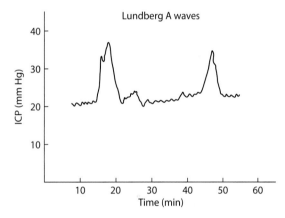

Lundberg A waves

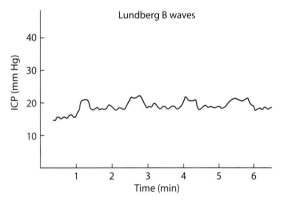

Lundberg B waves

Figure 2.3 Schematic diagram depicting Lundberg A and B waves.

- Indicate a very low CPP and ischemia, but when present they are an ominous sign for the development of brain herniation if ICP is left untreated.

- *Lundberg B waves*: These are sharply peaked rhythmic oscillations. They
  - Occur every 1–2 min.
  - Increase ICP in a crescendo manner to 20–30 mmHg from a variable baseline.
  - Are not sustained.
  - Reflect vasomotor changes.
  - Are associated with an unstable ICP.
- *Lundberg C waves*: These correspond to Traube–Hering–Meyer fluctuations in arterial pressure. They
  - Are documented in healthy adults.
  - Have no clinical significance.

Indications of ICP monitoring

1. Head injury[8]
2. Poor-grade subarachnoid hemorrhage (SAH)
3. Stroke
4. Intracerebral hematoma
5. Meningitis
6. Acute liver failure—hepatic encephalopathy
7. Hydrocephalus
8. Benign intracranial hypertension
9. Craniosynostosis
10. Intraoperatively—during resection of lesions that are at an increased risk of developing postoperative cerebral edema and perfusion pressure breakthrough, such as large brain tumors with mass effect or arteriovenous malformations.

The Brain Trauma Foundation (BTF) guidelines (2007) support ICP monitoring in traumatic brain injury (TBI) in the following conditions:

- Salvageable patients with severe TBI with a GCS between 3 and 8 after resuscitation, and an abnormal computed tomography (CT) scan, that is, one showing hematomas, contusion, swelling, herniation, or compressed basal cisterns (level II evidence)
- In patients with a GCS between 3 and 8 but a normal CT scan, ICP should be monitored if two or more of the following conditions are present:
  - Age over 40 years
  - Unilateral or bilateral motor posturing
  - Systolic blood pressure under 90 mmHg. (level III evidence)

Methods of ICP monitoring

Noninvasive techniques

The most accurate way to reliably diagnose elevated ICP is via a direct measurement approach with an invasive ICP monitor. Alternative noninvasive methods to assess ICP have however been sought because of the following reasons:

- Invasiveness of these monitoring techniques (which require insertion of an ICP sensor into the ventricles or brain parenchyma)
- Additional risks that they may pose to the patient (e.g., hemorrhage and infection)
- High costs associated with ICP sensor implantation
- Limited access to trained personnel, that is, a neurosurgeon/neurointensivist in suburban locations
- Invasive techniques may not be feasible in patients with severe coagulopathy

---

A detailed clinical examination along with imaging modalities (e.g., CT head and magnetic resonance imaging [MRI]) forms the basis for all ICP monitoring techniques.

Clinical examination: A thorough neurological evaluation may indicate an increased ICP:

- Symptoms: headache, nausea, vomiting
- Glasgow Coma Score: to assess the level of consciousness
- Pupillary reactivity
- Cushing's triad: bradycardia, hypertension, and respiratory depression
- Papilledema on fundoscopic examination

Imaging modalities

Noncontrast CT scan

This is the fastest and the most cost-effective. Findings suggestive of a high ICP[9] include

- Cerebral edema
- Midline shift
- Effacement of basal cisterns

- Loss of gray–white differentiation
- Loss of normal gyri and sulci pattern

Magnetic resonance imaging

This technique is costly and time consuming, and hence not the first-line investigation in the acute care setting.

A magnetic resonance imaging (MRI)-based method of measuring ICP (the MR-ICP method) has been recently developed. It integrates human neurophysiology and fluid dynamic principles with dynamic MRI techniques to measure intracranial elastance (inverse of compliance) and ICP.[10] It, however, provides a single time-point measurement and is useful in clinical settings in which a *snapshot* of the ICP may be beneficial.

Transcranial Doppler ultrasonography

This technique applies ultrasound to detect the velocity of blood flow through the major intracranial vessels, most commonly the middle cerebral artery. Elevated ICP can be estimated from the transcranial Doppler (TCD) measurements because it impedes the CBF and consequently decreases the blood flow velocity.[11] However, it requires training, has inter- and intraobserver variations, and may be difficult in 10%–15% patients who do not have an adequate bone window.

Tympanic membrane displacement

Because the CSF and perilymph communicate through the cochlear aqueduct, an increase in the ICP is directly transmitted to the footplate of the stapes, changing its initial position. Inward displacement of the eardrum in response to a sound (negative peak pressure on audiogram) is suggestive of high ICP, and outward displacement of the eardrum is suggestive of normal or low ICP.[12,13]

Optic nerve sheath diameter

The space between the optic nerve and its sheath is a continuation of the subarachnoid space, filled with CSF, whose pressure is equal to the ICP. The diameter of the nerve sheath, which increases with the increase in ICP, can be conveniently measured using a transocular ultrasound.[14,15] It is a cheap and efficient technique, and has been validated as a screening method for identification of patients with raised ICP requiring treatment, in several large studies. An optic nerve sheath diameter (ONSD) >5 mm corresponds to an ICP of 20 mmHg or higher.

Invasive methods of ICP monitoring

Modern ICP monitors can be classified on the basis of pressure transduction method into the following:

1. *Strain gauge* pressure transduction monitors: external (intraventricular drains) or internal (catheter tip microchip)
2. *Fiber-optic* technology-based monitors

Another classification may be into *fluid-coupled* devices (connected to an external strain gauge) or *non-fluid-coupled* devices (fiber-optic or catheter tip microstrain gauge).

Current ICP monitors can be placed in intraventricular, intraparenchymal, subarachnoid, subdural, or epidural locations.

> The intraventricular and the intraparenchymal catheter-tipped microtransducers are the most commonly used methods for monitoring the ICP.

Intraventricular devices

- The external ventricular drain (EVD) technique is considered the gold standard for ICP monitoring.[16–19]
- A catheter (EVD) is placed into one of the lateral ventricles through a burr hole connected to an external strain gauge (fluid coupled) to measure the ICP.
- The reference point for the external transducer is the foramen of Monro, 2 cm above the pterion on surface marking (external auditory meatus taken for convenience).
- It can be recalibrated in vivo against an external reference at any time.

Advantages

- Most reliable method of ICP monitoring.
- Minimal expense with maximum accuracy.

- Also suitable for therapeutic CSF drainage intermittently to control the ICP and to instill medications intrathecally (antibiotics in ventriculitis, thrombolytics in intraventricular hemorrhage).

Disadvantages

- Most invasive of all ICP monitoring methods— risk of bacterial transmission through the fluid coupling. The documented risk of infection varies between <1% and 27% (mean infection rate ~8%–9%).[20,21]
- Difficult to place in young patients with compressed or slitlike ventricles due to cerebral edema.[22]
- Overshunting may lead to aneurysmal rebleed in patients with poor-grade SAH, or hemispheric shifts and herniation in patients with unilateral mass lesions.[23,24]
- Hemorrhage—the rate of clinically significant hemorrhages (i.e., the ones causing neurological deficits, requiring surgical intervention, or resulting in fatality) varies from ~0.91% to 1.2%.[25,26]
- Chances of misplacement or obstruction of the catheter.[27]
- Frequent repositioning of the transducer level with each change in head position is required.

> Strict adherence to aseptic technique during insertion, use of antibiotic-impregnated catheters, subcutaneous tunneling of the catheter, sterile occlusive dressing over the incision points, minimal manipulation, and flushing or accessing of the CSF drainage tubing have all been known to reduce EVD-associated infection rates.[28–30]

Subarachnoid devices

- The subarachnoid bolt (or Richmond screw) is a hollow screw that can be quickly and easily placed without invading the brain, thus lowering the infection rates.
- It is inserted into the skull abutting the dura. The dura is perforated to fill the bolt with CSF, which is connected to closed fluid-filled tubing and a pressure transducer.

Advantages

- Less invasive as compared to intraventricular devices
- Lower infection rates

Disadvantages

- ICP underestimation
- Misplacement of the screw
- Occlusion by debris[31]

Pneumatic sensor (Spiegelberg brain pressure monitor)

- This is a fluid-filled catheter transducer system (internal strain gauge transducer system) that uses a distal air-filled balloon-tipped catheter to measure ICP.[32]
- Classically used for epidural and subdural ICP measurements: a newer version using a double-lumen intraventricular catheter system is also available.

Advantages

- Low cost
- Capable of doing automatic zero drift correction in vivo—obviates the problem of re-zeroing and drift

Disadvantages

- Its limited bandwidth makes most of the methods used for ICP waveform analysis impossible.

Intraparenchymal devices

- They can be divided into the following two subtypes:
  1. *Fiber-optic devices*, for example, Camino ICP monitor, InnerSpace ICP monitor
  2. *Strain gauge devices*, for example, Codman MicroSensor, Raumedic Neurovent-P ICP sensor, Pressio sensor
- They are non-fluid-coupled devices.
- They can be intraparenchymally inserted in the right frontal region at a depth of approximately 2 cm.

Advantages

- Accurate: close correlation observed between the ICP measured by them and the intraventricular drainage devices[33]
- Easy to transport; recordings are independent of patient positioning
- Measurement artifacts and damping of pressure waveform not seen
- Low risk of infection: they are non-fluid-coupled and do not require irrigation
- Incidence of clinically significant hemorrhage negligible

Disadvantages

- In vivo recalibration not possible
- Localized pressure measured, which may not be reflective of global ICP
- Therapeutic CSF drainage not possible
- Possibility of drift when used for long periods

Fiber-optic catheter tip transducers (Camino ICP monitor)

- They transmit light via a fiber-optic cable toward a displaceable diaphragm. The light is reflected off the diaphragm and change in light intensity is interpreted in terms of pressure.[34]

Disadvantages

- Costly system: disposable catheters.
- Daily baseline drift (~0.3 mmHg) if monitoring continued for >5 days; cannot be recalibrated once inserted.
- Fragile catheters: they can get damaged if acutely bent during insertion or maintenance, or if the patient is restless.[35]

Implanted microchip transducers (Codman sensors)

- They consist of a miniature solid-state pressure transducer mounted on a titanium case at the end of a 100 cm flexible nylon tube.
- Transducer tip contains a silicon microchip with diffuse piezoelectric strain gauges.
- Microsensor monitors ICP at the source; information relayed electronically rather than through a hydrostatic system or fiber optics (Figure 2.4).

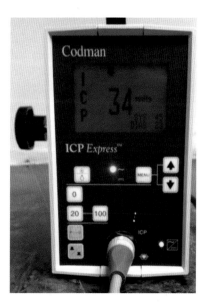

Figure 2.4 **Codman ICP monitor.**

Advantages

- Accurate and stable: daily drift of -0.13 to 0.11 mmHg per day.
- Simultaneous drainage of CSF when incorporated into a ventricular catheter along with ICP recording possible.
- Flexible: it can be tunneled beneath the scalp, preventing it from being easily broken.
- Small size: outer diameter 0.7 mm for the nylon vent tube, 1.2 mm for the transducer case, which enable it to be used in pediatric population.
- Absence of a fluid column: precludes dampening by blood clots, debris, or air bubbles, which makes it less prone to infections.
- Microsensor at the tip eliminates the need for constant realignment of the transducer with the patient's head and repeated re-zeroing.[36,37]

Which system to use?

> An optimal ICP monitoring device should be reliable and accurate, cost-effective, and associated with minimal patient morbidity.

Direct intraventricular ICP monitoring is preferred if access to the ventricles is required, besides being reliable and cost-effective. However, this is not always feasible, especially in patients with severe head injury, due to the presence of slitlike ventricles. In such situations, fiber-optic methods (Camino or InnerSpace) or implantable transducers (Codman) may be used as they can be inserted intraparenchymally.[38]

The Association for Advancement of Medical Instrumentation (AAMI), in association with the Neurosurgery Committee, has developed the American Standard for ICP monitoring devices. According to their standards, an ICP device should have the following specifications:

1. Pressure range from 0 to 100 mmHg
2. Accuracy of ± 2 mmHg within the range of 0–20 mmHg
3. Maximum error of 10% in the range of 20–100 mmHg[39]

Limitations of ICP monitoring

An important consideration that needs to be made in patients with traumatic brain injury (TBI) is the danger of localized elevations of ICP due to compartmentalized pressure gradients caused by mass lesions.[40,41] Care should therefore be exercised in the evaluation of patients where ICP and clinical symptoms differ markedly.

Conclusion

ICP monitoring is a robust brain monitoring modality that can be used to predict outcome and guide treatment. In the present-day scenario, additional neuromonitoring techniques should supplement ICP in the critical care setting to increase patient safety.

References

1. Czosnyka M, Hutchinson PJ, Balestreri M, Hiler M, Smielewski P, Pickard JD. Monitoring and interpretation of intracranial pressure after head injury. *Acta Neurochir Suppl* 2006;96:114–118.
2. Miller JD, Stanek A, Langfitt TW. Concepts of cerebral perfusion pressure and vascular compression during intracranial hypertension. *Prog Brain Res* 1972;35:411–432.
3. Ratanalert SN, Phuenpathom N, Saeheng S, Oearsakul T, Sripairojkul B, Hirunpat S. ICP threshold in CPP management of severe head injury patients. *Surg Neurol* 2004;61:429–435.
4. Saul TG, Ducker TB. Effects of intracranial pressure monitoring and aggressive treatment on mortality in severe head injury. *J Neurosurg* 1982;56:498–503.
5. Antoni N. Pressure curves from the cerebrospinal fluid. *Acta Med Scand* 1946 (Suppl. 170):431–462.
6. Bering EA, Ingraham FD. Arterial pulsation of the cerebrospinal fluid. *Trans Amer Neurol Assoc* 1953;3:49–54.
7. Lundberg N, Troupp H, Lorin H. Continuous recording of the ventricular-fluid pressure in patients with severe acute traumatic brain injury. A preliminary report. *J Neurosurg* 1965;22:581–590.
8. Bratton SL, Chestnut RM, Ghajar J, McConnell Hammond FF, Harris OA, Hartl R, et al. Guidelines for the management of severe traumatic brain injury. VI. Indications for intracranial pressure monitoring. *J Neurotrauma* 2007;24(Suppl. 1):S37–44.
9. Miller MT, Pasquale M, Kurek S et al. Initial head computed tomographic scan characteristics have a linear relationship with initial intracranial pressure after trauma. *J Trauma* 2004;56:967–973.
10. Alperin N, Mazda M, Lichtor T, Lee SH. From cerebrospinal fluid pulsation to noninvasive intracranial compliance and pressure measured by MRI flow studies. *Curr Med Imaging Rev* 2006;2:117–129.
11. Bellner J, Romner B, Reinstrup P, Kristiansson KA, Ryding E, Brandt L. Transcranial Doppler sonography pulsatility index (PI) reflects intracranial pressure (ICP). *Surg Neurol* 2004;62:45–51.
12. Reid A, Marchbanks RJ, Burge DM et al. The relationship between intracranial pressure and tympanic membrane displacement. *Br J Audiol* 1990;24:123–129.
13. Shimbles S, Dodd C, Banister K, Mendelow AD, Chambers IR. Clinical comparison of tympanic membrane displacement with invasive intracranial pressure measurements. *Physiol Meas* 2005;26:1085–1092.

14. Soldatos T, Karakitsos D, Chatzimichail K, Papathanasiou M, Gouliamos A, Karabinis A. Optic nerve sonography in the diagnostic evaluation of adult brain injury. *Crit Care* 2008;12:R67.

15. Rajajee V, Vanaman M, Fletcher JJ, Jacobs TL. Optic nerve ultrasound for the detection of raised intracranial pressure. *Neurocrit Care* 2011;15:506–515.

16. Zhong J, Dujovny M, Park HK, Perez E, Perlin AR, Diaz FG. Advances in ICP monitoring techniques. *Neurol Res* 2003;25:339–350.

17. March K. Intracranial pressure monitoring: Why monitor? *AACN Clin Issues* 2005;16:456–475.

18. Steiner LA, Andrews PJD. Monitoring the injured brain: ICP and CBF. *Br J Anaesth* 2006;97:26–38.

19. Smith M. Monitoring intracranial pressure in traumatic brain injury. *Anesth Analg* 2008;106:240–248.

20. Beer R, Lackner P, Pfausler B, Schmutzhard E. Nosocomial ventriculitis and meningitis in neurocritical care patients. *J Neurol* 2008;255:1617–1624.

21. Lozier AP, Sciacca RR, Romagnoli MF, Connolly ES Jr. Ventriculostomy-related infections: A critical review of the literature. *Neurosurgery* 2002;51:170–182.

22. Lundberg N. Continuous recording and monitoring of ventricular fluid pressure in neurosurgical practice. *Acta Psychiatr Neurol Scand* 1960;36(Suppl. 149):1–193.

23. Fountas KN, Kapsalaki EZ, Machinis T, Karampelas I, Smisson HF, Robinson JS. Review of the literature regarding the relationship of rebleeding and external ventricular drainage in patients with subarachnoid hemorrhage of aneurysmal origin. *Neurosurg Rev* 2006;29:14–18.

24. Bloch J, Regli L. Brain stem and cerebellar dysfunction after lumbar spinal fluid drainage: Case report. *J Neurol Neurosurg Psychiatry* 2003;74:992–994.

25. Binz DD, Toussaint III LG, Friedman JA. Hemorrhagic complications of ventriculostomy placement: A meta-analysis. *Neurocrit Care* 2009;10:253–256.

26. Gardner PA, Engh J, Atteberry D, Moossy JJ. Hemorrhage rates after external ventricular drain placement: Clinical article. *J Neurosurg* 2009;110:1021–1025.

27. Saladino A, White JB, Wijdicks EFM, Lanzino G. Malplacement of ventricular catheters by neurosurgeons: A single institution experience. *Neurocrit Care* 2009;10:248–252.

28. Dasic D, Hanna SJ, Bojanic S, Kerr RSC. External ventricular drain infection: The effect of a strict protocol on infection rates and a review of the literature. *Brit J Neurosurg* 2006;20:296–300.

29. Abla AA, Zabramski JM, Jahnke HK, Fusco D, Nakaji P. Comparison of two antibiotic-impregnated ventricular catheters: A prospective sequential series trial. *Neurosurgery* 2011;68:437–442.

30. Harrop JS, Sharan AD, Ratliff J et al. Impact of a standardized protocol and antibiotic-impregnated catheters on ventriculostomy infection rates in cerebrovascular patients. *Neurosurgery* 2010;67:187–191.

31. Miller JD, Bobo H, Kapp JP. Inaccurate pressure readings from subarachnoid bolts. *Neurosurgery* 1986;19:253–255.

32. Lang JM, Beck J, Zimmermann M, Seifert V, Raabe A. Clinical evaluation of intraparenchymal Spiegelberg pressure sensor. *Neurosurgery* 2003;52:1455–1459.

33. Gelabert-González M, Ginesta-Galan V, Sernamito-García R, Allut AG, Bandin-Diéguez J, Rumbo RM. The Camino intracranial pressure device in clinical practice. Assessment in a 1000 cases. *Acta Neurochir* 2006;148:435–441.

34. Piper I, Barnes A, Smith D, Dunn L. The Camino intracranial pressure sensor: Is it optimal technology? An internal audit with a review of current intracranial pressure monitoring technologies. *Neurosurgery* 2001;49:1158–1164.

35. Bekar A, Dogan S, Abas F et al. Risk factors and complications of intracranial pressure monitoring with a fiberoptic device. *J Clin Neurosci* 2009;16:236–240.

36. Koskinen LOD, Olivecrona M. Clinical experience with the intraparenchymal intracranial pressure monitoring Codman microsensor system. *Neurosurgery* 2005;56:693–698.

37. Fernandes HM, Bingham K, Chambers IR, Mendelow AD. Clinical evaluation of the Codman microsensor intracranial pressure monitoring system. *Acta Neurochir Suppl* 1998;71:44–46.

38. Czosnyka M, Czosnyka Z, Pickard JD. Laboratory testing of three intracranial pressure microtransducers: Technical report. *Neurosurgery* 1996;38:219–224.

39. Bratton SL, Chesnut RM, Ghajar J et al. Guidelines for the management of severe traumatic brain injury. VII. Intracranial pressure monitoring technology. *J Neurotrauma* 2007;24(Suppl. 1):S45–S54.

40. Mindermann T, Gratzl O. Interhemispheric pressure gradients in severe head trauma in humans. *Acta Neurochir Suppl* 1998;71:56–58.

41. Weaver DD, Winn HR, Jane JA. Differential intracranial pressure in patients with unilateral mass lesions. *J Neurosurg* 1982;56:660–665.

3

Cerebral perfusion pressure

NICOLE COLLINS and ALAA ABD-ELSAYED

Overview

Cerebral perfusion pressure (CPP) is of concern to anesthesiologists in the setting of both acute and chronic cranial pathologies. The importance of CPP in a given situation is largely dependent upon its use by the provider as an estimate of balance between brain tissue metabolic needs and by-product excretion. This is often described in terms of cerebral blood flow (CBF) and cerebral metabolic oxygen requirement ($CMRO_2$). While similar basic physiologic principles of supply and demand apply to most peripheral organ systems, the cranium represents a unique physiologic space to manage (Table 3.1). When addressing an injury, not only is there the usual tissue and vascular considerations to contend with, but in addition to a rigid encapsulating body (the cranium) there is also a semiflexible fluid column as represented by the dural-contained cerebrospinal fluid (CSF). Increase in any of these elements (tissue, blood, CSF volume) that is not met by adequate compensation can lead to increased intracranial pressure (ICP) and possible herniation. The ability of the brain to manage blood flow over a wide range of blood pressure levels is called *autoregulation*[1-3] and is an important adaptation of the brain to counter increased ICP. Taken together, the unusual and complex localized tissue environment of the cranium can make anesthetic management a challenge. CPP is both a measurement tool and an important conceptualization that can help us to simplify and direct treatment strategies in these patients.

Table 3.1 Cranial Components

Cranial components	Changeable	Inflexible
Cranium (skull) and dura		x
Intraparenchymal tissue		x
Blood volume	x (fast)	
CSF	x (slow)	

CSF, cerebrospinal fluid.

Measurement

Formally, CPP is measured as the difference between mean arterial pressure (MAP) and either ICP or central venous pressure (CVP), whichever is highest. In its simplest form, CPP obeys the rule of what goes in must come out; following this, CPP becomes a numerical representation of that principle. A second and equally important rule about CPP is to appreciate that the brain wants what it wants, and up until the point where it cannot manage anymore (a dire point at which to find a patient), it will change the body's entire physiology to meet its own needs. The brain is very good at manipulating CBF and can maintain a steady supply of oxygen-rich blood over a wide range of peripherally controlled pressure levels. This phenomenon, called autoregulation, is typically represented by the graphs of MAP versus CBF that we all become familiar with during our anesthesia training.[4]

Important *normal values* are listed in Table 3.2, but they must be viewed with caution by the clinician when dealing with cranial physiology altered by injury or treatment attempts. *Normal* ranges typically expect normal $PaCO_2$ and PaO_2, resting metabolic needs, perfect and symmetric vascular anatomy without recruitment of collateral flow,

functional kidneys, and blood that is neither too viscous nor too dilute, hardly the standard picture in most cranial pathology. As anesthesia providers, we try to wrest some of the control of CPP from the brain when managing intracranial injury, but it is crucially important that we recognize that what the brain is altering it is likely doing for a reason. Where intracranial injury management is concerned, mimicry really can be the most profound form of physiologic flattery, at least in the short term. In other words, normal CBF and blood pressure become whatever the brain tissue needs at that time to meet its current metabolic demands.

Within an ideal vascular and intracranial system, CPP measurement is as simple as subtracting ICP (ICP to be overcome to exit the cranium) from MAP (MAP pushing into the brain necessary to maintain adequate CBF for $CMRO_2$). The assumption of a peripheral MAP being the same as that which the internal carotid or major cerebral vasculature experiences is an extrapolation that requires varying amounts of leniency on the part of the provider as they take into account chronic disease processes (e.g., carotid stenosis, hypertension) and acute injury (e.g., hemorrhage, shock, cardiogenic processes). While CPP measurement is a mathematically derived number meant to help guide management, it is up to the clinician to account for and

Table 3.2 Normal Ranges for Various Cranial Components

Total CBF	50 mL/100 g/min (~15% total cardiac output)
"Safe" carotid clamp CBF	20–40 mL/100 g/min
Ischemic potential	<20 mL/100 g/min
General anesthesia CBF	>20 mL/100 g/min (autoregulation is preserved ≤1MAC)
Cell death	<10 mL/100 g/min
CPP	
Normal range	60–90 mmHg
Autoregulation range	50–110 mmHg
MAP for normal CPP	>60 mmHg
MAP for ischemic CPP	>70 mmHg
ICP	5–20 mmHg
$CMRO_2$	3.5 mL/100 g/min (~20% of resting oxygen consumption)
CSF	
Total volume	150–250 mL
Daily production	600–700 mL/day

CBF, cerebral blood flow; CPP, cerebral perfusion pressure; ICP, intracranial pressure; $CMRO_2$, cerebral metabolic oxygen requirement; CSF, cerebrospinal fluid.

accommodate physiologic variables that are not otherwise addressed by an idealized derivation of CPP.

Mean arterial pressure measurement

The most common source for obtaining MAP in an intracranial patient is a peripheral arterial catheter, usually from a radial source though other arterial sites may be used as well. While MAP can be measured by a blood pressure cuff, this is considered less than ideal for the management of all but the most stable intracranial processes (e.g., shunt placement for chronic hydrocephalus). Patients that are severely obtunded with evidence of acute herniation, children, and other emergency scenarios may require rapid intervention in order to relieve pressure on the intracranial contents. These patients may require placement of arterial lines after induction with frequent peripheral blood pressure readings in the interim. Ideally, however, any patient at risk for acute changes in CPP during induction or surgery should have an arterial blood pressure catheter placed prior to anesthetic or surgical insult.

Intracranial pressure measurement

ICP can be measured using various devices, and it is up to the anesthesia provider to be familiar with those common to their institution. ICP measurement devices can be placed to assess pressure changes at epidural, subdural, intraparenchymal, and ventricular locations. Of the options available for therapeutic intervention, ventricular and lumbar drains for CSF removal are the most common ones encountered in the OR. Care must be taken by the anesthesiologist when both interpreting the ICP measured by these devices, and when using a drain to remove CSF. Swollen parenchymal tissue can cause compartmentalization of CSF (a precursor to localized herniation in some instances) or occlude a drain. These scenarios can yield both falsely low and falsely elevated values. Draining of CSF, particularly from a lumbar catheter, must be performed with caution in a closed cranial system as rapid removal can form a vacuum effect that pulls cerebral and cerebellar tissue down toward the narrow canal housing the brain stem and its cranial nerves. Most often, in the operative environment, CSF is removed only after discussion between the neurosurgical team and the anesthesia provider.

Central venous pressure as a consideration

As already mentioned, CPP measurement in its most basic form is just a gross estimation of the blood flow that needs to go into the brain to satisfy metabolic needs, and the pressure needed to ensure venous drainage from the enclosed cranial vault into the extracranial circulation. Usually ICP is the greatest force to be overcome but there are occasions when CVP may be the deciding factor for venous drainage. This is especially true when there has already been a decompressive surgical event and yet the CPP as determined through calculation with ICP values does not correlate with the clinical picture. If that is the case, placement of a central venous catheter may yield a CVP that is more representative of the threshold pressure needed for adequate intracranial drainage. Therapies directed toward decreasing CVP rather than ICP could prove beneficial in such cases.

Vascular considerations

In practice, due to the rigidity and limited fenestrations of the cranium, the blood volume entering the brain can be estimated by measuring blood flow through the internal carotids as these supply the majority of the forebrain (the vertebral and medullary arteries provide ~20% of total CBF and are primary suppliers of the brain stem and spinal cord).[5,6] The CBF remains proportional between the internal carotid and vertebral arteries throughout life though there is a steady decline in overall CBF of roughly 15% by the age of 85. This may be of some consideration when directing management of the elderly patient.[7]

As with perfusion, cerebral drainage is primarily undertaken via multiple perforations in the skull base following collection and organization into large, semi-rigid venous tracts called sinuses that run along the underside of the skull. Due to the size, location, and lack of ready compression of some of the largest of the sinus tracts, injury to them can result in substantial morbidity not usually seen in a venous injury; the anesthesiologist should anticipate aggressive resuscitation efforts if such an injury is suspected. The largest sources of venous drainage from the brain are the internal jugular veins (~80% of intracranial drainage).

Jugular venous bulb monitoring was frequently used for management of cranial ischemia over a decade ago, but it has since largely fallen out of favor due to its complication profile and questionable utility. In current practice, jugular bulb monitors are rarely seen outside of a critical care environment and so their use in venous and intracranial monitoring will not be discussed here.

Factors that affect arterial perfusion and venous drainage are key in determining the modifiable components of CPP in a patient. When addressing the patient with acute cerebral injury in the OR, the factors that determine CPP can be divided into two categories of management: physiologic and pathologic. Physiologic issues often have chronic pathology associated with them, but they are typically something that can be surgically addressed; that is, they can be the immediate reason you are seeing the patient operatively. Pathologic issues are those in which there is a disease diagnosis with some known cranial etiology. These get lumped into chronic or soon to be chronic conditions. Events such as subarachnoid hemorrhage (SAH) have a tendency to fall between the two groupings. Except for conditions involving active intracranial bleeding, it is almost always better to err on the side of driving the MAP and CPP up to the patient's normal range, or even slightly greater, during treatment. Hypoxic ischemic damage is poorly tolerated by the brain tissues and is often the greatest contributor to morbidity in these patients.

Physiologic conditions with CPP alterations

From an arterial perspective, the internal carotid arteries are the primary vascular suppliers of the forebrain. Embolic stroke from sloughing of carotid atherosclerotic plaques is the leading cause of ischemic stroke in humans. Furthermore, development of carotid stenosis necessitates higher MAP to meet the CBF and metabolic demands of the brain. This means that these patients have an altered autoregulation curve, sometimes called a right-shifted curve. When treating these patients in the neuroangiography suite, the goal is for higher than *normal* CPP to perfuse what you can of the ischemic brain through collateral circulation while the interventionalist works on the emboli. How high the MAP should be is an area of debate among those who study and treat ischemic stroke,[8] but considering the vasorelaxant effects of most anesthetics aiming to maintain even a normal awake blood pressure can be challenging. Often these patients will come in with higher than average MAP as part of their chronic disease pathology. If you know an MAP at which the patients showed improved symptoms during the course of their acute ischemic event, you should aim for that or higher assuming that other organ systems, particularly the heart, are tolerating the increase in blood pressure. Of note, other types of arterial vascular ischemic pathologies (e.g., moyamoya and arteriovenous malformations) that are not embolic in nature frequently require specialized CPP management and manipulation of the CPP should be undertaken only after discussion with the neurosurgical or neurointerventional team caring for the patient.

Hemorrhagic cerebral events (i.e., AVM, aneurysms, bleeding tumors, intracranial hemorrhage) require maintenance of a stable blood pressure both during induction and intraoperatively to minimize transmural pressure variation across weakened vessel walls. Increased ICP from displaced tissue and blood must be closely monitored for herniation potential in the enclosed cranium. Intraoperatively intracranial hemorrhagic events (whether epidural, subdural, ventricular, or intraparenchymal) require clear communication between the surgical team and the anesthesia provider as alternating episodes of hypotension and hypertension may both be necessary during vascular clamping and bypass. In addition, a careful balance between adequate clotting and thrombosis (especially in the peripheral venous system) should be addressed by the management team as both scenarios can lead to devastating consequences in these patients.

Finally, venous drainage should be assessed in the patient receiving intracranial intervention, especially in the surgical suite. Positioning of the head for prone and lateral approaches to the cranium can result in significant occlusion of the internal jugular vein as well as regional nerve injuries. While ultrasound can be used to judge flow (and take note of dominant vasculature) prior to sterile preparation of the field, often a visual survey of the eyes, face, and head is sufficient to determine whether there is venous congestion. When in doubt, discuss repositioning of the head with the surgeon sooner rather than later; it is almost impossible to alter the arrangement after the cranium is open. As already discussed, if there are concerns for high CVP (ICP must be greater than CVP to allow for adequate drainage, especially when supine or prone), efforts should be made to lower this value (i.e., fluid restriction, cardiac optimization, minimizing/eliminating positive end-expiratory pressure [PEEP], decreasing pulmonary hypertension).

CSF and hydrocephalus in CPP management

In the face of elevated ICP, the brain typically alters the volume components over which it has control, namely CBF and CSF. Acute management of CSF volume by the brain is dependent upon shift of the CSF from the intracranial to the extracranial thecal sac. This can occur as a simple pressurized fluid shift in the supine position or with the aid of gravity in a recumbent posture. From the standpoint of an anesthesia provider managing the CSF component of an acute ICP event, the first thing to accomplish is optimization of the patient into a sitting position if possible so as to displace CSF into the lumbar cistern. If an externalized drain is in place, this too can be cautiously used to remove CSF volume and allow space for expanding tissue or hemorrhagic mass, keeping in mind the potential for herniation if CSF is too aggressively removed. Note that in an enclosed and sterile collecting system, once the CSF is drained from the patient, it is no longer considered acceptable to return it to intracranial circulation. Judicious removal is therefore advised as CSF is important for circulating nutrients, regulating ion concentration, transporting hormones, and providing support to the brain structure.[9] That being said, CSF is one of two components that the anesthesia provider can alter when attempting to optimize CPP with effects that can be immediate and lifesaving in some emergent situations.

Less acute changes to the CSF involve alterations in the synthesis, reuptake, and osmotic properties of the CSF as overseen by the choroid plexus and arachnoid villi. Most often there is an increase in overall CSF volume, a condition termed hydrocephalus. There are many different varieties of hydrocephalus that range from high to normal pressure, and from obstructive to communicating. Acute hydrocephalus is most often secondary to a localized event that has infringed upon the normal pathways of CSF flow (i.e., it is usually obstructive). On imaging,

collections of the CSF are often disproportionate between the ventricles surrounding the obstruction. This type of hydrocephalus is best managed by addressing the source of obstruction or by placing an internally or externally draining shunt.

Chronic hydrocephalus is host to a number of physiologic changes in the choroid plexus and arachnoid villi, and the provider should carry a high index of suspicion in any patient who has a history of infection, inflammation, or hemorrhage within the intracranial compartment. Foreign material can induce fibrotic change to the arachnoid villi that leads to decreased function, including reuptake of CSF. Patients who have survived an SAH are a classic group for this sort of communicating hydrocephalus. Another significant patient group with chronic hydrocephalus is the elderly who may display minimal notable symptoms due to a slow decline that is often attributed to age and medical comorbidities rather than altered ICP.

While the surgical procedure for shunt placement in patients with chronic hydrocephalus is fairly routine, as with any procedure the elderly and very young may require special attention by the anesthesiologist for management of comorbid conditions. Otherwise a single peripheral IV and adequate muscle relaxation for the placement of shunt are usually all that is needed.

Developing a management strategy using CPP

The CPP is a useful conceptual tool for the clinician managing the patient with intracranial pathology if the key principles that go into its measurement are accounted for: namely maintaining adequate forward CBF and allowing for ready venous and CSF drainage. Every management strategy undertaken, however, can be boiled down to altering these parameters and trending the results of your efforts with CPP. Common conditions with altered CPP encountered by the anesthesia provider are listed in Table 3.3.

Following are key principles of care when managing intracranial pathology:

- *Acute ischemic cranial pathologies generally benefit from a higher than normal CPP.*
  - If a blood pressure is known at which a patient showed improved mentation or physical exam findings that is the

Table 3.3 Conditions Altering the Cerebral Perfusion Pressure

Conditions that alter CPP	Arterial	Venous	CSF	Mass effect	Notes
Physiologic					
Carotid stenosis	x				Embolic stroke most common pathologic sequelae
Sinus thrombosis		x			Usually medically managed
Cervical flexion/ extension	x	x			Extreme positions of the neck can damage nerves, arteries, and veins of the neck
Trauma	x	x		x	Intracranial trauma, spinal cord injury, and peripheral trauma carry ischemic shock risk
Spinal injury[10]	x	x			Autonomic dysreflexia and hypotension
Pathologies					
Chronic HTN	x				Autoregulation is shifted towards a higher baseline MAP
Pulmonary hypertension	x	x			High CVP in the setting of chronic hypoxia
Chronic apnea[11]	x				
MS[12,13]	x	x			Dysautonomia has been associated with decreased IJ drainage and decreased CBF
Parkinsons[14,15]	x				Dysautonomia, particularly hypotension
SAH			x		Acute hemorrhagic bleeding followed by vasospasm and scarring of the CSF drainage system
Arteriopathies	x				
Hydrocephalus			x		Chronic hydrocephalus is often managed with ventricular-peritoneal or other similar shunts
Tumor/ inflammation				x	Intracranial hemorrhage can be a risk, especially with certain metastasized tumors

CPP, cerebral perfusion pressure; CSF, cerebrospinal fluid; HTN, hypertension; MS, multiple sclerosis; SAH, subarachnoid hemorrhage.

minimum pressure you should aim for. Trust the brain knowing what it wants over what your normal ranges are.

- *Chronic ischemic cranial pathologies generally carry with them a higher baseline blood pressure to start with; you will need to attempt maintenance of the patient's typical range of blood pressure while under general anesthesia to ensure adequate CPP.*
- *Intracranial hemorrhage requires that you determine the etiology (is it still bleeding?) and also treat evidence of high ICP.*

- Elevated ICP: treat what you can to prevent herniation while moving (rapidly) toward definitive intervention.
- Traumatic: major cerebrovascular versus localized intraparenchymal hemorrhage (IPH), venous sinus involvement, ischemia due to hemorrhage, compromise of CBF due to systemic shock?
- SAH: prompt intervention if the aneurysm is bleeding (expect a sympathetic picture in these patients with high MAP and CVP initially). Coiling or clipping procedures may be performed for known aneurysms and require controlled blood pressure during induction and surgical intervention; periodic hyper- and hypotension is frequently requested by the surgeon. Once the aneurysm is secured, inducing an elevated CPP is usually warranted for the treatment of subsequent vasospasm.
- IPH: often from a tumor, sometimes due to vascular malformations (i.e., AVM, arteriopathies, and aneurysm). There is a high risk for edema and herniation in these patients. Low to normal CPP goals should be correlated to hemorrhagic potential.
- *Hydrocephalus* is typically chronic in the elderly and acute in the pediatric or trauma patient. Treat any elevation in ICP that is concerning for herniation (i.e., apneic episodes in the pediatric patient, altered mental status in the adult). The definitive treatment is a CSF drain or a shunt.

The following steps are involved in acute management of high ICP:

1. Elevate head of bed (if possible) to increase venous drainage (get CVP < ICP).
2. Hyperventilate ($PaCO_2$ < 10 mmHg from patient's normal); this causes vasoconstriction (ischemic risk) so only use acutely.
3. Osmotic therapy: mannitol or hypertonic saline.
4. Diuretic therapy: for less acute settings, monitor electrolytes and kidney function, especially if used with osmotic agents.
5. Surgical intervention: craniotomy, intraventricular drain.

References

1. Lassen N. Cerebral blood flow and oxygen consumption in man. *Physiol Rev* 1959;39:183–238.
2. Tzeng YC, Ainslie PN. Blood pressure regulation IX: Cerebral autoregulation under blood pressure challenges. Eur J Appl Physiol 2014;114:545–559.
3. Numan T, Bain AR, Hoiland RL, Smirl JD, Lewis NC, Ainslie PN. Static autoregulation in humans: A review and reanalysis. *Med Eng Phy* 2014;36:1487–1495.
4. Gao E, Young WL, Pile-Spellman J, Ornstein E, Ma Q. Mathematical considerations for modeling cerebral blood flow autoregulation to system arterial pressure. *Am J Physiol* 1998;274:H1023–H1031.
5. Boyajian R, Schwend RB, Wolfe MM, Bickerton RE, Otis SM. Measurement of anterior and posterior circulation flow contributions to cerebral blood flow. An ultrasound-derived volumetric flow analysis. *J Neuroimaging* 1995;5:1–3.
6. Alexandrov AV. The Spencer's curve: Clinical implications of a classic hemodynamic model. *J Neuroimaging* 2007;17:6–10.
7. Scheel P, Ruge C, Petruch UR, Schöning M. Color duplex measurement of cerebral blood flow volume in healthy adults. *Stroke* 2000;31:147–150.
8. Jordan JD, Powers WJ. Cerebral autoregulation and acute ischemic stroke. Am J Hypertens 2012;25:946–950.
9. Spector R, Keep RF, Robert Snodgrass S, Smith QR, Johanson CE. A balanced view of choroid plexus structure and function: Focus on adult humans. *Exp Neurol* 2015;267:78–86.
10. Phillips A, Ainslie P, Krassioukov A, Warburton D. Regulation of cerebral blood flow after spinal cord injury. *J Neurotrauma* 2013;15:1551–1563.
11. Yadav S, Kumar R, Macey P et al. Regional cerebral blood flood alterations in obstructive sleep apnea. *Neurosci Lett* 2013;555:159–164.
12. Mancini M, Lanzillo R, Liuzzi R et al. Internal jugular vein blood flow in multiple sclerosis patients and matched controls. *PLoS One* 2014;9:e92730.

13. D'haeseleer M, Hostenbach S, Peeters I et al. Cerebral hypoperfusion: A new pathophysiologic concept in multiple sclerosis?. *J Cereb Blood Flow Metab* 2015;35:1406–1410.

14. Camargo C, Martins E, Lange M et al. Abnormal cerebrovascular reactivity in patients with Parkinson's disease. *Parkinsons Dis* 2015;2015:e523041.

15. Ko J, Lerner R, Eidelberg D. Effects of levodopa on regional cerebral metabolism and blood flow. *Mov Disord* 2015;30:54–63.

4

Brain protection

JUDITH DINSMORE and REBECCA CAMPBELL

Introduction

Acute brain injury is one of the leading causes of death and disability in the developed world. Brain injury may occur secondary to ischemia or hypoxia such as following a stroke or cardiac arrest. Traumatic brain injury (TBI) typically occurs following accidents but may also occur as a result of iatrogenic intraoperative damage. Whatever is the etiology or mechanism of injury, a cascade of pathophysiological processes is initiated resulting in neuronal damage and cell death. The primary injury occurs as a direct result of the initial trauma or ischemic event and can only be altered by preventative measures. However, neurological injury then progresses over hours and days, resulting in a secondary injury. Inflammatory and neurotoxic processes result in vasogenic fluid accumulation within the brain contributing to raised intracranial pressure (ICP), hypoperfusion, and cerebral ischemia. Secondary injury also occurs as a result of further physiological insults with hypoxia, hypotension, hyper- or hypocapnia, and hyper- or hypoglycemia all shown to increase the risk of secondary brain injury. Much of this secondary injury may be amenable to intervention and, given the long-term medical, social, and economic consequences of brain injury, neuropreventative strategies are of obvious importance. Despite the identification of many neuroprotective agents that appear to work in the laboratory in terms of limiting secondary injury or improving functional outcome, the translation of this work into clinical practice has been less successful.[1]

Brain injury can occur secondary to:
- Direct surgical injury
- Imbalance between oxygen/glucose supply and demand within brain tissue

these processes is ultimately cell death, which may lead to irreversible and functionally significant neurological impairment.[2] It is hoped that by identification of the various processes that lead to cell death, we will be able to identify an array of targets for neuroprotection (Figure 4.1).

Mechanisms of neuronal cell death

Interruption of the continuous supply of glucose and oxygen to the brain initiates a cascade of events that, unchecked, leads to neuronal cell death. The switch from aerobic to anaerobic respiration produces a lactic acidosis, which in turn inhibits presynaptic glutamate reuptake, thus increasing excitotoxic neuronal cell damage. The less efficient anaerobic respiration results in a deficiency of ATP and the subsequent failure of energy-dependent ion pumps. This in turn leads to increased amounts of intracellular sodium, calcium, chloride, and water, resulting in cytotoxic edema. The reuptake of excitatory amino acids is also energy dependent and the accumulation of these contribute to further worsening of excitotoxic cell damage. The increased level of intracellular calcium triggers a cascade of enzymes leading to the breakdown of mitochondria, the cellular cytoskeleton, and cell membranes. There is also an associated increase in the production of oxidative free radicals and release of inflammatory mediators. The end product of all

Strategies for intraoperative neuroprotection

New neurological dysfunction after surgery is one of the most serious adverse effects of anesthesia and surgery. Patients undergoing neurosurgical and cardiovascular procedures, and those with preexisting risk factors such as previous stroke, cardiac, renal disease, and diabetes are particularly at risk. Despite a wide variety of strategies for intraoperative neuroprotection, there is a limited evidence base supporting their use. There is a much greater body of evidence for specific areas such as the use of reperfusion strategies in ischemic stroke and manipulation of physiological variables such as cerebral blood flow (CBF), cerebral perfusion pressure (CPP), and ICP in TBI. The main approaches can be classified as

- Pharmacological
- Physiological
- Ongoing experimental research

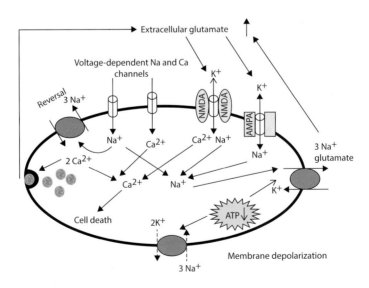

Figure 4.1 Representation of excitotoxic cell damage occurring following ischemia (adapted from Alzheimer C).[3]

Pharmacological strategies for neuroprotection

Numerous drugs with a variety of mechanisms of action have been tested for pharmacological neuroprotection over the years, but all with conflicting results. Agents investigated include anesthetic agents, sex hormones, erythropoietin (EPO), calcium channel blockers, magnesium, remifentanil, and lidocaine.[4]

Anesthetic agents

Anesthetic agents appear to have neuroprotective properties. A key property, potentially conferring protection, is the profound reduction of cerebral metabolic rate (CMR) and thus the demand for oxygen and glucose. In addition, anesthetic agents reduce ICP, and suppress seizures and sympathetic discharge. Theoretical benefits include the inhibition of excitatory neurotransmission and a reduction in accumulation of intracellular calcium and free radicals. However, despite promising animal studies demonstrating the protective effects of anesthetic agents in neuronal injury, clinical studies have been disappointing.

Volatile anesthetic agents

Volatile anesthetic agents have neuroprotective properties irrespective of the agent used. However, cerebral vasodilatation occurs with all agents, particularly at higher concentrations. In addition, higher doses will reduce arterial pressure. When considering the use of any volatile anesthetic agent for neuroanesthesia, the recommendation is to maintain the concentration less than 1 minimum alveolar concentration (MAC). This provides optimal reduction in CMR while minimizing the impact of changes in CBF and carbon dioxide reactivity. Sevoflurane appears to have the best neurophysiological profile in terms of maintaining this balance. Isoflurane has been shown to provide neuroprotection when administered before and after brain ischemia in animal models. However, despite theoretical benefits, this work has not been translated into clinical studies because of concerns regarding potential adverse effects on CBF and increases in ICP.

Barbiturates

Thiopentone was the induction agent of choice for neuroanesthetists for many years. It has the ability to produce an isoelectric electroencephalogram (EEG), reducing ICP, CMR, and oxygen demand profoundly. Animal studies have suggested that thiopentone has the ability to reduce infarct size in focal ischemia provided all other physiological variables are maintained. However, the clinical evidence is less convincing with conflicting results and no conclusive evidence of neuroprotection. Despite this, it may provide temporary benefits and is often still used as an adjunct during short periods of partial or complete artery occlusion intraoperatively. It is also used in the medical treatment of refractory intracranial hypertension. However, it is associated with cardiovascular depression and delayed wakening.

Propofol

Propofol appears to have the ability to attenuate brain injury following an ischemic insult, the mechanism for which is likely to be multifactorial. However, there is no clear clinical evidence that propofol has an improved neuroprotective profile over other anesthetic agents. A recent review article comparing propofol with volatile agents for maintenance of anesthesia for elective craniotomy[5] found that there was inadequate evidence to conclude whether there was any difference in neurological outcome, morbidity, or mortality. The only statistically different outcomes between the groups were in secondary outcome measures such as lower ICP, higher CPP, fewer periods of hypotension, and a reduced incidence of postoperative nausea and vomiting in the propofol group. The heterogeneity of the samples, anesthesia, and outcome measures made meta-analysis and summative recommendations a difficult task.

Etomidate

Etomidate reduces CMR without increasing CBF, hence reducing oxygen demand of vulnerable tissue; however, it has been dogged by criticism regarding the effects of adrenocortical suppression.[6] In addition, there is some evidence from animal studies that shows that etomidate use in the setting of focal cerebral ischemia in rats worsens outcome.[7]

Ketamine

The use of ketamine in neuroanesthesia has seen resurgence in recent times. Previous concerns about cerebral vasodilatation and raised ICP have been challenged with several studies suggesting that, when used as an adjuvant to other neuroanesthetic agents and with maintenance of normocapnia by mechanical ventilation, ICP remains stable.[8] In addition, ketamine antagonizes extrasynaptic N-methyl-D-aspartate receptor (NMDA) receptors, which under ischemic conditions can be stimulated by excess glutamate as part of the cascade, leading to neuronal cell death. This process is complex but does appear to be a potential target for neuroprotection. Certainly ketamine has become the induction agent of first choice for prehospital care and trauma within the United Kingdom, even in those with likely TBI. Its hemodynamic stability and sympathomimetic properties support its use in potentially shocked and multiple injured patients. Maintenance of adequate mean arterial pressure (MAP) is a key component of neuroprotection and will be discussed further under potential physiological strategies.

Dexmedetomidine (alpha-2 agonists)

Alpha-2 agonists, such as dexmedetomidine, have emerged in recent years as an alternative for sedation, analgesia, and anesthesia with the potential to attenuate excitotoxic brain injury. Their sympatholytic properties have been proposed as a potential neuroprotective mechanism through a reduction in free radicals, reduced sensitivity to excitatory amino acids such as glutamate, and improvement in both perfusion of the ischemic penumbra, and balance of oxygen supply with demand. However, there have also been concerns from animal models that any reduction in CBF may be out of proportion with decreases in CMR, potentially putting vulnerable neuronal tissue at risk.[9] Further clinical trials are required to elucidate the use of alpha-2 agonists in clinical practice.

Remifentanil

There is some evidence from animal studies that remifentanil may have neuroprotective effects in reducing infarct size and improving neurological function following ischemia. However, the clinical work is ongoing and no recommendations can be made at this point of time.[10]

Other agents
Hormones

Early administration of estrogen or progesterone appears to have both anti-inflammatory and antioxidant properties in animal models with the potential to accelerate reparative processes and improve neurological function. Several clinical trials have recently been completed in TBI. Unfortunately, there seems to be no benefit of intravenous progesterone over placebo in patients with moderate to severe TBI.[11] The safety and feasibility of administering a single dose of intravenous conjugated estrogens in patients with severe TBI has been investigated but no results are yet available. Glucocorticoids reduced peritumoral edema and improved the outcome in bacterial meningitis. However, they did not reduce neurological injury following TBI, stroke, or cardiac arrest but worsened the outcome.

Erythropoietin

Both hypoxia and ischemia are important regulators of EPO production in the brain, and in animal models EPO appears to have a neuroprotective effect in reducing both focal and global cerebral infarction. Although a restrictive red blood cell transfusion strategy is usually recommended in critically ill patients, in patients with severe brain injury brain tissue oxygenation may be compromised at higher hemoglobin levels than in other patients. However, the results of the Erythropoietin in Traumatic Brain Injury (EPO-TBI)[12] study failed to demonstrate any benefit with no reduction in the number of patients with severe neurological dysfunction and no difference in transfusion rate between the two groups. The effect of EPO on mortality remains uncertain.

Magnesium

Magnesium showed much potential for neuroprotection in animal studies and continues to show promise as a possible neuroprotective agent. However, as with so many other agents, this has so far failed to translate convincingly into clinical studies. Magnesium has been shown to be neuroprotective during procedures associated with ischemia such as coronary artery bypass graft and carotid endarterectomy.[13] However, early magnesium administration in stroke failed to improve outcome and no beneficial effect was observed regarding the incidence of delayed ischemic deficit following subarachnoid hemorrhage.[14] However, magnesium sulfate was found to be associated with a lower incidence of postoperative cognitive dysfunction (POCD) on the first postoperative day when compared with control patients and in patients undergoing vascular surgery. Questions remain about the optimum dosage and timing of administration.

Potential physiological strategies

Hypothermia

Induced hypothermia for neuroprotection would appear to be potentially beneficial. For each degree centigrade reduction in temperature, there is an associated 5% reduction in the CMR, which in turn reduces the oxygen demand of the vulnerable brain tissue. At times of reduced oxygen delivery secondary to physical or physiological changes, this may reduce ischemic damage. Multiple animal studies have demonstrated the potential for induced hypothermia to attenuate ischemic injury and reduce cerebral edema. It was first investigated as a potential neuroprotective strategy in the 1950s,[15,16] but its use was associated with complications. Nevertheless, the theoretical evidence of its benefit appears so convincing that clinical studies have continued. Therapeutic hypothermia is now accepted practice in patients post cardiac arrest[17] and following neonatal hypoxia.[18] It also forms part of some clinical guidelines for the management of TBI.[19] A Cochrane Collaboration in 2015 reviewed the use of therapeutic hypothermia in neurosurgical patients.[20] It focused on four randomized controlled trials[21-24] and reconfirmed the conclusion of their earlier 2011 review; there was still no evidence that induced hypothermia was associated with a significant reduction in mortality or severe neurological disability. Equally, there was no evidence of increased harm as a result of the intervention. The only caveat was a small but statistically significant increase in rates of infection in those patients in which cooling was commenced postoperatively. The four studies reviewed were heterogeneous in terms of study size, patient population, surgical procedures, and cooling strategies. Further studies to investigate therapeutic hypothermia as a tool for neuroprotection in neurosurgery are still ongoing.[25] The Eurotherm 325 trial targeted hypothermia as a Stage 2 therapy in TBI when ICP was >20 mmHg. It was found that hypothermia controlled ICP but led to excess mortality at 6 months. The trial was stopped early due to harm.[26]

- No current evidence for use of therapeutic hypothermia for neuroprotection during neurosurgery
- No current evidence of increased harm as a result of therapeutic hypothermia during neurosurgery
- Evidence of harm when hypothermia used as a Stage 2 therapy in TBI

Optimization of CPP and MAP

Cerebrovascular autoregulation describes the ability of the brain to maintain a constant CBF throughout a range of CPP. It is one of the key mechanisms by which the brain protects itself in response to changing arterial pressure, allowing maintenance of flow through a wide range of MAPs from approximately 50 to 150 mmHg. However, autoregulation may become impaired secondary to intracerebral pathology or as a result of surgical intervention. In addition, a raised ICP secondary to tumor, hemorrhage, hydrocephalus, or edema can further affect the CPP and CBF with the result that a higher MAP will be required to maintain adequate cerebral perfusion. Evidence for the preservation of CPP as a neuroprotective strategy has been extrapolated from studies looking at TBI and subarachnoid hemorrhage. Suggested CPP targets from the Brain Trauma Foundation were approximately 70 mmHg, but these have more recently been reduced to approximately 60 mmHg when studies showed that excessive fluid and vasopressor use to achieve these targets carried a higher risk of pulmonary complications.[27] Clinical studies have repeatedly shown that episodes of hypotension with systolic blood pressure <90 mmHg are associated with worse outcomes.

More recent studies, again focused on patients with TBI, have introduced the concept of an individualized optimal CPP.[28] This study by Aries and colleagues suggests that each patient has their own ideal perfusion pressure, which may result in better outcomes than simply targeting a *one-size-fits all* MAP, as described previously. Continuous monitoring of MAP and ICP, and subsequent calculation of variables including cerebrovascular reactivity enable us to identify each individual's optimal CPP range. Early results targeting these individual parameters have been promising. This model is mainly being used in the critical care setting, but as technology and experience develop, this strategy may be extended to the operating room.

- Clinical guidelines suggest aiming for CPP of 60–70 mmHg
- If ICP is likely to be raised, aim for MAP >80–90 mmHg
- Episodes of systolic hypotension <90 mmHg are associated with worse outcome
- Future strategies may evolve to aim for an individual optimized cerebral perfusion pressure

Alternative therapeutic and experimental strategies

Preconditioning

It may be possible to protect the brain by enhancing its tolerance to ischemia using a process called preconditioning. This refers to a physiological mechanism by which exposure of a tissue or organ to an ischemic insult can provide protection against a future insult. Most preconditioning experiments to date have involved the heart but the brain is an important current target. Ischemic conditioning can be applied before (preconditioning), during (per-conditioning), or after (postconditioning) an ischemic event. It is thought that preconditioning induces humoral factors that prevent reperfusion injury through modification of intracellular kinase activity, decreasing mitochondrial permeability, enhancing DNA restorative capacity, and attenuating the inflammatory response.

Remote preconditioning

Remote preconditioning would appear to be a more practical alternative in the clinical setting. Brief episodes of ischemia are produced by repeatedly inflating a limb cuff to pressures much greater than systolic blood pressure for 5–10 min. This is repeated in cycles prior to the potential ischemic event. Again, most research has been carried out on cardiac protection. In animal models, short repeated episodes of peripheral vascular occlusion before the induction of coronary ischemia reduced myocardial infarct size. However, in a similar manner, it is hoped that with preconditioning the brain would develop a tolerance toward a subsequent similar ischemic injury. Remote preconditioning appears to be a well-tolerated and noninvasive strategy that shows promise. However, clinical studies on the neuroprotective effects of preconditioning are awaited.[29]

Neuroreparative strategies

The central nervous system has limited ability for repair following insults. Neuroregenerative processes such as neurogenesis, gliogenesis, angiogenesis, synaptic plasticity, and axonal sprouting are stimulated by endogenous growth-related factors. Although these processes can facilitate functional and structural recovery, they are largely ineffective for the severity of damage typically encountered following TBI or stroke. Possible strategies being considered in these situations include stem cell therapies; mesenchymal stem cells can improve structural and functional outcomes in different brain injury models.[30] However, these interventions are at a very early stage and their safety and consistency need to be confirmed in clinical studies.

Conclusion

Despite much work characterizing the pathological mechanisms contributing to neuronal injury and many promising animal studies, the quest for clinically successful neuroprotective strategies continues. Both pharmacological and physiological perioperative neuroprotection are associated with conflicting results. However, given the complex pathophysiology of cerebral ischemia, it would be unlikely if one single intervention strategy would provide the answer. Although some interventions and specific agents appear to show potential in terms of contributing to a reduction in the incidence of new postoperative dysfunction, there is currently no evidence that any of them will provide a long-term effect on functional outcome or mortality. Despite this, major advances in clinical outcomes have been observed in recent years. The anesthetist and intensivist have played a vital role in this by the use of a package of clinical measures, including the prevention of secondary insults in the early phases after injury, multimodality monitoring, and maintenance of CPP.

References

1. Badenes R, Gruenbaum SE, Bilotta F. Cerebral protection during neurosurgery and stroke. *Curr Opin Anaesthesiol* 2015 Oct;28(5):532–536.
2. Core topics in neuroanaesthesia and neurointensive care. In: Matta BF, Menon DK, Smith M, editors. *Chapter 3 Mechanisms of Neuronal Injury and Cerebral Protection*. Kristin Engelhard and Christian Werner: Cambridge University Press; 2011.
3. Molecular and Cellular biology of Neuroprotection in the CNS. In: Alzheimer C, editor. *Chapter 5 Na+ Channels and Ca2+ Channels of the Cell Membrane as Targets of Neuroprotective Substances*. Christian Alzheimer: Plenum Publishers & Landes Bioscience. New York; 2002.
4. Bilotta F, Gelb AW, Stazi E, Titi L, Paoloni FP, Rosa G. Pharmacological perioperative brain neuroprotection: A qualitative review of randomized clinical trials. *Br J Anaesth* 2013 Jun;110(Suppl. 1):i113–i120.
5. Chui J, Mariappan R, Mehta J, Manninen P, Venkatraghavan L. Comparison of propofol and volatile agents for maintenance of anesthesia during elective craniotomy procedures: Systematic review and meta-analysis. *Can J Anaesthesiol* 2014;61:347–356.
6. Wagner RL, White PF, Kan P, Rosenthal MH, Feldman D. Inhibition of adrenal steroidogenesis by the anesthetic etomidate. *N Engl J Med* 1984;310:1415–1421.
7. Drummond JC, McKay LD, Cole DJ, Patel PM. The role of nitric oxide synthase inhibition in the adverse effects of etomidate in the setting of focal cerebral ischemia in rats. *Anesth Analg* 2005 Mar;100(3):841–846.
8. Bowles ED, Gold ME. Rethinking the paradigm: Evaluation of ketamine as a neurosurgical anesthetic. *AANA J* 2012 December;80(6):445–452.
9. Farag E, Argalious M, Sessler D, Kurz A, Ebrahim Z, Schubert A. Use of alpha-2 agonists in neuroanaesthesia: An overview. *Ochsner J* 2011;11:57–69.
10. Jeong S, Kim SJ, Jeong C et al. Neuroprotective effects of remifentanil against transient focal cerebral ischemia in rats. *J Neurosurg Anesthesiol* 2012;24:51–57.
11. Skolnick BE, Maas AI, Narayan RJ et al. A clinical trial of progesterone for severe traumatic brain injury. *N Engl J Med* 2014;371:2467–2476.
12. Nichol A, French C, Little L et al. Eryrthopoietin in Traumatic Brain Injury (EPO-TBI): A double-blind randomized controlled trial. *Lancet* 2015;386(10012):2499–2506.
13. Chang JJ, Mack WJ, Saver JL, Sanossian N. Magnesium: Potential roles in neurovascular disease. *Front Neurol* 2014;5:52.
14. Golan E, Vasquez DN, Ferguson ND et al. Prophylactic magnesium for improving neurologic outcome after aneurysmal subarachnoid hemorrhage: Systematic review and meta-analysis. *J Crit Care* 2013;28:173–181.
15. Hendrick EB. The use of hypothermia in severe head injuries in childhood. *Arch Surg* 1959;79:362–364.
16. Lougheed WM, Sweet WH, White JC, Brewster WR. The use of hypothermia in surgical treatment of cerebral vascular lesions: A preliminary report. *J Neurosurg* 1955;12(3):240–255.
17. Silverman MG, Scirica BM. Cardiac arrest and therapeutic hypothermia. *Trends Cardiovasc Med* 2015 Oct 22;26:337–344.
18. Davidson JO, Wassink G, van den Heuji LG, Bennet L, Gunn AJ. Therapeutic hypothermia for neonatal hypoxic-ischemic encephalopathy—Where to from here? *Front Neurol* 2015;6:198.

19. Helmy A, Vizcaychipi M, Gupta AK. Traumatic brain injury: Intensive care management. *Br J Anaesthesiol* 2007;99:32–42.

20. Galvin IM, Levy R, Boyd JG, Day AG, Wallace MC. Cooling for cerebral protection during brain surgery (review). The Cochrane Library 2015 Issue 1.

21. Els T, Oehm E, Voigt S, Klisch J, Hetzel A, Kassubek J. Safety and therapeutical benefit of hemicraniectomy combined with mild hypothermia in comparison with hemicraniectomy alone in patients with malignant ischemic stroke. *Cerebrovasc Dis* 2006;21(1–2):79–85.

22. Hindman BJ, Todd MM, Gelb AW et al. Mild hypothermia as a protective therapy during intracranial aneurysm surgery: A randomized prospective pilot trial. *Neurosurgery* 1999;44(1):23–32.

23. Qiu W, Zhang Y, Sheng H, Zhang J, Wang W et al. Effects of therapeutic mild hypothermia on patients with severe traumatic brain injury after craniotomy. *J Crit Care* 2007;22(3):229–235.

24. Todd MM, Hindman BJ, Clarke WR, Torner JC. Intraoperative Hypohermia for Aneurysm Surgery (HAST) Investigators. Mild intraoperative hypothermia during surgery for intracranial aneurysm. *N Engl J Med* 2005;352(2):135–145.

25. Neugebauer H, Kolmar R, Nielsen WD et al. DEcompressive surgery Plus hypoTHermia for Space-Occupying Stroke (DEPTH-SOS): A protocol of a multicenter randomized controlled clinical trial and a literature review. *Int J Stroke* 2013;8(5):383–387.

26. Andrews PJD, Sinclair HL, Rodriguez A et al. Hypothermia for intracranial hypertension after traumatic brain injury. *N Engl J Med* 2015;373:2403–2412.

27. Brain Trauma Foundation. Guidelines for the management of severe traumatic brain injury. Available online at https://www.braintrauma.org/uploads/06/06/Guidelines_Management_2007w_bookmarks_2.pdf.

28. Aries MJ, Czosnyka M, Budohoski KP et al. Continuous determination of optimal cerebral perfusion pressure in traumatic brain injury. *Crit Care Med* 2012;40(8):2456–2463.

29. Zwerus R, Absalom A. Update on anesthetic neuroprotection. *Curr Opin Anesthesiol* 2015;28:424–430.

30. Laroni A, Novi G, de Kerlero RN, Uccelli A. Towards clinical application of mesenchymal stem cells for treatment of neurological diseases of the central nervous system. *J Neuroimmune Pharmacol* 2013;8:1062–1076.

PART II

Examining the neurosurgical patient

5

Preanesthetic evaluation

SRILATA MONINGI

Introduction

A safe and sound anesthesia practice integrates four main components:

1. Preanesthesia evaluation, counseling, and informed consent
2. Planning, proper execution, and timely intervention
3. Airway and hemodynamic management
4. Postoperative care

Preanesthesia evaluation in neurosurgical practice is an integral base component for conduct of safe neuroanesthesia practice and patient management, to reduce perioperative morbidity and to boost the overall outcome.[1] The physical and functional status of the patient determines the short- and long-term outcomes in patients undergoing intracranial elective neurosurgery.[2] This even reduces the overall cancellation rates of cases, allays anxiety, reduces the complication rate, and makes the patient familiar with the perioperative management. The prerequisites for

effective care include good communication and a team approach in the preoperative period.[3]

Preanesthetic checkup

Preanesthetic checkup (PAC) covers the following:

- Wide aspects of history taking.
- Detailed examination.
- Neurological status.
- Rapport building with patients and their families.
- Counseling and education regarding surgery and anesthesia.
- Premedication and mode of analgesia.
- Getting written informed consent.
- Patient planning and preparation.
- Optimization of modifiable risk factors and identification of high risk cases.
- Specific referrals as and when required.
- Risk stratification.
- Explanation of the surgical procedure, its approach, and its anesthesia requisites

including airway, hemodynamic monitoring, and positioning of the patient during surgery. This also includes providing knowledge regarding postoperative care, intensive care unit (ICU) stay, ventilator management, nutrition, pain management, postoperative nausea and vomiting (PONV), and placement of drains with their associated complications.

- Awareness regarding specific anesthesia procedures and invasive monitoring and the risks involved.
- Investigations and interventions and their requisites.
- Recommendations and guidelines.

- Availability of ventilator, high dependency unit, or ICU bed, as and when required.

A stepwise evaluation avoids any missing elements and guides us to secure management of neurosurgical patients in both elective and emergency situations.[1] A PAC clinic along with the primary care targets to achieve the maximum benefit following surgery.

Components of history taking

History taking is an art. It should help us in determining the actual problem or disease the patient has. The predisposing factors to the presentation

Chief complaints	Presenting symptoms
	Other nonspecific (stated in patient's own words)
Patient characteristics	Age, gender, handedness (right or left)
History of present illness	Character of the presenting symptoms
Past medical history	Previous medical illness: diabetes, hypertension, stroke, myocardial infarction (MI)/coronary artery disease (CAD), infection, trauma, chronic obstructive pulmonary disease (COPD), allergy, blood transfusion
	Previous medical/surgical history, type of anesthesia, any complications, postponement of surgery hospital or ICU stay, e.g., neonates with spina bifida and hydrocephalus undergoing multiple surgeries
	Other specific problems that may be related to the patient's complaints
Family history	Diabetes, hypertension, dementia, CAD, cancer, stroke, arthritis, inherited conditions, prolonged apnea, unexplained death, malignant hyperpyrexia
Review of systems	Brief details about each system, specifically concentrating on those systems related to the presenting complaints:
	• General symptoms, e.g., fever, weight loss
	• Neurological and psychologic
	• Eye, nose, ear, mouth, and neck
	• Thorax
	• Cardiovascular
	• Respiratory
	• Gastrointestinal and genitourinary
	• Skin and musculoskeletal
	• Psychiatric
	• Allergic, immunologic, and hematologic
	• Endocrine, including hormonal
Social history	Marital status, menstrual history, occupation, hours of work, exercise, diet, alcoholism, smoking, addiction history, hobbies
Medications history	Both current and previous medications
	Most commonly: anticonvulsants, aspirin, and other anticoagulants; diuretics, steroids, pregabalin, and gabapentin; allergy or hypersensitivity to drugs; allergy to food, contrast drugs or dyes, or latex; radiotherapy or chemotherapy history and their effects

and the specific examination required can also be determined by proper history taking.[4,5] The components of history taking are tabulated as follows:

Each presenting complaint needs to be characterized by the following:

- Symptoms
- Duration
- Frequency
- Precipitating factors
- Alleviating factors
- Previous related problems
- Family history of similar or related problems

The symptomatology and its presentation vary with the type of intracranial pathology.[6] This gives us information about the disease process and the current neurological state. In emergency situations such as trauma and collapse, we must gather information from the people involved in resuscitation, standby witnesses, and relatives.

We will discuss the evaluation specific to various neuropathologies. A detailed description of each parameter and collaborating the findings help us in diagnosing the pathology in almost half of the cases.[1]

Neurosurgical pathologies: Presentation

The site and size of the lesion, rate of growth, the side involved, and its effects on intracranial pressure (ICP) determine the type of clinical presentation.

Pathology	Presenting complaints	Specific considerations
Intracranial tumors[7]	Symptoms and signs (s/s) of ICP: • Nausea and emesis • Headache • Altered mental status • Diminished alertness • Hypertension • Seizures • Visual disturbances • Papilledema • Unilateral pupillary dilation • Abducens or oculomotor palsy • Neck rigidity With increasing ICP, the symptomatology changes to an emergency setting of • Apnea • Dilated and unreactive pupils • Contralateral hemiplegia • Decreased consciousness • Bradycardia	Other associated comorbid illnesses and congenital anomalies need to be looked for
Pituitary tumors[7,8]	Hypertension, CAD, hypertrophy, diabetes, thyroid, changes in mental status, muscle weakness, headache, visual loss	Endocrine function: diabetes, thyroid, Cushing's Cardiac Fluid and electrolyte status Medications: corticosteroids, diuretics, and anticonvulsants

(Continued)

(*Continued*)

Pathology	Presenting complaints	Specific considerations
Neurosurgical vascular lesions: intracranial aneurysms and arteriovenous malformations[7]	Nonspecific: headaches, orbital pain, dizziness, and mild sensory or motor abnormalities Rupture of aneurysm: s/s of ICP secondary to hemorrhage, focal neurological signs, depressed level of consciousness, nausea and vomiting, hypothermia, the triad of meningeal irritation (photophobia, headache, and meningismus), cranial nerve palsies, and seizures Rarely may present with high output cardiac failure	Hypertension, CAD
Carotid artery disease	s/s of transient ischemic attack (TIA) or a completed stroke: • Paresthesia or numbness in the contralateral arm, leg or face weakness • Dysphasia • Contralateral monocular visual loss • Hyperreflexia • Affected side, extensor plantar response - Symptoms may be elicited with certain head and neck positions; h/o severe cervical arthritis and spondylosis; carotid bruit	• Hypertension • CAD • Valvular heart disease • Diabetes • Management: optimal control of blood pressure; cardiovascular evaluation: ECG (comparison with previous findings); precautions: careful positioning of head and neck to avoid cervical ischemia; avoid palpation of carotid artery (plaque dislodgment and embolization is a possibility)
Vertebrobasilar arterial disease	s/s of TIA or a completed stroke: • Paresthesia, weakness, or numbness in either or both sides • Dysarthria • Diplopia, decreased visual acuity, or blurring • Drop attacks or falling to floor from leg weakness • Vertigo	

Cerebral and lacunar infarction
Symptoms:

- Related to the particular vessel involved
- Extent of collateral circulation

TIAs: usually last from 30 min to 2 h; may have normal findings at the time of their examination
Completed stroke: may have additional signs of increased ICP, cerebral edema, coagulopathy, stupor, or coma

Pathology	Presenting complaints	Specific considerations
Spinal lesions: injury, tumor, spinal stenosis, aging	s/s attributed to spinal cord or nerve root compression; e.g., localized spinal segmental pain ± radiation to the extremity or weakness and atrophy in muscle groups of the affected extremity; bladder involvement indicates sacral nerve dysfunction	Motor function; sensory function; semi-emergent condition
Spinal dysraphism (pediatrics)	Associated Arnold–Chiari malformation, congenital cardiac anomalies, hydrocephalus, VP shunts, multiple surgeries, neurological deficit, bladder and bowel disturbances	Pediatric population, difficult intubation, difficulty in positioning, cerebrospinal fluid (CSF) leakage
Head injury • extent of injury • open or closed skull trauma	Mild-to-severe form s/s of increased ICP: seizures, decreasing level of consciousness, hypertension or hypotension	Primary survey: Assessment of breathing, circulation and airway (BCA) Glasgow Coma Scale (GCS) scoring Management of seizures, hypertension or hypotension; treatment of shock Associated injuries: abdominal injuries, long bone fractures, cervical spine fracture, calcaneal fracture

Details of comorbid illnesses

Some medical conditions poses the risk of perioperative complications like surgical infections, hemodynamic instability and respiratory morbidity. They affect the anesthetic management and should be optimized before surgery. These include:

- Diabetes: duration, type, medications (oral hypoglycemic and/or insulin), lifestyle, complications
- Hypertension: duration, complications, medications (angiotensin-converting enzyme [ACE] inhibitors, diuretics, angiotensin receptor blockers)
- Respiratory: asthma, COPD, medications, lifestyle modifications; smoking: duration, pack-years, duration of abstinence
- Cardiovascular: chest pain, breathlessness, medications, interventions
- Gastrointestinal: abdominal pain, jaundice, alcoholism, gastroesophageal reflux, acid peptic disease, bladder and bowel disturbances

- History of tuberculosis: duration, type, treatment, deranged liver parameters, infective or not
- History of blood transfusion: any complications

Physical examination (elective scenario)

- Demographic parameters: name, age, weight, height, body mass index (BMI), built, nutritional status, mobility, occupation, language, residence.

General examination

- Check for pallor, icterus, clubbing, lymphadenopathy, tremor, cyanosis, gingival hyperplasia, and edema.
- Vitals: pulse—rhythm, volume, peripheral pulses; blood pressure (noninvasive)—palpatory/auscultatory; respiration.

Neurological examination

(Refer to Chapter 6)

Examination of pupils

Checking pupils gives a clue to the diagnosis with other positive findings (described in Chapter 6).

Airway examination

This is performed to identify patients with difficult airway/mask ventilation.[5,9] Assessment should include the following:

- Obesity
- Face: bearded
- Snoring history
- Neck: circumference, neck length (short); neck movement (normal neck flexion, 25°–30°; atlanto-occipital joint extension, 85°)
- Inter-incisor gap
- Temporomandibular joint function
- Upper lip bite test
- Mallampati grading
- Sternomental distance, thyromental distance, and mentohyoid distance
- High arched palate: associated with difficult intubation
- Teeth: dentures, missing teeth, loose teeth, artificial

Cardiovascular system examination

- Heart rate: rhythm, rate, ectopics, pulse difference, any murmurs
- Blood pressure
- New York Heart Association (NYHA) grading: to grade exercise capacity
- Cardiopulmonary exercise testing: shuttle walk test
- To identify the risk factors, determine the need for optimization, and modify the risk by preoperative interventions

Respiratory system examination

- Respiration: rate, pattern of breathing, dyspnea
- Any fresh complaints of upper respiratory infection/cough (wet or dry)
- Lungs: bilateral air entry, vesicular/bronchial; any crepitations or other added sounds, wheeze

- Signs of lung collapse/consolidation/effusion
- Trachea: position, any deviation
- Identification of risk factors: smoking, elderly, COPD, congestive heart failure (CHF), functional dependence, prolonged duration of surgery, American Society of Anesthesiologists (ASA) classification III or more, long-term steroid usage

Gastrointestinal, hepatic, and renal system examination

- Any abnormal swelling/pain, jaundice; other associated findings, such as ascites, peripheral edema
- Identification of risk factors: alcoholism, hypertension, CAD, diabetes
- The Child–Turcotte–Pugh classification and model for end-stage liver disease (MELD) scoring: used for predicting mortality in patients with liver dysfunction

Endocrine system examination

- Diabetes: associated renal and cardiac disease; tests for autonomic dysfunction; difficult airway; identify complications, such as diabetic ketoacidosis, hyperosmolar nonketotic coma (HONC)
- Hypothyroidism: enlarged tongue, large goiter, tracheal compression; hypothermia, hypoglycemia, lethargic, delayed menstruation
- Hyperthyroidism: sleeping pulse rate, irregular rhythm, progressive weight gain, tremor

Skeletal system examination

- Stature/gait
- Spine: gibbus/kyphosis/scoliosis (using the Cobb angle)
- On traction/collar

Physical examination (emergency scenario)

- With head trauma: watch for vitals along with level of consciousness (GCS); look for other major injuries, such as abdominal, thoracic, vascular, and long bone injuries.
- With large posterior fossa tumors and basilar artery aneurysm: check for signs of increased

ICP, such as papilledema, cranial nerve IV and VI palsies; bradycardia, coma.

- Cerebrovascular accidents: watch for vitals, along with extent of neurological insult.
- Pituitary apoplexy: sudden loss of vision can occur.

Investigations and other specific tests

Most of the patients attend the PAC clinic after initial screening by the treating physician. Depending upon the surgical pathology, approach, and the associated complications, the investigations are asked for with respect to surgical and anesthetic implications.

Depending upon the age, presenting complaints, and other comorbids, chest roentgenogram and electrocardiogram are recorded to exclude any pathology. Specific investigations include computed tomography and magnetic resonance imaging of the brain to define the pathology, size, and extent of the lesion, midline shift, and involvement of vital structures. Correlations of clinical findings with findings of investigations guide us in planning the perioperative management and help us in comparing the pre- and postoperative neurological conditions (Table 5.1).[10]

Table 5.1 Investigations and implications

Investigations	Indications	Implications
Hemogram (Hb, Hct)	Craniotomies Malignancy Vascular malformations Vascular tumors; meningiomas Infants <1 year of age Associated chronic cardiovascular, pulmonary, renal, or hepatic disease	*Hemoglobin* (10 g/dL): carries the risk of cardiac and cerebral ischemia *Higher Hb levels*: carry the risk of thrombosis
Total leucocyte count	Infection On steroid therapy	To exclude any infection Patients susceptible to infection
Blood grouping and screening	All intracranial and major spinal surgeries	To replenish blood loss (when required)
Sickle cell screening		Susceptible patients
Pregnancy test............................ Susceptible patients Coagulation tests (BT, CT, PT, aPTT) Platelet counts	Craniotomies On anticoagulant therapy Liver disease Risk of bleeding/diathesis	To exclude any coagulation disorder
Renal parameters (blood urea, serum creatinine) and electrolytes (sodium, potassium), chloride, total CO_2, calcium	Hypertension Renal disease Diabetes Pituitary or adrenal disease On diuretic therapy Seizures, malignancy, elderly patients	*Changes in electrolyte status*: affect the fluid balance and cerebral dynamics

(Continued)

Table 5.1 Investigations and implications (*Continued*)

Investigations	Indications	Implications
Endocrine profile		
Blood sugar, Hb1aC	All craniotomies	Hyperglycemia aggravates neuronal ischemia
Thyroid	Spine surgeries	Sensitive to effects of opioids and inhalational agents
Liver function tests	*On anticonvulsant therapy*: phenytoin	Titration of dose is required in patients with deranged liver function tests
Electrocardiograph	Heart disease, hypertension, diabetes, elderly patients Subarachnoid hemorrhage, intracranial hemorrhage, cerebrovascular accident, head injury, vascular malformations	Any abnormality helps in identification of the pathology; guides in establishing the diagnosis
Echocardiograph	Coronary or valvular heart disease Surgery in sitting position	Guides the anesthetist in perioperative hemodynamic management of the patients Also helps in differentiating the changes incurred by subarachnoid hemorrhage with that of actual heart disease
Stress ECG, exercise thallium, dipyridamole thallium scans, coronary angiography	High risk conditions like previous myocardial infarction >6 weeks, compensated congestive heart failure, mild stable angina, low functional capacity, diabetes	To assess the significance of ECG changes/chest pain and to establish the severity of the pathology Risk stratification
Chest roentgenogram	Cardiac disease Pulmonary disease Malignancy Any critical care patient	To exclude any major pathology, thus avoiding any respiratory complications
Spirometry	Respiratory disease Cervical pathology Scoliosis	To assess the respiratory reserve and accordingly optimize
Arterial blood gas analysis	Significant pulmonary disease	For assessment of respiratory reserve
Sleep apnea testing	Markedly obese patients with h/o sleep apnea	Advised to have their continuous positive airway pressure (CPAP) machines available in the postoperative period Titration of anesthetic drugs Avoid drugs that impair respiratory drive Postoperative SpO_2 monitoring mandatory

Investigations	Indications	Implications
Specific neurodiagnostic studies[7]		
Computed tomography (CT) and magnetic resonance imaging (MRI)	*Head injury*: detects extra-axial hemorrhage (subdural, extradural, and subarachnoid), parenchymal bleeds, cerebral contusions, and skull fractures *Tumors*: site, extent of the lesion, associated hydrocephalus, vascularity, and tumoral edema	*Hemorrhage*: seen as areas of white density in CT *CT*: most preferred imaging modality in patients with head injury This helps in planning for the position required for surgical approach; CSF drainage options for deep lesions; blood conservation techniques; and arrangement of blood and blood products
	Cerebral edema: appears as decreased density (black) in CT; in MRI, seen as decreased signal (black) on T1-weighted studies and as increased signal (white) on T2-weighted studies Detects herniation syndromes and hydrocephalus (both communicating and noncommunicating)	
	Also detects pneumocephalus	*Pneumocephalus*: after skull fractures, postoperatively, after pneumocephalograms and lumbar punctures; use of nitrous oxide is avoided
	Raised ICP: seen as effaced cortical sulci, basal cisterns and interhemispheric fissures, compressed ventricles, and herniation syndromes	
Plain skull films	Fractures, investigating penetrating injuries, foreign bodies, site, and relationship of depressed skull fractures	
Positron emission tomography	In vivo evaluation of brain physiology and biochemistry Identifies grades of glioma and recurrent tumor from radiation induced necrosis	

(Continued)

Table 5.1 Investigations and implications (*Continued*)

Investigations	Indications	Implications
Angiography	Identifies vascular lesions, the site of origin, vessels at risk, vascularity of the lesion, presence of cross-filling, risk of bleeding (in arteriovenous malformations [AVMs]), etc. *Embolization of feeding vessels*: in highly vascular tumors and AVMs to decrease the risk of bleeding, to plan surgical access, to prepare for transfusion of blood and blood products, and for temperature management *Balloon occlusion test*: (awake patient) to test for any neurological changes at the time of occlusion; e.g., in cases of cavernous sinus aneurysm *Wada test*: to identify the dominant lobe for language and memory	
Ultrasound of carotids	To detect the degree of stenosis in both the carotids To assess the collateral circulation in times of carotid occlusion	If severe, hypotension may precipitate cerebral ischemia
Transcranial Doppler	To detect vasospasm; indicated by increased flow rate; seen in subarachnoid hemorrhage	Avoids induced hypotension in patients with vasospasm; may precipitate ischemia
Tests for visual field	Pituitary tumors	

Source: Committee on Standard and Practice Parameters, Apfelbaum JL, Connis RT, et al., *Anesthesiology*, 2012, 116, 522–538.

Preoperative evaluation is followed by optimization of modifiable conditions if any, stratification of risk explaining the anesthesia procedure, formulation of anesthesia planning, informed consent, and finally issuing of preoperative orders.

Risk scoring scales such as preoperative ASA physical status classification, the Karnofsky Performance Score (KPS), the Charlson comorbidity index score, and the modified Rankin Scale use preoperative variables to predict the postoperative outcome following intracranial surgery.[2,11] Other scoring systems such as the SKALE score (sex, KPS, ASA physical status classification, location, and edema) and the Helsinki ASA are also used in assessing postoperative outcome in cranial neurosurgery.

Preoperative orders

Preoperative orders are written that assure completion of the final steps in the preparation of the patient before operation. These orders usually include the following:[7,10]

1. Nothing by mouth for solids,[12] 6 h; for breast milk, 4 h; and for clear liquids, 2 h.
2. Medications: prescription of anti-anxiety medications is controversial; patients with low GCS are not advised.

a. Antihypertensive medications to be continued except for angiotensin receptor blockers and ACE inhibitors.

b. Patients on steroids and anti-epileptic medications to be continued on the day of surgery.

c. Patients on anti-parkinsonian drugs undergoing deep brain stimulation surgery, ideally to stop to facilitate target placement of electrodes.

d. Patients on anti-epileptic medications undergoing epilepsy surgery with monitoring of seizure activity, ideally to discontinue to facilitate monitoring of epileptic foci.

3. Communication skills: multidisciplinary team approach and planning plays an important role in the perioperative management, especially in patients with complex surgeries or those requiring a specific position for the surgical approach.

4. In cases of difficult intubation and compromised cervical spine: procedure for awake fiber-optic intubation is explained.

5. Incentive spirometry, cessation of smoking, and deep breathing exercises: advised in patients with respiratory compromise.

6. Arrangement for blood and blood products as and when required.

7. Explaining the procedure: anesthesia, pain, drain, and ventilator management.

8. Informed risk consent.

Comprehensive knowledge and awareness of the pathophysiological characteristics of neuro-surgical disorders in preanesthetic evaluation is vital for the formulation of an anesthetic sketch for perioperative patient management.

References

1. Fischer SP. Preoperative evaluation of the adult neurosurgical patient. *Int Anesthesiol Clin* 1996;34:21–32.

2. Reponen E, Tuominen H, Korja M. Evidence for the use of preoperative risk assessment scores in elective cranial neurosurgery: A systematic review of the literature. *Anesth Analg* 2014;119:420–432.

3. Gupta A, Gupta N. Setting up and functioning of a preanaesthetic clinic. *Indian J Anaesth* 2010;54:504–507.

4. Misulis KE, Head TC. *Netter's Concise Neurology*. Vol. 1. Philadelphia, PA: Saunders Elsevier; 2007.

5. Petranker S, Nikoyan L, Ogle OE. Preoperative evaluation of the surgical patient. *Dent Clin North Am* 2012; 56:163–181, ix.

6. Sappenfield JW, Martz DG, Jr. Patients with disease of brain, cerebral vasculature, and spine. *Med Clin North Am* 2013;97:993–1013.

7. Barnett SR, Nozari A. The preoperative evaluation of the neurosurgical patient. *Int Anesthesiol Clin* 2015;53:1–22.

8. Horvat A, Kolak J, Gopcevic A, Ilej M, Zivko G. Anesthetic management of patients undergoing pituitary surgery. *Acta Clin Croat* 2011;50:209–216.

9. Langeron O, Birenbaum A, Le Sache F, Raux M. Airway management in obese patient. *Minerva Anestesiol* 2014;80:382–392.

10. Committee on Standard and Practice Parameters, Apfelbaum JL, Connis RT et al. Practice advisory for preanesthesia evaluation: An updated report by the American Society of Anesthesiologists Task Force on Preanesthesia Evaluation. *Anesthesiology* 2012;116:522–538.

11. Reponen E, Korja M, Niemi T, Silvasti-Lundell M, Hernesniemi J, Tuominen H. Preoperative identification of neurosurgery patients with a high risk of in-hospital complications: A prospective cohort of 418 consecutive elective craniotomy patients. *J Neurosurg* 2015;123:594–604.

12. American Society of Anesthesiologists Committee. Practice guidelines for preoperative fasting and the use of pharmacologic agents to reduce the risk of pulmonary aspiration: Application to healthy patients undergoing elective procedures: An updated report by the American Society of Anesthesiologists Committee on Standards and Practice Parameters. *Anesthesiology* 2011;114:495–511.

6

Neurologic examination

SRILATA MONINGI

Introduction

Neurologic examination is the most vital examination to guide the diagnosis of any neurosurgical pathology. The main objectives and rationales behind neurologic examinations are the following:

1. To ascertain the site and magnitude of the lesion.
2. To document in the anesthesia records the physical and neurological states preoperatively and to compare them postoperatively.
3. To prepare a plan for perioperative anesthesia management.

This includes evaluation of function of both peripheral and central nervous systems. The order of examination should follow higher to lower levels of integration to avoid missing any steps. All patients without any neurological disease undergo neurological evaluation briefly. This includes the following, which can be termed as SRM^{2}C:

1. The sensory system: pain, touch, and vibration
2. Reflex test: both superficial and deep tendon

3. The musculoskeletal system: gait, walking with toe or heel, ability to maintain the arms forward, strength of the grip
4. Mental status: the level of consciousness and other tests for cerebral function
5. Cranial nerve: patient's history and observation

Enhanced neurologic examination is performed especially in patients presenting with symptoms relevant to neurologic abnormality. This comprises a detailed description and examination starting from consciousness to small reflexes. Detailed description of the neurological symptoms and the presentation is an important aspect of history taking, which forms a strong base for clinical guidance. This was already discussed in the "Preanesthetic evaluation," Chapter 5.

Level of consciousness

First and foremost is the level of consciousness. The Glasgow Coma Scale is the most commonly and widely used scale for grading the consciousness level though its predictive value is very limited mainly due to observer variability.[1,2] This is scored and interpreted as given in Table 6.1:

Other states of altered consciousness:

Brain death: An irreversible and permanent failure of cortical and brainstem activity

Persistent vegetative state: A condition of altered state following severe cerebral injury that becomes chronic or persistent

Locked-in syndrome: A condition where there is paralysis of the voluntary muscles but with preservation of full consciousness and cognition.

Tests for cerebral function

Tests for higher cerebral function measure any changes in the following:

* Emotional status
* Communication
* Intellectual performance
* Behavior
* Orientation
* Memory
* Language
* Speech

The Mini Mental State Examination is the most commonly used routine test for cerebral function.

It tests the orientation, memory, attention and calculation, recall, and language of the patient.[3] The patients are categorized based on their ability to perform various components of cerebral function tests. This is again repeated in the postoperative period and compared with the baseline characteristics. The Montreal Cognitive Assessment and Mini-Cog are other tools to assess cerebral function.[4,5]

Cranial nerve evaluation

This evaluation gives us knowledge regarding the specific cranial nerves involved, the site of the lesion, interference with anesthesia management if any, and other postoperative complications (Table 6.2).[6,7]

Testing vision

Testing vision includes the following:[7]

1. *Visual acuity*:

Step 1. Test the ability of each eye to read small and large print or with the Snellen chart (kept at a distance of 6 m) using normal refractive correction.

Table 6.1 Glasgow Coma Scale

Eye opening response (E)	Score	Motor response (M)	Score	Verbal response (V)	Score
Spontaneous	4	Obeys	6	Oriented	5
To command	3	Localizes	5	Confused conversation	4
To pain	2	Withdraws (flexion)	4	Inappropriate words	3
No response	1	Abnormal flexion	3	Incomprehensible sounds (moans, groans)	2
		Extensor response	2	No response	1
		No response	1		

E (4) + M (6) + V (5) = Minimum of 3 to Maximum of 15

3–8: Severe head injury; airway protection is lost with severe hemispheric dysfunction—requires intubation

9–12: Moderate head injury

≥13: Mild head injury

Table 6.2 Cranial nerve evaluation and interpretation

Cranial nerve	Function	Tests	Interpretation	Implications
Olfactory nerve	Smell	To smell coffee grounds (avoid mint)	*Loss of smell or smell disorders*: head injury, frontal lobe or pituitary lesion, meningitis, hydrocephalus, or an anterior fossa skull fracture	Increased ICP, cerebral hemorrhage, s/s of meningeal infection
Optic nerve	Vision	Eye testing with visual fields	*Monocular*: optic nerve lesion *Homonymous hemianopia*: optic lesion behind the chiasm *Incongruous deficits (e.g., bitemporal hemianopia)*: lesion around the chiasm (pituitary tumors)	–
Oculomotor nerve	Eye movements	Pupil size; response to light; comparison with PO data	Diplopia, ptosis, divergent squint, pupillary dilation, loss of accommodation and light reflexes: compression in the midbrain and surrounding areas, cavernous sinus or orbit	Complete oculomotor involvement including the peripheral fibers of the nerve bundle (supplies pupil)
Trochlear nerve	Downward movement of the eye	Diplopia Head rotated to opposite side	Lesions in and around the cavernous sinus	3rd and 4th cranial nerve palsies are usually associated because of the proximity of these nerves within the cavernous sinus and superior orbital fissure

(Continued)

Table 6.2 Cranial nerve evaluation and interpretation (*Continued*)

Cranial nerve	Function	Tests	Interpretation	Implications
Trigeminal nerve	Chewing action Sensation in V1, V2, and V3 areas Corneal reflex	*Motor:* ask the patient to clench his or her teeth *Sensory:* same distribution check with alcohol swab	Loss of sensation on one side of the face Trigeminal neuralgia with pain Idiopathic lesions in the CP angle or cavernous sinus	Pain may precipitate with face mask ventilation, triggers zones around the lips or buccal cavity, difficult to open the mouth during PAC or during induction
Abducens nerve	Abduction of the eye	Diplopia	*Convergent squint:* lesions in and around the cavernous sinus, raised ICP, and fractures of the base of the skull	–
Facial nerve	Muscles for facial expression Symmetry of the face; taste sensation	Evaluate patient's ability to raise eyebrows, frown and smile, close eyes tight, and puff cheeks	*Facial weakness:* on one side *Loss of taste:* lesion in the facial canal *Both upper and lower face involvement:* facial nerve lesion *Pred. lower facial involvement:* cerebral lesions, Bell's palsy, CP angle lesions	*Chances of damage:* pressure by face mask, surgery, or positioning *Documentation pre- and postoperative:* important
Vestibulococh-lear nerve	Hearing	*Weber's test:* tuning fork is placed on the forehead; patient is asked where the sound is heard; midline or lateralized *Rinne's test:* tuning fork is placed on the mastoid	Tumors	–

(*Continued*)

Table 6.2 Cranial nerve evaluation and interpretation (*Continued*)

Cranial nerve	Function	Tests	Interpretation	Implications
Glossopharyngeal nerve	*Sensory*: pharynx and soft palate	*Palatal reflex*: stroke each side of the mucous membrane of the uvula. If the side touched rises, it indicates that the nerve is intact *Pharyngeal gag reflex*: to elicit gag, touch the posterior pharynx with a tongue depressor	*Glossopharyngeal dysfunction*: severe pain almost like trigeminal neuralgia *Trigger point*: posterior pharynx and tonsillar area	Placement of an oral airway or laryngoscope blade stimulates the trigger zone; severe pain radiating to the angle of the jaw and ear; sometimes may result in reflex bradycardia and hypotension Absence of gag reflex increases the chances of regurgitation
Vagus nerve	*Motor*: pharynx, soft palate, larynx, and trachea *Sensory*: larynx and trachea	Ask the patient to swallow and speak Check gag reflex Watch for symmetrical movement of the soft palate when saying "ah"	*Hoarseness of voice*: vocal cord paralysis	Unopposed sympathetic output in the form of tachycardia—seen with vagus nerve damage
Accessory nerve		Ask the patient to turn his or her head Watch for the movement of sternocleidomastoid muscles	*Weakness of the sternocleidomastoid muscle on the same side*: extracranial compressive lesions	–
Hypoglossal nerve		Ask the patient to protrude his or her tongue	Ipsilateral weakness of the tongue is seen as deviation of the tongue to the side of the lesion	–

ICP, intracranial pressure; CP, cerebellopontine; PAC, preanesthetic check
*

Step 2. If step 1 fails, lower levels of acuity will be tested by counting fingers.

Step 3. If step 2 fails, perception of light is tested by switching on and off of a pen light.

2. *Visual fields*: All four quadrants for each eye will be tested individually. The tests include the following:

   a. Qualitative tests: moving finger test, red pin confrontation test, and binocular test.

      i. Moving finger test: the patient is asked to sit or stand in front of you. Both the eyes are tested alternatively. By closing one eye, ask the patient to fix his or her gaze on your eye. Slowly bring one of your fingers (midway between the patient and you) into the patient's view from the outer quadrant. All four quadrants are tested separately. This is helpful in the diagnosis of pituitary tumors.

      ii. Red pin confrontation test: the procedure is same as "Moving finger test" except that a large red hatpin (head 0.5 cms in diameter) is used in place of the examiners finger. Assumin the examiner's visual field as control, the patients visual field is compared with the examiner's.

      iii. Binocular test: the patient is asked to report the number of fingers seen, when fingers are presented on both sides of the visual field at the same time. In cases of hemisensory neglect (non dominant parietal lobe), patients do no report seeing the finger on the affected side.

   b. Quantitative tests: Perimetry quantifies the visual field mapping.

3. Color vision testing: this tests the functioning of the macular field. Colored plates with patterns of colored spots, some forming single or double digit numbers are used for identifying the numbers. Color blind patients identify the number wrongly or fail to identify.

4. *Fundoscopic examination*: Look for papilledema (increased ICP), optic atrophy (plaques), or retinopathy (hemorrhage, exudates).

5. *Pupillary examination:*[8]

   a. Check for size, shape and regularity.

      i. Pinpoint pupils: overdose with opiates, pontine hemorrhage

      ii. Mid position and not reacting: damage to midbrain

      iii. Dilated and fixed (not reacting), bilateral: severe anoxia or ischemia, death, anticholinergic drugs

      iv. Ovoid shape: intracranial hypertension, early sign of transtentorial herniation (transitional phase between normal pupils and bilateral, dilated, and fixed pupils)

      v. Keyhole: post-iridectomy, sluggish reaction to light

      vi. Large and irregular: traumatic orbital injury

   b. Reaction to light: direct light reflex and consensual light reflex. Patient is asked to look straight at a distant object in a shady room. A bright pen light is shone into the eye from the side. Pupil constricts to direct illumination (direct light reflex) and to illumination of the opposite eye (consensual light reflex).[6]

   c. Accommodation to light: Ask the patient to look straight at a distance and then at a finger brought nearby to the eye. Normal: pupils will constrict.[6] Pupillary responses and their interpretations were tabulated in Table 6.3.

6. *Eye movements:*[7] The cardinal actions of the extraocular muscles are depicted in Figure 6.1. The tests are conducted with both eyes open. A finger is held at about 1 m away from the patient.

   a. The finger is moved slowly in a large "H" pattern. Check for any double vision and for range of movements.

   b. Here the finger is moved slowly in a "+" pattern. Check for smooth pursuit and nystagmus.

Abnormal eye movements also guide in understanding the involvement of the cranial nerve and other parts of the brain in the pathology (Table 6.4). Some of the movements related to cranial nerve lesions have been discussed in the "Cranial nerve evaluation" section.

Table 6.3 Pupillary responses and their interpretations

Pupillary response	Interpretation
Direct light reflex: absent Consensual light reflex: present Affected eye is blind	Disruption of the afferent limb of the light reflex, e.g., prechiasmal lesion
Both direct and consensual reflex absent with dilated pupils	Disruption of the efferent arc of the light reflex, e.g., third nerve palsy
Sluggish reaction	Also seen with third nerve compression, e.g., cerebral edema, herniation
Direct response is weaker than the consensual response: the affected pupil dilates a little or oscillates when light is shone in the two eyes alternatively (Marcus Gunn pupil)	Optic neuritis
Light near dissociation:	
• Accommodation reaction (constriction) is better than light reaction • Light reaction better than accommodation response	• Partial third nerve lesions • Midbrain syndromes, e.g., encephalitis lethargica
Argyll Robertson pupil:	Neurosyphilis affecting the pretectal region of the mesencephalon
• Irregular and small pupil • Reacts briskly to accommodation • Both direct and consensual light reflexes lost • Bilateral	
Horner's syndrome:	Lesion in the ipsilateral central or peripheral sympathetic pathway
• Tonically constricted pupil with failure to dilate on shading the eye • Associated with partial ptosis, enophthalmos	
Hippus phenomenon:	
• The pupil dilates and contracts alternately (with uniform illumination of the pupil)	Early signs of transtentorial herniation, seizure activity

Cerebellar function

This includes balance and coordination. Any abnormality in physical movements such as dysdiadochokinesis, ataxia, and tremor indicates cerebellar lesion, for example, tumor, ischemia, or infarction.[9] Tests for coordination include the following:

Finger nose test: Patient is asked to move his or her finger between the examiner's finger and patient's nose quickly with eyes closed. The accuracy is lost in patients with cerebellar involvement.

Heel knee shin test: With the eyes closed, the patient is asked to move his or her heel of one side to run from the knee down the shin of the tibia of other side and make up and down movements. Wavering of the heel down the shin was observed in patients with cerebellar lesion.

Rapid alternating movements: Patient is asked to his or her slap the thigh with the front and back of the hand alternately. Cerebellar dysfunction leads to inaccurate alternating movements.

Finger tapping: The patient is asked to tap his or her thumb and index finger repeatedly with good excursions. Extrapyramidal lesions, for example, parkinsonism, present with reduced excursions, yet rapid and irregular.

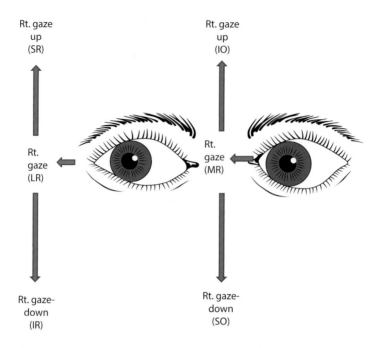

Figure 6.1 The fundamental positions of eye gaze (example: to the right) depicting the action of the six extraocular muscules (IO, inferior oblique; SO, superior oblique; SR, superior rectus; IR, inferior rectus; LR, lateral rectus; MR, medial rectus).

Table 6.4 Abnormal eye movements, its interpretations and implications

Findings on examination	Anatomic localization and implications
Muscles supplied by more than one cranial nerve are involved in both the eyes	Defect in the neuromuscular transmission: myasthenia gravis
Skew deviation where one eye is highly placed	Thalamomidbrain hemorrhage, vestibular or other midbrain lesions
Reflex movements relatively preserved compared to command movements	Supranuclear palsy (lesion affecting the fibers from cerebrum to brainstem): degenerative conditions or extensive cerebral dysfunction
Gaze palsy to one side	Same side of the gaze: hemispheric lesion; opposite side of the gaze: pontine lesion
Oculomotor palsy with sparing of the pupil	Oculomotor nerve lesion sparing the peripheral fibers of the nerve bundle supplying the pupil; microvascular disease—diabetes and hypertension
Conjugate gaze palsy (loss of abduction of ipsilateral eye and adduction of contralateral eye)	Lesion of the ipsilateral sixth nerve nucleus: brainstem disorders
Loss of adduction of one eye (internuclear ophthalmoplegia)	Lesions of the medial longitudinal fasciculus: brainstem lesions, e.g., multiple sclerosis, vascular disease
One and a half syndrome = conjugate gaze palsy + failure of adduction to opposite side	A large lesion of the medial longitudinal fasciculus involving the sixth nerve nucleus as well

(Continued)

Findings on examination	Anatomic localization and implications
Dilated and nonreactive to pupils, not able to look upward	Midbrain lesions, pineal tumors causing compression; Parinaud's syndrome
Unilateral horizontal nystagmus	Brainstem or cerebellar lesions (stroke or tumor)
Miotic pupil, ptosis, and anhidrosis on one side	Horner's syndrome, carotid occlusive disease
Vertical nystagmus (downward fast phase)	Involvement of the craniocervical junction (tumors, chiari malformation)

Dysdiadochokinesis: Abnormal movements. Ask the patient to tap your hand with his or her finger both in supination and pronation. Incoordination of the movements is called dysdiadochokinesis.

Gait: Once the patient enters the examination room, identification of the gait while standing and walking explains and provides us with relevant information. The patient is also asked to stand from a chair, walk a lap, and then turn around. The patient is watched for any wavering and side step.[6]

Romberg's test: The patient is initially asked to stand with eyes open and then to close. Then the patient is pulled backward, off balance. Observe for any fall or side stepping.

Heel–toe walking: The patient is asked to walk heel–toe and observed for side stepping while the walk is evaluated.

The following types have been identified:

1. *Stance*: narrow based, with eyes wide open and looking ahead. Observe for wavering of stance.
2. *Normal*: walks for more than one lap for a linear distance and then turns.
3. *Tandem*: not able to walk heel–toe; side stepping +

Positive Romberg: involvement of the dorsal column

Wide-based stance with broad-based gait: cerebellar disorder, hydrocephalus (occasionally)

Narrow-based stiff gait (spasticity) with short steps: lesions in the corticospinal tract (unilateral— brain; bilateral—spinal cord)

Narrow based with short steps and stooped posture: Lesions in the frontal lobe or basal ganglia (parkinsonism).

Motor function

Consists of three components: muscle tone, muscle strength, and muscle consistency.[10]

1. *Muscle tone*: This is tested by moving the joints and assessing the stiffness and resistance offered.
2. *Muscle strength*: Each representative muscle is tested for strength as per their functional activity. Muscles from both sides are tested for symmetry. This is graded as follows:
   5/5: movement against both gravity and resistance
   4/5: movement against gravity with little resistance
   3/5: movement against gravity alone
   2/5: movement with gravity eliminated
   1/5: muscle contraction that is palpable but no movement
   0/5: no contraction
3. *Muscle consistency*: difficult to evaluate
4. *Muscle wasting*: Long-term nonusage of muscles may lead to wasting

This is carried out for the muscles of all four limbs and compared. The characteristic of the findings and the neural innervations to the affected muscles guide the physician in interpreting the diagnosis (Table 6.5).[6,7]

Interpretations

Implications: Administration of succinylcholine in patients with upper motor neuron lesions hemiplegia and paraplegia may precipitate a hyperkalemic response.

Patients may have different presentations depending upon the site of lesion such as monoparesis, hemiparesis, and paraparesis.

Table 6.5 Interpretations of muscle strength and tone

Muscle strength	Muscle tone	Interpretation
Weakness	Decreased	Peripheral lesions, acute central lesions
Weakness	Increased	Corticospinal involvement
Normal	Increased	Muscular dystrophy, parkinsonism, repetitive intramuscular injections
Normal	Decreased	Cerebellar lesions (+impaired coordination)

Sensory examination

All the modalities of sensory such as touch, pinprick (sharp), temperature, position sense, and vibration are tested along with Romberg's test. This gives us an idea about the level of damage caused by spinal cord lesions or compressions. A good understanding of the dermatomes and their correlation with the clinical findings is critical to diagnosis and proper perioperative care[6] (Figure 6.2).

Altered sensory perception: Patients may also present with altered sensory presentations such as hyperpathia (pain), sensory hallucinations, paresthesias, dysesthesias, or unilateral facial pain.

Diaphragmatic breathing and respiratory reserve: Patients with low cervical lesions have impaired assistance from abdominal and intercostal muscles for respiratory drive. But this is maintained due to the intact diaphragmatic action supplied by C3, 4, and 5. Lesions above and at C5 level impair respiratory drive and may result in prolonged ventilator support and at times lead to respiratory arrest.

Tests for different modalities

Touch sensation: A cotton swab is commonly used to test for light touch sensation.

Sharp/pinprick sensation: A single use sharp device is used to check for sharp sensation. One should differentiate a light touch from a sharp sensation.

Position sense: With eyes closed, a joint is moved while stabilizing the proximal bone. The patient is asked to sense the direction of movement.

Vibration sense: A vibrating tuning fork is placed on the skin to elicit a vibration sense. Sensory modalities and their interpretations are displayed in Table 6.6.

Reflex examination

There are three modalities of reflexes:[6,7] tendon reflexes, plantar reflexes, and release signs.

Tendon reflexes (monosynaptic stretch reflexes)

The reflex is elicited by tapping the tendon of a slightly stretched muscle. This stimulates the spindle receptors of the muscles followed by Ia sensory afferent axons. Then, the motor efferent axon is activated via a synapse and finally leads to stimulation of the extensor muscles and inhibition of flexor muscles and generation of the reflex activity.

Grading of tendon reflex activity:

0: Absent
1: Present
2: Brisk
3: Very brisk
4: Clonus

Interpretation:

Loss of reflexes, such as observed in radiculopathy and mononeuropathy, suggests lesion of the sensory nerve or root.

Exaggerated activity suggests upper motor neuron or corticospinal tract lesion (unopposed activity of the anterior horn cells due to loss of descending inhibition), for example, that seen after a stroke, head injuries, brain tumors, cerebral, and brainstem disorders.

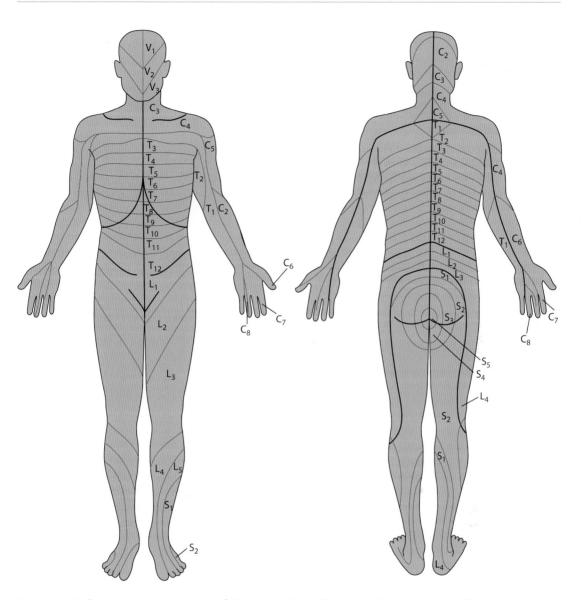

Figure 6.2 Schematic representation of dermatomal distribution and demarcation of sensory innervation.

Table 6.6 Sensory modalities and their interpretations

Sensory presentation	Interpretation
Sensory loss in a nerve distribution	Peripheral nerve lesion
Sensory loss in a dermatomal distribution	Disk lesion, inflammation, or osteophyte
Loss of sensation on one side of the body	Thalamic or spinothalamic tract involvement
Sensory loss at and below a spinal dermatome level	Lesion at spinothalamic tract or above the respective level in the spinal cord
Sensory loss of face	Trigeminal nerve lesion

Absence of all reflexes suggests peripheral neuropathy and Guillain–Barré syndrome (subacute presentation)

Following are the commonly used tests and nerve roots involved: (Table 6.7)

Superficial reflexes

Superficial reflexes are polysynaptic reflexes elicited in response to stimuli of the skin. All superficial reflexes are lost in upper motor neuron lesions above their spinal level.

1. *Corneal reflex and palatal reflex*:

Test for corneal reflex: The corneal surface (at its margin with the conjunctiva) is touched with a wisp of cotton to check for corneal reflex.

Afferent arc: Trigeminal nerve

Efferent arc: Facial nerve

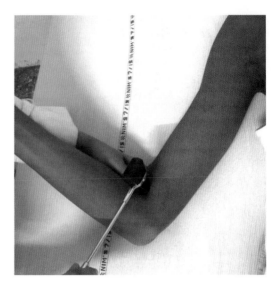

Figure 6.3 **Testing the biceps jerk.**

Table 6.7 Tendon reflexes and its interpretation

Tendon reflexes	Nerve root	Method	Interpretation
Jaw jerk	Trigeminal nerve	With the jaw half open and relaxed, tap the finger lightly placed on the chin below the lower lip	Corticobulbar (UMN) lesion
Biceps jerk (Figure 6.3)	Musculocutaneous (C6 root)	Keeping the patient's elbow at a right angle with the forearm in semi-pronation, tap the finger placed on the biceps tendon	Cervical myelopathy (midcervical lesions): supinator or biceps jerks may be absent, instead brisk flexion of the fingers may occur—inversion of the reflex; hyperexcitability of anterior horn cells below the affected level
Supinator jerk (Figure 6.4)	C5, C6	Keeping the patient's elbow slightly flexed and slightly pronated, tap the styloid process of the radius	
Triceps jerk (Figure 6.5)	C6, C7	Keeping the patient's elbow flexed and the forearm resting across the chest, tap the tendon above the olecranon	–
Knee jerk (Figure 6.6)	L2, L3, L4	With the knee flexed at a little less than 90°, tap the patellar tendon	–
Ankle jerk	S1, S2	With slight dorsiflexion of the ankle, tap the Achilles tendon on its posterior surface	–

UMN, upper motor neuron

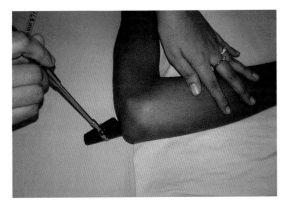

Figure 6.4 Testing the supinator jerk.

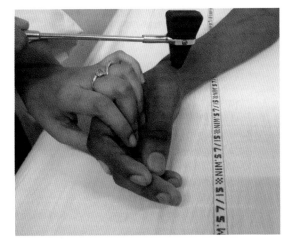

Figure 6.5 Testing the triceps jerk.

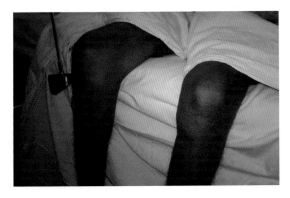

Figure 6.6 Testing the knee jerk.

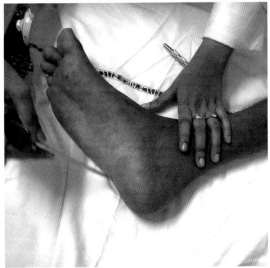

Figure 6.7 Testing the Babinski response.

Test for palatal reflex: discussed in Cranial nerve evaluation section

2. *Scapular reflex (C5–T1):*
Stimuli: The skin between the scapulae is stroked.
Response: The scapular muscles will contract.

3. *Superficial abdominal reflexes (T7–12):*
Stimulus: The abdominal skin is stroked in a dermatomal plane from the loin toward the midline.
Response: Contraction of the underlying abdominal musculature is observed.

4. *Cremasteric reflex (L1/2):*
Stimulus: The skin is stroked at the upper inner part of the thigh.
Response: The testicle moves upward.

5. *Plantar reflex (L5/S1) or Babinski response (Figure 6.7):*
Stimulus: The outer edge of the sole of the foot is stroked from the heel toward the little toe.
Response: Flexion of the four outer toes (flexor response).
Interpretation: Extensor plantar response—upper motor neuron (corticospinal) lesion
Bilateral extensor response—spinal cord lesion (compression or infarction)
Unilateral extensor response—cortical lesion (stroke, mass, abscess)

Release signs

Release signs are the reflexes given below numbers 1–4.

- Usually not seen in adults and may be seen in pediatric population.
- Indicative of cerebral damage.
- Most common lesions are frontal lobe and basal ganglia lesions, which produce abnormal signs.
- Include glabellar, palmomental, snout, and grasp.

1. *Grasp reflex*:
   Stimulus: The palmar aspect of the hand is stroked with fingers.
   Response: Hands close around the examiner's fingers.
   Afferent: Palmar nerves to spinal cord and frontal lobes.
   Efferent arc: Descending fibers of the corticospinal tract supplying to the arm, median, and ulnar nerves.
2. *Palmomental reflex*:
   Stimulus: Same as grasp reflex.
   Response: Contraction of the perioral muscles on the same side.
   Afferent: Palmar nerves to spinal cord and frontal lobes.
   Efferent: Facial nerve supplying the face.
3. *Snout reflex*:
   Stimulus: The skin between the upper lip and nose is tapped.
   Response: Pursing of the lips is seen.
   Afferent: Trigeminal nerve—brainstem.
   Efferent: Facial nerve.
   Positive response of these three reflexes indicates frontal lobe disorders, for example, dementia, any tumor, hydrocephalus, and subdural hematoma.
4. *Glabellar reflex*:
   Stimulus: The skin between the eyebrows is tapped, keeping the hand away from the line of sight.
   Response: The eye blinks.
   Afferent arc: Trigeminal nerve—brainstem.
   Efferent arc: Muscles for eye blink.
   Positive response indicates abnormality in the subcortical areas, for example, Parkinson's disease, dementia, or frontal lobe dysfunction.

Examination findings specific to increased intracranial pressure (ICP): Altered vitals, increase in head circumference (series of measurement), full fontanelle, drooping of eyelids, sunset sign, Macewen's sign (on percussion—cracked pot sign), change in respiration pattern, coma.

Detailed examination, understanding of the pathology, and correlation of the findings guide the physician in conducting proper diagnosis, planning the perioperative management, and monitoring the neurologic condition.

References

1. Teasdale G, Jennett B. Assessment of coma and impaired consciousness. A practical scale. *Lancet* 1974;2:81–84.
2. Rowley G, Fielding K. Reliability and accuracy of the Glasgow Coma Scale. *Lancet* 1991;337:535–538.
3. Lancu I, Olmer A. [The Mini Mental State Examination—an up-to-date review]. *Harefuah* 2006;145:687–690, 701.
4. Rosli R, Tan MP, Gray WK, Subramanian P, Chin AV. Cognitive assessment tools in Asia: A systematic review. *Int Psychogeriatr* 2016;28:189–210.
5. Mitchell AJ, Malladi S. Screening and case finding tools for the detection of dementia. Part I: Evidence-based meta-analysis of multidomain tests. *Am J Geriatr Psychiatry* 2010;18:759–782.
6. McAuley J, Swash M. Nervous system. In: Swash M, Glynn M, editors. *Hutchinson's Clinical Methods*, 22nd ed. Philadelphia, PA: Saunders Elsevier; 2007, pp. 178–247.
7. Misulis KE, Head TC. *Netter's Concise Neurology*. Vol. 1. Philadelphia, PA: Saunders Elsevier; 2007.
8. Barnett SR, Nozari A. The preoperative evaluation of the neurosurgical patient. *Int Anesthesiol Clin* 2015;53:1–22.
9. Fischer SP. Preoperative evaluation of the adult neurosurgical patient. *Int Anesthesiol Clin* 1996;34:21–32.
10. Reponen E, Korja M, Niemi T, Silvasti-Lundell M, Hernesniemi J, Tuominen H. Preoperative identification of neurosurgery patients with a high risk of in-hospital complications: A prospective cohort of 418 consecutive elective craniotomy patients. *J Neurosurg* 2015;123:594–604.

PART III

Monitoring the neurosurgical patient

7

Electrocardiography

BHAVNA HOODA

Introduction

Burch et al. described the classical CVA-T pattern and suggested a possible brain–heart connection as early as 1954. Over the years, these changes in the CVA-T pattern have been noticed in a gamut of neurologic conditions, for example, ischemic stroke, intracranial hemorrhage, head trauma, neurosurgical procedures, acute meningitis, intracranial space-occupying tumors, limbic encephalitis, multiple sclerosis, and epilepsy. These changes are noted in almost 49%–100% patients following an acute brain insult.

The most common electrocardiogram (ECG) morphologic abnormalities in the central nervous system (CNS) disorders involve ventricular repolarization in the form of elevated or depressed ST segment, flat or inverted T waves, prolonged QT interval, and prominent U waves. Cardiac conduction abnormalities also have a high incidence (>75%) with both tachy- and bradyarrhythmias noted. Though rhythm disturbances are usually benign (sinus tachycardia, premature atrial ectopics, and ventricular contractions), clinically important dysrhythmias may also be observed. Supraventricular rhythms (particularly atrial fibrillation) are reported in almost 30%–35% of patients with acute cerebrovascular accident (CVA) and all degrees of atrioventricular (AV) block have been reported. Malignant ventricular tachyarrhythmias (torsade) have been detected in 4% of patients with subarachnoid hemorrhage (SAH).

Sympathetic overactivity is suggested as the mechanism causing tall P waves, premature beats, and QT prolongation, whereas sinus arrhythmia with a fixed or wandering pacemaker and nodal rhythms are attributed to parasympathetic stimulation in various intracranial pathologies.

Pathogenesis of cardiovascular changes in neurologic conditions

There is a growing understanding of the brain–heart connection for homeostasis (the so-called field of Neurocardiology). On one hand, the pathologic effects of cardiovascular disorders on the brain are being delineated; on the other hand, the concept of cerebrogenic cardiac injury is being appreciated. It is this aspect of the cerebrovascular dysfunction-induced cardiac insult that is the core of our discussion about electrocardiographic manifestations of CNS disorders (Figure 7.1).

There are three mechanisms implicated:

1. Sympathetic storm-induced neurogenic stunned myocardium (NSM): Neurogenic stunned myocardium or neurocardiogenic syndrome (NCS) is defined as a triad of transient left ventricular (LV) dysfunction, ECG changes, and elevated levels of cardiac enzymes, often mimicking a myocardial infarction in the absence of coronary occlusion. Pathophysiologic mechanisms postulated are sympathetic storm following acute insult to the hypothalamus, the insular cortex, and the amygdala with associated parasympathetic dysfunction. The myocardial stunning occurs due to release of catecholamines locally in the myocardium, causing contraction band necrosis and myocardial dysfunction. This reversible cardiomyopathy is reported in almost all neurologic settings that induce stress, for example, in SAH, hemorrhagic cerebral contusion, ischemic cerebrovascular accident, status epilepticus, reversible posterior leukoencephalopathy, limbic encephalitis, or even in acute panic attacks. The typical LV dysfunction that occurs is described as the broken heart syndrome, Takotsubo cardiomyopathy, apical ballooning syndrome, neurogenic stress cardiomyopathy, and transient LV dysfunction syndrome.
2. Neuroinflammation: Intense release of inflammatory mediators such as cytokines, adhesion molecules, and peptides induces a systemic inflammatory response syndrome (SIRS) with resultant dysrhythmias.
3. Cortical rhythm control: This theory proposes the presence of a cardiac cortical rhythm control site probably lying in the anterior cingulate cortex, that is, middle cerebral artery (MCA) territory and ischemic/hemorrhagic stroke in this area causes disinhibition of the right insular cortex (right hemispheric stroke) with resultant sympathetic surge and cardiac dysrhythmias. Tachycardia and hypertensive responses are more common after lesions of the right insular cortex (or the left vagus that innervates the AV node) whereas bradycardia occurs with left insular cortical lesions (or the right vagus nerve that is the nerve supply to the sinoatrial (SA) node) or as a response of Cushing effect.

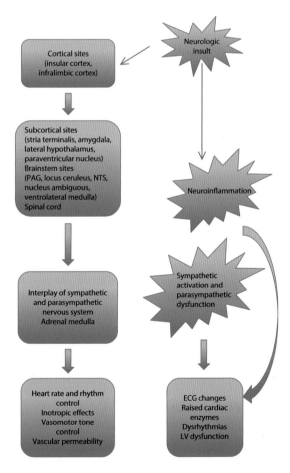

Figure 7.1 Brain–heart connection in physiologic and pathologic states.

ECG changes in subarachnoid hemorrhage

Mild LV dysfunction is observed in about 15% of patients after SAH, usually within 48–72 h of the ictus. Characteristically, it involves the basal and middle portions of the anteroseptal and anterior ventricular walls, with relative apical sparing reflecting the distribution of sympathetic nerves rather than specific coronary territories. Some patients develop a pattern of transient apical LV dysfunction (but in the absence of significant coronary artery disease), a condition known as Takotsubo cardiomyopathy or transient LV apical ballooning syndrome. Other variants have also been recognized, including an inverted Takotsubo pattern of severe basal hypokinesis that typically spares the apex.

- In SAH, the incidence of ECG abnormalities ranges from 49% to 100%.
- ECG changes occur most commonly in the first few days after injury and are often transient because repolarization normalizes as the neurological insult resolves. They may, however, persist for up to 8 weeks in some cases.

Morphologic changes

The most frequently encountered electrocardiographic changes are QT prolongation (observed on an average in 41% SAH patients) and ST-T changes. Benign changes such as nonspecific ST depression, T wave inversion (CVA-T pattern), appearance of U waves to more sinister QT prolongation, ST elevation, and pathologic Q waves have all been reported (Box 7.1).

Cardiac rhythm disturbances

Noted in 35% of patients after SAH within the first week of insult, but only 5%–8% are life-threatening. The incidence is also high in acute ischemic stroke (25%).

The most common arrhythmias are sinus bradycardia and supraventricular tachycardia (SVT), especially atrial fibrillation (AF). Sinus tachycardia, AF, premature atrial and ventricular contractions, AV dissociation, ventricular tachycardia (VT), Torsades, and ventricular fibrillation (VF) have all been noticed.

Clinical peril

The amount of intracranial blood (Fischer grades 3 and 4) correlates with the magnitude of ECG changes. Though these ECG changes may well produce a management dilemma in view of likelihood of myocardial dysfunction, only the cases with a high degree of suspicion should undergo cardiac enzyme levels and echocardiography. Rebleeding being a major determinant of morbidity and mortality, this should not cause unnecessary delay in neurosurgical intervention.

As a general rule, repolarization and ischemic-like ECG changes in SAH are mainly direct consequences of the cerebral insult and the absence of these changes virtually rules out structural heart disease. Contrary to this, in ischemic stroke and intracerebral hemorrhage, ECG abnormalities most often represent a preexisting coronary artery disease and the incidence is only 4% after excluding the preexisting structural heart disease.

BOX 7.1: Electrographic changes in SAH

Electrographic change	Incidence (%)
High R waves	19
ST depression	15–51
T-wave abnormalities	32
Large U waves (> 1 mm amplitude)	4–47
Prolonged QT	11–66
Pathologic Q waves	<1
Atrial arrhythmias (AF, atrial flutter)	4

Intracerebral hemorrhage

Electrocardiographic changes occur with a frequency of 60%–70% in ICH as compared to 15%–40% in ischemic CVA.

Supratentorial bleeds

ECG changes are commonly seen in basal ganglia and thalamic bleeds, particularly if there is intra-ventricular (IV) extension. The most common morphologic change is QT prolongation followed by sinus bradycardia, ST segment alterations, and T inversions. Insular cortex and IV bleeds with hydrocephalus particularly show QT prolongation.

Posterior fossa bleeds

Pontine and cerebellar bleeds show similar ECG findings as supratentorial hemorrhage, for example, QT prolongation, ST depression, inverted or flat T waves, tall R waves, and prominent U waves. Again pathogenesis is likely a centrally mediated catecholamine storm induced by hypoperfusion of posterior hypothalamus causing a contraction band necrosis.

CNS tumors

Electrocardiographic changes are observed in almost 42% of patients with brainstem tumors and 56% with supratentorial tumors. The causation is obvious in limbic structure lesions. Craniopharyngiomas may present with ST-T alterations due to anteromedial hypothalamic stimulation.

Other causes may be related to raised intracranial pressure (ICP), cranial nerve manipulation, and brainstem retraction.

Traumatic brain injury

The cardiac effects of traumatic brain injury (TBI) are mediated by the same mechanism of increased sympathetic nervous system activity and catechol-amine surge from the hypothalamus and the insular cortex producing NSM. Additionally, these may be compounded by presence of electrolyte and acid–base disturbances and hypoxia. The dysautonomia may last for up to 3 months after the primary insult.

- Prolonged QT and nonspecific ST/T changes are reported in 90% and 53% patients, respectively. Another feature may be the appearance of tall P waves.
- The most common rhythm disturbances are SVT and sinus tachycardia.

Carotid endarterectomy

- Periprocedural complications of stroke, myocardial infarction, unstable angina, and dysrrythmias are key concerns during carotid revascularisation.
- Perioperative MI occurs in 2.2% cases undergoing carotid endarterectomy (CEA).
- There is a fairly high incidence of perioperative rhythm changes such as bradycardia, asystole, and SVTs due to carotid sinus abnormalities.

Venous air embolism

Diagnosing acute embolism on the electrocardi-ography is a difficult feat. Electrocardiographic alterations rank low in sensitivity for VAE detection. An early reported change in animal studies is peaked P waves. However, the earliest clinical change observed is ST-T alterations followed by supraventricular and ventricular dysrhythmias. VAE may be suspected if there is a suggestive clinical setting with one or more of the following conditions:

- Sinus tachycardia
- Right ventricular strain
- $S_I Q_{III} T_{III}$ pattern as a consequence of RV dilatation: S in lead I with Q in lead III accompanied by T inversion
- Right axis deviation (RAD)
- ST depression suggestive of subendocardial ischemia
- ST elevation suggestive of transmural isch-aemia (coronary air embolism)
- Right bundle branch block (RBBB; rSr' in V1)

Clinical peril

Though ECG changes appear very late with poor sensitivity and specificity in acute embolism, it may be worthwhile to be aware of these patterns in the clinical scenario of intracranial surgery with a high incidence of venous air embolism (VAE), especially sitting craniotomy.

ECG in raised ICP

A variety of electrocardiographic changes are reported in patients with raised ICP depending on the etiology (SAH, Cushing reflex, cardioarrhythmogenic effects of limbic pathology):

- Tall P waves, prominent U waves, inverted U waves, ST-T changes
- Sinus bradycardia

Intraopeartive ECG abnormalities in common neurosurgical procedures

Morphologic and rhythm disturbances occur intraoperatively during neurosurgical procedures consequent to cranial nerve stimulation, brainstem manipulation or enhanced sympathetic outflow. Though most of these changes are innocuous and self limiting with removal of surgical stimuli; a watchful attention is warranted to prevent untoward events (Box 7.2).

Supratentorial surgery

- Trigeminocardiac reflex (TCR) following any stretch stimulus, such as skull pin application,

---

BOX 7.2: Summary of various ECG changes encountered in day-to-day neuroanesthesia practice

Neurologic disorder/procedure	Cause	Morphologic change	Rhythm disturbance
SAH	NSM	Prolonged QT ST segment depression Neurogenic T waves (giant T inversions) Prominent U waves	Sinus bradycardia SVT (AF, AFl) Sinus tachycardia VPBs
Hemorrhagic stroke	NSM Concomitant structural heart disease	Prolonged QT ST segment changes T inversions	Sinus bradycardia
Ischemic CVA	NSM Concomitant structural heart disease	Prolonged QT ST-T changes Prominent U waves	AF Ventricular ectopy AV blocks
TBI	NSM	Prolonged QT ST-T changes Tall P waves	SVT Sinus bradycardia
Neuroendoscopy	Irrigation with cold/warm saline or jet directed to hypothalamic nuclei/ICP changes	–	Sinus arrest Sinus bradycardia Ventricular irritability (VPBs, VT)
Pituitary surgery	TCR due to cavernous sinus stimulation Hypothalamic manipulation Pituitary apoplexy	ST-T changes	Sinus bradycardia Tachyarrhythmias (ST, SVT,VPBs)
Intracranial hypertension	Cushing reflex due to medullary ischemia	Tall P waves Prominent U Inverted U waves ST-T changes	Sinus bradycardia

Neurologic disorder/procedure	Cause	Morphologic change	Rhythm disturbance
Venous air embolism	Right heart dilatation	Right ventricular strain $S_I Q_{III} T_{III}$ pattern RAD P pulmonale ST depression Occasionally ST elevation T inversion in V1–V5 RBBB (rSr' in V1)	Sinus tachycardia SVT Ventricular dysrhythmias
Supratentorial surgery	TCR Raised ICP Insular cortex lesions	Changes due to raised ICP	Brady-asystole (left insular stimulation) Tachyarrhythmias (right insular stimulation)
Infratentorial procedures	TCR/brainstem or cranial nerve manipulation/GVR	Changes due to VAE	Bradycardia Asystole VPBs Sinus tachycardia
CEA	Carotid sinus stimulation Concomitant CAD	Perioperative MI	Brady-asystole SVT
Spinal cord transection	NSM Neurogenic shock Autonomic hyperreflexia	Transient ST-T changes with prolonged QT	Sinus bradycardia, sinus arrest/pause
Interventional neuroradiology (INR) procedures	Contrast induced Glue embolization of AVM Balloon dilatation in CAS Aneurysm rupture/leak	Prolonged QT Widened QRS ST changes Inverted T Peaked T in inferior chest leads	Sinus brady Asystole

dural stretch, skin traction, and in the sensory distribution of the trigeminal nerve

- Increased parasympathetic outflow in response to insular cortex stimulation, limbic, amygdala, or brainstem stimulation
- Elevated ICP
- Intracranial hypotension subsequent to rapid cerebrospinal fluid (CSF) drainage or application of suction to external ventricular drain/drain
- Irrigation with warm or cold saline as in endoscopic surgery may cause sinus arrest and bradycardia (41%) and ventricular irritability (28%–32%) secondary to posterior

hypothalamus distortion, irrigation jets directed to the hypothalamic nuclei, or brain shifts subsequent to irrigation/CSF drainage

Skull base surgery

During transnasal transsphenoidal approach to pituitary tumors, rhythm disturbances may occur as a result of TCR (observed in 10%–12% cases) due to cavernous sinus stimulation or anterior hypothalamic stimulation, causing parasympathetic outflow. An abrupt onset of tachyarrhythmias may occur in pituitary apoplexy due to midbrain compression. Similar changes may be observed in microvascular decompression for trigeminal neuralgia.

Posterior fossa surgery

Rhythm alterations as bradyarrhythmias, tachyarrhythmias, VPCs, and asystole may occur during infratentorial surgery due to:

- TCR
- Brainstem traction
- Cranial nerve traction
- Tumor manipulation
- Tentorium traction
- Glossopharyngeal vagal reflex (GVR)
- Vagal nerve rootlet stimulation
- Venous air embolism
- *Most of these changes are usually self-limiting with removal of surgical stimulus, and treatment is rarely required.*

Cerebrovascular surgery

Any of the stretch stimuli may cause TCR. Posterior fossa aneurysms may require cranial nerve or brainstem manipulation and cause rhythm alterations. Raised ICP may manifest as bradycardia in the event of rebleeding. In the interventional neuroradiology suite, embolization of arteriovenous malformations (AVMs) may present with bradyasystole after glue injection.

Spine procedures

Complete spinal cord injury may manifest with:

- NSM-induced ECG changes.
- Neurogenic shock with persistent bradycardia that resolves over 3–5 weeks is observed in 71% and hypotension in 68% of patients. Other ECG findings of sinus tachycardia, sinus pauses, wandering pacemaker, junctional ectopic beats (JEBs), AF, ventricular ectopic beats (VEBs), VT, and ST-T changes have all been reported.
- Autonomic hyperreflexia (2–3 weeks post insult) manifesting with episodic bradyarrhythmias in response to noxious stimuli in sympathetically transected distribution.

- A variety of rhythm disturbances are observed in various spine surgeries due to the following:
- Thoracoscopicsympathectomy
- VAE
- Upper cervical spine surgery due to reduced sympathetic activity

Apart from spinal cord injury induced changes, rhythm disturbances have been reported in spinal procedures. Implicated mechanisms are:

> Nerve root irritation
> Vagal response to dural traction
> Thoracic sympathectomy
> VAE
> Poor sympathetic control with

overactive parasympathetic system in upper cervical spine procedures.

Use of contrast agents

There is a likelihood of contrast agent cardiotoxicity mediated by hyperosmolarity and potentiated by contrast-induced hypocalcemia. Electrocardiographic changes such as QRS prolongation, prolonged QT, ST segment changes, T-wave inversion, and peaked T in inferior leads have been frequently reported during cardiac catheterization procedures. Rhythm changes as transient bradycardia or various degrees of AV block or sinus arrest have also been reported. Life-threatening arrhythmias, such as VF, have also been reported in 0.6%–1.3% of patients. This potential adverse effect should be borne in mind in the neuroradiology suite, though the incidence is reduced with low osmolar agents used nowadays.

Conclusion

ECG is a highly informative noninvasive screening test for underlying cardiac conditions. This is of utmost usefulness to the anesthesiologist who is tasked with delineating the preoperative cardiac risk and stratification while monitoring the cardiac and electrolyte milieu intraoperatively and continued care postoperatively. Therefore a detailed knowledge of ECG is paramount. A stepwise analysis of the ECG is conducted in terms of the following descriptors:

- Standardization and calibration
- Measurements
  - Heart rate
  - PR interval
  - QRS duration
  - QT interval
  - QRS axis
- Rhythm analysis: Sinus tachycardia/brady-cardia, atrial ectopics or atrial flutter/fibrilla-tion, junctional ectopics, ventricular ectopic beats (VEBs), Ventricular tachycardia (VT) or Ventricular Fibrillation.
- Conduction analysis: Normal conduction implies normal SA, AV, and IV conduction.
- Waveform description:
  - P waves: tall or wide notched
  - QRS complexes: look for pathologic Q waves, abnormal voltage
  - ST segments: abnormal ST elevation and/or depression
  - T waves: inverted T waves or unusually tall T waves
  - U waves: prominent or inverted U waves
- ECG interpretation: Interpret the ECG as *normal*, or *abnormal*. Once these findings are in place, a diagnosis to fit the description should be attempted in the relevant clinical setting.

Brain injury-induced cardiac dysfunction

This needs to be carefully and judiciously differentiated from structural heart disease to avoid an unnecessary battery of investigations and delay in neurosurgical intervention. Certain points need to be borne in mind in favor of a neurogenic cause of cardiac dysfunction:

- No history of structural heart disease
- Temporal relationship between brain injury and cardiac dysfunction
- ECG changes in absence of clinical correlation
- Modest elevations in cardiac biomarkers of injury (cTnI)
- New-onset LV dysfunction
- Cardiac wall motion abnormalities not conforming to coronary vascular territories
- Inconsistent echocardiographic and ECG findings

- Inconsistent cardiac enzyme biomarkers and LV ejection fraction findings (e.g., cTI < 2.8 µg/l in association with LVEF <40%)
- Spontaneous, early resolution

Suggested reading

1. Burch GE, Myers R, Abildskov JA. A new ECG pattern observed in cerebrovascular accidents. *Circulation* 1954;9:719–23.
2. AlGhatrif M, Lindsay J. A brief review: History to understand fundamentals of electrocardiography. *J Community Hosp Intern Med Perspect* 2012;2(1). doi:10.3402/jchimp.
3. Goldberger Ary L. *Clinical Electrocardiography: A Simplified Approach*, 6th ed. St. Louis, MO: Mosby; 2009.
4. Longo DL, Fauci AS, Kasper DL, Hauser SL, Jameson JL, Loscalzo J, editors. *Harrison's Principles of Internal Medicine*, 18th ed. New York: McGraw-Hill; 2012. ISBN 978-0-07174889-6; MHID 0-07-174889-X.
5. Cottrell JE, Young WL. *Cottrell and Young's Neuroanesthesia*. 5th ed. Philadelphia, PA: Mosby; 2010. ISBN: 978-0-0323-05908-4.
6. Matta BF, Menon DK, Smith M. *Core Topics in Neuroanaesthesia and Neurointensive Care*. New York: Cambridge University Press; 2011.
7. Gregory T, Smith M. Cardiovascular complications of brain injury. *Cont Educ Anaesth Crit Care Pain* Dec 2011;1–5.
8. Mieghem CV, Sabbe M, Daniel Knockaert D. The clinical value of the ECG in noncardiac conditions. *Chest* 2004;125:1561–1576.
9. Cheung RTF, Hachinski V. The insula and cerebrogenic sudden death. *Arch Neurol* 2000;57(12):1685–1688.
10. Togha M, Sharifpour A, Ashraf H et al. Electrocardiographic abnormalities in acute cerebrovascular events in patients with/without cardiovascular disease. *Ann Indian Acad Neurol* 2013 Jan–Mar;16(1):66–71.
11. Chatterjee S. ECG changes in subarachnoid haemorrhage: A synopsis. *Neth Heart J* 2011;19:31–34.
12. Van der Wall EE, Van Gilst WH. Neurocardiology: Close interaction between heart and brain. *Neth Heart J* 2013 Feb;21(2):51–52.

8

Oxygenation

MATTHEW J. HAMMER and LAURA B. HEMMER

Introduction

Ensuring adequate delivery of oxygen is crucial in perioperative patient management. The clinician must seek to achieve a balance between the deleterious extremes of hypoxemia and hyperoxia. The harmful effects of hypoxemia are well-established and warrant special consideration in neurosurgical patients, especially in those who have sustained a brain injury and are at risk for compromised cerebral blood flow (CBF). However, indiscriminate use of increased inspired oxygen fractions can lead to detrimental consequences as well, particularly with regard to pulmonary function and central nervous system toxicity. This chapter discusses the rationale for administering increased oxygen concentrations in neurosurgical and non-neurosurgical patients alike, as well as the harms of doing so. We also comment on high-acuity situations in neurosurgery and neurocritical care, and how tailoring oxygen therapy in these populations can affect patient outcomes.

Oxygen and cerebral blood flow

For normal metabolic function, the brain accounts for about 20% of the body's energy consumed.[1] Since the brain has very high metabolic demand for oxygen, one of the most critical and fundamental goals of patient management during neurosurgical procedures is the maintenance of CBF. CBF has multiple determinants including arterial blood pressure, partial pressure of carbon dioxide, and arterial oxygen content. The effect of PaO_2 on CBF is modest, between 60 and 300 mmHg. This finding is because CBF is influenced by blood oxygen content as opposed to partial pressure, and the shape of the oxygen–hemoglobin dissociation curve indicates that the arterial oxygen content is relatively constant within the aforementioned parameters.[2]

Outside these parameters, however, oxygen exerts a more substantial effect on CBF, particularly on the lower end. When PaO_2 falls below 60 mmHg, there is an abrupt increase in CBF, owing to a vasodilatory effect that is likely mediated by multiple mechanisms, including humoral influences and hyperpolarization of vascular smooth muscle caused by hypoxia.[3] The rostral ventrolateral medulla (RVM) senses oxygen levels in the brain. Hypoxia stimulates this center and the result is increased CBF.[3] The increased CBF is synergistic with the effect of hypercapnia.[2]

A review article by Johnston et al.[2] summarizes multiple studies that have investigated the effects of hyperoxia on CBF. While the methods of measuring CBF varied among them and the clinical relevance is uncertain, the studies did show a decrease in CBF under hyperoxic conditions. The authors hypothesize that the cerebral vasoconstriction in the face of hyperoxia may be a protective mechanism to prevent the formation of oxygen free radicals, which are known to cause central nervous system toxicity.[2] This ability to modulate cerebral vasomotor tone in response to inhalation of 100% oxygen appears to decrease in the setting of multi-infarct dementia, potentially placing older patients at risk for adverse effects of hyperoxia.[4]

Potential benefits of increased perioperative concentrations

Postoperative nausea and vomiting

The effect of increased FiO_2 on the incidence of postoperative nausea and vomiting has been widely investigated, but results are conflicting. A recent meta-analysis by Hovaguimian et al.[5] evaluated 11 trials, and, with all data combined, high FiO_2 decreased late nausea with statistical significance in patients who received an inhalational anesthetic and no prophylactic antiemetics. However, the number-needed-to-treat for this benefit to be seen was found to be approximately 15. In contrast, a number-needed-to-treat of 3–5 is expected for an effective antiemetic medication. Furthermore, with respect to other endpoints, including the composite endpoint of postoperative nausea and vomiting (PONV), there was no benefit to increased FiO_2.[5] In addition, the Society for Ambulatory Anesthesia in 2007 did not recommend using increased FiO_2 to prevent PONV.[6] In neurosurgical patients, in which postoperative vomiting can be particularly harmful, supplemental oxygen should not be considered

a reliable antiemetic therapy, and standard first-line antiemetics should still be administered.

Surgical site infections and wound healing

Another purported benefit of increased perioperative oxygen concentrations is a decreased incidence of surgical site infections, a complication that results in considerable morbidity. The hypothesis behind a possible benefit derives from an enhanced oxidative killing intensity with increased oxygen tension.[7] Furthermore, tissue oxygenation has been shown to be decreased in surgical wounds.[8] The efficacy of increased FiO_2 has been recently investigated in various populations. A randomized controlled trial by Wadhwa et al.[9] did not find any decrease in surgical site infections in gastric bypass patients who received approximately 80% supplemental oxygen compared to patients who received 2 L supplemental oxygen by nasal cannula from the time of tracheal extubation until the first postoperative morning (all patients received 80% inspired oxygen intraoperatively). In contrast, in a randomized controlled trial by Schietroma et al.,[10] patients undergoing colorectal surgeries who received 80% supplemental oxygen during and for 6 h following surgery had a decreased incidence of surgical site infections and anastomotic dehiscence. The aforementioned meta-analysis by Hovaguimian et al.[5] also showed a borderline statistically significant decrease in surgical site infections, although methodological concerns have been voiced regarding this study. There is a dearth of studies specific to neurosurgical populations investigating the possible benefits of hyperoxia on surgical site infections.

Potential adverse effects of hyperoxia

Free radical formation

The detrimental effects of hyperoxia are arguably better described than the advantages. Proteins, DNA, and lipids are all susceptible to damage by reactive oxygen species. Furthermore, neurons, glial cells, and myelin demonstrate increased vulnerability.[11] Reactive oxygen species produced in excess have the capacity to overwhelm the mitochondrial antioxidant defenses, causing damage to

DNA and even hastening apoptosis.[11] The clinical significance of free radical formation during exposure to increased FiO_2 for the duration of a surgical procedure, even a lengthy neurosurgical procedure, is unclear.

Pulmonary effects

Another unintended, often clinically relevant untoward effect of increased FiO_2 is absorption atelectasis. Patients with preexisting low ventilation to perfusion ratios are especially susceptible. These lung units have low PAO_2 at baseline, and when they are faced with a markedly increased FiO_2, such as with preoxygenation for general anesthesia, the net flow of oxygen can sharply favor its exodus into blood, and the lung unit decreases in size.[3] Under certain circumstances such as high FiO_2, low V/Q ratio, and prolonged time of exposure to high FiO_2, absorption atelectasis can occur in the face of inspired oxygen concentrations as low as 50%.[3] In these areas, exchange of both oxygen and carbon dioxide becomes abnormal.[12] The effects of absorption atelectasis can manifest during the early post-extubation period as well. Benoit et al.[13] demonstrated that patients receiving 40% oxygen before extubation had less atelectasis on computed tomography scans compared to patients who received 100% oxygen.

Special neurosurgical and neurocritical care issues

Traumatic brain injury

Patients who had traumatic brain injury are at risk of cerebral ischemia. In recent years, several modalities have emerged for measuring cerebral oxygenation in this population. Among them is the brain tissue PO_2 monitor. This catheter is inserted via a Burr hole directly into brain parenchyma.[14] This monitor provides information on the oxygen supply and demand balance at the local level.[15] Although data derived from this monitor reflect only the local area being sampled, if it is positioned in undamaged brain tissue, it can reflect global cerebral oxygenation.[15] However, the information obtained from this catheter may be more useful if placed in an area at risk of ischemia, in which case one must use caution in interpreting the data.

Given the invasive nature of this monitor, patients are at risk of brain tissue damage, though this damage has been shown to be minimal. Computed tomography guidance can help aid placement as well as assess the responsiveness by short-term increases in FiO_2.[15]

Jugular bulb oximetry offers a more global assessment of cerebral oxygenation. In this method, a catheter is inserted into the jugular vein and placed at the skull base in the jugular bulb. Sampling of jugular venous blood can be performed continuously or intermittently. Normal values for jugular venous blood saturation are in the 65%–75% range.[14] Higher oxygen extraction results in lower jugular venous saturation and is indicative of ischemia. However, if there is significant infarction and brain tissue ceases to drain blood, the value may not change.[15] Furthermore, as this method is a global measurement of oxygenation, it may fail to miss changes in regional flow.

Given that CBF diminishes following traumatic brain injury, it has been rationalized that hyperoxia could improve outcomes in this population. Given the mitochondrial damage that is sustained in head injury, it is theorized that increasing the delivery of oxygen to brain tissue could enhance mitochondrial function.[16] However, Obrist et al.[17] demonstrated that in closed head injury patients whose CBF has been reduced, there is little or no evidence of global cerebral ischemia. That is, there remains coupling between CBF and metabolism. Furthermore, a study by Diringer et al.[18] assessed the effect of normobaric hyperoxia on brain metabolism in a small group of patients with severe traumatic brain injury. In contrast to previous studies that assessed indirect physiologic measures, Diringer et al. directly measured brain metabolism using positron emission tomography and found that cerebral metabolic rate for oxygen did not change after ventilation with 100% oxygen. These data suggest that increased oxygen tension does not translate into increased use of oxygen by damaged brain.

Carotid endarterectomy

Patients undergoing carotid endarterectomy are at risk for cerebral ischemia. Increasing the FiO_2 may be of benefit, as these patients may have compromised delivery of oxygen due to distal migration of preexisting plaque or arterial clamping. A study by Stoneham et al.[19] showed consistent increases in regional cerebral oxygenation, evaluated using near-infrared cerebral oximetry, in patients receiving 100% oxygen compared to patients receiving 28% oxygen.[19] While this study was performed on awake patients, the results may be relevant for patients undergoing asleep carotid endarterectomy as well.

Venous air embolism

Optimizing oxygenation is of critical importance when a venous air embolism is suspected as many of these patients are on the verge of cardiopulmonary deterioration. If a patient had been receiving nitrous oxide, it should immediately be discontinued, as its presence can rapidly increase the volume of entrained air. Patients should be immediately placed on 100% FiO_2. In the short term, this is a measure to maximize oxygen content and delivery in a patient who is at risk of sudden cardiovascular collapse, as well as to enhance nitrogen elimination and reduce embolus volume.[20] Furthermore, hyperbaric oxygen therapy has been reported to demonstrate benefit in venous air embolism in multiple case studies. The underlying theory is that this therapy causes increased nitrogen resorption and increases the blood oxygen content, thereby reducing the size of the air bubbles.[20] A retrospective case review by Blanc et al.[21] reported improved neurologic outcomes in patients receiving hyperbaric oxygen therapy within 6 h as opposed to later. However, in the review of 86 patients who had an embolism, only 4 cases occurred in the context of a neurosurgical procedure and all of them had poor neurologic outcomes.[21]

Neurogenic pulmonary edema

Patients who had a traumatic brain injury or cerebral hemorrhage are at risk of developing neurogenic pulmonary edema. A sudden increase in sympathetic tone causes increased pulmonary capillary permeability, leading to fluid leak into the surrounding alveoli. A concomitant increase in pulmonary capillary hydrostatic pressure places these patients at risk for hypoxemia.[22] While there is a lack of studies elucidating clear oxygenation goals in the setting of neurologic pulmonary edema, supplemental oxygen therapy should be initiated to correct for hypoxemia. In some patients, this may involve initiation of mechanical ventilation.[23]

Spurious pulse oximetry readings

Inaccurate pulse oximetry readings that do not correctly state the arterial oxygen saturation may be encountered in certain neurosurgical populations. Errors arise from the presence of alterations in hemoglobin species or other light absorbers in the blood.[24] Methemoglobinemia, which, at high enough levels, causes a pulse oximetry reading around 85%, can be encountered in neurosurgical patients with unstable cervical spines where awake fiber-optic intubation was achieved with certain local anesthetics for topicalization.[24,25] More often, when indocyanine green is used for video angiography during intracranial neurovascular surgeries, a transient decrease in oxygen saturation appears.[26]

Conclusion

The overwhelming majority of patients will be exposed to increased oxygen concentrations during the perioperative period, even if for a short time such as in preoxygenation prior to induction of general anesthesia. The consequences of a prolonged exposure to high oxygen concentrations can be clinically significant, although not always immediately apparent. Oxygen toxicity is not an all-or-nothing phenomenon, that is, there is not a specific FiO_2 value that guarantees that the patient will not incur adverse events. Instead, the anesthesiologist should tailor the inhaled oxygen fraction on a patient-by-patient basis to maintain normal, but not excessive, arterial oxygen saturation. Patients undergoing certain neurosurgical procedures or having certain intracranial pathologies warrant further consideration and monitoring to decrease the likelihood of adverse outcomes from both hypoxemia and hyperoxia. If signs of impaired oxygen delivery, such as a change in neurophysiological monitoring, develop then the need to adjust the FiO_2 to possibly improve oxygen delivery should again be reassessed.

References

1. Buzsaki G, Kaila K, Raichle M. Inhibition and brain work. *Neuron* 2007;56(5):771–783.
2. Johnston AJ, Steiner LA, Gupta AK, Menon DK. Cerebral oxygen vasoreactivity and cerebral tissue oxygen reactivity. *Br J Anaesth* 2003;90(6):774–786.
3. Wilson WC, Benumof JL. Respiratory physiology and respiratory function during anesthesia. In: Miller RD, Fleisher LA, Johns RA, Savarese JJ, Wiener-Kronish JP, Young WL, editors. *Miller's Anesthesia*, Vol. 1–2, 6th ed. Philadelphia, PA: Churchill Livingstone; 2009, pp. 679–722.
4. Amano T, Meyer JS, Okabe T, Shaw T, Mortel KF. Cerebral vasomotor responses during oxygen inhalation. Results in normal aging and dementia. *Arch Neurol* 1983;40(5):277–282.
5. Hovaguimian F, Lysakowski C, Elia N, Tramer MR. Effect of intraoperative high inspired oxygen fraction on surgical site infection, postoperative nausea and vomiting, and pulmonary function: Systematic review and meta-analysis of randomized controlled trials. *Anesthesiology* 2013;119(2):303–316.
6. Gan TJ, Meyer TA, Apfel CC et al. Society for Ambulatory Anesthesia Guidelines for the management of postoperative nausea and vomiting. *Anesth Analg* 2007;105(6):1615–1628.
7. Babior BM. Oxygen-dependent microbial killing by phagocytes (first of two parts). *N Engl J Med* 1978;298(12):659–668.
8. Hopf HW, Holm J. Hyperoxia and infection. *Best Pract Res Clin Anaesthesiol* 2008;22(3):553–569.
9. Wadhwa A, Kabon B, Fleischmann E, Kurz A, Sessler DI. Supplemental perioperative oxygen does not reduce surgical site infection and major healing-related complications from bariatric surgery in morbidly obese patients: A randomized, blinded trial. *Anesth Analg* 2014;119(2):357–365.
10. Schietroma M, Cecilia EM, Sista F, Carlei F, Pessia B, Amicucci G. High-concentration supplemental perioperative oxygen and surgical site infection following elective colorectal surgery for rectal cancer: a prospective, randomized, double-blind, controlled, single-site trial. *Am J Surg* 2014;208(5):719–726.
11. Smith KJ, Kapoor R, Felts PA. Demyelination: The role of reactive oxygen and nitrogen species. *Brain Pathol* 1999;9(1):69–92.
12. Lumb AM, Walton LJ. Perioperative oxygen toxicity. *Anesthesiol Clin* 2012;30(4):591–605.
13. Benoit Z, Wicky S, Fischer JF et al. The effect of increased FIO_2 before tracheal extubation on postoperative atelectasis. *Anesth Analg* 2002;95(6):1777–1781.
14. Dagal A, Lam AM. Anesthesia for neurosurgery. In: Barash PG, Cullen BF, Stoelting RK, Calahan MK, Stock MC, editors. *Clinical Anesthesia*, 7th ed. Philadelphia, PA: Wolters Kluwer/Lippincott Williams & Wilkins; 2013, pp. 1006–1007.
15. Haitsma IK, Maas AI. Monitoring cerebral oxygenation in traumatic brain injury. *Prog Brain Res* 2007;161:207–216.
16. Diringer MN. Hyperoxia—good or bad for the injured brain? *Curr Opin Crit Care* 2008;14(2):167–171.
17. Obrist WD, Langfitt TW, Jaggi JL, Cruz J, Gennarelli TA. Cerebral blood flow and metabolism in comatose patients with acute head injury. Relationship to intracranial hypertension. *J Neurosurg* 1984;61(2):241–253.
18. Diringer MN, Aiyagari V, Zazulia AR, Videen TO, Powers WJ. Effect of hyperoxia on cerebral metabolic rate for oxygen measured using positron emission tomography in patients with acute severe head injury. *J Neurosurg* 2007;106(4):526–529.
19. Stoneham MD, Lodi O, de Beer TC, Sear JW. Increased oxygen administration improves cerebral oxygenation in patients undergoing awake carotid surgery. *Anesth Analg* 2008;107(5):1670–1675.

20. Mirski MA, Lele AV, Fitzsimmons L, Toung TJK. Diagnosis and treatment of vascular air embolism. *Anesthesiology* 2007;106(1):164–177.

21. Blanc P, Boussuges A, Henriette K, Sainty JM, Deleflie M. Latrogenic cerebral air embolism: Importance of an early hyperbaric oxygenation. *Intensive Care Med* 2002;28(5):559–563.

22. Vespa PM, Bleck TP. Neurogenic pulmonary edema and other mechanisms of impaired oxygenation after aneurysmal subarachnoid hemorrhage. *Neurocrit Care* 2004;1(2):157–170.

23. Baumann A, Audibert G, McDonnell J, Mertes PM. Neurogenic pulmonary edema. *Acta Anaesthesiol Scand* 2007;51(4):447–455.

24. Barker SJ, Curry J, Redford D, Morgan S. Measurement of carboxyhemoglobin and methemoglobin by pulse oximetry: A human volunteer study. *Anesthesiology* 2006;105(5):892–897.

25. Chowdhary S, Bukoye B, Bhansali AM et al. Risk of topical anesthetic-induced methemoglobinemia: A 10-year retrospective case–control study. *JAMA Intern Med* 2013;173(9):771–776.

26. Baek HY, Lee H, Kim JM, Cho S, Jeong S, Yoo KY. Effects of intravenously administered indocyanine green on near-infrared cerebral oximetry and pulse oximetry readings. *Korean J Anesthesiol* 2015;68(2):122–127.

9

End-tidal carbon dioxide

RYAN J. VEALEY and LAURA B. HEMMER

Introduction

Monitoring of carbon dioxide (CO_2) is a standard of practice endorsed by the American Society of Anesthesiologists (ASA). The analysis of CO_2 in a single exhaled breath provides real-time information regarding CO_2 production and elimination, metabolism, circulation, and ventilation.[1] Specifically, CO_2 plays a diverse role in the intraoperative and critical care management of patients undergoing neurosurgical procedures. End-tidal carbon dioxide (ET-CO_2) values and capnography can provide useful diagnostic information concerning critical events in the operating room, including those that may be life-threatening. Through manipulation of CO_2 levels, the anesthesia provider is able to facilitate reductions in cerebral blood flow (CBF) and intracranial pressure (ICP). Mild hyperventilation is routinely requested during craniotomies by neurosurgeons to take advantage of this phenomenon and theoretically optimize surgical conditions. The levels of CO_2 also have proven to influence autoregulation and play an important role in the recovery from traumatic brain injury (TBI). Knowledge of how ET-CO_2 values are obtained and the role of CO_2

in the intraoperative management of patients are indispensable tools for the neuroanesthesiologist.

Gas sampling and capnogram analysis

The analysis of expired respiratory and anesthetic gases has become a vital component of modern anesthetic practice. Current ASA standard monitoring guidelines include continuous monitoring of CO_2 when possible, stating "Continual monitoring for the presence of expired carbon dioxide shall be performed unless invalidated by the nature of the patient, procedure or equipment."[2] Assuming a normal alveolar/arterial gradient (5 mmHg in healthy, supine patients), ET-CO_2 obtained via capnometry provides a real-time, continuous assessment of ventilation.[1] Determination of this gradient has a particular relevance in neurosurgical procedures. To enhance brain relaxation, mild-to-moderate intraoperative hyperventilation is often requested and knowledge of each individual's alveolar/arterial gradient is necessary to provide this without inadvertently raising or lowering the CO_2 excessively. This is accomplished by sending a baseline arterial blood gas at the beginning of the procedure and noting the ET-CO$_2$ value at that time. A patient-specific gradient is then generated.

The clinical interpretation of changes to the capnogram and the numerical ET-CO$_2$ value displayed during a surgical procedure can alert the anesthesia provider to a variety of critical perioperative events (Table 9.1).

Overview of autoregulation and CO$_2$ reactivity

The concepts of autoregulation and CO$_2$ reactivity are important to the care of patients undergoing neurosurgical procedures. Autoregulation is classically defined as the maintenance of a constant CBF over a range of mean arterial blood pressures. As mean arterial pressure (MAP) rises or falls, cerebrovascular resistance (CVR) continually adapts to ensure a constant CBF.

The autoregulation curve in an unanesthetized adult is shown in Figure 9.1.

Autoregulation in a normal brain has historically been quoted as between MAP values of approximately 60 and 150 mmHg. This is depicted as the flat, plateau portion of the autoregulation curve between those MAP values. Below or above these autoregulatory limits, CBF becomes pressure dependent. Below the lower autoregulatory limit, cerebral blood vessels have reached maximal dilation and flow is pressure dependent; CBF will fall as MAP values decrease beyond that point. Above the upper autoregulatory limit, maximal vasoconstriction occurs and pressure-dependent flow is again observed. That is, CBF will increase directly with further increases in MAP values.

These autoregulatory values, however, are the means of various study groups and may markedly underestimate or overestimate true values in any individual patient.[3] For example, a lower limit range of 40–110 mmHg has been reported![4] The position of the lower limit has also been noted to

Table 9.1 Clinical Events Associated with ET-CO$_2$ Changes

Elevated ET-CO$_2$		Decreased ET-CO$_2$	
Hyperthermia	Fever	Hypothermia	Extubation
Sepsis	CO$_2$ embolism	Decreased cardiac output	Circuit disconnect
Malignant hyperthermia	Tourniquet release	Pulmonary embolism	Apnea
Shivering	Increased cardiac output	Air embolism	
Hypoventilation	Airway obstruction	Hyperventilation	
Hyperthyroidism	Ventilator malfunction	Hypothyroidism	
Rebreathing		Cardiac arrest	

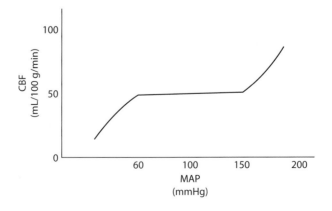

Figure 9.1 Autoregulation curve.

depend partly on the mechanism of hypotension. That is, there may be differences in the lower autoregulatory limit not only from patient to patient, but also depending on what the specific etiology of the hypotension is (i.e., acute hemorrhage and drug-induced).[5]

Within the normal autoregulatory range, CVR varies with blood pressure to ensure that CBF remains constant. However, this response is not immediate. Following an abrupt change in blood pressure, it may take 1–2 min for CVR and CBF to adjust accordingly. The autoregulatory curve is individualized to a patient's baseline blood pressure values. The curve is shifted to the right for a patient with chronic hypertension, necessitating a higher MAP for a given CBF as compared to a patient with no hypertension.[3,4]

Another important mediator of cerebral vasomotor tone and CBF is the arterial tension of carbon dioxide ($PaCO_2$), termed *cerebrovascular CO_2 reactivity*. CBF has a linear relationship with $PaCO_2$ at certain partial pressures and will change 1–2 mL/100 g/min for every 1 mmHg change in $PaCO_2$ between the ranges of 20 and 60 mmHg.[6] This is the principle that underlies common practice of using moderate hyperventilation to reduce CBF and subsequently ICP in patients with intracranial mass lesions.

The mechanism of $PaCO_2$ changes affecting cerebral vasomotor tone is thought to be due to alterations in the hydrogen ion concentration on the brain side of the blood–brain barrier. In the case of hypercapnia, CO_2 diffuses easily across the blood–brain barrier and lowers the pH of the periarteriolar cerebrospinal fluid (CSF) within 20–30 s. The decreased pH of CSF directly affects the endothelial cells via voltage-gated potassium channels that hyperpolarize the endothelial cell and lead to a reduction in vascular tone. In the case of hyperventilation, within 6–8 h the pH of CSF will normalize as bicarbonate crosses the blood–brain barrier and hyperventilation-induced vasoconstriction will cease.[7]

TBI, mass lesions, and ischemia may all decrease CO_2 responsiveness, which is a particularly poor prognostic indicator. Autoregulation is impaired in patients with ischemic insults to the brain, mass lesions, following TBI and during episodes of hypercapnia or hypoxemia.[7]

Autoregulation and CO_2 reactivity are interrelated principles. Each is an important mediator

of CBF, but they should not be thought of as two distinct processes operating parallel to one another. In fact, the $PaCO_2$ level significantly affects the autoregulation curve by altering vascular tone in and of itself, in addition to changes seen with a changing perfusion pressure.

With available literature, Meng and Gelb have recently proposed that the effect of hypercapnia on the autoregulatory curve shifts the plateau portion (i.e., CBF) upward, the lower limit of autoregulation (LLA) is shifted to the right, and the upper limit of autoregulation (ULA) is shifted to the left.[3] This is because the dilation in response to a reduced cerebral perfusion pressure (CPP) occurs at a higher CPP than normal due to concurrent hypercapnia-induced dilation. Similarly, vasoconstriction in response to an increased CPP is blunted by hypercapnic vasodilation.[3] Studies have found that a $PaCO_2$ of approximately 55–60 mmHg is the threshold at which hypercapnia impairs autoregulation in human subjects under anesthesia.[8]

Meng and Gelb have also proposed that the effect of hypocapnia on the autoregulation curve shifts the plateau portion downward and has little effect on the lower autoregulatory limit.[3] Studies have shown that CBF is reduced during the combination of hypocapnia and hypotension.[3,9,10] It remains unclear what happens to the upper autoregulatory limit.[3]

Influence of anesthetic agents and other factors on CO_2 reactivity

Given that the $PaCO_2$ values are very commonly manipulated in neurosurgical procedures and in the setting of neurosurgical emergencies, it is important to have an understanding of what conditions or circumstances may affect the vascular reactivity in response to intentional $PaCO_2$ changes. A recent systematic review examined anesthetic and patient-related factors that have been postulated to affect cerebrovascular reactivity to CO_2.[11] Within clinically relevant ranges, cerebrovascular reactivity to CO_2 seems to remain intact with both inhaled and intravenous anesthetic agents. For medical comorbidities, cerebrovascular reactivity to CO_2 can be impaired by diabetes mellitus, and its impairment varies with severity correlating with the glycosylated hemoglobin concentration and insulin dependency.

There is no definitive effect from the presence of hypertension or cerebrovascular attack (CVA), at least when CVA occurred more than 6 months ago. Reactivity was not impaired by the presence of intracranial tumors or arteriovenous malformations (AVMs). These findings are, however, limited in generalizability due to wide variation in CBF measurement technique, CO_2 manipulation, and anesthetic technique, and due to a lack of randomized, controlled studies.[11]

Hyperventilation during routine craniotomy

Mild-to-moderate hyperventilation is very commonly requested during routine neurosurgical procedures. By taking advantage of an induced decrease in CBF and ICP, neurosurgeons hope to reduce brain bulk and optimize operating conditions. A *relaxed* brain minimizes the need for aggressive retraction to provide adequate exposure and thus limits the potential damage to adjacent neural structures.

A recent randomized, crossover trial was conducted to determine the efficacy of moderate hyperventilation on patients undergoing elective craniotomy for resection of supratentorial tumors with either propofol or isoflurane anesthesia. Moderate hyperventilation ($PaCO_2 = 27 \pm 2$ mmHg) improved operating conditions, decreased ICP by 24%, and decreased risk of brain swelling as compared to eucapnia ($PaCO_2 = 37 \pm 2.6$ mmHg). The anesthetic regimen had no effect on surgeon-assessed operating conditions or ICP.[12]

Other studies have suggested that routine moderate hyperventilation may in fact be harmful to patients where it may not be truly necessary.[13] Patients with brain tumor undergoing craniotomy for resection with hyperventilation have been observed to have jugular venous oxygen saturations ($SjvO_2$) of less than 50%, but how this ischemic threshold should be applied to an anesthetized patient remains unclear.[14]

Current data and recommendations seemingly support the use of intraoperative moderate hyperventilation to improve operating conditions, even in patients undergoing scheduled, routine craniotomy for brain tumor resection where elevated ICP may not be a significant concern.[12]

Hyperventilation following traumatic brain injury

One of the more controversial debates in neurocritical care has been the CO_2 management of patients who have had severe TBI. Aggressive hyperventilation (target $PaCO_2$ of 25 mmHg) historically had a pivotal role in management of severe TBI.[15] Since brain swelling and increased ICP are among the leading causes of morbidity and mortality in this population, hyperventilation seemingly rapidly reduced ICP via cerebral vasoconstriction. However, subsequent research has revealed that this aggressive hyperventilation may cause excessive cerebral vasoconstriction to the point of ischemia, particularly harmful in these patients who already have an injured brain and may even need augmented brain perfusion.[16] Worsened outcomes in patients with severe TBI undergoing hyperventilation were presumably from the reduction of CBF to ischemic levels and the impairment of cerebral oxygen extraction. Further, the benefits from hyperventilation are short-lived as the pH of CSF equilibrates after 6–8 h and cerebral vasoconstriction relaxes.[15,16]

Research has shown sustained hyperventilation is potentially harmful for the patient with a severely injured brain, based on neurologic outcomes at 3–6 months after injury.[15] A review of all available randomized controlled trials using hyperventilation in this patient population suggests that there is no definitive benefit from sustained hyperventilation following head injury and again suggests that there may be some harm.[16]

Despite the available data, study limitations and confounding factors have prevented the neurocritical care community from treating patients with TBI in a standard, evidence-based manner. A recent survey described a wide variety of practice patterns in UK intensive care units for the monitoring and management of severe TBI,[17] including hyperventilation practices, underscoring the lack of consensus there is when treating these patients. The most recent 2007 Brain Trauma Foundation guidelines suggest limiting the use of hyperventilation to combat elevated ICP in TBI to avoid the morbidity of iatrogenic cerebral ischemia. Hyperventilation is recommended to be used only as an acute temporizing therapy for increased ICP after the first 24 h of TBI.[18]

This phenomenon does not appear to be limited to TBI. Intraoperative hypocapnia has also been shown to have worse outcomes at 90 days following endovascular treatment for acute ischemic stroke,[19] again suggesting that CO$_2$-mediated vasoconstriction may be the underlying etiology.

Role of CO$_2$ in the trigeminocardiac reflex

The trigeminocardiac reflex (TCR) is a brain stem reflex, and it is defined as the sudden onset of cardiac rhythm perturbations (bradycardia, asystole), hypotension, apnea, and/or gastric hypermotility during stimulation of any of the sensory branches of the trigeminal nerve. The TCR has occurred in all surgical procedures where a branch of the trigeminal nerve is surgically manipulated, including transsphenoidal surgery, cerebellopontine angle (CPA) and skull base surgery, ocular surgery, craniomaxillofacial surgery, and microvascular trigeminal decompression.[20]

The trigeminal nerve may be stimulated either along its intracranial course or peripherally outside the cranium in any of the three main sensory branches. Sensory branches are stimulated and afferent signals are transmitted to the Gasserian ganglion and then to the sensory nucleus of the trigeminal nerve in the caudal pons. Small fibers connect the afferent pathway to an efferent pathway with the motor nucleus of the vagus nerve. This efferent pathway activates a cardioinhibitory parasympathetic vagal response, producing the clinically observed bradycardia and hypotension.

Among the known risk factors for eliciting the TCR are light anesthesia, hypoxemia, acidosis, and hypercapnia.[20] These abnormalities are corrected prior to surgical manipulation of the nerve and direct trauma is minimized to avoid eliciting the response. If the reflex is observed, then the surgeon should be informed and instructed to discontinue manipulating the nerve. This is typically the only intervention that is needed, but, if persistent, a small dose of an anticholinergic (atropine, glycopyrrolate) is effective. Particularly severe cases may require the use of epinephrine.

Afferent pathway blockade, such as a peribulbar block for ocular surgery patients, may decrease the incidence of the TCR but is not effective all of the time and certainly not for procedures that involve manipulating the central portions of the nerve. There is no current role for the use of prophylactic anticholinergics.[20]

End-tidal CO$_2$ and vascular air embolism

Vascular air embolism (VAE) is the entrainment of air (or exogenously delivered gas) from the surgical field or environment into the arterial or venous vasculature that produces systemic effects. A large volume of air immediately produces a clinical situation known as an *air lock* where the volume of air in the right ventricle completely obstructs outflow to pulmonary circulation. Right-sided failure and cardiovascular collapse occur rapidly. Smaller, nonlethal volumes of air produce incomplete right ventricular outflow obstruction with subsequent hypotension, myocardial and cerebral ischemia, pulmonary hypertension, a systemic inflammatory response, and lung injury. The morbidity and mortality from a VAE are determined by both the volume of air entrained and the rate at which the air is accumulated. Animal models and case reports have determined that the lethal volume of air is approximately 200–300 mL or 3–5 cc/kg. Smaller volumes may be lethal as well if the source of entrainment is close to the right side of the heart. The rate of entrainment is important because the alveolar interface provides a means for absorption and even larger volumes of air may be tolerated if entrained over longer periods.[21]

The true incidence of VAE is difficult to determine since many events are likely minor and go unnoticed, but is believed to be 35% in highest-risk procedures. In the neurosurgical setting, an air embolism occurs when the surgical site is above the level of the heart. When the open vasculature is exposed to air and cannot readily be collapsed, such as opening of the dural sinuses, air moves into the vasculature by a gravitational gradient and relative negative pressure. The classic surgical procedure with the highest concern and risk for VAE is a craniotomy in the sitting position. These procedures are performed for posterior fossa and upper cervical spine pathology. Other neurosurgical procedures, such as spine fusion surgery, may also be associated with VAE.[21]

The diagnosis of VAE during modern anesthetics is made with the use of real-time monitors. It is a clinical diagnosis that requires an understanding of at-risk patients, the timing of key surgical events, and vigilance to detect monitoring changes. Prompt diagnosis is key to treatment and a successful outcome. The most sensitive methods for entrained air detection are transesophageal echocardiography (TEE) and precordial Doppler, which can detect air volumes as small as 0.01–0.02 and 0.05 cc/kg, respectively.[21] Transcranial Doppler examination and pulmonary artery catheters are also sensitive methods but both require specific expertise to interpret, and pulmonary artery catheters are invasive in nature. Changes in pulse oximetry, electrocardiogram, and hemodynamics are late signs of VAE and are typically present after a large volume of air has already been entrained.

The values of ET-CO_2 and the capnogram are useful in aiding with the diagnosis of VAE. ET-CO_2 is a convenient and practical method, although it is relatively insensitive when compared to some of the other modalities. Anesthetized patients will demonstrate a decreased ET-CO_2 value, decreased arterial oxygen saturation, and hypercapnia. There will be an enlarging gradient between the recorded ET-CO_2 value (falling) and $PaCO_2$ value (rising) as less blood reaches the lungs for CO_2 elimination. An appropriately timed decrease in ET-CO_2 value of 2 mmHg may be an indicator of VAE. Limitations include a lack of specificity, questionable reliability with hypotension, and lack of use in spontaneously breathing patients. For surgical procedures with an elevated risk for VAE, monitoring recommendations include continuous ET-CO_2 monitoring and precordial Doppler placement when feasible.[21]

Treatment includes promptly alerting the surgeon that air is being entrained so that they may stop entrainment by flooding the surgical field with saline, by applying bone wax, or by altering the patient position to decrease the gravitational gradient (left lateral decubitus or Trendelenburg when possible). The fraction of inspired oxygen should be increased to enhance oxygenation. Circulation should be supported with vasopressors and inotropes as needed. If a multiorifice aspiration catheter is in place, air can potentially be aspirated from the right side of the heart, although this technique has been described as only modestly effective with success rates of 6–16% reported.[21] In the event of cardiac arrest and dysrhythmias, there should always be rapid availability of a defibrillator and resources to beginning advanced cardiac life support (ACLS), if needed.

Conclusion

With a myriad of clinical implications relevant to patients undergoing neurosurgical procedures and procedures, an understanding of ET-CO_2 is imperative for the anesthesiologist. Important, real-time data can be obtained regarding a patient's ventilation, hemodynamics, and metabolism. Manipulation of the $PaCO_2$ values and cerebrovascular reactivity can modify CBF and ICP, and can impact patients' neurological comorbidities and operating conditions. ET-CO_2 also serves as a monitor for a variety of important intraoperative events that are common to neurosurgical procedures.

References

1. Connor CW. Commonly used monitoring techniques. In: Barash PG, Cullen BF, Stoelting RK, Callahan MK, Stock MC, Ortega R, editors. *Clinical Anesthesia*. 7th ed. Philadelphia, PA: Lippincott Williams & Wilkins; 2013, pp. 699–722.
2. American Society of Anesthesiologists. Standards for basic anesthetic monitoring. Affirmed October 2015. http://www.asahq.org/quality-and-practice-management/standards-and-guidelines. Accessed 17 December 2015.
3. Meng L, Gelb AW. Regulation of cerebral autoregulation by carbon dioxide. *Anesthesiology* 2015;122:196–205.
4. Drummond JC. The lower limit of autoregulation: Time to revise our thinking? *Anesthesiology* 1997;86:1431–1433.
5. Fitch W, Ferguson GG, Sengupta D, Garibi J, Harper AM. Autoregulation of cerebral blood flow during controlled hypotension in baboons. *J Neurol Neurosurg Psychiatry* 1976;39:1014–1022.
6. Kety SS, Schmidt CF. The effects of altered arterial tensions of carbon dioxide and oxygen on cerebral blood flow and cerebral oxygen consumption of normal young men. *J Clin Invest* 1948;27:484–492.

7. Joshi S, Ornstein E, Young WL. Cerebral and spinal cord blood flow. In: Cottrell JE, Young WL editors. *Cottrell and Young's Neuroanesthesia*. 5th ed. Philadelphia, PA: Mosby Elsevier; 2010, pp. 17–59.

8. McCulloch TJ, Visco E, Lam AM. Graded hypercapnia and cerebral autoregulation during sevoflurane or propofol anesthesia. *Anesthesiology* 2000;93:1205–1209.

9. Artu AA. Partial preservation of cerebral vascular responsiveness to hypocapnia during isoflurane-induced hypotension in dogs. *Anesth Analg* 1986;65:660–666.

10. Artu AA, Katz RA, Colley PS. Autoregulation of cerebral blood flow during normocapnia and hypercapnia in dogs. *Anesthesiology* 1989;70:288–292.

11. Mariappan R, Mehta J, Chui J, Manninen P, Venkatraghavan L. Cerebrovascular reactivity to carbon dioxide under anesthesia: A qualitative systematic review. *J Neurosurg Anesthesiol* 2015;27(2):123–134.

12. Gelb AW, Craen RA, Umamaheswara Rao GS et al. Does hyperventilation improve operating condition during supratentorial craniotomy? A multicenter randomized crossover trial. *Anesth Analg* 2008;106(2):585–594.

13. Peterson KD, Landsfeldt U, Gold GE et al. Intracranial pressure and cerebral hemodynamics in patients with cerebral tumors: A randomized, prospective study of patients subjected to craniotomy with propofol-fentanyl, isoflurane-fentanyl or sevoflurane-fentanyl anesthesia. *Anesthesiology* 2003;98:329–336.

14. Jansen GF, van Praagh BH, Kendaria MB, Odoom JA. Jugular venous bulb saturation during propofol and isoflurane/nitrous oxide anesthesia during brain tumor surgery. *Anesth Analg* 1999;89:358–363.

15. Muizelaar JP, Marmarou A, Ward JD et al. Adverse effects of prolonged hyperventilation in patients with severe head injury: A randomized clinical trial. *J Neurosurg* 1991;75:731–739.

16. Roberts I, Schierhout G. Hyperventilation therapy for acute traumatic brain injury. *Cochrane Database Syst Rev* 1997;(4):CD 000566.

17. Wijayatilake DS, Talati C, Panchatsharam S. The monitoring and management of severe traumatic brain injury in the United Kingdom: Is there a consensus? A national survey. *J Neurosurg Anesthesiol* 2015;27(2):241–245.

18. Bratton SL, Chestnut RM, Ghajar J et al. Guidelines for the management of severe traumatic brain injury. I. Blood pressure and oxygenation. Brain Trauma Foundation; American Society of Neurological Surgeons; Congress of Neurological Surgeons; Joint Section on Neurotrauma and Neurocritical Care, AANS/CNS. *J Neurotrauma* 2007;24 (Suppl. 1):S7–S13.

19. Takahashi CE, Brambrink AM, Aziz MF et al. Association of intraprocedural blood pressure and end tidal carbon dioxide with outcome after acute stroke intervention. *Neurocrit Care* 2014;20:202–208.

20. Chowdhury T, Mendelowith D, Golanov E et al. Trigeminocardiac reflex: The current clinical and physiologic knowledge. *J Neurosurg Anesthesiol* 2015;27(2):136–147.

21. Mirski MA, Lele AV, Fitzsimmons L, Toung TJ. Diagnosis and treatment of vascular air embolism. *Anesthesiology* 2007;106:164–177.

10

Arterial blood pressure

NIDHI GUPTA

Introduction

Arterial blood pressure (ABP) is one of the fundamental cardiovascular vital signs included in the mandated standards for basic anesthetic monitoring. It is the simplest and most reproducible monitoring modality to ensure the adequacy of the patient's circulatory function during all anesthetics.

Indications for arterial blood pressure monitoring

Maintenance of hemodynamic stability and optimal cerebral perfusion pressure (CPP) are crucial to the treatment of patients with intracranial pathology. To maximize cerebral perfusion, it is imperative that optimal respiratory and preload conditions are achieved. Invasive ABP monitoring allows continuous real-time beat-to-beat monitoring of heart rate and blood pressure along with uninterrupted display of pulse contour. It also provides access to frequent sampling of serial blood

gases, electrolytes, hematocrit, and serum osmolality. It, thus, may guide manipulation of blood pressure and arterial blood gases to optimize cerebral perfusion and oxygenation.

In neurosurgery, noninvasive blood pressure monitoring is appropriate for minor cases. However, during major intracranial and complex spine surgery, invasive ABP monitoring is quintessential in view of sudden hemodynamic instability due to hemorrhage, venous air embolism, herniation syndromes, or cranial nerve manipulation (Table 10.1). Given the unreliability of sphygmomanometers at blood pressure extremes, invasive ABP monitoring is also indicated in patients who are hemodynamically unstable and in patients with significant comorbidities.

In patients with low intracranial compliance, a rise in arterial partial pressure of carbon dioxide ($PaCO_2$) may lead to cerebral vasodilatation, thereby causing an increase in intracranial pressure (ICP). End-tidal carbon dioxide often correlates poorly with the $PaCO_2$, especially in patients

Table 10.1 Indications for Invasive Arterial Blood Pressure Monitoring

Continuous beat-to-beat monitoring of ABP
Serial sampling of arterial blood gases
Inability to obtain noninvasive blood pressure measurements (e.g., in polytrauma patient with all extremities affected)
Assessment of cardiac preload through analysis of the cyclic variation in arterial pressure

with pulmonary disease. Therefore, $PaCO_2$ should preferably be monitored in patients at risk of intracranial hypertension. In addition, intraoperative fluid administration can be facilitated by examining systolic variation in ABP with the respiratory cycle, which acts as a sign of preload reserve and correlates with fluid responsiveness.

An arterial catheter should also be preserved in neurocritically ill patients requiring elective ventilation, and in patients showing lateralizing signs and/or deterioration in consciousness to allow frequent estimation of arterial blood gas values. Invasive ABP monitoring also allows precise blood pressure control within the limits specified by the neurosurgeon, depending on whether the goal is to prevent postoperative hematoma formation (e.g., in patients operated for intracranial tumors or after arteriovenous malformation embolization) or to preserve perfusion (e.g., during hypertensive therapy for management of cerebral vasospasm).

Percutaneous arterial cannulation

In elective neurosurgical cases, invasive arterial line placement is performed soon after induction of anesthesia. However, in patients with ruptured aneurysm, it may be prudent to institute invasive arterial monitoring before induction of anesthesia to allow accurate beat-to-beat observation of blood pressure and optimum drug titration.

Common sites of placement of an arterial cannula include radial, femoral, brachial, axillary, and dorsalis pedis arteries. The radial artery is the most common site for invasive ABP monitoring. It is technically easy to cannulate and complications are uncommon because of extensive collateral circulation provided via the ulnar artery and palmar arch.[1-3]

Although the ulnar artery is usually of larger diameter, it is relatively inaccessible percutaneously compared to the radial artery. The dorsalis pedis artery, although popular for pediatric patients and easily accessible during neurosurgical cases, should be avoided in patients with peripheral vascular disease.

Before attempting percutaneous radial artery cannulation, an Allen test should be performed to identify patients at increased risk for ischemic complications from arterial occlusion or embolization of the debris or clot from the catheter tip. The Allen test is the simplest and most practical method to assess patency of the collateral circulation to the hand.[2]

The examiner compresses both the radial and the ulnar arteries and asks the patient to tighten fist, exsanguinating the palm. The patient then opens the hand, avoiding hyperextension of the wrist or fingers. As occlusion of the ulnar artery is released, the color of the open palm is observed. Normally, the color will return to the palm within several seconds; severely reduced ulnar collateral flow is present when the palm remains pale for more than 6–10 s (positive Allen test).

An abnormal finding from an Allen test, however, does not preclude radial artery access as it has poor predictive value for ischemic injuries.[4,5] Hence, use of this test as a predictor of ischemic complications is still a matter of controversy.

A modified Allen test can also be performed under pulse oximetry guidance. The pulse oximetry sensor is placed on the tip of the thumb of the selected hand and baseline oxygen saturation is noted. Compression of both the radial and ulnar arteries is sustained until the oxygen saturation reading falls to zero. The pressure on the ulnar artery is then released and the time for the oxygen saturation to return to the baseline value is recorded. Failure of the oxygen saturation to return to the baseline value within 10 s indicates being positive to the test.

A peripheral perfusion index (PI), which is the ratio between the pulsatile and the nonpulsatile components of the pulse oximetry signal, has been found to be a reliable indicator of peripheral perfusion.[6]

Placing an arterial line

Arterial cannulation can be performed with a standard 20-G IV cannula, a 20-G arterial cannula with flow switch, or an integrated guidewire–catheter assembly using the Seldinger technique. The wrist and hand are immobilized in mild dorsiflexion and secured with the wrist resting across a soft pad. Extreme wrist dorsiflexion should be avoided to prevent injury to the median nerve.[7]

Three common techniques for cannulation include direct arterial puncture, guidewire-assisted cannulation (Seldinger technique), and the transfixion–withdrawal method. The technique of cannulation per se, however, is not associated with a more frequent rate of complications or failure.

Arterial catheterization with the help of palpation of the artery alone is sometimes insufficient in patients who are hemodynamically unstable, obese, or have edema. Furthermore, palpation alone often fails in pediatric patients. In adults, ultrasound-guided percutaneous radial arterial catheterization improves first-attempt and overall catheterization success and shortens insertion time, irrespective of experience.[8]

In pediatric patients aged less than 3 years, subcutaneous radial artery depth between 2 and 4 mm is associated with fastest ultrasound-guided catheterization and greatest overall catheterization success.[9] For patients in whom the radial artery is located at a depth of less than 2 mm, increasing the depth to 2–4 mm by subcutaneous saline injection improves catheterization time and the success rate.

Arterial line flush

The flush device provides a continuous, slow (1–3 mL/h) infusion of normal saline to purge the monitoring system and prevent thrombus formation within the arterial catheter. Using incorrect arterial line fluid infusions, especially dextrose-containing solutions, is a common error in intensive care settings.

Sodium chloride 0.9%, with or without heparin, should be the only solution to be used for arterial line infusion and flushing.[10] Addition of heparin (1–2 units heparin/mL saline) has been used to further reduce the incidence of catheter thrombosis, but it increases the risk of heparin-induced thrombocytopenia, and hence, should be avoided.

Invasive arterial blood pressure monitor setup

In current clinical practice, the system most commonly used for invasive ABP monitoring consists of an intravascular catheter connected to an electronic transducer via low-compliance, saline-filled tubing. The stopcocks in the system provide sites for blood sampling and allow the transducer to be exposed to atmospheric pressure to establish a zero reference value.

The electronic transducer contains a deformable diaphragm connected to a Wheatstone bridge, which converts the mechanical energy of the pressure waves into electric signals. The signals are then amplified, displayed, or recorded. The pressure monitoring system should be constructed of short lengths of stiff tubing with a limited number of stopcocks and other connections that are free of air bubbles and blood clots to maximize its natural frequency. Lines and stopcocks must be clearly labeled and manipulated with care to avoid unintentional intra-arterial injection of drugs or air.

To avoid measurement errors, one must always consider three things before instituting invasive ABP monitoring: the pressure transducer must be zeroed, calibrated, and leveled to the appropriate position relative to the patient. The current disposable pressure transducers meet accuracy standards established by the American National Standards Institute. As such, formal bedside transducer calibration is no longer performed.

Zeroing the transducer

Intravascular pressures are referenced against ambient atmospheric pressure by exposing the pressure transducer to air through an open stopcock and pressing the zero-pressure button on the monitor. Zeroing refers to adjustment of the Wheatstone bridge in the transducer so that starting pressure is atmospheric pressure and has a value of zero. When a significant or unexpected change in pressure occurs, the zero reference value can be rechecked quickly by opening the stopcock and noting that the pressure value on the bedside monitor is still zero.

Leveling the transducer

After zeroing the catheter system, the transducer system should remain fixed relative to the patient. For arterial catheters, the midpoint of the right atrium is used as the reference. The position of the pressure transducer relative to the patient must be considered in interpreting blood pressure measurements. Monitoring of CPP, defined as the difference between ABP and ICP, requires that the transducer be placed at the level of the brain, approximating the position of the circle of Willis. Hence, in patients with brain injury the reference point for arterial catheters should ideally be at the level of the tragus.[11]

Similarly, if the transducer is placed at the standard thoracic level during sitting position, then the arterial pressure at the level of the heart will be recorded. Hence, during sitting craniotomies, the arterial line transducer should be located and zeroed at the level of the tragus to estimate the CPP correctly.[12,13]

In the lateral decubitus position, one arm is necessarily higher than the other. However, as long as the pressure transducer remains fixed at the level of the heart, the location of the arms or the vessel in which the catheter resides has no influence on the measured arterial pressure.

Errors are, however, common when pressure transducers are fixed and the patient's bed height is adjusted. Raising the height of the bed relative to the transducer will cause overestimation of ABP, whereas lowering the patient below the transducer will lead to underestimation.

Arterial pressure waveform analysis

Normal arterial waveform morphology

The systemic arterial pressure waveform results from ejection of blood from the left ventricle into the aorta during systole, followed by peripheral runoff during diastole.

The normal arterial waveform recorded in the radial artery follows the ECG R wave by approximately 120–180 ms and consists of a steep systolic upstroke, peak, and decline (Figure 10.1). The down slope is interrupted by the dicrotic notch which is sharply defined when recorded in the aorta and undoubtedly represents aortic valve closure. It is however, delayed and slurred when pressure is recorded more peripherally and is related to arterial wall properties. The arterial pressure wave continues to decline following the dicrotic notch and the electrocardiogram (ECG) T-wave, reaching its lowest point at end diastole.

Compared with central ABPs, peripheral arterial pressures have steeper systolic upstrokes,

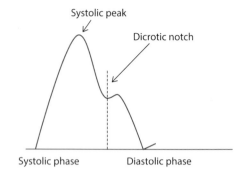

Figure 10.1 Normal arterial blood pressure waveform.

higher systolic peaks, slurring (femoral) or loss (dorsalis pedis) of the dicrotic notch, prominent diastolic wave, and lower end-diastolic pressures. As a result, compared with central aortic pressure, peripheral arterial waveforms have higher systolic, lower diastolic, and wider pulse pressures.

In contrast, as blood flows from the aorta to the radial artery, mean arterial pressure (MAP) decreases only slightly because there is little resistance to flow in the major conducting arteries. Therefore, clinical therapy is often better guided using radial artery MAP than radial artery systolic blood pressure.

Abnormal arterial pressure waveforms

Various pathologic conditions such as aortic stenosis, aortic regurgitation, and cardiac tamponade can influence arterial pressure waveform morphology.[5] Hence, detailed examination of the morphologic features of individual arterial pressure waveforms and observation of how arterial waveform patterns change over time can provide important diagnostic information.

Dynamic/functional hemodynamic monitoring

Until recently, it has been unclear as to which hemodynamically unstable patients are volume-responsive and likely to benefit from fluid resuscitation (i.e., fluid boluses). However, during the past decade, a number of dynamic tests of volume responsiveness (defined as the hemodynamic response to a fluid load) have been reported.

Dynamic variables such as systolic pressure variation (SPV) and pulse pressure variation (PPV) derived from the analysis of the arterial waveform and the stroke volume variation (SVV) derived from the pulse contour analysis estimate preload dependence, the key factor in predicting fluid responsiveness.[14,15]

These variations demonstrate cardiopulmonary interactions that result from changes in intrathoracic pressure and lung volume. With the onset of positive-pressure inspiration, the rise in lung volume effectively squeezes the pulmonary venous bed, increases drainage of blood from the pulmonary veins into the left atrium, and augments left ventricular preload. Concurrently, left ventricular afterload decreases because of the increased intrathoracic pressure. The increase in left ventricular preload and decrease in afterload lead to an increase in both left ventricular stroke volume (SV) and ABP. At the same time, the increase in intrathoracic pressure observed in early inspiration reduces systemic venous return and decreases both right ventricular preload and right ventricular SV. Toward the end of inspiration or during early expiration, the reduced right ventricular SV that occurred during inspiration leads to reduced left ventricular filling and, as a result, decreased left ventricular SV and systemic ABP. Systolic ABP thus varies cyclically during a positive-pressure mechanical breath being maximal at end inspiration and minimal at end expiration.

This cyclic variation in ABP may be measured and quantified as the SPV, which is defined as the difference between the maximum inspiratory and minimum expiratory systolic pressures during one mechanical breath. Normally, a patient on mechanical ventilation will have a total SPV of <10 mmHg.

PPV is the difference between the maximal and minimal pulse pressures during the mechanical breath cycle. SVV is continuously displayed by the pulse index continuous cardiac output (PiCCO) monitor and is defined as the percentage change between the maximal and minimal SV divided by the average of the minimum and maximum over a floating period of 30 s.

According to a meta-analysis, arterial pressure variation is sensitive and specific in predicting volume responsiveness (with PPV performing slightly better than SVV), and outperforms static measures of preload such as central venous pressure.[16]

Several clinical trials have documented that an SVV greater than 10% or a PPV greater than 13%–15% on a tidal volume of 8 mL/kg or greater is highly predictive of volume responsiveness.[15–20] In clinical practice, use of arterial pressure variation as a marker of volume responsiveness has become quite helpful in hemodynamic assessment, volume management, and institution of more specific goal-directed fluid therapy in critically ill patients, which has decreased many complications, including organ failure.[17]

In neurosurgical patients, SVV-directed fluid therapy has been shown to result in optimal fluid management.[12,18,19] These dynamic markers are able to predict fluid responsiveness even in sitting[12] and prone position.[19,20] Such a goal-oriented therapy is especially helpful in patients with reduced cardiovascular reserves (such as elderly patients) who also have decreased brain compliance.

Limitations of arterial blood pressure monitoring

Atherosclerosis or pathologic conditions such as arterial dissection, stenosis, or embolism may preclude accurate pressure monitoring from affected sites. In addition, unusual patient positions during surgery may produce regional arterial compression, thereby distorting the arterial pressure waveform.

The functional hemodynamic monitoring parameters derived from arterial waveform analysis have their own limitations. They have been validated as predictors of fluid responsiveness only in patients on mechanical ventilation with adequate tidal volume (at least 8 mL/kg).[14] The values are further confounded by the presence of arrhythmias, changes in chest wall and lung compliance, addition of positive end-expiratory pressure, or other pulmonary pathology.

Complications of direct arterial pressure monitoring

Complications of arterial cannulation, including hemorrhage, infection, vascular insufficiency, ischemia, thrombosis, embolization, and neuronal or adjacent structure injury, have been recognized since the introduction of the technique into practice (Table 10.2).[2]

Table 10.2 Complications of Direct Arterial Pressure Monitoring

Equipment misuse

Data misinterpretation

Distal ischemia

Pseudoaneurysm

Arteriovenous fistula

Hemorrhage

Arterial embolization

Infection

Peripheral neuropathy

Factors associated with an increased risk of complications include prolonged cannulation, pre-existing vasculopathy, extracorporeal circulation, protracted shock, high-dose vasopressor administration, female gender, and multiple insertion attempts.

These iatrogenic injuries contribute to morbidity, prolonged length of stay, financial burden, and appreciable long-term injury of medicolegal significance.

However, such complications are rare (<0.1%).[1] Equipment misuse and data misinterpretation are still the most frequent complications of arterial catheterization.

Hence, careful placement technique and catheter care, as well as proper equipment use and data interpretation, are primary issues to avoid many complications related to arterial pressure monitoring.

References

1. Mandel MA, Dauchot PJ. Radial artery cannulation in 1000 patients: Precautions and complications. *J Hand Surg Am* 1977;2:482–485.
2. Wilkins RG. Radial artery, cannulation and ischaemic damage: A review. *Anaesthesia* 1985;40:896–899.
3. Scheer B, Perel A, Pfeiffer UJ. Clinical review: Complications and risk factors of peripheral arterial catheters used for haemodynamic monitoring in anaesthesia and intensive care medicine. *Crit Care* 2002;6:199–204.
4. Martin C, Sauz P, Papazian L, Gouin F. Long term arterial cannulation in ICU patients using the radial artery or dorsalis pedis artery. *Chest* 2001;119:901–906.
5. Schroeder B, Barbeito A, Baryosef S, Mark JB. Cardiovascular monitoring. In: Miller RD, editor. Miller's Anesthesia. 8th ed. Churchill Livingstone/Elsevier, Publishers, 2014; pp. 1345–1395.
6. Lima AP, Beelen P, Bakker J. Use of a peripheral perfusion index derived from the pulse oximetry signal as a noninvasive indicator of perfusion. *Crit Care Med* 2002;30:1210–1213.
7. Chowet AL, Lopez JR, Brock-Utne JG, Jaffe RA. Wrist hyperextension leads to median nerve conduction block: Implications for intra-arterial catheter placement. *Anesthesiology* 2004;100:287–291.
8. Shiver S, Blaivas M, Lyon M. A prospective comparison of ultrasound-guided and blindly placed radial arterial catheters. *Acad Emerg Med* 2006;13:1275–1279.
9. Nakayama Y, Nakajima Y, Sessler DI et al. A novel method for ultrasound-guided radial arterial catheterization in pediatric patients. *Anesth Analg* 2014;118:1019–1026.
10. Sprint Working Party, Woodcock TE, Cook TM, Gupta KJ, Hartle A. Arterial line blood sampling: Preventing hypoglycaemic brain injury 2014: The association of anaesthetists of great Britain and Ireland. *Anaesthesia* 2014;69:380–385.
11. Bijker JB, Gelb AW. Review article: The role of hypotension in perioperative stroke. *Can J Anesth* 2013; 60:159–167.
12. Lindroos AC, Niiya T, Silvasti-Lundell M, Randell T, Hernesniemi J, Niemi TT. Stroke volume-directed administration of hydroxyethyl starch or Ringer's acetate in sitting position during craniotomy. *Acta Anaesthesiol Scand* 2013;57: 729–736.
13. Feigl GC, Decker K, Wurms M et al. Neurosurgical procedures in the semisitting position: Evaluation of the risk of paradoxical venous air embolism in patients with a patent foramen ovale. *World Neurosurg* 2014;81:159–164.

14. Marik PE, Monnet X, Teboul JL. Hemodynamic parameters to guide fluid therapy. *Ann Intensive Care* 2011;1:1.

15. Marik PE, Cavallazzi R, Vasu T, Hirani A. Dynamic changes in arterial waveform derived variables and fluid responsiveness in mechanically ventilated patients. Asystematic review of the literature. *Crit Care Med* 2009;37:2642–2647.

16. Marik PE, Baram M, Vahid B. Does central venous pressure predict volume responsiveness? A systematic review of the literature and the tale of seven mares. *Chest* 2008;134:172–178.

17. Benes J, Giglio M, Brienza N, Michard F. The effects of goal-directed fluid therapy based on dynamic parameters on post-surgical outcome: A meta-analysis of randomized controlled trials. *Crit Care* 2014;18:584.

18. Berkenstadt H, Margalit N, Hadani M et al. Stroke volume variation as a predictor of fluid responsiveness in patients undergoing brain surgery. *Anesth Analg* 2001;92:984–989.

19. Lindroos AC, Niiya T, Randell T, Niemi TT. Stroke volume-directed administration of hydroxyethyl starch (HES 130/0.4) and Ringer's acetate in prone position during neurosurgery: A randomized controlled trial. *J Anesth* 2014;28:189–197.

20. Biais M, Bernard O, Ha JC, Degryse C, Sztark F. Abilities of pulse pressure variations and stroke volume variations to predict fluid responsiveness in prone position during scoliosis surgery. *Br J Anaesth* 2010;104:407–413.

11

Central venous pressure

NIDHI GUPTA

Introduction

Central venous pressure (CVP) is the measure of right atrial pressure (RAP), which can be estimated noninvasively by measuring the jugular venous pressure (JVP) or invasively by transducing a central venous catheter (CVC) with its tip placed in the superior vena cava or right atrium (RA).

The terms CVP, RAP, and JVP are used synonymously as normally there is only minimal resistance along the great vessels. However, there are certain situations, such as sclerosis of a central vein, that can increase the resistance along the major veins, and the pressures may not always be the same.

Normal CVP in a spontaneously breathing patient is 0–5 mmHg whereas the generally accepted normal upper limit in mechanically ventilated patients is 10 mmHg. Like arterial pressure waveforms, CVP waveform morphology can provide important information about clinical pathophysiology.[1] In contemporary practice, the CVP waveform is used simply to extract the CVP value at end expiration.

Indications for central venous cannulation in neurosurgical patients

There are a number of indications for central venous cannulation in neurosurgical patients (Table 11.1). In general, placement of the CVC is considered essential in patients with neurogenic or cardiovascular instability, those undergoing sitting craniotomy, and when substantial blood loss is anticipated. The main indications include monitoring of CVP, aspiration of entrained air embolus, absence of peripheral veins, and need for administration of vasoactive drugs, antibiotics, or hypertonic solutions during or after surgery.

In a postal questionnaire sent to all UK consultant members of the Neuroanaesthesia Society regarding any consensus on indications for use and route of insertion of the CVC in elective neuroanesthesia practice, 98% indicated that they would insert a CVC into patients requiring excision of an acoustic neuroma in the sitting position, 76% indicated that they would use it for clipping of an intracranial aneurysm, and 75% indicated that they would use it for resection of an arteriovenous malformation.[2]

Table 11.1 Indications for Central Venous Cannulation

Monitoring of central venous pressure

Aspiration of air emboli

Administration of vasoactive drugs

Administration of fluids or drugs that can cause peripheral vein sclerosis (e.g., hypertonic saline, potassium infusion, total parenteral nutrition, chemotherapeutic agents, and prolonged antibiotic therapy)

During active resuscitation of critically ill or polytrauma patients in addition to peripheral venous access

To obtain venous access when peripheral venous access is not obtainable

Transvenous cardiac pacing

Temporary hemodialysis

Sampling site for repeated blood testing

The antecubital fossa was the preferred route of insertion for 43.5% of respondents with 36.5% preferring the internal jugular vein (IJV) approach. The subclavian vein (SCV) and femoral vein (FV) were the unpopular first-choice approaches.

Measurement of central venous pressure to guide fluid management

Traditionally, CVP has been considered an important tool to guide fluid management based on the assumption that the CVP reflects intravascular volume. It was widely believed that patients with a low CVP are volume-depleted whereas patients with a high CVP are volume-overloaded. However, CVP is the back-pressure to, and not a synonym for, venous return. Independent of the blood volume returning to the right heart, factors affecting cardiac performance and structure can influence CVP.

As CVP determines RA pressure, it is a good indicator of right ventricle (RV) preload. Furthermore, because RV stroke volume determines left ventricle (LV) filling, the CVP is assumed to be an indirect measure of LV preload. However, due to the changes in heart compliance, venous tone, and high intrathoracic pressures that occur in critically ill patients, there is a poor relationship between the CVP and RV end-diastolic volume. In addition, the RV end-diastolic volume may not reflect the patients' position on the Frank–Starling curve, which determines the preload reserve.

To date, more than 100 studies have been published, which demonstrate that there is no relationship between the CVP (or change in CVP) and fluid responsiveness in various clinical settings.[3,4] Except for extremely low values, static levels of CVP are often unreliable in predicting fluid responsiveness.[4]

Overall, it is best not to use a single value of CVP to predict volume responsiveness, and some kind of dynamic test should be used. However, conflicting evidence exists regarding the use of CVP variation in response to fluids or in relation to the respiratory cycle as a predictor of fluid responsiveness because it can be altered by a number of factors including changes in tidal volumes, abdominal pressure, and vascular tone.[5,6]

Aspiration of venous air embolus

During venous air embolism (VAE), aspiration of air through a CVC has both diagnostic and therapeutic roles. Aspiration of air confirms VAE and is probably the only management strategy with demonstrated clinical efficacy. Two large series of patients have reported a success rate of 43%–52%.[7,8] However, accurate placement of a CVC tip is quintessential for aspirating air from the circulation should an embolism occur (discussed in the section "Ideal catheter tip location").

Neurointensive care units

Central venous cannulation is often required in neurointensive care unit patients as they often have lengthy stays and require an extended vascular access. Central venous access is also recommended for hypertonic saline infusions (greater than 2% concentration) to prevent peripheral vein thrombosis, except for bolus or short-term hyperosmolar therapy.

CVP monitoring is essential in neurosurgical patients with hemodynamic instability and for accurate assessment of the volume status of the patients with disorders of water homeostasis.[9] Measurement of CVP is the only reliable indicator for differentiating syndrome of inappropriate antidiuretic hormone secretion (SIADH) from cerebral salt-wasting syndrome. For the diagnosis of SIADH to be made, the patient must be clinically euvolemic.

CVP monitoring is also recommended to ensure normovolemia in patients with subarachnoid hemorrhage to prevent cerebral vasospasm and for effective fluid management of patients with pathological polyuria due to diabetes insipidus.

Central venous cannulation

The decision to perform central venous cannulation before or after induction of anesthesia is guided most often by individual patient and physician preferences or institutional practice. However, in neurosurgical patients, it is safer to place a CVC in an anesthetized patient preoperatively than that in a cerebrally compromised postoperative patient.[2] Practice guidelines have been published to

provide guidance regarding placement and management of CVCs and reduce infectious, mechanical, thrombotic, and other adverse outcomes associated with central venous catheterization.[10]

Proper positioning of the pressure transducer is extremely important because seemingly small errors in transducer height amplify errors in measuring cardiac filling pressure. The consensus is that this level should be at the midpoint of the RA, because at this location blood comes back to the heart before being ejected again.[11] More commonly, the level is taken at the mid-axillary or mid-thoracic line in the fourth intercostal space.

Choosing the catheter and site for central venous cannulation

The decision to choose the type of CVC, as well as the approach used, depends on the clinical indications for its placement balanced against the potential complications associated with the particular route of insertion. Each approach has advantages and disadvantages, which must be considered while choosing the insertion site (Table 11.2).

Table 11.2 Advantages and Disadvantages of Various Routes of Central Venous Cannulation

Insertion approach	Advantages	Disadvantages
Right internal jugular	High success rate with less catheter malposition[12] Low risk of pneumothorax and hemothorax as compared to the subclavian route[13]	The most common complication is carotid puncture[1,13]—of particular hazard in neurosurgical patients as the pressure needed for hemostasis will almost inevitably lead to reduced cerebral perfusion pressure. Should be avoided in cervical spine fractures and penetrating neck injury. Head-down tilt traditionally used during insertion is also a disadvantage in neurosurgical patients (increases ICP).
Subclavian	Most suitable for long-term intravenous therapy or dialysis and for emergency volume resuscitation Easy to insert in trauma patients who may be immobilized in a cervical collar Less frequent risk of infection compared with femoral sites[14]	As with the IJV route, the time spent with head-down tilt for placement should be kept to a minimum. Risk of serious complications on insertion, notably pneumothorax and hemothorax is higher than for any other route.[1,13] Avoid ipsilateral placement in case of chest wall trauma or deformities.

(continued)

Table 11.2 Advantages and Disadvantages of Various Routes of Central Venous Cannulation (Continued)

Insertion approach	Advantages	Disadvantages
Antecubital Fossa	No reported major insertion-related complications Does not require the patient to be placed head-down during cannulation Best suited to intra- and immediate postoperative CVP measurement[2]	Higher risk of catheter-related large vein thrombosis.[15,16] Length of the catheter is not ideal for the rapid withdrawal of large volumes of air. Unsuitable for multiple drug therapy postoperatively because of large dead space and limited number of lumens available (maximum two).
Femoral	Useful when the more common IJV and SCV sites are not accessible (in patients with burns, with trauma, during surgical procedures that involve the head, neck, and upper thorax, and if CVC is needed for resuscitation from shock)[13] Relatively easy and uncomplicated insertion Added advantage of avoiding head-down positioning during insertion	High risk of infectious and thrombotic complications.[14] Damage to large vessels that may lead to intraabdominal or retroperitoneal hemorrhage[13] and more rarely, the femoral nerve. Misplaced catheters can enter the ascending lumbar vein, internal iliac vein, left renal vein, and the contralateral iliac vein, giving rise to potential toxicity from venous perfusion if inotropes are used. To be avoided in cases of abdominal trauma, significant trauma to the lower extremity, or presence of deep venous thrombosis.

ICP, intracranial pressure

Many different types of CVCs exist, for example, tunneled or nontunneled, mono-lumen or multi-lumen, dialysis catheters, and peripherally inserted central venous catheters (PICCs). The most commonly used catheter is a 7-Fr, 20-cm multiport catheter that makes simultaneous CVP monitoring and infusion of drugs and fluids possible.

Centrally inserted central venous catheters:
Centrally inserted CVCs are generally 20–30 cm long nontunneled venous devices placed in a deep central vein (IJV, SCV, axillary vein, or innominate vein) as well as in the FV.

In critically ill neurologic patients, centrally inserted CVCs have been found to have a better risk profile compared to PICCs, with significantly lower risk of catheter-related large vein thrombosis

(CRLVT) and no statistically significant difference in central line-associated bloodstream infection or line insertion-related complications.[16]

Decades ago, it was advocated that IJV cannulation should be avoided in neurosurgical patients as IJV represents the main cerebral venous output and any reduction in its flow could create an increase in cerebral blood volume and intracranial pressure (ICP). However, ultrasound and ICP monitoring studies have confirmed that IJV cannulation does not cause significant reduction in cerebral venous flow drainage[17] and there is no increase in ICP.[18] Hence, IJV access can be considered safe in patients with risk for cerebral hypertension.

Peripherally inserted central venous catheters:
PICCs are 50–60 cm long nontunneled central catheters placed via an antecubital vein, preferably the basilic vein, which is generally more

successfully catheterized than the cephalic vein due to its more linear course. PICCs are increasingly being used in intensive care unit (ICU) patients for their ease of insertion and lack of insertion-related complications. In addition, PICC placement is appropriate to avoid postprocedural hemorrhage in patients with decreased platelet count or coagulation abnormalities.

However, in recent studies, PICCs, have been found to be associated with a higher risk of CRLVT and possible pulmonary emboli.[15,16] This is particularly important in neurological ICU patients who often have strong contraindications for anticoagulation, putting them at a significant risk for morbidity or mortality when deep venous thrombosis occurs.

Various risk factors for CRLVT associated with PICC lines include placement in a paretic arm, mannitol therapy during the dwell time of the line, surgery lasting longer than 1 h during dwell time of the line, and a history of venous thromboembolism.

Role of ultrasound in central venous cannulation

Real-time two-dimensional ultrasound guidance for IJV cannulation is recommended as the method of choice in both elective and emergency settings, in adult and pediatric patients.[19,20]

In patients with head and neck trauma or previous cervical spine fusion, ultrasound guidance allows easy cannulation of IJV, keeping neck in neutral position with similar complications and access time as a normal cannulation with 45° neck rotation.[21]

It has been suggested that when using ultrasound, a study of IJV diameters and flows should be conducted in every patient with intracranial hypertension or when bilateral cannulation of the IJV has to be performed (e.g., for jugular bulb oxygen saturation monitoring) to avoid cannulating the vein with the wrong-sized CVC and worsening cerebral damage.[17,20]

Ultrasound-guided central vein catheterization of the SCV and FV is also superior to the landmark method as it prevents complications (arterial puncture, hematoma formation) and increases success on the first attempt and hence should be the method of choice.[22]

Ideal central venous catheter tip placement

Ideal catheter tip location

Optimal positioning of the tip of a CVC is a complex and controversial subject.[23] Misplaced catheter tips not only lead to inaccurate measurement of the CVP but may also increase the risk of chemical and bacterial thrombophlebitis, arrhythmias, and myocardial perforation, leading to cardiac tamponade. In patients undergoing neurosurgical procedures, the use of hyperosmolar agents (mannitol or hypertonic saline) further increases the risk of venous thrombosis.

To prevent the rare but lethal complication of cardiac tamponade, the tip should ideally lie proximal to the boundaries of the pericardial sac; however, too proximal placement of the tip increases the risk of thrombosis.

In general, it is widely accepted that the tip of the catheter should be in superior venae cava (SVC), ideally outside the pericardial sac, and parallel with the long axis of the vein such that the tip does not abut the vein or heart wall at an acute angle or end on and move freely within the vascular lumen.[24]

For aspirating an air embolus, the ideal location for multi-orifice catheters is 2 cm below the junction of the SVC and RA at an inclination of 80° for maximal efficacy (up to 80%).[25] A single-orificed catheter gives a maximum yield of 45%–50% aspiration when the tip is positioned 3.0 cm above the SVC and arterial chamber junction.[25]

Malposition of central venous catheter

Malposition of CVC is more common with the SCV approach compared to the IJV approach.[12] Rath et al.[26] have described a simple bedside saline flush test for detection of a misplaced SCV catheter into ipsilateral IJV. Even if the CVC lies in the designated course of vein, the tip of the catheter is not in a fixed location but shows a range of motion as the patient changes body position. In the majority of patients, the catheter tip shows a range of movement extending 2–3 cm depending on the catheter insertion site and the patient's body habitus. Hence, it is imperative that the catheter tip is readjusted and reconfirmed after final patient positioning.

A catheter tip placed deliberately in the RA for aspiration of air should be withdrawn once the risk of air embolism is over.

In the supine position, the mediastinal structures, including the central veins, are compressed by the abdominal contents. When the patient moves to an upright position, there is descent of the abdominal contents and diaphragm, thereby causing a relative change in the position of the catheter tip with respect to the SVC and RA. Hence, when a patient moves from a supine to a sitting position, the catheter tip moves upward (cephalad) in relation to the RA. Similarly, the final position of the tip of a PICC is dependent on the specific insertion site and the position of the patient's arm. If the PICC is inserted with the arm abducted, the tip of the catheter will move lower (caudal) when the arm is moved to the patient's side (adducted).

Appropriate placement of a CVC can be confirmed by plain chest X-ray (CXR), real-time X-ray imaging, intravascular electrocardiography (ECG; point of large negative P complex),[25] or transesophageal-guided placement,[27] or by withdrawing the catheter after eliciting a right ventricular waveform on a pressure transducer.

Plain CXR can be used to confirm catheter position within the chest. However, in view of its two-dimensional projection, it is not possible to reliably state whether the tip of the catheter is in an artery, vein, pleura, or mediastinum in the chest. The most reliable radiographic landmark to delineate the borders of the SVC and the SVC/RA junction is the right tracheobronchial angle. This angle is created as the right main bronchus bifurcates from the trachea. Cadaveric studies have also confirmed that the tracheal carina is always more cephalad than the pericardial reflection on the SCV, suggesting

that a CVC tip should always be located superior to this radiographic landmark (Figure 11.1).[28]

Real-time X-ray imaging uses an image intensifier. However, without the injection of contrast, it has similar limitations as those of a plain CXR. Intravascular ECG guidance also has limitations as the characteristics P wave changes in ECG may be observed whenever a guidewire or conducting catheter is close to the right or left atrium irrespective of whether it is in a vein, an artery, a mediastinum, or in another structure.[29] Use of ultrasound during CVC insertion enables identification of the target vein and detection of anatomical variations or thrombosis at the site of insertion but does not prevent catheter tip misplacement distal to the site of insertion.

Complications of central venous cannulation

Although serious complications are rare in experienced hands, complications do exist for central venous catheterization, which can lead to serious morbidity and mortality.[13] These are classically divided into mechanical, thromboembolic, and infectious etiologies.[1,13] Ultrasound guidance for CVC insertions dramatically reduces insertion-related mechanical complications and is most likely to become the standard of care in the future.

A noncentral tip location of a CVC greatly increases the risk of complications including thrombosis, vascular erosion, cardiac erosion, tamponade, and arrhythmias.[23] Catheter-related thrombosis can be prevented by using ultrasound guidance with appropriate match of vein diameter and catheter diameter and the appropriate *central* position of the tip.

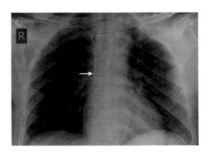

Figure 11.1 Plain chest X-ray film showing tip of subclavian vein central venous catheter.

Among major complications during IJV cannulation, carotid artery puncture is the most common and considered one of the most severe complications. It has been reported to be relatively common despite ultrasound guidance and can cause neck hematoma leading to airway obstruction, stroke in the case of carotid artery dissection, or brain ischemia from the lack of blood flow because of hematoma or dislodged emboli.[30]

Management of carotid artery puncture

If arterial puncture occurs with a small needle, the needle should be removed immediately and external pressure should be applied for several minutes to prevent hematoma formation. However, such a practice may increase the risk of cerebral ischemia in neurosurgical patients with compromised cerebral perfusion.

When an unintended cannulation of an arterial vessel with a dilator or large-bore catheter occurs, then the dilator or catheter should be left in situ due to the risk of complications, in particular uncontrolled hemorrhage. Advice from a vascular surgeon or interventional radiologist and further imaging should be undertaken. With regard to misplaced CVCs, the most important thing to remember is: *If in doubt, don't take it out!*

References

1. Schroeder B, Barbeito A, Baryosef S, Mark JB. Cardiovascular monitoring. In: Miller RD, editor. *Miller's Anesthesia.* 8th ed. Philadelphia, PA: Churchill Livingstone/Elsevier; 2014, pp. 1345–1395.
2. Mills SJ, Tomlinson AA. The use of central venous cannulae in neuroanaesthesia. A survey of current practice in the UK. *Anaesthesia* 2001;56:465–470.
3. Marik PE, Baram M, Vahid B. Does central venous pressure predict fluid responsiveness? A systematic review of the literature and the tale of seven mares. *Chest* 2008;134:172–178.
4. Marik PE, Cavallazzi R. Does the central venous pressure predict fluid responsiveness. An updated meta-analysis and a plea for some common sense. *Crit Care Med* 2013;41:1774–1781.
5. Teboul JL, Monnet X. Prediction of volume responsiveness in critically ill patients with spontaneous breathing activity. *Curr Opin Crit Care* 2008;14:334–339.
6. Magder S, Lagonidis D, Erice F. The use of respiratory variations in right atrial pressure to predict the cardiac output response to PEEP. *J Crit Care* 2001;16:108–114.
7. Young ML, Smith DS, Murtagh F, Vasquez A, Levitt J. Comparison of surgical and anesthetic complications in neurosurgical patients experiencing venous air embolism in the sitting position. *Neurosurgery* 1986;18:157–161.
8. Girard F, Ruel M, McKenty S et al. Incidences of venous air embolism and patent foramen ovale among patients undergoing selective peripheral denervation in the sitting position. *Neurosurgery* 2003;53:316–319.
9. Hannon MJ, Finucane FM, Sherlock M, Agha A, Thompson CJ. Clinical review: Disorders of water homeostasis in neurosurgical patients. *J Clin Endocrinol Metab* 2012;97:1423–1433.
10. American Society of Anesthesiologists Task Force on Central Venous Access, Rupp SM, Apfelbaum JL et al. Practice guidelines for central venous access: A report by the American Society of Anesthesiologists Task Force on Central Venous Access. *Anesthesiology* 2012;116:539–73
11. Magder S. Central venous pressure: A useful but not so simple measurement. *Crit Care Med* 2006;34:2224–2227.
12. Ruesch S, Walder B, Tramer MR. Complications of central venous catheters: Internal jugular versus subclavian access—A systematic review. *Crit Care Med* 2002;30:454–460.
13. McGee DC, Gould MK. Preventing complications of central venous catheterization. *N Engl J Med* 2003;348:1123–1133.
14. Merrer J, De Jonghe B, Golliot F et al. Complications of femoral and subclavian venous catheterization in critically ill patients: A randomized controlled trial. *JAMA* 2001;286:700–707.

15. Wilson TJ, Brown DL, Meurer WJ, Stetler Jr WR, Wilkinson DA, Fletcher JJ. Risk factors associated with peripherally inserted central venous catheter-related large vein thrombosis in neurological intensive care patients. *Intensive Care Med* 2012;38:272–278.

16. Fletcher JJ, Wilson TJ, Rajajee V et al. A randomized trial of central venous catheter type and thrombosis in critically Ill neurologic patients. *Neurocrit Care* 2016;25(1):20–28.

17. Vailati D, Lamperti M, Subert M, Sommariva A. An ultrasound study of cerebral venous drainage after internal jugular vein catheterization. *Crit Care Res Pract* 2012;2012:685481.

18. Woda RP, Miner ME, McCandless C, McSweeney TD. The effect of right internal jugular vein cannulation on intracranial pressure. *J Neurosurg Anesthesiol* 1996;8:286–292.

19. Dolu H, Goksu S, Sahin L, Ozen O, Eken L. Comparison of an ultrasound-guided technique versus a landmark-guided technique for internal jugular vein cannulation. *J Clin Monit Comput* 2015;29:177–182.

20. Lamperti M, Caldiroli D, Cortellazzi P et al. Safety and efficacy of ultrasound assistance during internal jugular vein cannulation in neurosurgical infants. *Intensive Care Med* 2008;34:2100–2105.

21. Lamperti M, Subert M, Cortellazzi P et al. Is a neutral head position safer than 45-degree neck rotation during ultrasound-guided internal jugular vein cannulation? Results of a randomized controlled clinical trial. *Anesth Analg* 2012;114:777–784.

22. Brass P, Hellmich M, Kolodziej L, Schick G, Smith AF. Ultrasound guidance versus anatomical landmarks for subclavian or femoral vein catheterization. *Cochrane Database Syst Rev* 2015;1:CD011447.

23. Vesely TM. Central venous catheter tip position: A continuing controversy. *J Vasc Interv Radiol* 2003;14:527–534.

24. Gibson F, Bodenham A. Misplaced central venous catheters: Applied anatomy and practical management. *Br J Anaesth* 2013;110:333–346.

25. Bunegin L, Albin MS, Helsel PE, Hoffman A, Hung TK. Positioning the right atrial catheter: A model for reappraisal. *Anesthesiology* 1981;55:343–348.

26. Rath GP, Bithal PK, Toshniwal GR, Prabhakar H, Dash HH. Saline flush test for bedside detection of misplaced subclavian vein catheter into ipsilateral internal jugular vein. *Br J Anaesth* 2009;102:499–502

27. Reeves ST, Bevis LA, Bailey BN. Positioning a right atrial air aspiration catheter using transesophageal echocardiography. *J Neurosurg Anesthesiol* 1996;8:123–125.

28. Albrecht K, Nave H, Breitmeier D, Panning B, Tröger HD. Applied anatomy of the superior vena cava—The carina as a landmark to guide central venous catheter placement. *Br J Anaesth* 2004;92:75–77.

29. Schummer W, Schummer C, Schelenz C et al. Central venous catheters—The inability of "intra-atrial ECG" to prove adequate positioning. *Br J Anaesth* 2004;93:193–198.

30. Blaivas M, Adhikari S. An unseen danger: Frequency of posterior vessel wall penetration by needles during attempts to place internal jugular vein central catheters using ultrasound guidance. *Crit Care Med* 2009;37:2345–2349.

12

Neuromonitoring

ELIZABETH A. M. FROST

Introduction

The choice of monitors in neuroanesthesia depends in large measure on the procedure and the needs of the surgeon. While trauma victims may require considerable effort to control intracranial pressure (ICP), the elderly patients in interventional radiology undergoing vertebroplasty have quite different needs. Similarly, the patient requiring implantation of electrodes for deep brain stimulation is awake but needs sedation at different stages, often in different locations of the hospital. Thus, communication with the surgical team at the outset is essential for best patient outcome.

General overview of neuromonitoring

Monitoring is divided roughly into three areas: systemic, central nervous system, and biomarkers including laboratory studies as shown in Table 12.1.

Systemic monitoring

Standard American Society of Anesthesiologists (ASA) monitors including oxygenation, electro-cardiography, capnography, and temperature are indicated in all patients. Cannulation of an artery affords valuable information as to wave forms, systemic pressures, and laboratory values and is indicated in most craniotomies. Vessels in either the wrist or the feet may be easily cannulated. While central venous pressure continues to be used as a monitor, it does not indicate circulating blood volume or vascular responsiveness to a fluid challenge.[1] It should not be used to make clinical decisions regarding fluid administration. Moreover, a recent study looked at a database of 110 claims for injuries related to central catheters (1.7% of 6449 claims).[2] Claims for central catheter injuries had a higher severity of injury, with an increased proportion of death (47%) compared with other claims in the database (29%, $p < 0.01$). Most common complications included wire/catheter embolus ($n = 20$), cardiac tamponade ($n = 16$), carotid artery puncture/cannulation ($n = 16$), hemothorax ($n = 15$), and pneumothorax ($n = 14$). Cardiac tamponade, hemothorax, and pulmonary artery rupture had a higher proportion of death ($p < 0.05$). The proportion of claims for vascular access injury

Table 12.1 Neuroanesthesia Monitoring May Be Divided into Three Main Areas

Systemic	Cerebral	Laboratory
Standard ASA monitors	Neurologic exam (including awake)	Glucose
Arterial and venous pressures	Intracranial pressure	Coagulation profile
Fluid and electrolyte balance	Transcranial Doppler sonography	Sodium
Pulse pressure variation	Stump pressure	Lactate
Stroke volume variation	Jugular venous bulb oxygenation	Hemoglobin
Transesophageal echocardiography	Electroencephalogram/evoked potentials/spectral edge	White cell counts
Respiratory parameters	Cerebral blood flow	Blood gas analyses
	Cerebral oxygenation	Biomarkers: SCD40L,
	Cerebral microdialysis	GFAB/S100B

increased (47%–84%) in 1994–1999 compared with 1978–1983 ($p < 0.05$). Other complications include infection, disruption of the glycocalyx, and thrombosis, all of which question the risk–benefit ratio of central line insertion.

Maintenance of fluid balance is critical as excessive fluid administration results in increased interstitial fluid in vital organs, leading to impaired renal, hepatic, and cardiac function. Historically, anesthesiologists have cannulated a vein, connected the cannula to a flow system, and infused fluids hoping that the amount given will compensate for unknown losses and maintain hemodynamic stability. Given that the purpose of fluid administration is to maintain vascular volume, cardiac function, and tissue oxygenation, assessment of the adequacy of intravascular volume is essential to determine the amount, timing, and even type of fluid infused. Cardiac filling pressures have been used to guide volume therapy but have not been shown to reliably predict volume therapy.[3] An endotracheal (ET) cardiac output monitor incorporated in the cuff of an ET tube has been developed. On the basis of the principle that the electrical resistance of blood changes when it moves or changes in volume, flexible electrodes on the ET cuff use information from an arterial pressure line and thus continuously calculate stroke volume.[4] The transesophageal Doppler, supplying continuous real-time objective data, also monitors preload conditions and helps optimize cardiac contractility and the effect of afterload impedance on left ventricular performance.[5] But perhaps of even greater and more practical value is goal-directed fluid management based on pulse oximeter plethysmogram variations (pleth variability index [PVI]). The arterial pulse pressure variation induced by mechanical ventilation has been appreciated for decades as an indicator of hypovolemia. Computerized analyses have incorporated information from the pulse oximeter arterial wave form to provide a continuous display of arterial pressures, stroke volume, cardiac output, pulse pressure variation, and stroke volume variation. In one study, PVI-guided fluid therapy resulted in less crystalloid administered perioperatively and significantly reduced lactate levels.[6] Thus, fluid versus vasopressor therapy can be tailored to an individual patient's needs rather than general application of formulas.

The ability to assess neurologic status quickly postoperatively is very important in patients undergoing neurosurgical procedures. Thus, early extubation is desirable. However, excessive lung fluid may dictate continued ventilation and with it the risk of ventilation-associated pneumonia. Increased extravascular lung water (EVLW) is particularly lethal, leading to iatrogenic salt water drowning. Lung ultrasound (LUS) may be used to assess pulmonary congestion through the evaluation of vertical reverberation artifacts, known as B-lines. These handheld devices can easily indicate accumulation of EVLW.[7]

Neurologic monitoring

Although the best means to assess neurologic function is the awake patient, many neurosurgical procedures dictate general anesthesia. Thus, other monitors look at electrical activity, ICP, and cerebral blood flow (CBF) and oxygen availability among other parameters. No ideal single monitor is available.

Intracranial pressure

Blood (5%), cerebrospinal fluid (CSF) (10%), and brain bulk (85%) are contained within the closed box of the cranium. Any increase in any one of these compartments must result in a decrease in one of the other two or an increase in ICP. Normal ICP is around 7–10 mmHg. It is elevated in trauma, tumors, clot, hyperemia, hypoxia, and CSF disturbances. It may be measured invasively by insertion of a subarachnoid bolt, an intraventricular cannula (which has the added advantage of allowing CSF to be withdrawn), or an epidural sensor placed between the skull and the dural tissue.[8] Microchips may be incorporated in the tips of the catheters to relay pressure measurements. Noninvasive methods have been explored including two-depth transorbital Doppler sonography. This technique uses Doppler ultrasound and is based on a principle similar to that of sphygmomanometry. The ophthalmic artery (OA) is a unique vessel with intracranial and extracranial segments. Blood flow in the intracranial OA segment is affected by ICP, while flow in the extracranial (intraorbital) OA segment is influenced by externally applied pressure to the eyeball and orbital tissues. A special pressure cuff is used to compress the tissues surrounding the eyeball and the intraorbital tissues around the extracranial OA segment. External pressure changes the characteristics of blood flowing from inside the skull cavity into the eye socket. A Doppler ultrasound beam measures the blood flow pulsations in intracranial and extracranial OA segments. The noninvasive ICP meter gradually increases the pressure over the eyeball and intraorbital tissues so that the blood flow pulsation parameters in two OA segments are equal. At this pressure balance point, the applied external pressure equals ICP.

Transcranial Doppler

Transcranial Doppler (TCD) sonography assesses velocity and flow. A 2-MHz pulsed Doppler ultrasound is used to access the ipsilateral middle cerebral artery at a depth of 45–50 mm. The method can predict stroke better than the processed electroencephalogram (EEG) and may detect emboli that benefit from a change in surgical technique. Interpretation is subject to observer variability.

Stump pressure

Stump pressure measures back flow after clamping of the carotid artery prior to carotid endarterectomy. It has been used to determine whether selective shunting is indicated. However, although it is simple to perform, there is no evidence of efficacy and it may increase the risk of perioperative stroke as unnecessary shunts are inserted.

Jugular venous bulb oxygenation

For this monitor, a catheter is inserted into the jugular bulb under fluoroscopic control, a far from simple maneuver. An artery is also cannulated. The difference between the oxygen content in arterial and cerebral venous blood ($A - VDO_2$) is then determined and can be used to determine the rate of flow across the brain:

$$A - VDO_2 = \frac{CMRO_2}{CBF}$$

where $CMRO_2$ is the metabolic rate of oxygen utilization and CBF is cerebral blood flow. The values higher than 10 indicate cerebral ischemia and increased ICP is better managed with decease of brain bulk, while lower values suggest that CBF is adequate. The monitor is more likely to be used in an intensive care setting.

Electroencephalogram and evoked potential monitors

The EEG directly measures cortical recordings to identify seizure activity. Grids may be placed over the brain during awake craniotomies or over the scalp. Four types of waves are identified and occur in varying percentages at all times:

1. Alpha (8–10 Hz): Predominating at rest with eyes closed
2. Beta (13–30 Hz): Normal waves
3. Theta (4–8 Hz): Mainly during sleep
4. Delta (0–4 Hz): During sleep and coma or deep anesthesia

Placement of the leads is determined by the International 10–20 System, which is an internationally recognized method to describe and apply the location of scalp electrodes (Figure 12.1). This method was developed to ensure standardized reproducibility to compare a patient's own study results over time and make a comparison with other patients. This system is based on the relationship between the location of an electrode and the underlying area of cerebral cortex. The "10" and "20" refer to the fact that the actual distances between adjacent electrodes are either 10% or 20% of the total front–back or right–left distance of the skull. The letters F, T, C, P, and O stand for frontal, temporal, central, parietal, and occipital lobes, respectively. The letter codes A, Pg, and Fp identify the earlobes, nasopharyngeal, and frontal polar sites, respectively. Odd numbered leads are on the left side and even numbered ones are placed on the right side.

Evoked potential monitoring

Several types of evoked potential (EP) monitoring may be used intraoperatively during both spinal and intracranial surgeries to detect ischemia and/or identify nerves, including sensory, auditory, visual, and motor. Generally, anesthetic agents increase latency and decrease amplitude of the waves generated, and a close communication with the other members of the surgical team is essential. Somatosensory evoked potentials (SSEPs) warn of ischemia if there is more than 60% decrease in signal amplitude, which equates to CBF of 14 mL/100 g/min. At this level, changes are still reversible. The changes are slower than those seen with EEG monitoring due to signal averaging. SSEP tracts follow the dorsal columns. Peripheral stimulation is recorded in the cortex. Brain stem evoked responses (BAERs) are monitored during surgery of the acoustic nerve and involve the use of earphones that deliver controlled clicks. Visual evoked potentials (VEPs) are monitored during surgery around the optic chiasma and use light-emitting diodes from glasses covering the eyes. Motor evoked potentials (MEPs) involve transcranial direct cortical stimulation and are often combined with SSEPs. They map the motor cortex and are recorded from peripheral nerves (the opposite of SSEPs).

Compressed arrays are used as simple noninvasive means to assess awareness and depth during anesthesia (Bispectral Index™ [BIS™]). They use the power spectrum and bispectrum from one EEG channel to calculate a number, with numbers close to 100 indicating completely awake and below 70 as unconscious. Increasing synchrony indicates deepening anesthesia. Entropy monitoring is another method of assessing anesthetic depth. It relies on a method of assessing the degree of irregularities in the EEG. The principle behind this theory is that the irregularity within an EEG signal decreases with increasing brain levels of anesthetic drugs assigning an entropy score.

The signal is captured via a forehead mounted sensor, in a similar way to that used by BIS™.

Some recent devices are used to monitor cervical nerves. Leads can be placed on ET tubes to detect recurrent laryngeal nerve irritation and monitor the vagus nerve. Use is mainly during skull-based procedures and head and neck surgery. Electrodes may be implanted in ET tubes (NIM®

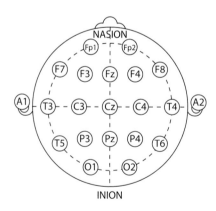

Figure 12.1 The 10–20 International scalp placement system for EEG monitoring.

electromyographic [EMG] tube) or added as an attachment to regular tubes (Dragonfly®).[9]

Cerebral blood flow

CBF is determined by several factors, such as viscosity, degree of vasodilation, and cerebral perfusion pressure. Cerebral vessels control blood flow over changing situations by altering their diameters (autoregulation). In the face of hypertension and hypocarbia, they constrict and dilate with hypotension and hypercarbia. Means to directly and continuously monitor CBF are mainly restricted to the laboratory. Functional magnetic resonance imaging and positron emission tomography are neuroimaging techniques that can be used for one-time assessments. These techniques are also used to measure regional CBF (rCBF) within a specific brain region. rCBF at one location can be measured over time by thermal diffusion.[10]

Cerebral oximetry/near-infrared spectroscopy

Cerebral oximetry has been around for some three decades but has had a somewhat checkered history regarding application and reliability. Recently, several monitors have been approved in the United States and elsewhere and the technique is emerging as a useful tool for assessing not only adequate cerebral oxygenation but also tissue oxygenation and perfusion in other organs. Cerebral oximetry alerts the clinician to changes in oxygen delivery. It is a noninvasive technology using near-infrared spectroscopy (NIRS) to monitor regional cerebral tissue oxygen saturation (rSO_2) and has been widely used to assess cerebral tissue oxygenation in a variety of populations, including the fields of neonatology, anesthesiology, neurology, and cardiac surgery.

Cerebral oximetry estimates regional tissue oxygenation by transcutaneous measurement of the cerebral cortex, an area of the brain that is most susceptible to changes in oxygen supply and demand and has limited oxygen reserve. Measurement is based on the ability of light to penetrate the skull and determine hemoglobin oxygenation according to the amount of light absorbed by hemoglobin.[11] NIRS cerebral oximetry uses two photodetectors with each light source, allowing selective sampling of tissue beyond a specified depth beneath the skin.

Near-field photodetection can then be subtracted from far-field photodetection to provide selective tissue oxygenation measurement. Adhesive pads are applied over the frontal lobes that both emit and capture reflected near-infrared light passing through the cranial bone to and from the underlying cerebral tissue.

Tissue sampling is mainly from venous (70%–75%) rather than arterial (25%) blood and does not depend on pulsatile flow. Monitoring is noninvasive and can provide an early warning of decreased oxygen delivery. The technique can provide continuous intraoperative insight into brain perfusion and oxygenation dynamics. A decrease in rSO_2 has been shown to correlate with cognitive dysfunction, perioperative cerebrovascular accident, increased hospital stay, postoperative nausea and vomiting, prolonged ventilation, and renal failure.[12] Cerebral desaturation is indicated by a decrease of more than 20% for more than 1 min. Intervention including ensuring normocapnia, increased oxygen delivery, hypertension, transfusion, and head elevation is required when rSO_2 is less than 75% for more than 15 s. It is important to note the different baseline values for cerebral rSO_2 of each of the commercially available cerebral oximeters. Bilateral room air baseline rSO_2 values should be established prior to the induction of general anesthesia or measurement by secure adherence of the pads to the skin. Values must be interpreted in the context of available clinical information as many factors alter measurements, including cardiac output, blood pressure, hypo/hypercapnia, arterial pH, inspired oxygen concentration, temperature, local blood flow, hemoglobin concentration, hemorrhage, embolism, preexisting disease (e.g., cerebral infarction), and position changes among others. Given that the technology of several devices differs, individual validation is required. It may be reasonable to suggest that invasive and direct measurement of regional tissue oxygen pressure ($tiPO_2$) might be equivalent to rSO_2, but these are not the same parameters although some correlations may exist.

Cerebral microdialysis

Used mainly in intensive care units to follow the course of traumatic brain injury (TBI) and subarachnoid hemorrhage, and in research, microdialysis involves placement of fine double-lumen probes, lined with semipermeable membranes into the brain to analyze brain tissue biochemistry. Measurements include glucose, lactate, pyruvate, glycerol, and glutamate among others. Impending ischemia may also be identified as lactate levels rise.

Laboratory studies

Several laboratory studies should be monitored and followed in the patient undergoing neurosurgical procedures. While glucose is essential for brain metabolism, producing energy via the Krebs or citric acid cycle, it depends on oxygen. In a hypoxic situation, glucose is metabolized via anaerobic pathways, resulting in the formation of lactate that can convert an ischemic area into an infarct. As blood glucose levels tend to rise with stress and especially with steroid administration, it is essential that frequent assessments of blood glucose are made and necessary corrections taken.

The brain is a rich source of thromboplastin. In addition, brain tumors can produce both pro- and anticoagulant substances. Perioperative knowledge of the coagulation status can give advanced warning of the need for reversal agents.

The brain is particularly sensitive to changes in serum sodium levels, operating within a narrow range. Awareness that changing intracranial dynamics can alter levels of this electrolyte quickly is important to allow corrective action.

As noted, the brain requires oxygen, carried by hemoglobin. Adequate numbers are essential. Increasing white cell counts may herald infection that can adversely affect cerebral metabolism.

Cerebral contusion releases leukocytes and chemokines. Several biomarkers have been identified including SCD 40L, a membrane glycoprotein that is activated in severe injury. It is part of the tissue-necrotizing factor superfamily of molecules. Glial fibrillary acidic protein/astroglial protein or GFAB/S100B is also released in contusion. Levels may be used to indicate degree of damage and as prognostic indicators. Biomarkers of neuronal, axonal, and astroglial damage from either peripheral blood or CSF are used to diagnose mild TBI and predict the need for further studies and/or hospital admission. Usefulness on the sports field is also under consideration.

Conclusion

The brain is a complex organ that controls and is controlled by the rest of the body. Thus, monitoring requires comprehensive and coordinated input from all systems. No single monitor suffices and information must be taken from multiple sources to ensure safe patient outcome.

References

1. Marik PE. Iatrogenic salt water drowning and the hazards of a high central venous pressure. Ann Intensive Care 2014;4:21.
2. Domino KB, Bowdle TA, Posner KL, Spitellie PH, Lee LA, Cheney FW. Injuries and liability related to central vascular catheters: A closed claims analysis. Anesthesiology 2004;100(6):1411–1418.
3. Cavallaro F, Sandroni C, Antonelli M. Functional hemodynamic monitoring and dynamic indices of fluid responsiveness. Minerva Anesthesiol 2008;74:123–135.
4. Wallace AW, Salahieh A, Lawrence A, Spector K, Owens C, Alonso D. Endotracheal cardiac output monitor. Anesthesiol 2000;92:178–189.
5. Chytra I, Pradl R, Bosman R, Pelnár P, Kasal E, Zidková A. Esophageal Doppler-guided fluid management decreases blood lactate levels in multiple-trauma patients: A randomized controlled trial. Crit Care 2007;11(1):R24.
6. Forget P, Lois F, de Kock M. Goal-directed fluid management based on the pulse oximeter-derived pleth variability index reduces lactate levels and improves fluid management. Anesth Analg 2010;111(4):910–914.
7. Michard F. Bedside assessment of extravascular lung water by dilution methods: Temptations and pitfalls. Crit Care Med 2007;35(4):1186–1192.
8. Chesnut RM, Temkin N, Carney N et al. A trial of intracranial-pressure monitoring in traumatic brain injury. N Engl J Med 2012;367:2471–2481.
9. Randolph GW, Dralle H, International Intraoperative Monitoring Study Group et al. Electrophysiologic recurrent laryngeal

nerve monitoring during thyroid and parathyroid surgery: International standards guideline statement. *Laryngoscope* 2011;121:S1–S16.

10. Vajkoczy P, Roth H, Horn P et al. Continuous monitoring of regional cerebral blood flow: Experimental and clinical validation of a novel thermal diffusion microprobe. *J Neurosurg* 2000;93(2):265–274.

11. Ferrari M, Mottola L, Quaresima V. Principles, techniques and limitations of near-infrared spectroscopy. *Can J Appl Physiol* 2004;29:463–487.

12. Murkin JM, Adams SJ, Novick R et al. Monitoring brain oxygen saturation during coronary bypass surgery: A randomized, prospective study. *Anesth Analg* 2007:104(1):51–58.

13

Hemodynamic variations

CHARU MAHAJAN

Introduction

Hemodynamic variability refers to any abnormality in heart rate or blood pressure. This chapter mainly focuses on hemodynamic variations due to various neurologic causes during the early perioperative period.

Importance of blood pressure in relation to the brain

Cerebral blood flow (CBF) is maintained constant at cerebral perfusion pressure (CPP) of 60–160 mmHg by autoregulation. However in a diseased brain or beyond the autoregulatory limits, this does not hold true and CBF becomes pressure dependent. On the one hand, hypotension may result in decreased cerebral perfusion and ischemia. On the other hand, hypertension can lead to cerebral edema, bleeding, or hemorrhagic transformation of an infarcted area.

Hypertension

The risk of an adverse perioperative cardiac event is high in patients with hypertension. These patients are also more prone to hemodynamic lability perioperatively. Perioperative beta-blockers do not confer any benefit and may even increase the risk

of stroke.[1] In patients with chronic hypertension, the autoregulation curve is shifted toward the right side and thus a higher threshold should be considered for treatment. The management of hypertensive patients planned to undergo a neurosurgical procedure is an elaborate topic and will not be dealt with here. Our main aim is to understand and manage hemodynamic variations due to certain specific neurologic causes. Table 13.1 shows a list of conditions leading to hypertension in a neurologic/neurosurgical patient.

Cushing's reflex is a protective reflex in response to raised intracranial pressure (ICP). Instead of lowering blood pressure, measures to reduce ICP should be applied. Intraoperative hypertension is defined as a 20% increase in systolic blood pressure from baseline or mean arterial pressure (MAP) higher than 90 mmHg. Strict control of blood pressure is imperative during surgery to prevent cerebral edema or profuse bleeding from the surgical site. Noxious stimulation should be taken care of by transiently deepening the plane of anesthesia or an additional bolus of analgesic agent. Stimulation of brain stem may result in hypertension or hypotension and/or tachycardia or bradycardia. If this variability occurs in concurrence with a surgeon's handling of these structures, immediately inform the surgeon to stop the stimulation. Administration of drugs will reverse the abnormality but will also mask any further changes, and damage to vital structures may go unnoticed. Only in life-threatening situations should treatment be instituted. Vasodilators are usually not used for correcting hypertension in patients undergoing neurosurgical procedures, and beta-blockers and mixed alpha- and beta-adrenergic antagonist labetalol are commonly used.

Table 13.1 Conditions Leading to Hypertension in a Neurologic/Neurosurgical Patient

Causes of Hypertension	Management
White coat hypertension	Reassure and make patient comfortable
Essential hypertension	In known hypertensive patients, continue with anti-hypertensive treatment until the morning of surgery (except angiotensin receptor blockers). May administer short-acting anxiolytics (alprazolam) the night before surgery in patients having normal ICP
Laryngoscopy and intubation	Additional bolus of propofol or thiopentone/Esmolol/Xylocard before laryngoscopy
	Gentle and quick laryngoscopy
Incision	Maintain adequate depth of anesthesia
Pin fixation	Local infiltration at pin site, additional bolus of analgesic agent
Light level of anesthesia	Deepen depth of anesthesia and provide adequate analgesia
Tunneling of skin during VP shunt insertion	Deepen the plane of anesthesia and administer a bolus of fentanyl
Hypercarbia	Adjust ventilatory strategy
Raised intracranial pressure, e.g., tumor, intracranial hemorrhage, subarachnoid hemorrhage, acute ischemic stroke, traumatic brain injury	Hypertension may be part of Cushing's reflex, treat raised ICP
Brain stem handling	Inform surgeon immediately, will resolve once stimulation stops
Coughing on emergence	Smooth emergence, Short-acting, beta-blockers, lidocaine
Post-carotid endarterectomy	Reperfusion syndrome may occur even at normal blood pressure; strict control of blood pressure with the help of anti-hypertensives
Autonomic dysreflexia (SCI above T6)	Eliminate the precipitating stimulus, anti-hypertensives
Autonomic neuropathy (e.g., Guillain–Barré syndrome)	Adequate level of anesthesia, short-acting agents should be used
May be part of Cushing's disease, pheochromocytoma, thyroid storm	Treat underlying cause, symptomatic treatment according to disease
Bladder distension	Encourage spontaneous passage of urine if patient is awake or else catheterize

Hypotension

Hypotension is defined as a decrease of MAP to less than 20% below baseline or MAP less than 60 mmHg. In a patient with raised ICP, the CPP is already compromised, so hypotension may further reduce the perfusion resulting in ischemia and secondary brain injury. A single episode of systolic blood pressure less than 90 mmHg is known to be associated with poor outcome in patients with traumatic brain injury (TBI).[2,3] Table 13.2 lists common causes of perioperative hypotension and its management. There are no recommendations for using a particular vasopressor. Some authors have found norepinephrine to be more efficient for maintaining CPP, while others noted that patients who received phenylephrine had higher MAP and CPP than those who received dopamine and norepinephrine.[4-6] However, the effect of different agents on cerebral metabolism also needs to be ascertained. Friess et al.[7] studied the effect of phenylephrine and norepinephrine on ICP, CBF, brain tissue oxygen tension, and cerebral microdialysis. No difference was seen in ICP and CBF between the two groups. It was observed that animals who received norepinephrine had greater brain tissue oxygenation, but those animals who received phenylephrine had greater reduction in metabolic crisis and cell injury. The effect of various vasopressors on mitochondrial function requires further studies.

Table 13.2 Causes of Perioperative Hypotension and Its Management

Causes of Hypotension	Management
Systemic	
Preexisting cardiomyopathy	If an elective surgery, stabilize the patient before taking up for operation
Arrhythmias	Treat arrhythmias
Cardiac failure	Treat cardiac failure
Myocardial infarction (MI)	Treat MI
Pulmonary embolism (PE)	Oxygen and specific treatment
Hypovolemia due to decreased intake, diuretics, diabetes insipidus, cerebral salt wasting syndrome, hemorrhage from systemic injuries	Adequate replacement of fluids and blood
Anesthesia drugs (postinduction)	Lighten anesthesia plane, ephedrine bolus
Anaphylaxis	Manage along the lines of anaphylactic shock
Sepsis	Manage along the lines of septic shock
Tension pneumothorax	Resuscitation and needle thoracotomy
Cardiac tamponade	Pericardiocentesis
Hemothorax	Chest tube drainage
Embolism	Symptomatic treatment
Adrenal insufficiency	Steroid replacement
Autonomic neuropathy	Symptomatic treatment, vasoactive agents, fludrocortisone may help in orthostatic hypotension
Neurologic	
Neurogenic stunned myocardium	ICP control and symptomatic treatment
During positioning (especially sitting)	Preload with crystalloids, mephentermine bolus
Acute blood loss	Blood replacement
Massive venous air embolism VAE	Treat VAE along with symptomatic treatment
	Volume repletion and vasopressors

(continued)

Table 13.2 Causes of Perioperative Hypotension and Its Management (continued)

Causes of Hypotension	Management
Spinal shock	Increase blood pressure by administration of fluids and vasopressors
Carotid cross-clamping and carotid body stimulation during carotid endarterectomy (CEA)	Hemodynamic variability can be minimized by asking the surgeon to infiltrate local anesthetic into the adventitia over carotid bulb during CEA; during carotid body stimulation, bradycardia and hypotension may occur, administer atropine
Trigeminocardiac reflex (TCR)	Inform the surgeon to stop the stimulus
Brain stem handling	Inform the surgeon, usually corrects once stimulation is stopped
Hypothalamic lesions	Symptomatic treatment
Panhypopituitarism	Hormone replacement

Bradycardia and tachycardia

Bradycardia and tachycardia with or without blood pressure changes may often be encountered in neuroanesthesia practice. Tachycardia is defined as heart rate (HR) of more than 100 beats per minute and bradycardia as HR of less than 50 beats per minute. Tables 13.3 and 13.4 enumerate the causes of bradycardia and tachycardia along with their management.

Table 13.3 Bradycardia and Its Management

Bradycardia	Management
Systemic	
Cardiac conduction disturbances	Intravenous atropine or pacemaker
Drugs (calcium channel blockers, beta-blockers, digitalis, etc.)	Part of their therapeutic effect; if hemodynamically stable, continue same, otherwise stop drugs
Hypothyroidism	Treat underlying disease
Hypothermia	Rewarming
Hypoxia	Correct hypoxemia
Neurologic	
As part of Cushing's reflex (bradycardia, hypotension, and respiratory disturbances)	Control ICP
During neuroendoscopic procedures	Monitor fluid irrigation through endoscope, stimulation of floor of third ventricle or distortion of posterior hypothalamus may also result in bradycardia; inform surgeon immediately
Brain stem handling during surgery	Inform surgeon immediately, usually resolves promptly; anticholinergic treatment is not advisable as it may mask further handling; however, if symptomatic and impending arrest, atropine may be given as lifesaving intervention
As part of trigeminocardiac reflex	Inform surgeon immediately, usually resolves promptly on discontinuation of stimulation

(continued)

Bradycardia	Management
Vagus nerve stimulation during posterior fossa surgery	Inform surgeon immediately, usually resolves promptly
Intracranial hypotension	Sudden decompression of hydrocephalic ventricles; fill the ventricles with saline
	Extradural drains when connected to vacuum device; release the negative pressure
Acute spinal shock and autonomic dysreflexia	Eliminate the precipitating stimulus; sedate patient during tracheal suctioning; treat hemodynamically significant bradycardia with atropine; if refractory, consider temporary pacemaker

Table 13.4   Tachycardia and Its Management

Tachycardia	Management
Systemic	
Hypovolemia	Fluid repletion
Sudden blood loss	Blood transfusion
Pain	Analgesia
Fever	Active cooling, acetaminophen
Hypercarbia	Adjust ventilator strategies
Lighter plane of anesthesia	Deepen anesthesia
Cardiac arrhythmias	Arrhythmia-specific management
Drugs (anticholinergics, adrenaline, dopamine, etc.)	Stop inciting drugs, if possible
Thyroid storm	Active cooling, acetaminophen, beta-blockers, hydrocortisone, methimazole
Neurologic	
Brain stem handling	Inform surgeon immediately, usually resolves promptly
Transsphenoidal pituitary surgery	Tachycardia and hypertension on insertion of nasal speculum can be taken care of by deepening the plane of anesthesia, bolus of fentanyl, or beta-blockers
During deep brain stimulation surgery (stimulation of subthalamic nucleus)	Inform the surgeon
Dysautonomia, e.g., after TBI	Morphine, benzodiazepines, propranolol

Conclusion

This chapter highlights common causes of hemodynamic variability during neuroanesthesia practice and their management. It may be a harbinger of impending neurologic catastrophe or may be an important sign of ongoing CNS insult. So, before directly treating it, it is important to understand the underlying cause.

References

1. Devereaux PJ, Yang H, Yusuf S, POISE study Group. Effects of extended-release metoprolol succinate in patients undergoing non-cardiac surgery (POISE trial): A randomised controlled trial. *Lancet* 2008; 371:1839–1847.

2. Chestnut RM, Marshall LF, Klauber MR et al. The role of secondary brain injury in determining outcome from severe head injury. *J Trauma* 1993;34:216–222.
3. Marmarou A, Anderson RL, Ward JD et al. Impact of ICP instability and hypotension on outcome in patients with severe head trauma. *J Neurosurg* 1991;75: 159–166.
4. Steiner LA, Johnston AJ, Czosnyka M et al. Direct comparison of cerebrovascular effects of norepinephrine and dopamine in head-injured patients. *Crit Care Med* 2004;32:1049–1054.
5. Pfister D, Strebel SP, Steiner LA. Effects of catecholamines on cerebral blood vessels in patients with traumatic brain injury. *Eur J Anaesthesiol Suppl* 2008;42:98–103.
6. Sookplung P, Siriussawakul A, Malakouti A et al. Vasopressor use and effect on blood pressure after severe adult traumatic brain injury. *Neurocrit Care* 2011;15:46–54.
7. Friess SH, Bruins B, Kilbaugh TJ, Smith C, Margulies SS. Differing effects when using phenylephrine and norepinephrine to augment cerebral blood flow after traumatic brain injury in the immature brain. *J Neurotrauma* 2015;32:237–243.

Temperature

KAVITHA JAYARAM

Introduction

Temperature regulation remains a highly active area of research. Thermoregulation is the mechanism by which body temperature is maintained around 37°C. Hypothalamus is the center around which this function of the body revolves. Its importance in neuroanesthesia is always understated as several studies are still ongoing in this field.

Physiology and pathophysiology

Thermoregulatory physiological responses are subject to physiological variations such as gender, age, circadian variations, and exercise. They can also be modified by drugs and certain pathological conditions such as obesity, altered thyroid functions, hypothalamic–pituitary abnormalities, and dysautonomia.

1. The brain represents 2%–3% of body weight, but it uses 20% and 25% of body's total consumption of oxygen and glucose, respectively. Energy metabolism is mostly aerobic and approximately 60% of the energy is converted into heat.[1] This heat is not easily dissipated as the brain is protected by the skull.

2. Brain temperature depends on three factors: local production of heat, temperature of the blood vessels, and cerebral blood flow. Dissipation of the generated heat is improved by vascular anatomical specializations that permit heat exchange.[2]

3. Two neuronal models have been described with respect to temperature regulation:

   a. The *set-point model*, which includes an adjustable set point and signals from central and peripheral areas integrated and compared with a set point at the level of the hypothalamus. Any variation in the set point, such as fever or hypothermia, is corrected by a mechanism that reverses the original change and brings the system back to the set point.[3,4]

   b. The *null-zone model*, which hypothesizes that rather than a set point, body core temperature is defended around a null zone based on interaction between two variables and not on comparison of a variable with a constant set point. Reciprocal cross-inhibition between a cold sensor and a heat production effector and a warm sensor and a heat loss pathway forms the basis of this model.[5,6]

In this spectrum of temperature variation in the body, both the extremes occur in neuroanesthesia and critical care. Both these extremes have many advantages and disadvantages in the cerebral and body metabolism, which are detailed as follows.

Hypothermia

Hypothermia is characterized by a fall in the core body temperature by a minimum of 1°C from the normal and becomes clinically relevant if the body temperature is less than 36°C. The effects of hypothermia on different systems are given in the "Cerebrovascular system," Cardiovascular system," "Respiratory System," and "Excretory system" sections.

Cerebrovascular system

1. *Cerebral metabolic rate (CMR)*: The CMR reduces by 6%–7% per degree Celsius[7,8] Hypothermia at 18–20°C can cause complete suppression of an electroencephalogram (EEG).[9]
2. *Electrophysiology*: Synaptic transmission is temperature dependent. Mainly, the excitatory postsynaptic transmission has a more pronounced effect with reduction in temperature.[10,11] The somatosensory and auditory evoked potentials start reducing at <33°C. All the nerve conduction impulses reduce at <26°C with an increase in muscle tone and rigidity.
3. *Burst suppression in EEG*: This is different from the burst suppression induced by anesthetic agents. In EEG, the CMR continuously decreases even after the isoelectric EEG with a decrease in temperature whereas with anesthetic agents, the reduction is constant after the burst suppression. This is because anesthetic agents reduce the CMR associated with neuronal function whereas hypothermia reduces energy utilization for electrophysiologic function as well as the basal component associated with maintenance of cellular integrity.
4. *Cerebral blood flow (CBF)*: Hypothermia induces a decrease in brain temperature, thereby causing a reduction in cerebral metabolism as well as blood flow.[12] It occurs due to physiological coupling between metabolism and blood flow leading to a decrease in intracerebral vascular volume and intracranial pressure (ICP).[13] Thus, hypothermia is associated with improved ICP and cerebral perfusion pressure.
5. *Cerebral oxygenation*: Cerebral oxygenation is also improved.
6. *Carbondioxide*: The partial pressure of carbon dioxide in arterial blood depends on the solubility coefficient of the gas, which by itself is dependent on temperature. So in hypothermia, the amount of gaseous carbon dioxide decreases.[14] This gas crosses the blood–brain barrier and induces modifications in the extracellular environment, producing alkalosis in hypothermia. Alkalosis is an important factor regulating the arterial vascular tone.[15]

Cardiovascular system

1. There is a generalized increase in peripheral vascular resistance, hence an increase in the afterload. There is a reduction in heart rate as a compensatory mechanism.[16]
2. An increase in coronary vascular resistance and a reduction in coronary perfusion pressure occur, hence a tendency toward angina and ischemia.
3. There is an increase in contractility in order to maintain adequate stroke volume, which adds to the state of hypoperfusion to the heart.[17]
4. At <28°C, there is disruption of sinoatrial pacing, resulting in ventricular irritability and fibrillation.[18]
5. Hypothermia per se does not precipitate myocardial infarction, though coronary blood flow decreases as the reduction is in proportion to cardiac work.[19]
6. There is a threefold increase in morbid cardiac events such as low cardiac output, arrhythmias, and ventricular fibrillation.

Respiratory system

1. Owing to stimulation of the respiratory center, there is hyperventilation followed by hypoventilation in spontaneously breathing patients.
2. Overall reduction in oxygen demand, especially in tissues where oxygen consumption is high, such as the brain. Whole-body metabolic rate decreases at a rate of 8% per degree Celsius and almost to half at 28°C.[20]
3. Decrease in arterial blood flow delays the oxygen uptake and delivery to the tissues.
4. Leftward shift of the oxygen–hemoglobin dissociation curve causes an increase in oxygen affinity, thus precipitating hypoxia, anaerobic metabolism, and lactic acidosis. Oxyhemoglobin affinity increases by 5.7% per degree Celsius decrease in temperature.[18]

Excretory system

1. In hypothermia, blood flow to the kidney is reduced by an increase in the renovascular resistance.[18]
2. Urinary flow is maintained by inhibition of the tubular absorption.
3. As temperature decreases, reabsorption of sodium and potassium is progressively inhibited, causing antidiuretic hormone-mediated *cold diuresis*.
4. Plasma concentration of electrolytes remains normal despite excretion of these ions.

Pharmacology of drugs

1. Decreased hepatic and renal blood flow results in a decrease in metabolism of most drugs.
2. As pharmacokinetics and dynamics of most of the anesthetics (intravenous, inhalational agents, neuromuscular blockers, and opioids) are dependent on these organs, there is prolongation of recovery from anesthesia even when temperature is not a discharge criterion.

Coagulation system and rheology

1. Hypothermia directly impairs enzymes of the coagulation cascade.
2. Production of thromboxane B2 by platelets is decreased when temperature is <33°C, resulting in reversible platelet dysfunction. The anomaly in platelet function is more related to local temperature than core temperature.[21,22]
3. Increase in the viscosity and peripheral vascular resistance enhances stasis in the extremities. Therefore, patients are more prone to developing deep venous thrombus formation and pulmonary embolus.
4. Meta-analyses indicate that there is a significant increase in blood loss and transfusion requirements following hypothermia.[23,24]

Immunologic system

1. Impaired antibody and cell-mediated immunity[24]
2. Impaired leukocyte mobilization
3. Increased cortisol levels due to cold stress
4. Decreased oxygen delivery to wound site following thermoregulatory vasoconstriction[25]

All these factors contribute to impaired wound healing and enhance the chances of wound infection.

Primary therapeutic hypothermia

Primary therapeutic hypothermia (PTH) can be defined as the deliberate lowering of the core body temperature on the presentation of the patient to achieve a beneficial outcome. Induced mild hypothermia (32–34°C) reduces mortality and morbidity in patients who have had cardiac arrest, traumatic brain injury (TBI), stroke, and difficult aneurysm surgeries. But there is a considerable difficulty in the conduct of hypothermia, particularly in unanesthetized patients such as those managed in neurocritical care. Conventionally, several neurological and trauma centers use hypothermia as a treatment modality for several indications. These are as follows:

1. Severe TBI[26]
2. Giant intracranial aneurysm surgeries[27–29]
3. Post cardiac arrest[30]
4. Neonates who had hypoxic ischemic encephalopathy following cardiac arrest[31]

Induction of hypothermia is relatively easy during surgery as most of our anesthetic drugs impair thermoregulatory responses. Also, under anesthesia, it is easy to achieve tolerance to hypothermia pharmacologically and maintain patient comfort. These are particularly important in critically ill patients as the thermoregulatory responses such as shivering vasoconstriction can completely negate the advantages of hypothermia.

As with all other brain injuries, fever after a TBI can be related to the development of infection, occurrence of inflammatory responses, and hypothalamic dysfunction following the injury. Observational studies have found that the occurrence of fever in the first week after injury is associated with an increased ICP, neurologic impairment, and prolonged length of stay in intensive care.[32]

In nonanesthetized patients requiring PTH such as stroke, tolerance to hypothermia has to be induced pharmacologically. This becomes important as patients otherwise undergo vigorous responses to a decrease in temperature by shivering and vasoconstriction.[33] These responses have a tendency to nullify the advantages of hypothermia. Pharmacologically, the combination of meperidine and buspirone synergistically reduces the shivering threshold to less than 34°C without producing many respiratory adverse effects and sedation.[34] Inspite of multiple smaller trials, a recent meta-analysis failed to identify high-quality data to support the use of PTH in reducing neurological morbidity and mortality.[35]

Fever and hyperthermia

Fever is an adaptive response to a variety of infectious, inflammatory, and foreign stimuli. Fever results from a cytokine-mediated reaction leading to generation of acute-phase reactants and controlled elevation of core body temperature. The anterior hypothalamus coordinates the "febrile response" in reaction to the release of endogenous pyrogens and subsequent upregulation of prostaglandin synthesis. This change in hypothalamic set point ensues a synchronized physiologic response throughout the body, manifested as fever.

This differs from hyperthermia, which refers to heat retention attributable to unregulated readjustment of the thermoregulatory mechanism. Hyperthermia occurs when there are disturbances to the central mechanisms of thermoregulation and heat-dissipating mechanisms have been compromised. The exact mechanism of hyperthermia is unknown. This may persist for weeks with lack of diurnal variation and a plateau-like pattern of elevation and maintenance.[36]

Hyperthermia has an opposite effect on cerebral physiologic function, which is detrimental. Between 37°C and 42°C, CBF and CMR increase. However, above 42°C, a dramatic reduction in cerebral oxygen consumption occurs, which is an indication of a threshold for a toxic effect of hyperthermia that may occur as a result of protein (enzyme) denaturation.[37] Avoidance of fever and hyperthermia remains a major aim in the management of patients in neurointensive care units (NICUs).

The various causes for fever are enumerated in the flow chart given on the following page.

The neurosurgical patient having suffered a central nervous insult but lacking a documented source of fever has a central neurogenic fever or posttraumatic hyperthermia by definition.[38] To make the diagnosis of noninfectious unexplained fever (central neurogenic fever or posttraumatic hyperthermia), the clinician must have a high

Type	Definition
Fever	An abnormal elevation of body temperature, usually as a result of a pathologic process
Hyperthermia	Abnormally high temperature (>41°C) intentionally induced in living things regionally or whole body. It is most often induced by radiation (heat waves, infrared), ultrasound, or drugs

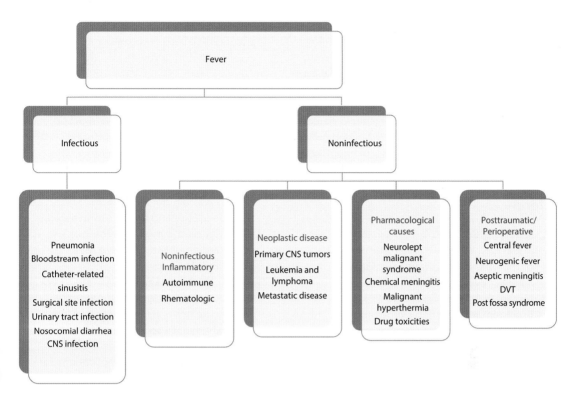

index of suspicion. Signs of fever are common in neurocritical care patients and antibiotics are often administered without proof of infection in almost all places. The clinical features of infectious and noninfectious fever markedly overlap and most of the biomarkers cannot differentiate infection and inflammation, especially after neurosurgery.

Monitoring

As per the American Society of Anesthesiologists guidelines, it is mandatory to monitor temperature, particularly in neurosurgeries, as most of them are of prolonged duration. The core temperature is more reliable than the skin surface and the common noninvasive sites of monitoring include the nasopharyngeal and tympanic membrane, which correlate well with brain temperature.[39-41] (Tympanic membrane temperature is close to the hypothalamus and responds well to the set temperature.) Other noninvasive sites include rectal, urinary bladder, and esophagus.

Invasive methods of core temperature monitoring include pulmonary artery catheter (PAC), jugular bulb thermistor, and brain tissue temperature, which involve placement of invasive lines or a burr hole.

Temperature management in the intraoperative period

Temperature loss in the intraoperative period has to be reduced to the minimum possible as shivering and vasoconstriction during extubation are more detrimental in neurosurgery patients. The various measures include the following:

1. Regulating operating room temperature particularly before and during induction Until the patient is draped.
2. Using warm fluids for intravenous and irrigation purposes.
3. Using forced air warming devices continuously.[42,43]
4. Using fluid-warming devices, particularly for blood and blood products.
5. Using active inspired air humidification with heating circuits to warm the inhaled gas mixture.[44]
6. Using amino acid infusions as they are found to be effective in maintaining temperature when given as continuous infusion in the intraoperative and early postoperative periods. They are found to reduce postanesthetic shivering and decrease the infection rate as well.[45]

Conclusion

Measurement of body temperature often underestimates brain temperature, especially when central nervous system is vulnerable. Usefulness of Therapeutic hypothermia in human beings is still debated though its being used in severe TBI, Subarachnoid hemorrhage, stroke. Fever management in the perioperative period as well in neurosurgical ICUs is of importance to avoid secondary insults.

References

1. Alberts B, Johnson A, Lewis J, Raff M, Roberts K, Walter P. *Molecular Biology of the Cell*, 4th ed. New York: Garland Science; 2002.
2. Mrozek S, Vardon F, Geeraerts T. Brain temperature: Physiology and pathophysiology after brain injury; 2012, Article ID989487. *Anesthesiol Res Pract* 2012;2012:989487.
3. Hammel HT, Jackson DC, Stolwijk JA, Hardy JD, Stromme SB. Temperature regulation by hypothalamic proportional control with an adjustable set point. *J Appl Physiol* 1963;18:1146–1154.
4. Boulant JA. Neuronal basis of Hammel's model for set-point thermoregulation. *J Appl Physiol* 2006;100(4):1347–1354.
5. Mekjavic IB, Sundberg CJ, Linnarsson D. Core temperature "null zone." *J Appl Physiol* 1991;71(4):1289–1295.
6. Bligh J. A theoretical consideration of the means whereby the mammalian core temperature is defended at a null zone. *J Appl Physiol* 2006;100(4):1332–1337.
7. Lanier WL. Cerebral metabolic rate and hypothermia: Their relationship with ischemic neurologic injury. *J Neurosurg Anesthesiol* 1995;7(3):216–221.
8. Rosomoff HL, Holaday DA. Cerebral blood flow and cerebral oxygen consumption during hypothermia. *Am J Physiol* 1954;179(1):85–88.
9. Patel PM, Drummond JC, Lemkuil BP. Cerebral physiology and the effects of anesthetic drugs. In: Miller RD, editor. *Miller's Anesthesia*, 8 ed. Philadelphia, PA: Elsevier Saunders; 2015, pp. 391, 392.
10. Volgushev M, Vidyasagar TR, Chistiakova M, Eysel UT. Synaptic transmission in the neocortex during reversible cooling. *Neuroscience* 2000;98(1):9–22.
11. Volgushev M, Kudryashov I, Chistiakova M, Mukovski M, Niesmann J, Eysel UT. Probability of transmitter release at neocortical synapses at different temperatures. *J Neurophysiol* 2004;92(1):212–220.
12. Bisschops LLA, Hoedemaekers CWE, Simons KS, van der Hoeven JG. Preserved metabolic coupling and cerebrovascular reactivity during mild hypothermia after cardiac arrest. *Crit Care Med* 2010;38(7):1542–1547.
13. Clifton GL, Miller ER, Choi SC et al. Lack of effect of induction of hypothermia after acute brain injury. *N Engl J Med* 2001;344(8):556–563.
14. Tremey B, Vigué B. Changes in blood gases with temperature: Implications for clinical practice. *Ann Fr Anesth Reanim* 2004;23(5):474–481.
15. Vigué B, Ract C, Zlotine N, Leblanc PE, Samii K, Bissonnette B. Relationship between intracranial pressure, mild hypothermia and temperature-corrected PaCO2 in patients with traumatic brain injury. *Intensive Care Med* 2000;26(6):722–728.
16. Frank SM, Fleisher LA, Breslow MJ et al. Perioperative maintenance of normothermia reduces the incidence of morbid cardiac events. A randomized clinical trial. *JAMA* 1997;277:1127–1134.
17. Weisser J, Martin J, Bisping E et al. Influence of mild hypothermia on myocardial contractility and circulatory function. *Basic Res Cardiol* 2001;96:198–205.
18. Daniel I. Sessler: Temperature regulation and monitoring. In: Ronald D. Miller, editor. *Miller's Anesthesia*, 8th ed. Philadelphia, PA: Elsevier Saunders; 2015, p. 1640.
19. Dae MW, Gao DW, Sessler DI, Chair K, Stillson CA. Effect of endovascular cooling on myocardial temperature, infarct size, and cardiac output in human-sized pigs. *Am J Physiol Heart Circ Physiol* 2002;282:H1584–H1591.

20. Hynson JM, Sessler DI, Moayeri A, McGuire J. Absence of nonshivering thermogenesis in anesthetized humans. *Anesthesiology* 1993;79:695–703.

21. Michelson AD, MacGregor H, Barnard MR, Kestin AS, Rohrer MJ, Valeri CR. Reversible inhibition of human platelet activation by hypothermia in vivo and in vitro. *Thromb Haemost* 1994;71(5):633–640.

22. Valeri CR, Khabbaz K, Khuri SF et al. Effect of skin temperature on platelet function in patients undergoing extracorporeal bypass. *J Thorac Cardiovasc Surg* 1992;104(1):108–116.

23. Rajagopalan S, Mascha E, Na J, Sessler DI. The effects of mild perioperative hypothermia on blood loss and transfusion requirement: A meta-analysis. *Anesthesiology* 2008;108(1):71–77.

24. Schmied H, Kurz A, Sessler DI, Kozek S, Reiter A. Mild intraoperative hypothermia increases blood loss and allogeneic transfusion requirements during total hip arthroplasty. *Lancet* 1996;347:289–292.

25. Van Oss CJ, Absolam DR, Moore LL Park BH, Humbert JR. Effect of temperature on chemotaxis, phagocytic engulfment, digestion and O_2 consumption of human polymorphonuclear leukocytes. *J Reticuloendothel Soc* 1980;27:561–565.

26. Sheffield CW, Sessler DI, Hopf HW et al. Centrally and locally mediated thermoregulatory responses alter subcutaneous oxygen tension. *Wound Rep Reg* 1997;4:339–345.

27. Kimberger O, Kurz A. Thermoregulatory management for mild therapeutic hypothermia. *Best Pract Res Clin Anaesthesiol* 2008;22(4):729–744.

28. Ponce FA, Spetzler RF, Han PP et al. Cardiac standstill for cerebral aneurysms in 103 patients: An update on the experience at the Barrow Neurological Institute. Clinical article. *J Neurosurg* 2011;114(3):877–884.

29. Mahaney KB, Todd MM, Bayman EO, Torner JC. Acute postoperative neurological deterioration associated with surgery for ruptured intracranial aneurysm: Incidence, predictors, and outcomes. *J Neurosurg* 2012;116:1267–1278.

30. Todd MM, Hindman BJ, Clarke WR, Torner JC. Mild intraoperative hypothermia during surgery for intracranial aneurysm. *N Engl J Med* 2005;352(2):135–145.

31. Shinada T, Hata N, Kobayashi N et al. Efficacy of therapeutic hypothermia for neurological salvage in patients with cardiogenic sudden cardiac arrest: The importance of prehospital return of spontaneous circulation. *J Nippon Med Sch* 2013;80:287–295.

32. Wassink G, Gunn ER, Drury PP, Bennet L, Gunn AJ. The mechanisms and treatment of asphyxial encephalopathy. *Front Neurosci* 2014;8:40.

33. Peterson K, Carson S, Carney N. Hypothermia treatment for traumatic brain injury: A systematic review and meta-analysis. *J Neurotrauma* 2008;25(1):62–71.

34. Zweifler RM, Sessler DI, Zivin JA. Thermoregulatory vasoconstriction and shivering impede therapeutic hypothermia in acute ischemic stroke victims. *J Stroke Cerebrovasc Dis* 1997;6:100–104.

35. Mokhtarani M, Mahgob AN, Morioka N et al. Buspirone and meperidine synergistically reduce the shivering threshold. *Anesth Analg* 2001;93(5):1233–1239.

36. Georgiou AP, Manara AR. Role of therapeutic hypothermia in improving outcome after traumatic brain injury: A systematic review. *Br J Anaesth* 2013;110(3):357–367.

37. Childers MK, Upright J, Smith DW. Posttraumatic hyperthermia induced brain injury rehabilitation. *Brain Inj* 1994;8(4):335–343.

38. Laws C, Jallo J. Fever and infection in the neurosurgical intensive care unit. *JHN J* 2010;5(2):5.

39. Sund-Levander M, Grodzinsky E. Assessment of body temperature measurement options. *Br J Nurs* 2013;22(16):944–950.

40. Drake-Brockman T, Hegarty M, Chambers N, von Ungern-Sternberg B. Monitoring temperature in children undergoing anaesthesia: A comparison of methods. *Anaesth Intensive Care* 2014;42(3):315–320.

41. El-Radhi AS, Barry W. Thermometry in paediatric practice. *Arch Dis Child* 2006;91(4):351–356.

42. Sessler DI, Moayeri A. Skin-surface warming: Heat flux and central temperature. *Anesthesiology* 1990;73(2):218–224.

43. Giesbrecht GG, Ducharme MB, McGuire JP. Comparison of forced-air patient warming systems for perioperative use. *Anesthesiology* 1994;80(3):671–679.

44. Bissonnette B, Sessler DI. Passive or active inspired gas humidification increases thermal steady-state temperatures in anesthetized infants. *Anesth Analg* 1989;69(6):783–787.

45. Moriyama T, Tsuneyoshi I, Omae T, Takeyama M, Kanmura Y. The effect of amino-acid infusion during off-pump coronary arterial bypass surgery on thermogenic and hormonal regulation. *J Anesth* 2008;22(4):354–360.

Urine output

KAVITHA JAYARAM

Introduction

Urine output forms the basis for assessment of intravascular volume status and for diagnosis of multiple diseases. This is the basic tool for volume replacement, particularly in neurosurgery patients. Multiple kinds of electrolyte imbalances present when there is a neurological problem in relation to urine output.

Physiological association of the kidney and brain

Two mutually dependent but opposing neurohormonal systems maintain blood pressure, intravascular volume, and salt and water homeostasis. The sympathoadrenal axis, the renin–angiotensin–aldosterone system, and arginine vasopressin (AVP) defend against hypotension and hypovolemia by promoting vasoconstriction and salt and water retention. The prostaglandins and natriuretic peptides defend against hypertension and hypervolemia by promoting vasodilation and salt and water excretion.[1]

Hypothalamic osmoreceptors are sensitive to increases in serum osmolality of as little as 1% above normal. The threshold for AVP secretion (and sensation of thirst) is between 280 and 290 mOsm/kg. Even mild dehydration results in rapid antidiuresis, and urine osmolality can increase from 300 to 1200 mOsm/kg as plasma AVP levels rise from 0 to 5 pg/mL. Decreases in intravascular volume also stimulate AVP secretion, mediated by stretch receptors with vagal afferents from the left atrium and pulmonary veins.

Antidiuretic hormone (ADH), presently known as AVP, plays a major role in the regulation of urinary volume and osmolality, and control of diuresis and antidiuresis. Synthesized by supraoptic and paraventricular nuclei of anterior hypothalamus, AVP undergoes neuroaxonal transport to posterior pituitary to be stored in granules.[2] Neural stimulation triggers exocytosis of AVP into circulation. AVP acts on V2 receptors in the collecting duct to increase water reabsorption and concentrate the urine. In the thick ascending loop of Henle, it increases sodium chloride absorption, thereby maintaining hypertonicity of medullary interstitium. The net effect is to increase urine osmolality and to decrease plasma osmolality without altering the solute excretion. Thus, AVP plays a major role in maintaining the urine concentrating ability of the kidney along with the countercurrent mechanism and urea recycling. At higher concentrations of AVP,

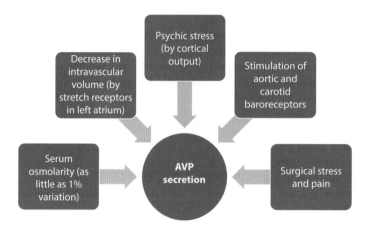

Figure 15.1 Regulation of arginine vasopressin (AVP) secretion and its various stimuli.

as occurs in severe hypotension, it predominantly acts on V1a receptors and causes vasoconstriction of the efferent arterioles to maintain effective glomerular filtration pressure in the renal cortex (Figure 15.1). The half-life of AVP is 5–15 min.

Brain–Kidney crosstalk

Any acute problems in the kidney resulting in acute kidney injury may originate from different organs such as the brain, heart, lungs, and liver. This is depicted as "organ crosstalk," as crosstalk works in both ways and one dysfunction can precede the other.[3] In Brain–Kidney crosstalk category, we have multiple diseases such as syndrome of inappropriate antidiuretic hormone (SIADH), cerebral salt-wasting syndrome (CSWS), and central neurogenic diabetes insipidus (CNDI) arising out of trauma to the hypothalamus and pituitary either directly or indirectly. The common problem with all three disorders is abnormalities in sodium concentration and water content, and osmolality of blood and urine. (Table 15.1).

Syndrome of inappropriate antidiuretic hormone secretion

The most common neurological causes of SIADH are subarachnoid hemorrhage (SAH), tumors, traumatic brain injury (TBI), meningitis, and encephalitis. Positive pressure ventilation, lung carcinomas, and medications such as morphine, chlorpromazine, acetaminophen, and carbamazepine can also cause it.

The clinical features are related to hyponatremia and resulting brain edema due to renal reabsorption of water, causing dilutional hyponatremia. These include weight gain, weakness, lethargy, mental confusion, obtundation, disordered reflexes, convulsions, and coma. The diagnostic criteria for SIADH are the following:

1. Urinary sodium greater than 20 mEq/L
2. Clinical euvolemia—absence of peripheral edema and dehydration
3. Serum sodium lower than 130 mEq/L (hypotonic hyponatremia)
4. Plasma osmolality lower than 270 mOsm/L
5. Urine hypertonic relative to plasma (urine osmolality > plasma osmolality)
6. Normal thyroid, renal, and adrenal function (Figure 15.2)

Absence of dehydration is a very important feature that differentiates SIADH from CSWS as treatment of both of them is entirely opposite. SIADH is suspected in any patient with hyponatremia excreting hypertonic urine in relation to plasma. Water loading is a useful way of assessing SIADH as patients are unable to excrete dilute urine even after water loading.

The condition is often self-limiting and treatment is initiated only in symptomatic patients. In mild-to-moderate disease, the intake of fluids is restricted to 800–1000 mL/day. This may be difficult to achieve as it may produce cardiovascular instability and worsen cerebral ischemia in brain-injured patients. When symptoms are severe, hypertonic saline (1.8%) is instituted intravenously slowly, particularly after SAH when fluid restriction is contraindicated. The increase in serum sodium level should not be more than 1 mEq/L/h.[4] Hypertonic saline is discontinued when the serum sodium level reaches 120–125 mEq/L and fluid restriction is followed. Too vigorous treatment of chronic hyponatremia can result in disabling demyelination.[4]

Pharmacological treatment is an option. Different drugs act by different mechanisms.

Table 15.1 Comparative Features of SIADH, CSWS, and DI

Feature	SIADH	CSWS	Diabetes insipidus
Definition	Persistent production of AVP resulting in water intoxication and volume expansion	Renal loss of sodium leading to true hyponatremia and a volume-contracted state in which the kidneys do not reabsorb sodium	Fluid imbalance due to decreased secretion of AVP or renal unresponsiveness to AVP
Etiology	Head trauma, brain tumor, abscess, subarachnoid hemorrhage, hydrocephalus, meningitis, encephalitis, Guillain–Barré syndrome, pneumonia, drugs associated with increased ADH secretion (oral hypoglycemic agents, nonsteroidal anti-inflammatories, opiates, anesthetics)	Cause unclear but often occurs in patients with intracranial abnormalities (head trauma, stroke, subarachnoid hemorrhage, brain tumors)	Hypotension, stress, pain, anxiety, and an upright position Trauma, surgery, or damage to the hypothalamus
Clinical features			
Mental status	Confusion Lethargy	Decreased level of consciousness, agitation, coma	Normal to impaired
Heart rate	Slow or normal	Resting or postural tachycardia	Tachycardia
Blood pressure	Hypertensive	Postural hypotension	Normal or mild hypertension
Extracellular fluid	Increased	Decreased	Decreased
Urine			
Output	Decreased (400–500 mL/day)	Decreased	Increased (>250 mL/h)
Specific gravity	>1.010 (concentrated, dark) Elevated (>100)	>1.010 (concentrated, dark) Elevated (>100)	<1.005 (very dilute)
Osmolality	Normal or >25	Increased (>25)	Decreased (<200)
Sodium (mEq/L)			Normal or decreased
Serum			
Sodium (mEq/L)	Low (<135)	Low (<135)	High (>145)

(Continued)

Table 15.1 Comparative Features of SIADH, CSWS, and DI (*Continued*)

Feature	SIADH	CSWS	Diabetes insipidus
Osmolality (mOsm/kg)	Low (<275)	Low (<275)	High (>295)
Treatment	Fluid restriction (800–1000 mL/24 h) Slow sodium replacement with normal saline or hypertonic (3%–5%) saline intravenously	Replacement of fluid volume and sodium No restriction of fluids Slow sodium replacement with hypertonic (3%) saline intravenously	Fluid replacement (0.45% saline intravenously replaced milliliter for milliliter, or greater) ADH replacement with desmopressin acetate intranasally or orally, lypressin intranasally, or aqueous vasopressin intravenously

1. Increase in excretion of water with furosemide or other diuretics: Simultaneous saline or salt supplementation should be administered to replace the associated sodium loss.
2. Inhibition of the renal responses of ADH by demeclocycline or lithium: Demeclocycline is the least toxic and an initial daily dose of 900–1200 mg should be reduced to 600–900 mg per day after the desired therapeutic effect is achieved, usually between 3 days and 3 weeks after starting treatment. It interferes with the ability of the renal tubules to concentrate urine, thereby causing excretion of isotonic or hypotonic urine and lessening the hyponatremia.
3. ADH receptor antagonists, such as conivaptan and lixivaptan, inhibit the binding of ADH to renal receptors. They have been shown to be effective in small clinical trials by inducing aquaresis, the electrolyte-sparing excretion of free water.

When a patient with SIADH comes to the operating room for any surgical procedure, fluids are managed by measuring the central volume status by CVP, pulmonary artery lines, or the cross-sectional left ventricular area at end diastole on transesophageal echocardiography and by frequent assays of urine osmolarity, plasma osmolarity, and serum sodium, including the period immediately after the surgical procedure.

Cerebral salt-wasting syndrome

Unlike SIADH, CSWS is characterized by true hypotremia caused by loss of both salt and water. The predominant features are polyuria, hyponatremia, hypovolemia, and natriuresis. It is predominantly associated with SAH, intracranial surgery, and TBI, but described in ischemic stroke and meningitis also. The precise mechanism behind it is unknown and multiple mechanisms are supposed to affect sodium and water balance. The primary pathogenic mechanism is renal loss of sodium, which leads to hyponatremia and a decrease in extracellular volume.[5]

Patients present with headache and increased thirst. They also have tachycardia, orthostatic hypotension, dehydration, weight loss, lethargy, decreased level of consciousness, convulsions, and coma. The primary difference between SIADH and CSWS is that the former is a state of volume expansion whereas the latter is that of volume depletion.

The biochemical criteria for CSWS are the following:

1. Low or normal serum sodium
2. High or normal serum osmolality
3. High or normal urine osmolality
4. Increased levels of hematocrit, urea, bicarbonate, and albumin as a consequence of hypovolemia (Figure 15.2).

The treatment of CSWS is appropriate volume replacement with normal saline, depending on the sodium levels. Hypertonic saline can be used for severe hyponatremia. In patients who can tolerate orally, salt supplementation in the form of tablets is given. It is important to note that some patients receiving fluid replacement may have increased natriuresis and water loss, worsening the clinical situation. Hence, it is important to monitor the fluid status, serum sodium concentration, and total sodium balance.

Central neurogenic diabetes insipidus

Central neurogenic diabetes insipidus is often associated with TBI, neurosurgeries, tumor, increased intracranial pressure, brain death, and central nervous system infections. Development of diabetes insipidus (DI) in nonpituitary surgery is associated with severe, preterminal cerebral edema. It is a common finding after brainstem death and also an important feature for management in organ donors.[6]

The pathophysiology occurs as a result of the failure of ADH release due to the disorder of hypothalamic–pituitary axis. The ability to concentrate urine is impaired, resulting in excess production of dilute urine. If the damage to the hypothalamus is above the median eminence, it results in permanent DI, whereas if it is below this level, DI is transient.

If there is a lack of renal response to ADH, there can be hypokalemia, hypercalcemia, obstructive uropathy, or renal insufficiency. In awake patients, the classical triad of polyuria, polydypsia, and

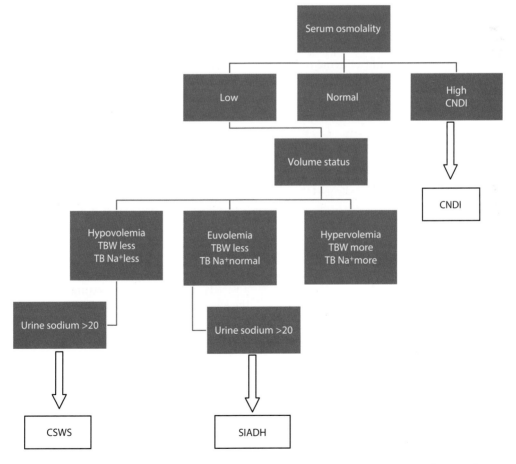

Figure 15.2 Flowchart for diagnosis of cerebral salt-wasting syndrome (CSWS), syndrome of inappropriate antidiuretic hormone (SIADH), and central neurogenic diabetes insipidus (CNDI) (TBW, total body water).

thirst are the presenting features (hyperglycemia has to be ruled out). Other causes of polyuria have to be ruled out in neurological patients such as prehospital fluid resuscitation, osmotic diuretics, hypertonic saline, and application of triple-H therapy to avoid vasospasm.

The diagnosis of DI is made in the presence of:

1. Increased urine volume (usually 3000 mL/24 h)
2. High serum sodium (>145 mmol/L)
3. High serum osmolality (>305 mmol/kg)
4. Abnormally low urine osmolality (<350 mmol/kg)
5. Urine-specific gravity <1.005 (Figure 15.2)

Measurement of plasma ADH concentration can distinguish between nephrogenic and central DI, but confirmation of the diagnosis ultimately comes with the observation of the response to synthetic ADH.

The aim of management is replacement and retention of water and replacement of ADH. In the acute phase, exogenous ADH is provided and fluid equivalent to the amount of urine output is given orally (if the patient can tolerate oral intake) or intravenously. Serum sodium should not be reduced more than 10 mmol/L/day as it can have harmful side effects such as pulmonary edema or cerebral edema. To calculate the body water deficit, the following formula is used:

$$\left(0.6\left[\text{weight in kilograms}\right]\right) \times \left(\text{serum sodium} - 140\right) \div 140 =$$

$$\text{body water deficit}\left(\text{in liters}\right)$$

Hypotonic solutions such as 0.45% saline or 5% dextrose are used for the replacement of the calculated fluid deficit intravenously.

If the urine output is >250 mL/h, then exogenous ADH in the form of desmopressin, aqueous vasopressin, or lypressin is administered: desmopressin, 5–200 µg intranasally or 5–40 µg intravenously; aqueous vasopressin, 100 milliunits bolus followed by 100–200 milliunits per hour infusion; lypressin, 5–20 units intranasally 3–7 times a day. Plasma osmolality has to be measured hourly during the acute phase. If such a patient presents for surgery, in the intraoperative period vasopressin infusion is continued and isotonic fluids are used for replacement. Because of harmful side effects, the dose of vasopressin should be limited to that necessary for control of diuresis. The oxytocic and coronary-artery-constricting properties of vasopressin make this limit especially applicable to patients who are pregnant or have coronary artery disease (CAD).

Fluid management in special situations

Rational management of fluids in neurosurgical patients should start with maintaining baseline blood volume and cerebral perfusion and avoiding significant decreases in serum Na^+, osmolality, and oncotic pressure. Special situations are as follows:

1. Increased intracranial pressure: Mannitol and hypertonic saline are mainstays in this area. Though their osmotic action is reduced when the blood–brain barrier is disrupted, they have other therapeutic effects also.[7] The benefit of one over the other has been proved and disproved by multiple studies and meta-analyses.[8–10]
2. Cerebral vasospasm: The triple-H therapy has entered practice without any evidence of randomized controlled trials, based on a few smaller trials.[11,12] Caution must be exercised against hypervolemia as it is potentially injurious in the presence of disrupted blood–brain barrier and could have extracranial side effects such as pulmonary edema.[13]
3. Any intracranial pathological conditions that produce syndromes such as SIADH, CSWS, or central neurogenic DI should be assessed and treated promptly.

Clear comparisons of crystalloid and colloid in a variety of neurosurgical settings are lacking. In the absence of more robust evidence, a mixture of isotonic crystalloids and colloids is advocated in other neurosurgical settings.[12,14]

References

1. Mcilroy D, Sladen RN. Renal physiology, pathophysiology, and pharmacology. In: Miller, RD, editor. *Miller's Anesthesia*, 8th ed. Philadelphia, PA: Elsevier Saunders; 2015, pp. 568–571.
2. Genuth SM. The adrenal glands. In: Berne RM, Levy EM, editors. *Physiology*, 4th ed. St Louis, MO : Mosby; 1998, pp. 930–964.

3. Li X, Hassoun HT, Santora R, Rabb H. Organ crosstalk: The role of the kidney. *Curr Opin Crit Care* 2009;15(6):481–487.

4. Rojiani AM, Prineas JW, Cho ES. Protective effect of steroids on electrolyte-induced demyelination. *J Neuropathol Exp Neurol* 1987;46(4):495–504.

5. Yee A, Burns J, Wijdicks E. Cerebral salt wasting: Pathophysiology, diagnosis, and treatment. *Neurosurg Clin North Am* 2010;21(2):339–352.

6. Smith M. Physiological changes during brain stem death—Lessons for management of the organ donor. *J Heart Lung Transplant* 2004;23:S217–S222.

7. Wijayatilake DS, Shepherd SJ, Sherren PB. Updates in the management of intracranial pressure in traumatic brain injury. *Curr Opin Anaesthesiol* 2012;25(5):540–547.

8. Kamel H, Navi BB, Nakagawa K, Hemphil JC, Ko NU. Hypertonic saline versus mannitol for the treatment of elevated intracranial pressure: A meta-analysis of randomized clinical trials. *Crit Care Med* 2011;39(3):554–559.

9. Bulger EM, May S, Brasel KJ et al. Out-of-hospital hypertonic resuscitation following severe traumatic brain injury: A randomized controlled trial. *JAMA* 2010;304(13):1455–1464.

10. Ryu JH, Walcott BP, Kahle KT et al. Induced and sustained hypernatremia for the prevention and treatment of cerebral edema following brain injury. *Neurocrit Care* 2013;19(2):222–231.

11. Velat GJ, Kimball MM, Mocco JD, Hoh BL. Vasospasm after aneurysmal subarachnoid hemorrhage: Review of randomized controlled trials and meta-analyses in the literature. *World Neurosurg* 2011;76:446.

12. Sen J, Belli A, Albon H, Morgan L, Petzold A, Kitchen N. Triple-H therapy in the management of aneurysmal subarachnoid haemorrhage. *Lancet Neurol* 2003;2(10):614–621.

13. Tummala RP, Sheth RN, Heros RC. Hemodilution and fluid management in neurosurgery. *Clin Neurosurg* 2006;53:238–251.

14. Van Aken HK, Kampmeier TG, Ertmer C, Westphal M. Fluid resuscitation in patients with traumatic brain injury: What is a SAFE approach? *Curr Opin Anaesthesiol* 2012;25(5):563–565.

Anaesthesia for the neurosurgical patient

Difficult airway

ANKUR LUTHRA

Introduction

Difficult airway

This is a clinical situation in which a conventionally trained anesthesiologist experiences difficulty with mask ventilation (MV), difficulty with tracheal intubation, or both.[1,2] It represents a complex interaction between patient factors, the clinical setting, and the skills of the practitioner.

Difficult airway: Spectrum

The difficult airway has three components that may or may not coexist:[2]

1. Difficult bag-MV
2. Difficult laryngeal MV
3. Difficult surgical airway

Difficult mask ventilation

As per the definition provided by the American Society of Anesthesiologists (ASA) Task Force on Management of the Difficult Airway, difficult mask ventilation is a situation that develops when

1. It is *not* possible for the unassisted anesthesiologist to maintain the peripheral oxygen saturation (SpO_2) > 90% using 100% oxygen and positive-pressure mask ventilation (PPMV) in a patient whose SpO_2 was >90% before anesthetic intervention.[1]
2. It is *not* possible for the unassisted anesthesiologist to prevent or reverse signs of inadequate ventilation during PPMV.

Difficult face mask ventilation

This is a condition that develops when

1. It is not possible for the anesthesiologist to provide adequate face MV due to one or more of the following problems: inadequate mask seal, excessive gas leak, or excessive resistance to the ingress or egress of gas.[2]
2. Signs of inadequate face MV include (but are not limited to) the following: *absent or inadequate chest movement, absent or inadequate breath sounds, auscultatory signs of severe obstruction, cyanosis, gastric air entry or dilatation, decreasing or inadequate SpO_2, absent or inadequate exhaled CO_2, absent or inadequate spirometric measures of exhaled gas flow, and hemodynamic changes associated with hypoxemia or hypercarbia (e.g., hypertension, tachycardia, and arrhythmia).*

Difficult laryngoscopy

This is not possible to visualize any portion of the vocal cords after multiple attempts at conventional laryngoscopy.

Difficult tracheal intubation

Tracheal intubation requires multiple attempts, in the presence or absence of tracheal pathology.

Failed intubation

Placement of the endotracheal tube (ETT) fails after multiple intubation attempts.

Difficult laryngeal mask ventilation

This is defined as the inability within three insertions to place the mask in a satisfactory position to allow clinically adequate ventilation and airway patency.

Clinical adequate ventilation

Indices of clinically adequate ventilation generally are delivered (expired) at tidal volume of >7 mL/kg and leak pressure of >15–20 cm H_2O.

Can't ventilate, can't intubate

Can't ventilate, can't intubate (CVCI) indicates failed face MV and failed intubation. Hypoxemia and death occur unless emergency transtracheal oxygenation is successful. When face MV fails, the laryngeal mask airway (LMA) may provide a satisfactory airway. A better term that indicates attempts to manage airway by face mask, laryngeal mask, and intubation have failed is can't intubate, can't oxygenate (CICO). It is rare in patients requiring elective surgical procedures. The current ASA Closed Claims Project database contains 8954 claims representing events that occurred from 1970 to 2007, with 5230 claims since 1990. Complications leading to anesthesia malpractice claims have changed considerably since the 1970s. With the introduction of modern respiratory monitoring in the mid-1980s as well as practice guidelines for management of difficult airway in 1993, death and brain damage have declined significantly.

How to avoid CVCI?

Before we even render a patient unconscious, we must ask ourselves the following four questions:

1. Will I be able to oxygenate/ventilate this patient using a mask?
2. Will I be able to place a supraglottic device (SAD) in this patient if required?
3. Will I be able to tracheally intubate this patient should the need arise?
4. Do I have access to this patient's trachea if a surgical airway is required?

The only way we can accurately answer these questions is if we do a thorough assessment of the airway.

Difficult airway in neurosurgery

Challenges

Following are the challenges faced with difficult airway in neurosurgery:

Patients with intracranial pathology respond poorly to even short periods of hypoxia or hypercarbia because of increase in intracranial pressure (ICP).

Airway anatomy is completely normal but the patient's head is fixed in a frame.

Patients associated with acromegaly for pituitary surgery.

Patients with unstable cervical spine.
Unanticipated difficult airway becomes an even greater challenge in patients at risk for cerebral aneurysm rupture.
After temporal craniotomy, pseudoankylosis of the temporomandibular joint (TMJ) can cause significant impairment of mouth opening in patients, resulting in difficult intubation (DI).
Patients may have reduced jaw movement after skull base surgery when a transtemporal surgical approach has been used.
Other challenges include considerations for extubation after prolonged surgery.

Airway management in patients with head injury

Indications: Following are the indications for emergency intubation in patients with traumatic brain injury (TBI):

- Glasgow Coma Scale (GCS) score of ≤8
- Risk of increase in ICP due to agitation, impending herniation
- Inability to control/protect the airway or loss of protective laryngeal reflexes

Ten percent of patients with TBI have associated cervical spine injuries. All patients with head injury should be assumed to have cervical spine injury until proven otherwise.

Standard approach: Rapid sequence induction + head and neck stabilization (manual in-line stabilization [MILS]) + defasciculation + cricoid pressure + induction agent (if hemodynamically stable).

Newer airway techniques: These include optical and video laryngoscopes and stylets.

Fiberoptic (FOB) laryngoscopy: This is the gold standard for difficult airway, especially if concomitant cervical spine injury is suspected.

Difficult airway scenarios

- Patients with cervical spine lesions are susceptible to both primary and secondary neurological injuries during intubation (Figure 16.1).
- Overall incidence of development of secondary neurological injury ranges from 2% to 10%.
- In addition, airway management is difficult in a patient who is obese, has facial fractures, has blood in the pharynx, or has oral soft-tissue injury.

Airway management techniques

Some techniques for the management of difficult airway are shown in Table 16.1.

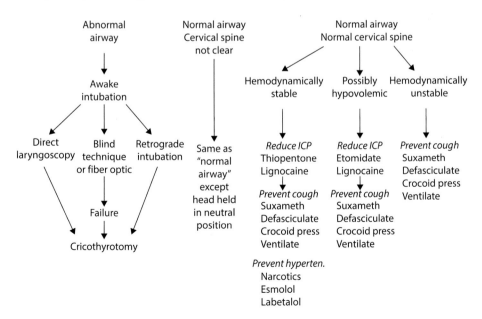

Figure 16.1 Airway management in patients with acute cervical spine injury.

Table 16.1 Airway Management Techniques

Maneuver	Condition	Results
Chin lift/jaw thrust	C5–C6 instability	>5-mm widening disk space at the level of injury
NP/oral airway	C5–C6 instability	≈2-mm widening disk space at the level of injury
Mask ventilation		Significant AP translation displacement with maximum flexion and extension of head
Cricoid pressure	Normal, anesthetized, in-line stabilization	Single-handed pressure causes vertical displacement of neck ≈5 mm, but no spine movement
Blind nasotracheal	C5–C6 instability	Up to 2-mm subluxation but no increase in disk space
		Intubation of >5-mm subluxation when neck is stabilized anteriorly by hand pressure

NP, nasopharyngeal; AP, anteroposterior.

Airway manoeuvres in cervical spine instability

This section discusses the airway management techniques for patients with cervical injury and their effect on spine immobilization (Table 16.2).

Cervical collar, sandbags, backboard, head tape: These are very effective methods of limiting flexion, extension, lateral bending; they make orotracheal intubation much more difficult if left in space at time of intubation.

Hard and soft collar: They have little effect on spine immobilization. The anterior collar interferes with mouth opening. It is to be removed during direct laryngoscopy (DL). Its removal also helps in increasing mouth opening and facilitates application of backward, upward, rightward pressure (BURP) and cricoid pressure (also called the Sellick maneuver). It increases incidence of Grade III or IV laryngoscopic view, if left in place. Their advantage is that they also alert medics to the possibility of cervical spine injury.

Manual in-line stabilization: This is a recommended method of reducing neck mobility during tracheal intubation (orotracheal/nasotracheal)—standard of care:

- DL and orotracheal intubation with MILS (Figure 16.2)
- Likely does not worsen cervical spine injury: cervical spine extension decreases by 60% when MILS was provided during endotracheal intubation (ETI)[3]

- Probably worsens laryngoscopic view[4]: Grade 3 or 4 CL view obtained on laryngoscopy in 22% patients

"Any beneficial effects of using MILS with direct laryngoscopy and orotracheal intubation must be balanced against the potential for the practice to contribute to clinically apparent and subtle hypoxic impairment in brain function."[5]

Axial traction: Excessive axial traction may cause distraction and subluxation, especially at the C5–C6 level causing deterioration of neurologic function. It has been reported to be associated with excessive traction during cervical spine stabilization procedures.

During ETT: Only MILS should be used and cervical traction should not be performed.

Halo brace: This is the most rigid immobilization technique of all spinal orthoses. It is highly effective in limiting upper cervical spine motion, thus limiting both flexion/extension and lateral bending movements of the cervical spine by 96% and axial rotation by 99%. But it makes DL very difficult. FOB intubation is recommended (awake or after induction).

In an emergency setting, early tracheostomy should be considered in patients with

- High cervical injury
- History of cardiac disease
- Age of >60 years
- Intubated on arrival
- History of DI
- Anticipated length of intubation >1 week

Table 16.2 Cervical Spine Immobilization Techniques

Maneuver	Condition	Result
Direct laryngoscopy	Normal, anesthetized	Extension at OA and C1–C2 articulation C2–C5 displaced only minimally
	C5–C6 instability	3–4 mm widening of disc space at level of injury
Straight vs. curved blade	Normal, anesthetized	No difference in cervical spine movement
GlideScope	Normal, anesthetized	Overall spine movement reduced 50% at C2–C5 as compared to curved blade
Intubating LMA and classical LMA		Exerts high pressure against upper cervical vertebrae with insertion and manipulation May produce posterior displacement of upper cervical spine Little movement of spine above C3

OA, occipitoatlantal; LMA, laryngeal mask airway

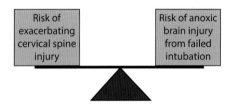

Figure 16.2 Direct laryngoscopy and orotracheal intubation with manual in-line stabilization.

In case of respiratory failure or airway obstruction, use of adjuncts such as intubating laryngeal mask airway (ILMA) or a Combitube may be lifesaving.

Stereotactic head frames: The early stereotactic frames produced by Lars Leksell provided head fixation but significantly interfered with airway access (Figure 16.3). Recent frames have crossbars that may (potentially) be directed cephalad for easier access to the nose and mouth. The crossbar can be removed by unscrewing two screws with an Allen wrench (which should always be available). Despite moderate access to the airway, the head positioning and fixation to the table make proper positioning for airway management extremely difficult.

Techniques to manage the airway in stereotactic surgeries

1. Spontaneous ventilation with oxygen supplementation
2. Awake or asleep LMA
3. Awake oral or nasal FOB intubation
4. Spontaneous intubation and blind nasal intubation

5. Awake or asleep FOB intubation by LMA
6. Awake or asleep lighted stylet intubation

Airway management in acromegaly

The factors that lead to airway difficulty in acromegaly patients are as follows:

1. Prognathism
2. Macroglossia
3. Osteophytes in cervical spine and decreased range of motion
4. Thickening of pharyngeal and laryngeal structures
5. Thickened vocal cords
6. Recurrent laryngeal nerve palsy
7. Decrease in width of cricoid arch
8. Central sleep apnea
9. Hypertrophied artytenoepiglottic cartilages and ventricular folds

The occurrence of difficult airway in acromegaly is well described, and the incidence of DI in these patients ranges from 10% to 30%. Hoarseness in a patient with acromegaly should alert the

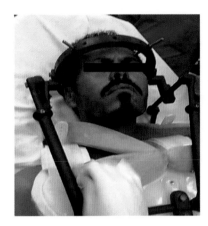

Figure 16.3 Stereotactic head frames.

physician to the possibility of laryngeal stenosis or RLN injury. A coexisting goiter occurs in 25% of patients with acromegaly, which may cause tracheal compression.

For suspected DI, perform FOB orotracheal intubation, with the patient either awake or asleep (if MV is easy).

ILMA is associated with a small (52.6%) first-attempt success rate in unparalyzed patients.[6]

Difficult airway management in pediatric patients

Incidence of *unanticipated* difficult pediatric airway is low. Most of the airway difficulties are associated with congenital syndromes. The principles outlined in ASA difficult airway management apply to pediatric patients as well (Figure 16.4). Evaluation, recognition, and preparation are key elements.

Difficulties unique to pediatric airway management

- Anatomical
- Physiological
  - Frequent upper airway obstruction under anesthesia
  - Higher metabolism, smaller functional residual capacity (FRC) lead to faster desaturation and subsequent bradycardia
  - Preoperative assessment
  - History

- Airway examination may be difficult to perform in uncooperative child
- Awake FOB and regional anesthesia usually not an option in children

History: Ask parents (vital source of information) about the following:

- Persistent snoring, episodes of apnea/obstruction
- Feeding problems, choking, breathlessness during feeding
- Airway noise, stridor, stertor, wheeze
- Hoarse voice, abnormal cry
- Past DI
- Syndromes related to pediatric difficult airway

Physical examination: Unable to cooperate
Look for predictors of DI such as the following:

- Micrognathia
- Macroglossia
- Loose teeth
- Facial (especially mandibular) asymmetry
- Limited mouth opening: preclude placement of SADs
- Limited neck movement
- Palate: narrow, high arched, cleft
- Abnormalities of the ear or the presence of ear tags: presence of bilateral microtia is used as an independent predictor of DI[6]
- Normal A-P distance from middle of inside of mentum to hyoid measured: >1.5 cm (neonates), >3 cm (adults)

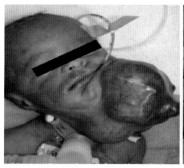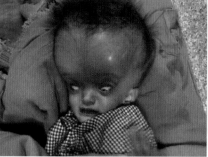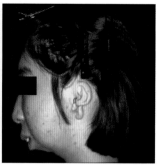

Figure 16.4 Difficult airway: pediatric patients.

Following are the signs of respiratory distress and increase in work of breathing (WOB):

- Tachypnea, grunting, sternal and subcostal recession
- Tracheal tug, nasal flaring, cyanosis, or agitation
- Lung fields: for a hoarse voice, abnormal cry, stridor, and other added sounds

The presence of cardiac lesions in syndromic craniosynostosis should also be taken into consideration.

Induction technique

Traditional approach

The traditional approach to the difficult pediatric airway is maintenance of spontaneous ventilation under inhalational anesthesia. Premedication includes oral or IV atropine (0.01–0.02 mg/kg) as it has vagolytic and antimuscarinic effects.

Inhalation induction includes use of halothane/sevoflurane in 100% O_2. Muscle relaxants/propofol are recommended after confirming adequate face MV.

Use of oropharyngeal airway (OPA)/nasopharyngeal airway (NPA) and application of continuous positive airway pressure (CPAP) is invaluable in helping to maintain a patent airway.

Awake/sedated technique

- Use of pharmacologic agents that are easily antagonized is recommended.
- Antisialagogue, midazolam, and fentanyl combination/remifentanil infusion.

Topical anesthesia

- Nebulizing, spraying, or swabbing local anesthetic (LA) solution or applying viscous gel to a gloved finger.
- FOB with suction ports can be used to spray LA on the vocal cords under direct vision.

FOB laryngoscopy

This is the *gold standard* for achieving tracheal intubation in children with airway abnormality. It includes

- Maintenance of spontaneous respiration
- LMA assistance if possible
- Assistant to pull the tongue out of the way: jaw lift given

Supraglottic airway devices

Following are the currently available SADs in pediatric sizes:

- Laryngeal tube
- Cobra perilaryngeal airway
- Esophageal tracheal combitube
- Air-Q intubating laryngeal airway

Video or optical laryngoscopes

Of these laryngoscopes, the following four are available in sizes appropriate for use in children less than 2 years of age:

- Airtrach disposable optical laryngoscope
- Glidescope
- Storz DCI video laryngoscope (Karl Storz, Germany)
- TruView infant

Syndromic craniosynostosis

This is associated with craniofacial abnormalities that impact both the skull vault and the facial skeleton. The upper airway obstruction (secondary to maxillary hypoplasia), exorbitism, and increase in ICP are common. The most common of the craniofacial-associated syndromes are Apert, Crouzon, and Pfeiffer syndromes. Difficult laryngoscopy is unusual in patients with midface hypoplasia—muscle relaxant can be safely given if able to MV with the help of OPA/NPA/LMA.

Hydrocephalus

This is associated with craniosynostosis syndromes (Apert and Pfeiffer syndrome) and mucopolysaccharidosis—one of the most difficult airways in pediatric patients.

Following are the airway challenges involved:

1. Interference with face MV
2. Large head/shoulder roll may be used
3. Raised ICP, vomiting, risk of aspiration— rapid sequence induction (RSI), intubation with cricoid pressure

Occipital encephalocele

Patients with occipital encephalocele may have associated airway abnormalities such as micrognathia, cleft lip or palate, and pulmonary hypoplasia. When large, they interfere with mask fit and laryngoscopy.

Intubation is performed

- In supine position (with sac placed in a doughnut)
- In right lateral position
- With head placed beyond the edge of the table with an assistant supporting it

References

1. ASA Difficult Airway Task Force. Practice guidelines for management of the difficult airway. A report by the American Society of Anesthesiologists Task Force on Management of the Difficult Airway. *Anesthesiology* 1993;78:597–602.
2. ASA Difficult Airway Task Force. Practice guidelines for management of the difficult airway: An updated report by the American Society of Anesthesiologists Task Force on Management of the Difficult Airway. *Anesthesiology* 2003;93:1269–1277.
3. Nolan JP, Wilson ME. Orotracheal intubation in patients with potential cervical spine injuries. An indication for the gum elastic bougie. *Anaesthesia* 1993;48:630–633.
4. Manoach S, Paladino L. Manual in-line stabilization for acute airway management of suspected cervical spine injury: Historical review and current questions. *Ann Emerg Med* 2007;50:236–245.
5. Law-Koune J, Liu N, Szekely B, Fischler M. Using the intubating laryngeal mask airway for ventilation and endotracheal intubation in anesthetized and unparalyzed acromegalic patients. *J Neurosurg Anesthesiol* 2004;16:11–13.
6. Uezono S, Holzman RS, Goto T, Nakata Y, Nagata S, Morita S. Prediction of difficult airway in school-aged patients with microtia. *Paediatr Anaesth* 2001;11:409–413.

17

Venous cannulation

ANKUR LUTHRA

Introduction

Intravenous (IV) cannulation is a technique whereby an intracath or IV cannula is placed inside a vein to provide venous access which allows blood sampling and administration of fluids, medications, parenteral nutrition, chemotherapy, and blood products.[1]

Venous channels have a three-layered wall consisting of an internal endothelium (intima) surrounded by a thin layer of muscle fibers (media) that is surrounded by an outer layer of connective tissue (adventitia). Venous valves allow unidirectional flow of blood thus preventing pooling of blood in the dependent portions of the extremities; they also can hinder the passage of a cannula through and into a vein. Venous valves are more numerous just distal to the points where tributaries join larger veins as well as in the lower extremities.[2]

Indications

Indications for IV cannulation include:

- Repeated blood sampling
- IV fluids and drug administration
- IV chemotherapy administration
- IV nutritional support (parenteral)
- IV blood or blood products administration

- IV administration of radiologic contrast agents for CT scan, magnetic resonance imaging (MRI), or nuclear imaging

Contraindications

There are no absolute contraindications to IV cannulation.

Peripheral venous access in a damaged, infected, or burned extremity should be avoided, if possible.

Some of the vesicant and irritant solutions (pH < 5, pH >9, or high osmolarity [>600 mOsm/L]) can cause blister formation and tissue necrosis if they leak into the tissue, including some sclerosing solutions, some chemotherapeutic agents, and inotropes. These solutions are better infused into a central vein. They should only be given through a peripheral vein in emergency conditions or when a central venous access is not readily available.

Peripheral venous cannulation

Veins with high internal blood pressure become engorged and are easier to access. The use of tourniquets, dependent positioning, and "pumping" through muscle contraction, and the local application of heat can contribute to venous engorgement and thus easy placement of IV cannula.

The superficial veins of the upper limbs are preferred to those of the lower limbs for peripheral venous access because cannulating upper-extremity veins is less likely to interfere with patient mobility and also reduces risk of phlebitis.[3] It is easier to insert a venous catheter where two tributaries merge into a Y-shaped form and also it is recommended to choose a straight portion of a vein to minimize the chance of hitting valves.

Sizes of IV cannula

The IV cannulas are available in various sizes which are color-coded for easy recognition; the flow allowed through the catheter channel is inversely proportional to the size (in gauge) and length of the catheter channel.

Placement of an IV catheter

In general, it is suitable to select the smallest gauge or size of catheter that can still effectively be used to deliver the prescribed therapy which will minimize the risk of damage to the vessel intima and ensure adequate blood flow through the catheter, which reduces the risk of venous inflammation (phlebitis).[4] But, if the situation is an emergency situation or if the patient requires large volumes of fluid to be infused over a short span of time, the largest-gauge and shortest catheter that is likely to fit the chosen vein should be used.

Recent advances in venous cannulation

The AccuVein AV400, a venous illumination system manufactured by AccuVein Inc. (Cold Spring Harbor, NY) is used for locating peripheral venous channels. The system displays a sort of map directly on the skin's surface, enabling clinicians to locate veins for intravenous cannulation, drawing blood,

sclerotherapy, general surgical purposes, and other medical procedures.

The AV400 uses a two-axis optical scanner system to sweep an infrared (IR) laser over a patient's skin, thus maximizing the contrast between veins and other tissues. Also, the device at the same time records the reflected light using photo-diodes tuned to the IR laser's wavelength. The laser beam illuminates only one spot at a time, thus generating data from a full image over the due course of one field. Then, after information about the vein is extracted using digital signal processing, the processed image is reprojected on the skin using a visible laser beam. Aligned with the data acquired in the infrared range, the image provides the practitioner with direct and immediate feedback for needle placements.

Ultrasound guided central venous cannulation

Ultrasound (US) guidance for the insertion of peripheral intravenous (PIV) catheters is a relatively new development. This technique offers the following advantages over the traditional method of gaining PIV access:

- Allows cannulation of veins that are neither visible nor palpable
- Reduces the need for a central line and its potential complications

The traditional method of PIV catheter insertion requires knowledge of vascular anatomy for estimation of the location of the target vessel and requires visualization or palpation of the vessel for accurate puncture.

The traditional approach carries numerous inherent problems that include the following:

- Location of vessels can vary considerably because of anatomic variability.

Size	Ext. diameter (mm)	Length (mm)	Color of the cap	Flow (ml/min)
14 gauge	2.1	45	Orange	300
16 gauge	1.7	45	Grey	172
18 gauge	1.3	45	Green	76
20 gauge	1	33	Pink	54
22 gauge	0.8	25	Blue	31
24 gauge	0.7	19	Yellow	14
26 gauge	0.6	19	Violet	13

- Veins can be distorted as a result of scarring from previous cannulation attempts or sclerosis.
- Veins are difficult to palpate in patients who are obese or edematous.
- Patients with difficult access are routinely subjected to multiple insertion attempts by different operators and are at increased risk of complications. In addition to increased discomfort, such patients often have their blood draw and laboratory test results delayed.

Studies have shown that ultrasound-guided PIV catheter placement results in higher overall and first-pass success rates and very low complication rates.

Indications for performing ultrasound-guided peripheral intravenous (PIV) cannulation include, but are not limited to, the following:

- Failure to cannulate by using the traditional technique.
- Cannulation of a patient who is severely dehydrated, obese patients, or in the presence of peripheral edema
- Cannulation in patients who use intravenous drugs or who have had multiple intravenous catheters placed in the past (e.g., patients with sickle cell disease) or long-term antibiotic usage
- Cannulation in the presence of burns that overlie the cannulation site

Venous cannulation in neurosurgery

Two large bore IV cannulas are usually inserted prior to most of the neurosurgical cases before various positions (sitting, park bench, supine, prone) are made.

The central venous cannulation is attempted post anaesthetic induction usually for neurosurgical cases that involve the sitting position (for air aspiration in venous air embolism), large brain tumours with significant midline shift which involve major blood loss, pediatric patients (craniosynostosis surgeries), fluid and electrolyte shifts and imbalances, pituitary surgeries (for postoperative diabetes insipidus), or in elderly ASA III patients, cardiac patients, or patients with prior neurosurgical interventions.

Usually emergency decompressive craniectomies can be undertaken with two large bore IV access unless patients are moribund, cardiac patients or those in whom major fluid shifts and electrolyte imbalances are expected.

CVP monitoring should be done in all such cases

For aneurysmal SAH (with or without cardiac changes), large AVM surgeries, CVP monitoring and central line insertion is mandatory not only for intraoperative course but even for postoperative periods where major complications like vasospasm, hydrocephalus are expected.

For major spine surgeries like scoliosis correction, large spinal tumours and instrumentations are carried out, central venous cannulation is usually advised. Patients with high cervical spine surgeries who are expected to have a prolonged ICU stay and mechanical ventilation and subsequent tracheostomies are also candidates for early central venous line insertion.

Difficult venous access in neurosurgical patients

Venous access can be difficult in a certain group of patients presenting for various neurosurgical procedures that include

1. Pediatric patients
2. Patients with Cushing's disease and acromegaly presenting for pituitary surgeries
3. Patients having recurrent brain tumours presenting for multiple surgeries within a short span of time
4. Elderly and obese patients
5. Patients in the neuro ICUs during a prolonged stay and repeated IV punctures

Pediatric patients

The most notorious and difficult intravenous access is of the pediatric age group, especially newborns, and infants who present with hydrocephalus for repeated shunt surgeries, encephalocele, medulloblastomas, brain stem gliomas, meningomyeloceles, and other paediatric neurosurgical procedures.

IV access in pediatric patients is usually inserted after inhalational induction with sevoflurane which also causes vasodilatation thus enabling an easier IV access. Most of the time, a 24 or a 22 G cannula is inserted (depending upon the age of the child).

When intravenous access is taken in such patients, because of the small calibre, the patency of the cannula should be maintained by repeated flushing of the IV cannula. Careful attention should be paid to the fixing of this IV cannula as it can easily get kinked while fixing on the child's skin.

Cushing's disease and acromegalic patients

In Cushing's disease, venous access becomes very difficult because of the fact that venous channels are highly fragile, tortous, and thin walled and the patients are obese with a lot of fat underneath the skin obscuring the venous channels from direct vision. Thus cannulation which appears easy may become very difficult because such veins get pricked easily; the threading of IV cannula becomes difficult.

In acromegaly, the skin is very thick thus pricking the vein for peripheral access becomes difficult. Central venous cannulation also becomes difficult in Cushing's as the patients are obese and the landmarks cannot be easily felt. Here comes the role of USG guided cannulation.

References

1. Scales K. Intravenous therapy: A guide to good practice. Br J Nurs. 2008 Oct 23-Nov 12. 17(19):S4-S12.
2. Feldman R. Venipuncture and Peripheral Intravenous Access. Reichman and Simon. Emergency Medicine Procedures. New York: Mcgraw Hill; 2004. 297-313.
3. Dougherty L. Peripheral cannulation. Nurs Stand. 2008 Sep 3-9. 22(52):49-56; quiz 58.
4. Roseman JM. Deep, percutaneous antecubital venipuncture: An alternative to surgical cutdown. Am J Surg. 1983 Aug. 146(2):285.

18

Brain relaxation

RAVI K. GRANDHI, SAMUEL Y. LEE, and ALAA ABD-ELSAYED

Introduction

Intracranial pressure (ICP), which refers to the pressure inside the skull and thus in the brain and cerebrospinal fluid (CSF), is a critical component to be managed preoperatively both in neurosurgical procedures and in head trauma situations. Elevated ICP can occur due to a variety of mechanisms, such as presence of a brain mass (tumor, edema, hematoma, abscess), generalized brain swelling (acute liver failure, hypertensive encephalopathy, hypercarbia), increase in venous pressure, obstruction to CSF flow and/or absorption, and increased production of CSF. At baseline, the body regulates ICP through alterations in absorption or production of CSF. ICP is normally 7–15 mmHg in a supine adult.[1] Once ICP raises to 20–25 mmHg, providers must consider management strategies to help lower it, particularly if it is an acute increase in the ICP. Elevated ICP is associated with very adverse outcomes, including, but not limited to, brain death or severe cognitive disabilities due to hypoperfusion of the brain as a result of the elevated ICP obstructing cerebral perfusion. In a study of 846 patients with traumatic brain injury (TBI), mortality rates were found to be 14% if the ICP was <20 mmHg by 48 h, but increased to 34%

if the ICP was >30 mmHg at 48 h.[2] This chapter discusses the importance of brain relaxation via management of ICP.

Pathophysiology

The cranium and vertebral canal are relatively inelastic parts, so any increase in volume of brain (approximately 80%), blood (approximately 12%), or CSF (approximately 8%) will increase the ICP.[3] The normal brain weighs 1400 g and contains 75 mL CSF and 75 mL blood. An additional 100–150 mL fluid can be absorbed in the cranium before ICP begins to rise.[4] The relationship between these variables (ICP, CSF volume, brain tissue, blood, and cerebral perfusion pressure) is known as the Monro–Kellie hypothesis, which states that the cranium and its constituents are in an incompressible compartment, so any increase in the volume of one of these cranial constituents must be compensated by a decrease in the volume of another.[5] When ICP is between 15 and approximately 25 mmHg, increases in one of the three components can be sufficiently compensated with changes in the amount of CSF in the cranium. Major compensatory mechanisms include an initial displacement of CSF from the cranial to the spinal compartment, increased absorption of CSF, decrease in CSF production, and decrease in cerebral blood volume (venous).[3] Although this autoregulation functions well in the normal brain, it is impaired in the injured brain. In addition, the time course of change also affects how ICP responds. A brain tumor that is slowly growing may often present normally or with a mild elevation in the ICP because the brain has time to accommodate. Conversely, even an intracranial bleed that occurs suddenly can produce a sharp and sudden rise in the ICP. Regardless of whether the progression is acute or insidious, elevated ICP will develop as compensatory mechanisms are exhausted. Once the amount of pressure exceeds 25 mmHg, every small change in volume can lead to marked increases in the ICP due to failure of the intracranial compliance. Such an increase in the ICP can decrease cerebral perfusion pressure (CPP), which is the pressure of the blood flowing to the brain; CPP (normally 80–100 mmHg) is equal to the mean arterial pressure (MAP) minus the ICP. CPP <60–70 mmHg worsens the outcomes.[4] Further, increased ICP is particularly concerning because, by decreasing CPP, it can lead to ischemia of the brain. The body's response to the fall in the CPP is to raise the systemic blood pressure and dilate the cerebral blood vessels. Although this may initially increase perfusion of the brain, the increased cerebral blood volume will further increase ICP and lower the CPP. This is a vicious cycle that leads to ischemia and brain infarction over time. If there are sustained pressures <25 mmHg, then there may be irreversible brain damage.[3] Symon et al.[6] further detailed the relationship between the ICP, cerebral blood flow (CBF), and functional effects:

CBF of 50 mL/100 g/min: normal
CBF of 25 mL/100 g/min: EEG slowing
CBF of 6–15 mL/100 g/min: ischemic penumbra
CBF of <6 mL/100 g/min: neuronal death

ICP can also be increased due to a space-occupying lesion such as a hematoma or a brain mass that can result in a midline shift. The midline shift can compress the ventricles and lead to hydrocephalus or it can be pushed against the skull or outside of the skull, causing a herniation. If there is any sort of brain stem compression, then it can be fatal due to respiratory depression.

Presentation

While significant morbidity due to infarction or respiratory depression is rare, there are other presentations that occur more frequently. Initially, patients are often asymptomatic. However, over time more symptoms develop, including headache, vomiting without nausea, ocular palsies, altered level of consciousness, back pain, and papilledema. Usually changes in consciousness occur at ICP >40. The headache is quite unique in that it is classically a morning headache that may wake the patient from sleep. This occurs due to a reduced oxygen supply of the brain at night secondary to relative hypoventilation during sleep or cerebral edema that may be exacerbated from recumbent positioning. The headache is worse with coughing and sneezing, and may worsen with time. There may also be various changes in personality and behavior. If there is any midline shift or herniation, then there may be changes associated with displacement of brain tissue, which may include pupillary dilation, abducens palsies, or Cushing's triad (widening pulse pressure, irregular respirations, and bradycardia).[7] In children, a low heart rate may indicate an elevated ICP. In infants and small children, since the fontanels are not closed, the soft spots on the head bulge when ICP increases significantly.

Management

Acute

The treatment or prevention of factors that may precipitate or exacerbate ICP is of utmost importance upon initial treatment of elevated ICP. Elevating the head of bed (HOB) and keeping the head in a neutral position is the standard of care to improve venous drainage and promote displacement of CSF from the intracranial compartment to the spinal compartment.[8] The primary complication with reducing blood flow to the brain is that it can cause ischemia. Optimal respiratory management to control ICP is imperative, as respiratory dysfunction is common in patients with elevated ICP. The resulting hypoxia and hypercapnia can increase ICP substantially. Controlled ventilation should be implemented with a goal of PaO_2 >100 mmHg and $PaCO_2$ 30–35 mmHg. MAP should be maintained at the preintubation level and the lowest possible airway pressure should be maintained so as not to impede the venous drainage.

Although pain and agitation may contribute significantly to increasing ICP, there is no sedative regimen that has clear advantages in patients with elevated ICP. Sedation should only be used in agitated or anxious patients.[9] This may increase metabolic demand, thus increasing oxygen consumption and increasing blood pressure.[10] In such cases, morphine (2–5 mg/kg/h) and vecuronium 10 (mg/h) may be used to decrease anxiety and response to pain, both of which contribute to increased ICP. In patients at risk for elevated ICP, fever should be controlled with antipyretics and cooling blankets. Fever can increase CBF due to increasing metabolic requirements and exacerbate elevated ICP due to dilation of cerebral vessels. Furthermore, fever has been shown to worsen neurologic injury in experimental models of TBI.[11]

Patients with intracranial hypertension commonly have systemic hypertension as well. While it is contraindicated to reduce systemic blood pressure in patients with untreated intracranial mass lesions, it is controversial whether systemic hypertension in patients without an intracranial mass lesion should be treated. In patients with untreated intracranial mass lesions, it is clear that cerebral perfusion is maintained by the higher systemic blood pressure. In patients without a mass lesion, particularly in those with impaired pressure autoregulation secondary to TBI, the systemic hypertension may increase CBF and ICP. The choice of antihypertensive agent is very important if the decision is made to treat systemic hypertension. Vasodilating drugs (nitroprusside, nitroglycerin, and nifedipine) should be avoided, as they can increase the ICP and may reflexively increase plasma catecholamines. Antihypertensive drugs that reduce blood pressure without affecting the ICP are preferred; these include beta-blockers (labetalol and esmolol) and central-acting alpha-receptor agonists (clonidine).[12]

In addition, in situations in which intubation is necessary, a neuromuscular blockade (NMB) and lidocaine should be given. An NMB reduces ICP by preventing the patient from coughing while lidocaine blunts the autonomic response to intubation, thus avoiding a further increase in the ICP. Paralysis allows the cerebral veins to be drained more easily; however, it can mask the signs of seizures. Another option to reduce the ICP is to reduce MAPs via administration of an antihypertensive. However, this is a rarely used option.

In situations of acute elevations of ICP, first oxygenate the patient appropriately and elevate the HOB up to 30°. If the patient needs to be intubated, then give an NMB and lidocaine.

Persistent elevation in ICP

Patients with sustained elevated ICP of 20–25 mmHg or higher need additional treatment measures to control it. If ICP continues to be elevated after initial treatment, heavier sedation and paralysis may be necessary. As previously discussed, routine paralysis is not indicated, but intracranial hypertension caused by agitation, posturing, or coughing can be prevented by sedation and nondepolarizing muscle relaxants that do not alter cerebrovascular resistance (CVR). Commonly, a regimen of morphine and lorazepam for analgesia/sedation and cisatracurium or vecuronium as a muscle relaxant is used, with the dose titrated by twitch response.[13] This regimen has been effective in lowering ICP, but it can be difficult to perform a neurologic physical examination; interrupting this regimen once per day before morning rounds to allow for the neurologic examination will not prevent this therapy from working effectively.

If there is an intact blood–brain barrier, osmotherapy can be performed using IV mannitol. Mannitol is the most commonly used hyperosmolar option for the treatment of elevated ICP. It should be administered in boluses at 0.25–1 g/kg; this is preferred over continuous infusion (continuous infusion can reverse the osmotic gradient because it may enter the CSF).[14] Mannitol decreases blood viscosity and decreases ICP by reducing cerebral parenchymal cell water. Onset of effect is 1–5 min with a peak total effect at approximately 20–30 min.[14] Vigorous and repetitive administrations of mannitol may lead to side effects such as excess diuresis, electrolyte abnormalities, and intraoperative hypovolemia if patients later undergo neurosurgical procedures. Normoglycemia needs to be maintained and, in some cases, insulin should be used. Maintenance fluids should be given judiciously, so as not to exacerbate cerebral edema. Isotonic saline (aiming to keep serum sodium above 135 mmol/L) is preferred to glucose-containing solutions.

In patients with elevated ICP resistant to mannitol, hypertonic 3% saline can be administered as an alternative. This saline (1–2 mL/kg) provides a similar osmotic effect as mannitol. In addition, it also enhances cardiac output, reduces inflammation, restores normal cellular resting membrane potential and cell volume, and stimulates the release of atrial natriuretic peptide. This may help counteract perioperative hypotensive effects.[15] There may even be the potential for use of hypertonic saline in situations where there are large fluid administrations leading to cerebral swelling and intracranial hypertension; however, this is not clearly proven yet.[15] Studies have also indicated the potential for hypertonic saline to have longer lasting effects.[16,17] Further studies are needed to fully compare the effectiveness of these two hyperosmotic agents.

Hyperventilation has been shown to lower ICP. While this is not the preferred method to control elevated ICP, it can be the method of last resort. While hyperventilation does decrease ICP, it is also known to decrease CBF by 3%–4% for every 1 mmHg decrease in PCO_2.[18] This treatment option is highly controversial as there is inadequate data to assess whether the benefit outweighs the harm.

In patients with refractory intracranial hypertension, inducing a barbiturate coma may be carefully considered. This therapy includes pentobarbital given in a loading dose of 10 mg/kg followed by 5 mg/kg each hour for 3 h. A maintenance dose of 1–2 mg/g/h is then continued and titrated to a serum level of 30–50 µg/mL. In a randomized multicenter study, Eisenberg et al.[19] have shown that the use of barbiturate coma in patients with refractory intracranial hypertension resulted in a twofold improvement in controlling ICP. Similar findings have also been reported by Bader et al.[20] However, other studies have not shown the benefits of high-dose barbiturate coma in the management of elevated ICP due to increased mortality.[21] As a result, more research has to be conducted to evaluate the use of barbiturates.

Other treatment options that require further study include hypothermia and steroids. A multicenter randomized clinical trial of moderate hypothermia was conducted in patients with severe TBI. Although it showed no significant benefit in neurologic outcomes, it did show that those randomized to moderate hypothermia had less intracranial hypertension.[22] A pilot randomized clinical trial was then conducted and showed similar findings.[23] Routine induction of hypothermia is not yet indicated, but it may be an important adjunctive option to consider in patients with refractory elevated ICP. Mild hypothermia may be protective, but extreme levels will exacerbate coagulopathy and bleeding. If there are concerns regarding coagulopathies or bleeding, then the abnormalities should be corrected. Steroids are commonly used to decrease vasogenic cerebral edema in patients with primary and metastatic brain tumors. This use of steroids has been shown to decrease intracranial hypertension over 2–5 days after initiating the treatment.[24] Of note, steroid therapy should not be implemented in patients with increased ICP secondary to TBI or spontaneous intracerebral hemorrhage; they have been shown to have no benefit,[24,25] and even exert detrimental effects.[26,27]

Clinical pearl

If the ICP remains elevated, then consider adding mannitol followed by hypertonic saline. The evidence for hyperventilation, barbiturate coma, hypothermia, and steroids is limited.

Neuroanesthesia

During surgical operations, ICP may be affected by four variables: hyperventilation, diuretics, head position, and anesthetic drugs. The first three have been discussed, so the focus of this section is regarding the use of anesthetic drugs. Volatile anesthetics produce direct vasodilation and thus have the potential to increase ICP. While this increase is usually not significant if the anesthetic concentration is below 1.2 MAC, it becomes a concern with elevated ICPs.[28–31] Hypocapnia blunts the increase in CBF and ICP that usually occurs with volatile anesthetics.[3]

Propofol- and volatile-maintained anesthesia were associated with similar brain relaxation scores, although mean ICP values were lower and CPP values were higher with propofol-maintained anesthesia.[32] Intravenous agents preserve autoregulation while inhalational agents impair it to varying degrees. As a result, in situations of extremely elevated ICP, some may prefer to use total intravenous anesthesia (TIVA). TIVA decreases CBF and cerebral metabolism while increasing CVR. This decrease in cerebral metabolism, redistribution of cerebral blood flow, and prevention of large increases in blood glucose may be neuroprotective. Intravenous induction agents (barbiturate, propofol) are the most potent depressants of cerebral metabolic rate (CMR), followed by inhalational agents (isoflurane, sevoflurane, desflurane), benzodiazepines (midazolam), and narcotics (fentanyl, alfentanil, sufentanil). All intravenous agents, with the exception of ketamine, decrease ICP.

Opioids also have a role to play. Remifentanil seems to be particularly suitable for neurosurgery because of its rapid onset and rapid offset of action and minimal effect on ICP. The important difference between remifentanil and other opioids is remifentanil's rapid offset of action that facilitates early response to verbal commands and rapid tracheal extubation.

Summary

When there is concern with elevated ICP intraoperatively, limit the use of volatile anesthetics and use TIVA if possible.

Conclusion

Elevated ICP is something all providers must be acutely aware of both inside and outside the operating room. Serious complications, including death, are associated with elevated ICP. Management varies based on the length of time since occurrence—immediate management includes ensuring adequate oxygenation and elevating the HOB. Soon thereafter, mannitol has an important role if the ICP continues to be a concern. Sedation or paralytics also has an important role. Further, operative considerations include the use of TIVA rather than volatile anesthetics.

References

1. Steiner LA, Andrews PJ. Monitoring the injured brain: ICP and CBF. *Br J Anaesth* 2006;97(1):26–38.
2. Jiang JY, Gao GY, Li WP, Yu MK, Zhu C. Early indicators of prognosis in 846 cases of severe traumatic brain injury. *J Neurotrauma* 2002;19(7):869–874.
3. Butterworth JF, Mackey DC, Wasnick JD, Morgan GE, Mikhail MS. *Morgan and Mikhail's Clinical Anesthesiology*. New York: McGraw-Hill; 2013.
4. Bouma GJ, Muizelaar JP. Cerebral blood flow, cerebral blood volume, and cerebrovascular reactivity after severe head injury. *J Neurotrauma* 1992;9(Suppl. 1):S333–S348.
5. Mokri B. The Monro–Kellie hypothesis: Applications in CSF volume depletion. *Neurol* 2001;56(12):1746–1748.
6. Symon L, Lassen NA, Astrup J, Branston NM. Thresholds of ischaemia in brain cortex. *Adv Exp Med Biol* 1977 Jul 4–7;94:775–782.
7. Sanders MJ, McKenna K. Head and facial trauma. In: *Mosby's Paramedic Textbook*. 2nd ed. St. Louis, MO: Mosby; 2001, p. 22.
8. Rosner MJ, Coley IB. Cerebral perfusion pressure, intracranial pressure, and head elevation. *J Neurosurg* 1986;65:636–641.
9. Hsiang JK, Chesnut RM, Crisp CB, Klauber MR, Blunt BA, Marshall LF. Early, routine paralysis for intracranial pressure control in severe head injury: Is it necessary? *Crit Care Med* 1994;22(9):1471–1476.
10. Bechtel K. Pediatric controversies: Diagnosis and management of traumatic brain injuries. Trauma Report. Supplement to Emergency Medicine Reports, Pediatric Emergency Medicine Reports, ED Management, and Emergency Medicine Alert. Volume 5, Number 3. Thomson American Health Consultants.
11. Dietrich WD, Alonso O, Halley M, Busto R. Delayed posttraumatic brain hyperthermia worsens outcome after fluid percussion brain injury: A light and electron microscopic study in rats. *Neurosurgery* 1996;38:533–541.
12. Robertson CS, Clifton GL, Taylor AA, Grossman RG. Treatment of hypertension associated with head injury. *J Neurosurg* 1983;59:455–460.
13. Schramm WM, Papousek A, Michalek-Sauberer A, Czech T, Illievich U. The cerebral and cardiovascular effects of cisatracurium and atracurium in neurosurgical patients. *Anesth Analg* 1998;86:123–127.
14. Sakowitz OW, Stover JF, Sarafzadeh AS, Unterberg AW, Kiening KL. Effects of mannitol bolus administration on

intracranial pressure, cerebral extracellular metabolites, and tissue oxygenation in severely head-injured patients. *J Trauma* 2007;62(2):292–298.

15. Shao L, Hong E, Zou Y, Hao X, Hou H, Tian M. Hypertonic saline for brain relaxation and intracranial pressure in patients undergoing neurosurgical procedures: A meta-analysis of randomized controlled trials. *PLoS One* 2015;10(1):e0117314.

16. Vialet R, Albanèse J, Thomachot L et al. Isovolume hypertonic solutes (sodium chloride or mannitol) in the treatment of refractory posttraumatic intracranial hypertension: 2 mL/kg 7.5% saline is more effective than 2 mL/kg 20% mannitol. *Crit Care Med* 2003;31(6):1683–1687.

17. Mirski MA, Denchev DI, Schnitzer MS, Hanley DF. Comparison between hypertonic saline and mannitol in the reduction of elevated intracranial pressure in a rodent model of acute cerebral injury. *J Neurosurg Anesthesiol* 2000;12(4):334–344.

18. Raichle ME, Posner JB, Plum F. Cerebral blood flow during and after hyperventilation. *Arch Neurol* 1970;23(5):394–403.

19. Eisenberg HM, Frankowski RF, Contant CF, Marshall LF, Walker MD. High-dose barbiturate control of elevated intracranial pressure in patients with severe head injury. *J Neurosurg* 1988;69:15–23.

20. Bader MK, Arbour R, Palmer S. Refractory increased intracranial pressure in severe traumatic brain injury: Barbiturate coma and bispectral index monitoring. *AACN Clin Issues* 2005;16:526–541.

21. Schwartz, ML, Tator CH, Rowed DW, Reid SR, Meguro K, Andrews DF. The University of Toronto head injury treatment study: A prospective, randomized comparison of pentobarbital and mannitol. *Can J Neurol Sci* 1984;11(4):434–440.

22. Clifton GL, Miller ER, Choi SC et al. Lack of effect of induction of hypothermia after acute brain injury. *N Engl J Med* 2001;344:556–563.

23. Adelson PD, Ragheb J, Kanev P et al. Phase II clinical trial of moderate hypothermia after severe traumatic brain injury in children. *Neurosurgery* 2005;56:740–754.

24. Saul T, Ducker T, Saleman M, Carro E. Steroids in severe head injury: A prospective, randomized clinical trial. *J Neurosurg* 1981;54:596–600.

25. Gudeman S, Miller J, Becker D. Failure of high-dose steroid therapy to influence intracranial pressure in patients with severe head injury. *J Neurosurg* 1979;51:301–306.

26. Edwards P, Arango M, Balica L et al. Final results of MRC CRASH, a randomised placebo-controlled trial of intravenous corticosteroid in adults with head injury—outcomes at 6 months. *Lancet* 2005;365:1957–1959.

27. Feigin VL, Anderson N, Rinkel GJ, Algra A, van Gijn J, Bennett DA. Corticosteroids for aneurysmal subarachnoid haemorrhage and primary intracerebral haemorrhage. *Cochrane Database Syst Rev* 2005;(3):CD004583.

28. Sponheim S, Skraastad Ø, Helseth E, Due-Tønnesen B, Aamodt G, Breivik H. Effects of 0.5 and 1.0 MAC isoflurane, sevoflurane and desflurane on intracranial and cerebral perfusion pressures in children. *Acta Anaesthesiol Scand* 2003;47(8):932–938.

29. Kaye A, Kucera IJ, Heavner J et al. The comparative effects of desflurane and isoflurane on lumbar cerebrospinal fluid pressure in patients undergoing craniotomy for supratentorial tumors. *Anesth Analg* 2004;98(4):1127–1132, table of contents.

30. Fraga M, Rama-Maceiras P, Rodiño S, Aymerich H, Pose P, Belda J. The effects of isoflurane and desflurane on intracranial pressure, cerebral perfusion pressure, and cerebral arteriovenous oxygen content difference in normocapnic patients with supratentorial brain tumors. *Anesthesiology* 2003;98(5):1085–1090.

31. Ravussin P, Guinard JP, Ralley F, Thorin D. Effect of propofol on cerebrospinal fluid pressure and cerebral perfusion pressure in patients undergoing craniotomy. *Anaesthesia* 1988;43 Suppl:37–41.

32. Chui J, Mariappan R, Mehta J, Manninen P, Venkatraghavan L. Comparison of propofol and volatile agents for maintenance of anesthesia during elective craniotomy procedures: Systematic review and meta-analysis. *Can J Anesth* 2014;61(4):347–356.

19

Anesthetic agents: Intravenous

INDU KAPOOR

Introduction

Anesthesia for neurosurgery requires not only understanding of the anatomy and physiology of the central nervous system (CNS) but also the possible changes occurring in response to infections, lesions, and trauma. To balance anesthesia with smooth induction and emergence, maintenance of an adequate cerebral perfusion pressure (CPP) and cerebral blood flow (CBF), avoidance of intracranial hypertension, and the provision of optimal surgical conditions need attention. The comprehensive knowledge of anesthetic drugs and their effects on cerebral metabolism, circulation, and intracranial pressure (ICP) is very important. The selection of a specific drug and its route of administration to produce general anesthesia is based on its pharmacokinetic properties and its secondary effect. Intravenous agents enter the highly perfused and lipophilic tissues in the brain and spinal cord where they produce anesthesia within a single circulation time. The drug is redistributed out of the brain into the blood and then it enters the less perfused tissues

such as muscles and viscera. Intravenous anesthetic agents decrease both CBF and cerebral metabolic rate of oxygen ($CMRO_2$) consumption (Table 19.1); however, $CMRO_2$ is decreased but CBF is increased by inhalational anesthetic agents. This decrease in CBF by intravenous agents may occur as a result of decreased cerebral metabolism secondary to depressed cerebral function. Among all intravenous anesthetic agents, ketamine is the only agent that produces an increase in CBF, $CMRO_2$, and ICP. This chapter discusses the most commonly used intravenous anesthetic agents and their anesthetic implications in patients undergoing brain tumor surgery (Table 19.2).

Barbiturates

Barbiturates are derivatives of barbituric acid (2,4,6-trioxohexahydropyrimidine). They are the central nervous system depressant drugs that can induce mild sedation to total anesthesia. They can also produce hypnosis and anxiolysis, and are also effective as anticonvulsants and analgesics.

Table 19.1 Cerebral Effects of Intravenous Anesthetic Agents

Anesthetic agents	ICP	CPP	CBF	CMRO$_2$	CSF dynamics	
					Resistance to resorption	CSF formation
Thiopentone sodium	--	++	---	---	0/-	+/0/-
Propofol	--	++	--	--	0	0
Etomidate	--	++	--	--	0/--	0/-
Ketamine	++	--	++	+	0/-	+

CSF, cerebrospinal fluid; +, increase; -, decrease; 0, no effect

Table 19.2 Physical Properties of Intravenous Anesthetic Agents

Drugs	Induction dose (intravenous)	Induction duration (min)	t$_{1/2}$ (h)	Clearance (mL/kg/min)	Protein binding (%)
Sodium thiopental	3–5 mg/kg	5–8	12.1	3.4	85
Propofol	2.0–2.5 mg/kg	4–8	1.8	23–50	95–99
Etomidate	0.2–0.4 mg/kg	4–8	2.9–5.3	18–25	76
Ketamine	0.5–1.5 mg/kg	10–15	3	19.1	12

t$_{1/2}$, half-life

The most commonly used barbiturate in clinical anesthesia is *sodium thiopental.* The formulation of barbiturates involves their preparation as sodium salts mixed with 6% anhydrous sodium carbonate by weight and then reconstituted with either water or normal saline to produce 2.5% solution of thiopental. Thiobarbiturates remain stable for 1 week after reconstitution.

Mechanism of action

These agents act primarily as an agonist of gamma-aminobutyric acid A (GABAA) receptors.[1] Their sedative and hypnotic effect is due to interaction with inhibitory neuron GABA. Like benzodiazepines, barbiturates potentiate the effect of GABA at this receptor. In addition to GABA receptors, they also act on glutamate receptors, adenosine receptors, and nicotinic acetylcholine receptors.

Pharmacokinetics

The clinically recommended dosage and pharmacokinetics of sodium thiopental are summarized in Table 19.2. The induction dosage of thiopental produces unconsciousness in 10–30 s and the duration of anesthesia is 5–8 min. However the elderly population requires a low induction dose (1–3 mg/kg) compared to neonates and infants (5–8 mg/kg).[2,3] Intravenous injection of barbiturates can produce a little pain, which can be eliminated by prior intravenous injection of lidocaine (0.5–1.0 mg/kg). Intra-arterial injection should be avoided as it might cause severe inflammatory reaction. Thiopental is eliminated by hepatic metabolism and renal excretion. In pediatric patients without intravenous access, anesthesia can be induced by giving these drugs rectally at tenfold intravenous dose.

Systemic effects

Sodium thiopentone produces a dose-dependent decrease in CBF, CMRO$_2$, and ICP. Decrease in CBF and CMRO$_2$ occurs until the electroencephalogram becomes flat. Thiopental produces significant reduction in infarct size on moderate doses.[4] Because of its neuroprotective effect, thiopental is considered a favorable drug for patients undergoing neurosurgical procedure. Its systemic effects on the central nervous system and other systems of human body are described briefly in Table 19.3.

Propofol

Propofol (2,6-diisopropylphenol) is also known as "milk of amnesia," because of its milklike appearance.[5] The presently available preparation of propofol is 1% (10 mg/mL), which contains 2.25% glycerol as a tonicity/stabilizing agent, 10% soybean oil, and 1.2% purified egg phospholipid as an emulsifier, with sodium hydroxide to adjust the pH. A local anesthetic such as lignocaine as well as an opioid such as fentanyl can be combined with propofol to decrease the pain.[6] A recently developed form of propofol, fospropofol, does not cause pain on intravenous administration like the traditional one.

Mechanism of action

The mechanism of action is either though activation of GABA receptors[7,8] or though blocking action on sodium channels.[9,10] However, propofol is assumed to exert its sedative and hypnotic effects through GABA receptor interaction.

Pharmacokinetics

The clinically recommended dosage and pharmacokinetics of propofol are summarized in Table 19.2. The induction dose of propofol in a healthy individual is 1.5–2.5 mg/kg. Because of its short half-life, propofol can also be used as total intravenous anesthesia in maintenance of anesthesia. The maintenance dose of propofol in patients <55 years is 0.1–0.2 mg/kg/min and in patients >55 years, it is 0.05–0.1 mg/kg. Recovery after propofol infusion or multiple doses is much faster than that after barbiturates.[11] In patients receiving propofol for prolonged duration, there is increased risk of developing "propofol infusion syndrome," which is a rare medical condition. It usually develops if infusion is continued for more than 48 h at a dose of 4 mg/kg/h.[12] This potentially lethal metabolic derangement has been more commonly found in children and critically ill patients on prolonged infusion of high-dose substance in combination with catecholamines or corticosteroids.[13] The signs and symptoms of propofol infusion syndrome include rhabdomyolysis, metabolic acidosis, cardiac failure, and renal failure.[12,14,15]

Systemic effects

Propofol also causes dose-related reduction in CBF and ICP along with decrease in $CMRO_2$.

Table 19.3 Systemic Effects of Sodium Thiopentone

Central nervous system	• Decreases CBF, $CMRO_2$
	• Decreases ICP
	• Decreases infarct volume
	• Exerts neuroprotective effect
	• Causes burst suppression on electroencephalogram
	• Is a proven drug for status epilepticus
Cardiovascular system	• Leads to a dose-dependent decrease in blood pressure
	• Is a venodilator: decreases LVEDV
	• Maintains myocardial oxygen demand and supply ratio
	• Is safe to use in patients with coronary artery disease or valvular heart disease
Respiratory system	• Acts like primarily respiratory depressants
	• Decreases respiratory rate, tidal volume, minute ventilation
	• Diminishes respiratory response to hypoxia and hypercarbia
Other systems	• Exerts no significant effect on renal, endocrine, and hepatic systems if used for shorter duration

LVEDV, left ventricular end diastolic volume

Its cerebral and metabolic effects are found to be similar to sodium thiopental. Many of the studies have reported the favorable effect of burst suppression by propofol.[16,17] The mechanisms that contribute to make propofol a neuroprotective agent include antioxidant activity, enhancement of GABA receptor actions, cerebral metabolic rate reduction, and prevention of mitochondrial swelling.[18] Systemic effects of propofol on various systems in the human body are described briefly in Table 19.4.

Etomidate

Etomidate (ethyl 3-[(1R)-1-phenylethyl]imidazo-5-carboxylate) is a short-acting anesthetic agent used for induction of general anesthesia as well as for sedation.[19] It is a clear colorless solution for injection containing 2 mg/mL etomidate in an aqueous solution of 35% propylene glycol. Etomidate is also used because of its limited suppression of ventilation, lack of histamine release, and protection from myocardial and cerebral ischemia.[20] Thus, it is considered a good inducing agent in patients who are hemodynamically unstable.

Mechanism of action

The drug acts primarily on $GABA_A$ receptors[21] and is highly protein bound. It is metabolized by hepatic and plasma esterases to inactive products.[22,23] Its elimination is through both biliary (22%) and renal (78%) routes.

Pharmacokinetics

The clinically recommended dosage and pharmacokinetics of etomidate are summarized in Table 19.2. Injection of etomidate has rapid onset and recovery. Its onset of action is 30–60 s and peak effect is achieved at 1 min. Intravenous administration of etomidate causes severe pain and myoclonic movement. This myoclonic activity can be reduced by prior administration of opioids. Etomidate also suppresses corticosteroid synthesis in the adrenal cortex by reversibly inhibiting 11-beta-hydroxylase, leading to primary adrenal suppression.[24,25] Another drawback of etomidate is that it has also been associated with vomiting.[26]

Systemic effects

Etomidate like sodium thiopental reduces $CMRO_2$ until there is an isoelectric EEG pattern. With a decrease in CBF, there is a parallel decrease in ICP but without affecting the CPP. Overall, it has cerebral depressant effect. The neuroprotective effect of etomidate is undetermined because of varied reports in the literature.[27-29] Further large studies are required to draw any conclusion on its neuroprotective effect. Systemic effects of etomidate on various systems are described briefly in Table 19.5.

Table 19.4 Systemic Effects of Propofol

Central nervous system	• Decreases CBF, ICP, $CMRO_2$ • Decreases IOP • Exerts neuroprotective effect • Exerts anticonvulsant effect
Cardiovascular system	• Causes dose-dependent decrease in blood pressure • Decreases myocardial blood flow, oxygen consumption • Reduces SVR • Blunts baroreceptor reflex
Respiratory system	• Acts like primarily respiratory depressants • Can cause frequent apnea • Produces profound reduction in tidal volume, minute ventilation, functional residual capacity, and respiratory rate • Can induce bronchospasm in patients with reactive airway disease
Other systems	• Has no significant effect on renal, endocrine, and hepatic system if used for shorter duration

IOP, intraocular pressure; SVR, systemic vascular resistance

Table 19.5 Systemic Effects of Etomidate

Central nervous system	• Decreases CBF, CMRO$_2$
	• Decreases ICP
	• Exerts neuroprotective effect
Cardiovascular system	• Is a cardiostable drug
	• Causes minimal or no fall in blood pressure
	• Exerts minimal effect on coronary perfusion pressure
	• Can cause slight increase in heart rate
Respiratory system	• Exerts minimal effect on respiratory system
	• Can cause short-duration apnea, hypoventilation, sometimes hyperventilation
	• Can also cause laryngospasm and hiccup
	• Preserves ventilatory response to carbon dioxide
Other systems	• Exerts no significant effect on renal, endocrine, and hepatic system if used for shorter duration

Ketamine

Ketamine is a phencyclidine derivative and its chemical formulation is arylcyclohexylamine. It produces the state called "dissociated anesthesia," which is characterized by the presence of dissociation between thalamocortical and limbic systems.[30] It is an anesthetic state in which the eyes remain open with slow nystagmus. Independent skeletal muscle movement often occurs after the administration of this drug. It also provides intense analgesia as well as amnesia. Because of the possibility of increased airway secretions and emergence delirium, it is advised to give antisialagogue (glycopyrrolate) and midazolam as a premedication in patients receiving ketamine.

Mechanism of action

Ketamine mainly binds to N-methyl-D-aspartate (NMDA) receptors. It also acts on other receptors such as opioid receptors, GABA receptors, muscarinic receptors, and voltage-sensitive sodium channels and calcium channels.

Pharmacokinetics

Ketamine can be administered through many routes: intravenous, intramuscular, oral, and per-rectal (PR). The induction dose of ketamine is 0.5–1.5 mg/kg intravenously, 4–6 mg/kg intramuscularly (IM), and 8–10 mg/kg through the PR route.[24] It is highly lipid soluble and has rapid onset of action and relative duration of action like barbiturates. For maintenance of anesthesia, ketamine is occasionally used in infusion at a dose of 25–100 µg/kg/min.[31] The patient can develop tolerance with continuous use. Ketamine is not highly bounded to plasma proteins, hence it is rapidly distributed to tissues. Because of high lipid solubility, it rapidly crosses the blood–brain barrier. Ketamine further increases the CBF, leading to increased concentration of drug in the brain. It is metabolized in liver, has high hepatic clearance, and is excreted by the kidney. Also, the volume of distribution is very high, leading to an elimination half-life of 2–3 h.

Systemic effects

In both humans and animals, ketamine is found to increase CBF, ICP, and CMRO$_2$. The maximum increase in regional CBF is in frontal and parieto-occipital areas. The increase in ICP is marked with ketamine. However, it can be reduced or blocked by benzodiazepine or induced hypocapnia. Its neuroprotective effect has been shown in various intracranial pathologies such as head trauma and ischemia; however, these findings have been reported only in studies with a short observation period.[32] At 6 months, ketamine failed to provide a beneficial effect on functional outcome.[33] The systemic effects of ketamine on various systems are described briefly in Table 19.6.

Table 19.6 Systemic Effects of Ketamine

Central nervous system	• Increases CBF, ICP, and CMRO$_2$
	• Increases IOP
	• Can induce emergence delirium
	• Increases the amplitude of somatosensory evoked potentials
Cardiovascular system	• Increases heart rate, blood pressure, and cardiac output
	• Increases myocardial oxygen consumption
	• Has indirect sympathomimetic activity
	• Increases arrhythmogenic effect of epinephrine
Respiratory system	• Causes less respiratory depression compared to other inducing agents
	• Preserves airway reflexes as well as airway tone
	• Preserves ventilatory response to carbon dioxide
	• Causes bronchodilation
Other systems	• Exerts no significant effect on renal, endocrine, and hepatic systems

References

1. Loscher W, Rogawski MA. How theories evolved concerning the mechanism of action of barbiturates. *Epilepsia* 2012;53:12–25.
2. Homer TD, Stanski DR. The effect of increasing age on thiopental disposition and anesthetic requirement. *Anesthesiology* 1985;62:714–724.
3. Jonmarker C, Westrin P, Larsson S, Werner O. Thiopental requirement for induction of anesthesia in children. *Anesthesiology* 1987;67:104–107.
4. Warner DS, Takaoka S, Wu B et al. Electroencephalographic burst suppression is not required to elicit maximal neuroprotection from pentobarbital in a model of focal cerebral ischemia. *Anesthesiology* 1996;84:1475–1484.
5. Euliano TY, Gravenstein JS. A brief pharmacology related to anesthesia. *Essential Anesthesia: From Science to Practice. Cambridge*, UK: Cambridge University Press; 2009, p. 173.
6. Miner JR, Burton JH. Clinical practice advisory: Emergency department procedural sedation with propofol. *Ann Emerg Med* 2007;50:182–187.
7. Trapani G, Latrofa A, Franco M et al. Propofol analogues. Synthesis, relationships between structure and affinity at GABA$_A$ receptor in rat brain, and differential electrophysiological profile at recombinant human GABAA receptors. *J Med Chem* 1998;41:1846–1854.
8. Krasowski MD, Jenkins A, Flood P, Kung AY, Hopfinger AJ, Harrison NL. General anesthetic potencies of a series of propofol analogs correlate with potency for potentiation of gamma-aminobutyric acid (GABA) current at the GABA(A) receptor but not with lipid solubility. *J Pharmacol Exp Ther* 2001;297:338–351.
9. Haeseler G, Leuwer M. High-affinity block of voltage-operated rat IIA neuronal sodium channels by 2,6 di-*tert*-butylphenol, a propofol analogue. *Eur J Anaesthesiol* 2003;20:220–224.
10. Haeseler G, Karst M, Foadi N et al. High-affinity blockade of voltage-operated skeletal muscle and neuronal sodium channels by halogenated propofol analogues. *Br J Pharmacol* 2008;155:265–275.
11. Doze VA, Westphal LM, White PF. Comparison of propofol with methohexital for outpatient anesthesia. *Anesth Analg* 1986;65:1189–1195.
12. Kam PC, Cardone D. Propofol infusion syndrome. *Anaesthesia* 2007;62:690.
13. Vasile B, Rasulo F, Candiani A, Latronico N. The pathophysiology of propofol infusion syndrome: A simple name for a complex syndrome. *Intensive Care Med* 2003;29:1417–1425.
14. Zaccheo MM, Bucher DH. Propofol infusion syndrome: A rare complication with potentially fatal results. *Crit Care Nurs* 2008;28:18–25.
15. Sharshar T. [ICU-acquired neuromyopathy, delirium and sedation in intensive care unit]. *Ann Fr Anesth Reanim* 2008;27:617–622.

16. Cervantes M, Ruelas R, Chávez-Carrillo I, Contreras-Gomez A, Antonio-Ocampo A. Effects of propofol on alterations of multineuronal activity of limbic and mesencephalic structures and neurological deficit elicited by acute global cerebral ischemia. *Arch Med Res* 1995;26:385–395.

17. Kochs E, Hoffman WE, Werner C, Thomas C, Albrecht RF, Schulte am Esch J. The effects of propofol on brain electrical activity, neurologic outcome, and neuronal damage following incomplete ischemia in rats. *Anesthesiology* 1992;76:245–252.

18. Adembri C, Venturi L, Pellegrini-Giampietro DE. Neuroprotective effects of propofol in acute cerebral injury. *CNS Drug Rev* 2007;13:333–351.

19. Vinson DR, Bradbury DR. Etomidate for procedural sedation in emergency medicine. *Ann Emerg Med* 2002;39:592–598.

20. Hohl CM, Kelly-Smith CH, Yeug TC, Sweet DD, Doyle-Waters MM, Schulzer M. The effect of a bolus dose of etomidate on cortisol levels, mortality, and health services utilization: A systematic review. *Ann Emerg Med* 2010;56:105–113.

21. Vanlersberghe C, Camu F. Etomidate and other non-barbiturates. *Handbook of Experimental Pharmacology.* 2008; vol. 182, pp. 267–282.

22. Gooding JM, Crossen G. Etomidate: An ultra-short acting nonbarbiturate agent for anesthesia induction. *Anesth Analg* 1976;55:286–289.

23. Heykant JJ, Meuldermans WE, Michiels LJ, Lewi PJ, Jansen PA. Distribution, metabolism and excretion of etomidate, a short-acting hypnotic drug, in the rat. Comparative study of (R)-(+)-(-)-Etomidate. *Arch Int Pharmacodyn Ther* 1975;216:113–129.

24. Wagner RL, White PF, Kan PB, Rosenthal, MH, Feldman D. Inhibition of adrenal steroidogenesis by the anesthetic etomidate. *N Engl J Med* 1984;310:1415–1421.

25. Archambault P, Dionne CE, Lortie G, LeBlanc F, Rioux A, Larouche G. Adrenal inhibition following a single dose of etomidate in intubated traumatic brain injury victims. *CJEM* 2012;14:270–282.

26. Fragen RJ, Caldwell N. Comparison of a new formulation of etomidate with thiopental-side effects and awakening times. *Anesthesiology* 1979;50:242–244.

27. Sano T, Patel PM, Drummond JC, Cole DJ. A comparison of the cerebral protective effects of etomidate, thiopental, and isoflurane in a model of forebrain ischemia in the rat. *Anesth Analg* 1993;76:990–997.

28. Guo J, White JA, Batjer HH. Limited protective effects of etomidate during brainstem ischemia in dogs. *J Neurosurg* 1995;82:278–283.

29. Hoffman WE, Charbel FT, Edelman G, Misra M, Ausman JI. Comparison of the effect of etomidate and desflurane on brain tissue gases and pH during prolonged middle cerebral artery occlusion. *Anesthesiology* 1998;88:1188–1194.

30. Kohrs R, Durieux ME. Ketamine: Teaching an old drug new tricks. *Anesth Analg* 1998;87:1186–1193.

31. White PF, Way WL, Travor AJ. Ketamine: Its pharmacology and therapeutic uses. *Anesthesiology* 1982;56:119–136.

32. Himmelseher S, Durieux ME. Revising a dogma: Ketamine for patients with neurological injury? *Anesth Analg* 2005;101:524–534.

33. Bourgoin A, Albanèse J, Wereszczynski N, Charbit M, Vialet R, Martin C. Safety of sedation with ketamine in severe head injury patients: Comparison with sufentanil. *Crit Care Med* 2003;31:711–717.

20

Anesthetic agents: Inhalational

INDU KAPOOR

Introduction

In patients undergoing neurosurgical procedures, the main goals of inhalational anesthetic agents are to provide good operative condition, rapid recovery, minimal interference with electrophysiological monitoring, and preservation of neurocognitive function. Intraoperative maintenance of cerebral perfusion pressure (CPP), cerebral blood flow (CBF), and intracranial pressure (ICP) makes them ideal anesthetic agents (Table 20.1). If the anesthetic drugs are not used properly, it can further deteriorate the intracranial pathological situation and can cause new injury. Despite theoretical benefits of intravenous anesthetic agents, inhalational agents remain more popular. Numerous studies have shown differential effects of inhalational anesthetic agents on cerebral hemodynamics. According to Holmstrom and Akeson,[1] on comparing desflurane, isoflurane, and sevoflurane in a porcine model of intracranial hypertension, at equipotent doses and normocapnia, CBF and ICP were greatest with desflurane and least with sevoflurane. They further demonstrated that sevoflurane caused the least vasodilatation.[2] In another study in healthy patients, isoflurane was found to impair autoregulation, although this was reversible with hyperventilation.[3] In this chapter, we discuss the most commonly used inhaled anesthetic agents in clinical practice such as nitrous oxide, and volatile liquids such as desflurane, sevoflurane, and isoflurane, and their importance in anesthesia management for patients undergoing neurosurgery or with any other brain disorders (Table 20.2).[4]

Nitrous oxide

Nitrous oxide (N$_2$O) is also known as laughing gas because of its euphoric effect. Its chemical formula is *dinitrogen monoxide*. It is a colorless gas with sweet odor.[4] It is a noninflammable gas but supports combustion.[5] It is available as a liquid gas in an anesthesia machine. Because of its poor blood solubility, alveolar and brain concentration are achieved very rapidly. It is used in many procedures and surgeries because of its analgesic and anesthetic effects. It is also considered a major air pollutant with high global warming probability.

Table 20.1   Cerebral Effects of Inhalational Agents

Anesthetic agents	ICP	CPP	CBF	CMRO$_2$	CSF dynamics	
					Resistance to resorption	CSF formation
Isoflurane	+/0	-/0	+/0	--	-/0/+	0
Sevoflurane	+/0	-/0	+/0/-	--	+	-
Desflurane	+/0	-/0	+/-	--	0	0/+
Nitrous oxide	++	--	++	+	0	0

ICP, intracranial pressure; CPP, cerebral perfusion pressure; CBF, cerebral blood flow; CMRO$_2$, cerebral metabolic rate of oxygen consumption; CSF, cerebrospinal fluid; +, increase; -, decrease; 0, no effect.

Table 20.2   Physical Properties of Inhalational Anesthetic Agents

	Desflurane	Sevoflurane	Isoflurane	Nitrous oxide
Odor	Pungent	Sweet	Pungent	Sweet
MAC	6.6	1.8	1.2	104
Blood–gas partition coefficient	0.42	0.69	1.46	0.46
Soda lime stability	Yes	No	Yes	Yes

MAC, minimum alveolar concentration.

Mechanism of action

The exact mechanism of action of N$_2$O is not well known. It partially blocks N-methyl-D-aspartate (NMDA) receptors, nicotinic acetylcholine (nACh) receptors, gamma-aminobutyric acid (GABA) receptors, and histamine (5-hydroxytryptamine [5-HT$_3$]) receptors, and it partially potentiates GABA and glycine receptors.[6,7] On reaction with oxygen, N$_2$O produces nitric oxide (NO) and its action on the central nervous system leads to analgesic and anxiolytic effects.[8]

Pharmacokinetics

As discussed in Table 20.2, N$_2$O is not very soluble in blood, produces rapid equilibrium between delivery and alveolar concentration of N$_2$O, and hence results in rapid induction and rapid recovery from anesthesia. This rapid alveolar concentration results in a *second gas effect* by concentrating the other simultaneously administered anesthetic agents. The patient should be ventilated with 100%

oxygen once N$_2$O is discontinued. On discontinuation, N$_2$O diffuses rapidly from blood to alveoli, leading to *diffusion hypoxia* because of alveolar oxygen dilution. The elimination half-life of N$_2$O is roughly 5 min.[9] It is excreted essentially unchanged via lungs and degraded in intestine. The prolonged use of N$_2$O can produce vitamin B$_{12}$ neuropathy.[10]

Systemic effects

N$_2$O is a subject for debate in neurosurgical anesthesia. It has been accepted that N$_2$O augments the CBF, cerebral metabolic rate of oxygen consumption (CMRO$_2$), and ICP as well. The maximal increase in CBF and ICP occurs when N$_2$O is administered alone or in combination with other anesthetic agents in minimal concentration. However, this increase does not seem to be only because of sympathetic overactivity. Also, N$_2$O does not have a direct vasodilating effect on cerebral vasculature.[11] The systemic effects of N$_2$O on the central nervous system and other systems of the body are described in Table 20.3.

Table 20.3 Systemic Effects of Nitrous Oxide

Central nervous system	• Increases CBF, ICP, and $CMRO_2$ • Increases IOP • Increases regional CBF and CBV in gray matter at 50% concentration
Cardiovascular system	• Has direct myocardial depressant action but stimulates the sympathetic nervous system • Has little effect on arterial blood pressure • Causes pulmonary vessel vasoconstriction, leading to increase in PVR that in turn increases right atrial pressure • With halogenated volatile agents increases heart rate, blood pressure, as well as cardiac output
Respiratory system	• Increases respiratory rate and decreases tidal volume • Maintains minute ventilation • Reduces ventilatory response to both hypoxia and hypercapnia
Other systems	• Has no significant effect on renal, endocrine, and hepatic systems

ICP, intracranial pressure; CBF, cerebral blood flow; CBV, cerebral blood volume; $CMRO_2$, cerebral metabolic rate of oxygen consumption; IOP, intraocular pressure; PVR, peripheral vascular resistance.

Isoflurane

Isoflurane is a halogenated volatile agent with chemical formula 2-chloro-2-(difluoromethoxy)-1,1,1-trifluoroethane. It is a volatile anesthetic agent with noninflammable and nonexplosive properties. It is liquid at room temperature but vaporizes very rapidly. Its pungent odor can irritate the airway leading to laryngospasm. Hence, it is not considered for induction of anesthesia in pediatric patients.

Mechanism of action

The exact mechanism of action of isoflurane has not been clearly explained. Similar to halothane, it binds to GABA and glycine receptors. It enhances the activity of glycine receptors resulting in decreased motor function. It has inhibitory action on NMDA receptors and potassium channels. It increases the membrane fluidity by activating calcium ATPase.

Pharmacokinetics

The blood–gas partition coefficient of isoflurane is low. As a result, the induction as well as recovery from isoflurane anesthesia is relatively rapid compared to the other two. Around 99% isoflurane is excreted via lungs and a small fraction is oxidatively metabolized by cytochrome P2E1 (CYP2E1).

However, it does not carry carcinogenic, mutagenic, or teratogenic activity.[12] It does not produce hepatic, renal, or endocrine toxicity in other organs.

Systemic effects

Isoflurane increases CBF and ICP accompanied by a decrease in $CMRO_2$. It introduces a greater degree of cerebral vasodilation compared to halothane. It has been reported to decrease whole brain metabolism by half.[13] Because of its depressive cerebral metabolic effect, isoflurane is considered to have neuroprotective effects. The various mechanisms contributing to its neuroprotective effects include inhibition of excitatory neurotransmitters, enhancement of actions of GABA receptors, and regulation of intracellular calcium response.[14] Its systemic effects on the central nervous system and other systems are described briefly in Table 20.4.

Sevoflurane

Sevoflurane has the chemical formula of fluoromethyl 2,2,2-trifluoro-1-(trifluoromethyl)ethyl ether. It is one of the most widely used volatile anesthetic agents for induction and maintenance of general anesthesia. It is a noninflammable agent with a sweet odor. Because of its nonpungent odor, sevoflurane is commonly used for induction of anesthesia in children and for outpatient anesthesia because of its rapid recovery.

Table 20.4 Systemic Effects of Isoflurane

Central nervous system	• Causes cerebral vasodilation • Increases CBF and ICP • Decreases $CMRO_2$ • Produces significant EEG ischemic changes
Cardiovascular system	• Decreases blood pressure and systemic vascular resistance • Maintains cardiac output • Produces mild rise in heart rate • May cause *coronary steal*, i.e., diversion of blood from less-perfused to well-perfused areas • Does not sensitize the myocardium on exogenous epinephrine
Respiratory system	• Is primarily a respiratory depressant • Decreases ventilation dose dependently • Decreases tidal volume, however respiratory rate remains unchanged • Depresses the ventilatory response to hypoxia and hypercapnia • Is an effective bronchodilator and airway irritant
Other systems	• Produces no significant effect on renal, endocrine, and hepatic systems, if used for shorter duration

ICP, intracranial pressure; CBF, cerebral blood flow; $CMRO_2$, cerebral metabolic rate of oxygen consumption; EEG, electroencephalogram.

Mechanism of action

The exact mechanism of action of sevoflurane has not been outlined. It acts on many receptors, including activation of GABA and glycine receptors, and inhibition of NMDA, nACh, and 5-HT$_3$ receptors.[15,16]

Pharmacokinetics

Because of low blood–gas partition coefficient, sevoflurane provides rapid induction as well as rapid recovery from general anesthesia. It is one of the anesthetic agents of choice for induction of anesthesia in pediatric patients. Its nonpungent odor does not cause coughing or airway irritation like desflurane or isoflurane. It is metabolized in the liver.[17] Its interaction with soda lime produces a major degradation product called compound A that could be nephrotoxic.[18]

Systemic effects

Sevoflurane demonstrated decrease or no change in CBF.[19,20] However, increase in CBF has also been reported in the literature.[21] Sevoflurane with or without N_2O produces either slight or no increase in ICP. The neuroprotective effects of sevoflurane

at present appear to be similar to those of isoflurane. Its effects on various systems in the human body including the central nervous system are described briefly in Table 20.5.

Desflurane

Desflurane (1,2,2,2-tetrafluoroethyl difluoromethyl ether) is a highly fluorinated inhalational anesthetic agent. It is a highly pungent inhalational agent with low potency. Because of its odor, desflurane can cause airway irritation, leading to its infrequent use to induce anesthesia. Another drawback of desflurane anesthesia is its high cost. Desflurane is a greenhouse gas producing much higher carbon dioxide than sevoflurane and isoflurane.[22] If desflurane is used for 1 h at 1 MAC, it causes 26.8 times the global warming of sevoflurane.[23,24]

Mechanism of action

The precise mechanism of action of desflurane by which it produces unconsciousness has not been clearly defined. It binds to membrane proteins and alters their functions and potentiates the activity of the inhibitory neurotransmitter GABA. Another theory is the *Meyer–Overton theory*, which suggests that the effect of these agents is because of their action on lipid matrix of neuronal membrane.[25]

Pharmacokinetics

Because of its very low blood–gas partition coefficient (0.42) and lower fat solubility, desflurane provides very rapid induction and rapid emergence from general anesthesia. Its time of emergence is half that of sevoflurane and halothane and does not exceed 5–10 min.[26] Most of the desflurane (99%) is eliminated via the lungs.

Systemic effects

Desflurane produces a dose-dependent increase in CBF and a decrease in $CMRO_2$[27] It also causes a greater increase in ICP compared to isoflurane at normocapnia, however at hypocapnia their effects are similar.[28] The degree of neuroprotection by desflurane at present is comparable to that of isoflurane. The systemic effects of desflurane on the central nervous system and other systems are described briefly in Table 20.6.

Table 20.5 Systemic Effects of Sevoflurane

Central nervous system	• Increases CBF and ICP • Decreases $CMRO_2$ • Leads to decrease, increase, or no change in MCA velocity • Has neuroprotective effect
Cardiovascular system	• Is a potent cardiostable agent • Does not cause increase in heart rate • Decreases myocardial contractility • Dose not sensitize the heart to catecholamines • Reduces baroreflex function
Respiratory system	• Increases respiratory rate dose dependently • Decreases tidal volume • Is a potent bronchodilator
Other systems	• Has no significant effect on hepatic system • May cause nephrotoxicity because of compound A

ICP, intracranial pressure; CBF, cerebral blood flow; $CMRO_2$ = cerebral metabolic rate of oxygen consumption; MCA, middle cerebral artery

Table 20.6 Systemic Effects of Desflurane

Central nervous system	• Increases CBF and ICP • Reduces $CMRO_2$ • Preserves cerebrovascular reactivity to carbon dioxide • Has neuroprotective effect
Cardiovascular system	• Decreases blood pressure concentration dependently • Decreases systemic vascular resistance • Preserves cardiac output well • Increases heart rate with sudden increase in concentration
Respiratory system	• Increases respiratory rate dose dependently • Decreases tidal volume • Can cause airway irritation, coughing, and laryngospasm • Is also a bronchodilator
Other systems	• Shows no significant effect on renal, endocrine, and hepatic systems

ICP, intracranial pressure; CBF, cerebral blood flow; $CMRO_2$, cerebral metabolic rate of oxygen consumption.

References

1. Holmstrom A, Akeson J. Desflurane increases the intracranial pressure more and sevoflurane less than isoflurane in pigs subjected to intracranial hypertension. *J Neurosurg Anesthesiol* 2004;16:136–143.
2. Holmstrom A, Akeson J. Sevoflurane induces less cerebral vasodilation than isoflurane at the same A-line autoregressive index level. *Acta Anaesthesiol Scand* 2005;49:16–22.
3. McCulloch TJ, Boesel TW, Lam A. The effect of hypocapnia on the autoregulation of cerebral blood flow during administration of isoflurane. *Anesth Analg* 2005;100:1463–1467.
4. Smith I, Nathanson M, White PF. Sevoflurane–a long awaited volatile anesthetic. *Br J Anaesth* 1996;76:435–445.
5. Sethi NK, Mullin P, Torgovnick J, Capasso G. Nitrous oxide "whippit" abuse presenting with cobalamin responsive psychosis. *J Med Toxicol* 2006;2:71–74.
6. Neuman GG, Sidebotham G, Negoianu E et al. Laparoscopy explosive hazards with nitrous oxide. *Anesthesiology* 1993;78:875–879.
7. Yamakura T, Harris RA. Effects of gaseous anaesthetics nitrous oxide and xenon on ligand-gated ion channels. Comparison with isoflurane and ethanol. *Anesthesiology* 2000;93:1095–1101.
8. Mennerick S, Jevtovic-Todorovic V, Todorovic SM, Shen W, Olney JW, Zorumski CF. Effect of nitrous oxide on excitatory and inhibitory synaptic transmission in hippocampal cultures. *J Neurosci* 1998;18:9716–9726.
9. Emmanouil DE, Quock RM. Advances in understanding the actions of nitrous oxide. *Anesth Prog* 2007;54:9–18.
10. Browne DR, Rochford J, O'Connell U, Jones JG. The incidence of postoperative atelectasis in the dependent lung following thoracotomy: The value of added nitrogen. *Br J Anaesth* 1970;42:340–346.
11. Reinstrup P, Ryding E, Algotsson L, Berntman L, Uski T. Effect of nitrous oxide on human regional cerebral blood flow and isolated pial arteries. *Anesthesiology* 1994;81:396–402.
12. O'Sullivan H, Jennings F, Ward K, McCann S, Scott JM, Weir DG. Human bone marrow biochemical function and megaloblastic hematopoiesis after nitrous oxide anesthesia. *Anesthesiology* 1981;55:645–649.
13. Alkire MT, Haier RJ, Shah NK, Anderson CT. Positron emission tomography study of regional cerebral metabolism in humans during isoflurane anesthesia. *Anesthesiology* 1997;86:549–557.
14. Fukuda S, Warner DS. Cerebral protection. *Br J Anaesthesia* 2007;99:10–17.
15. Eger EI II, White AE, Brown CL, Biava CG, Corbett TH, Stevens WC. A test of the carcinogenicity of enflurane, isoflurane, halothane, methoxyflurane, and nitrous oxide in mice. *Anesth Analg* 1978;57:678–694.
16. Brosnan RJ, Thiesen R. Increased NMDA receptor inhibition at an increased sevoflurane MAC. *BMC Anesthesiology* 2012;12:9.
17. Suzuki T, Koyama H, Sugimoto M, Uchida I, Mashimo T. The diverse actions of volatile and gaseous anesthetics on human-cloned 5-hydroxytryptamine3 receptors expressed in Xenopus oocytes. *Anesthesiology* 2002;96:699–704.
18. Kharasch ED, Armstrong AS, Gunn K, Artru A, Cox K, Karol MD. Clinical sevoflurane metabolism and disposition. II. The role of cytochrome P 450 2E1 in fluoride and hexafluoroisopropanol formation. *Anesthesiology* 1995;82:1379–1388.
19. Kitaguchi K, Ohsumi H, Kuro M, Nakajima T, Hayashi Y. Effects of sevoflurane on cerebral circulation and metabolism in patients with ischemic cerebrovascular disease. *Anesthesiology* 1993;79:704–709.
20. Conzen PF, Vollmar B, Habazettl H, Frink EJ, Peter K, Messmer K. Systemic and regional hemodynamics of isoflurane and sevoflurane in rats. *Anesth Analg* 1992;74:79–88.
21. Crawford MW, Lerman J, Saldivia V, Carmichael FJ. Hemodynamic and organ blood flow responses to halothane and sevoflurane anesthesia during spontaneous ventilation. *Anesth Analg* 1992;75:1000–1006.

22. Hanaki C, Fujii K, Morio M, Tashima T. Decomposition of sevoflurane by sodalime. *Hiroshima J Med Sci* 1987;36:61–67.

23. Sulbaek Andersen MP, Sander SP, Nielsen OJ, Wagner DS, Sanford TJ Jr, Wallington TJ. Inhalation anaesthetics and climate change. *Br J Anaesth* 2010;105:760–766.

24. Ryan SM, Nielsen CJ. Global warming potential of inhaled anesthetics: Application to clinical use. *Anesth Analg* 2010;111:92–98.

25. Koblin DD. Mechanisms of action. In: Miller RD, editor. *Anesthesia*, 4th ed. New York, NY: Churchill Livingston; 1994, pp. 67–99.

26. Smiley RM, Ornstein E, Matteo RS, Pantuck EJ, Pantuck CB. Desflurane and isoflurane in surgical patients: Comparison of emergence time. *Anesthesiology* 1991;74:425–428.

27. Lutz LJ, Milde JH, Milde LN. The cerebral functional, metabolic, and hemodynamic effects of desflurane in dogs. *Anesthesiology* 1990;73:125–131.

28. Artru AA. Intracranial volume/pressure relationship during desflurane anesthesia in dogs: Comparison with isoflurane and thiopental/halothane. *Anesth Analg* 1994;79:751–760.

21

Neuromuscular blockade and opioids

PRASANNA U. BIDKAR and NARMADHA LAKSHMI K

Introduction

A neuromuscular junction is a unit of motor nerve terminus and postsynaptic muscle end plate. The cell membranes of the motor nerve terminus and postsynaptic muscle end plate are separated by a 20-nm gap, known as the synaptic cleft. Acetylcholine is stored in the vesicles at the motor nerve terminus. As a nerve's action potential depolarizes its terminus, calcium ions influx through voltage-gated calcium channels into the nerve cytoplasm and allow storage vesicles to fuse with the terminal membrane and release their acetylcholine (ACh) contents into the synaptic cleft. The ACh molecules reach the muscle membrane where the motor end plate contains ligand-gated, nicotinic acetylcholine receptors (nAChRs), which convert the chemical signal (i.e., binding of two ACh molecules) into electrical signals (depolarization in the postsynaptic membrane of striated muscle).

Acetylcholine receptor

The normal junctional or mature ACh receptor consists of five protein subunits—two α-subunits and a single β-, δ-, and ε-subunit. Only the two identical α-subunits are capable of binding ACh molecules. If both binding sites are occupied by ACh, a conformational change in the subunits briefly (1 ms) opens an ion channel in the core of the receptor.

Electrical conduction at neuromuscular junction

When two ACh molecules bind at two α-subunits of a nicotinic ACh receptor, an opening is created in the center of the rosette, allowing sodium and calcium ions to enter the cell and potassium ions to exit,[1,2] generating an end-plate potential. The quantum of ACh release from a single vesicle (10^4 molecules per quantum) produces a miniature end-plate potential. The quanta released by each nerve impulse are very sensitive to extracellular ionized calcium concentration. When enough receptors are occupied by ACh, the end-plate potential is sufficiently strong to depolarize the perijunctional membrane. The resulting action potential propagates along the muscle membrane and T-tubule system, opening sodium channels and releasing calcium from the sarcoplasmic reticulum. This intracellular calcium allows the contractile proteins actin and myosin to interact, bringing about muscle contraction. The amount of ACh usually released and the number of receptors subsequently activated normally far exceed the minimum required for the initiation of an action potential. The nearly 10-fold margin of safety is overwhelmed in Eaton–Lambert myasthenic syndrome (decreased release of ACh) and myasthenia gravis (decreased number of receptors).

ACh is rapidly hydrolyzed into acetate and choline by the substrate-specific enzyme acetylcholinesterase. This enzyme (also called specific cholinesterase or true cholinesterase) is embedded into the motor end-plate membrane immediately adjacent to the ACh receptors. Eventually, the receptors' ion channels close, causing the end plate to repolarize. When generation of action potential ceases, the sodium channels in the muscle membrane also close. Calcium is resequestered in the sarcoplasmic reticulum, and the muscle cell relaxes.

Neuromuscular receptor blockers

Neuromuscular blockers are classically divided into two types—depolarizing and nondepolarizing blockers (Figure 21.1).

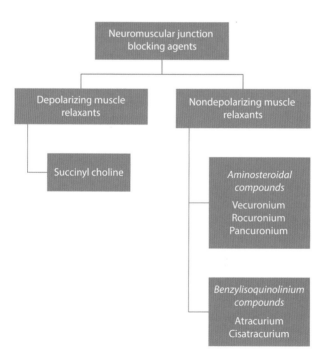

Figure 21.1 Currently used neuromuscular blocking agents.

Neuromuscular blocking agents in neurosurgical anesthesia

Succinylcholine and raised ICP

Succinylcholine is the only depolarizing neuromuscular blocking agent (NMBA) available that binds and activates ACh receptor sites. The quick onset and short duration of action of succinylcholine makes it a suitable NMBA in many intubating conditions, especially in difficult airway scenarios and rapid sequence induction (RSI).[3] Though transient, succinylcholine raises intracranial pressures (ICPs) to a variable extent, depending on the anesthetic plane and levels of carbon dioxide in the blood. In neurosurgical patients with raised ICP and anticipated difficult airway, the question about the priority of raised ICP or difficult airway management arises. The airway management and oxygenation is always a priority, and succinylcholine can be chosen for facilitating intubation as the increase in the ICP by succinylcholine is transient and minimal under optimal anesthetic plane. As the increase in ICP by succinylcholine is suspected to be due to the muscle fasciculations produced, defasciculating doses of nondepolarizing agent can be administered before succinylcholine to prevent raise in the ICP.[4] But there is sufficient evidence for the use of defasciculating doses in RSI, so the pretreatment with nondepolarizing NMBA is not routinely recommended and it should only be considered if it does not delay the establishment of a definitive airway. With the advent of sugammadex, rocuronium can replace succinylcholine as the muscle relaxant of choice in patients with difficult airway.

Succinylcholine and hyperkalemia

Another concern with the use of succinylcholine in neurosurgical patients is hyperkalemia in patients with certain neurological disorders such as spinal cord injury, stroke, demyelinating disorders, myotonia, muscular dystrophies, and upper or lower motor neuron injury. Under normal conditions, postjunctional membrane depolarization results in leakage of potassium that produces an increase of 0.5–1.0 mEq/L in serum potassium concentration. The risk of succinylcholine-induced hyperkalemia in these patients increases over time and the precise time of onset and the duration of the risk period are unknown. In the conditions like spinal cord injury, muscular dystrophies, and stroke, there will be increased proliferation of immature ACh receptors, which when depolarized by succinylcholine leads to an efflux of intracellular potassium into the plasma, leading to acute hyperkalemia. The magnitude of increase in serum potassium concentration may be much higher in patients with immature ACh receptors. Even cardiac arrests have been reported following acute increases in serum potassium concentration after succinylcholine administration. Hence, succinylcholine is generally avoided in patients who are bedridden for more than 24 h.

Succinylcholine and malignant hyperthermia

There is no clear evidence in the literature indicating that administration of succinylcholine alone induces malignant hyperthermia in susceptible individuals. But when used in combination with inhalational agents, there will be marked clinical response.[5] The resulting hyperkalemia from rhabdomyolysis can itself lead to cardiac arrest. It is advisable to continue with total intravenous anesthesia in patients who develop sustained masseter spasm following administration of succinylcholine.[6]

Nondepolarizing neuromuscular blocking agents

Vecuronium and rocuronium are the most commonly used intermediate-acting NMBAs in neurosurgical patients. Pancuronium is a long-acting, nondepolarizing compound. It is vagolytic, which limits its use in patients who cannot tolerate an increase in heart rate.[7] Accumulation of metabolite along with parent compound in patients with organ dysfunction may contribute to the prolonged duration of blockade. Hence, pancuronium is not being used routinely in neurosurgical practice.

Rocuronium is a monoquaternary steroidal compound that has rapid onset and intermediate duration of action. At a dose of 1–1.2 mg/kg, blockade is almost always achieved within 60–90 s. In neurosurgical conditions with raised ICP and in which risk of aspiration is present, rocuronium can be used as an NMBA for RSI due to early onset of action. In contrast to succinylcholine, rocuronium has no action on ICP. Rocuronium is not recommended in anticipated difficult intubation in RSI due to the prolonged duration of the blockade. But now with the availability of sugammadex, rocuronium can be used for difficult airways, with rapid reversal of neuromuscular blockade. The steroid-based NMBAs are associated with reports of prolonged recovery and myopathy.[8]

Atracurium is an intermediate-acting NMBA with minimal cardiovascular adverse effects and is associated with histamine release at higher doses. It undergoes ester hydrolysis and Hofmann elimination. ED_{90} of atracurium is 0.5 mg/kg. Laudanosine is a metabolite[9] of atracurium and cisatracurium that is shown to decrease seizure threshold. The concentrations required to produce seizures are not achieved in clinically administered doses. But caution is advised in elderly patients and in patients with hepatic failure (laudanosine is metabolized by the liver). There has been only one report of a surgical patient who had a seizure while receiving atracurium.[10]

With the exception of atracurium and cisatracurium, which need to be given continuously because of their short half-lives, bolus administration of other NMBAs with neuromuscular monitoring offers potential advantages for controlling tachyphylaxis, monitoring for accumulation, and limiting complications related to prolonged or excessive blockade. Laudanosine is a metabolite[9] of atracurium and cisatracurium that is shown to decrease seizure threshold in animal studies.

Though NMBAs facilitate ventilation and control ICP in patients with increased muscular activity, there is no direct effect on either of the conditions. Seizure patients under paralysis may not show active seizures, so electroencephalogram (EEG) monitoring has to be ensured to monitor any seizure activity in the brain. Chronic treatment with phenytoin or carbamazepine is associated with an increase in ACh receptor numbers and enzyme induction, which leads to reduced duration of action of nondepolarizing NMBAs.

NMBAs are given to prevent respiratory dyssynchrony, stop spontaneous respiratory efforts and muscle movement, improve gas exchange, and manage raised ICP. Nondepolarizing NMBAs do not exert any direct effect on ICP either by bolus dose or by continuous infusion.

Intense neuromuscular blockade in neurosurgery

The most common indications for NMBAs in neurosurgical anesthesia include facilitation of intubation and controlled mechanical ventilation, which helps prevent increases in ICP, by avoidance of coughing and movement of the patients. Also immobility is essential in patients with surgery being performed near vital areas like brainstem.

In neurosurgical patients, it is recommended that the clinician wait until the absence of simple twitch and the adequate depth of anesthesia is achieved before attempting laryngoscopy. The central muscles such as the diaphragm are less sensitive to NMBAs than peripheral muscles. So, intense paralysis with post-tetanic count of zero (PTC-0) in the thumb is recommended. This intense neuromuscular block is also called the "period of no response phase," characterized by TOF-0 and PTC-0. Many neurosurgeries such as endoscopic surgeries, posterior fossa tumors, brainstem lesions involving lower cranial nerves, cerebellopontine (CP) angle tumors, and spinal cord surgeries (especially in the cervical region) require intense or deep blockade with a PTC-0.

Avoidance of neuromuscular blocking agents

There are certain neurosurgeries where neuromuscular monitoring is recommended to prevent injury to neural structures in which muscle relaxants are generally avoided. Those surgeries include CP angle tumor, meningomyelocele, excision of lesion at motor cortex area, and spinal cord surgeries. Here, cranial nerve or spinal nerve monitoring is generally used to prevent injury. First, a bolus of NMBA can be used to facilitate intubation and subsequent doses are withheld to monitor the nerve function.

When the NMBAs are avoided, it is important to maintain adequate depth of anesthesia to prevent movement of the patient. Bispectral index (BIS) or entropy can be used to monitor and maintain the depth of anesthesia. The adequacy of depth of anesthesia can be maintained using inhalational agents, total intravenous anesthesia, or a combination of both techniques.

Reversal of neuromuscular blocking agent

Smooth extubation is preferred in neurosurgical anesthesia. Reversal of NMBA is usually carried out with an anticholinesterase inhibitor such as neostigmine or with a newer agent sugammadex. Neostigmine is administered along with glycopyrrolate or atropine to counteract the muscarinic effects. Sugammadex is a selective relaxant binding agent that is primarily used to reverse rocuronium-induced neuromuscular block. In a study comparing sugammadex and neostigmine, the authors found that sugammadex rapidly and effectively reverses rocuronium-induced NMB in pediatric patients undergoing neurosurgery when administered at reappearance of T2 of train of four (TOF) at a dose of 4 mg/kg.[11]

Monitoring neuromuscular blockade in neurosurgical patients

Peripheral nerve stimulation (PNS) resulted in a significantly lower total dose and lower mean infusion rate of NMBA as well as a faster time to recovery of neuromuscular function and spontaneous ventilation. The implementation of a protocol using PNS to monitor the level of blockade in patients receiving a variety of NMBAs found a reduction in the incidence of persistent neuromuscular weakness.[12] A prospective, randomized trial comparing TOF to standard clinical assessment showed decreased NMBA usage and faster return of spontaneous ventilation with TOF monitoring.[13] Compared to other methods of monitoring, TOF monitoring of PNS remains the easiest and most reliable method to assess the patient's muscle tone.[14–20]

Residual neuromuscular block in the postoperative recovery room leads to significant pulmonary morbidity,[21] impairs ventilatory response to hypoxia,[22] and increases the risk of airway obstruction and aspiration.[23] It is now thought that significant residual curarization is still present if the TOF ratio is <0.9.[24] So, quantitative assessment and monitoring of paralysis during neurosurgery to provide satisfactory operative conditions for the surgeon and to assess postoperative neuromuscular function during recovery are more important than clinical judgment.

Poor results of neuromuscular monitoring at times show the importance of the use of more than one method of monitoring; poor technique in using any device will invariably produce inaccurate results. In clinical practice, though the patients appear comfortable, there is always an overestimation of pain and sedation under NMBAs. So it is recommended to adjust sedative and analgesic drugs to provide adequate sedation and analgesia in accordance with the physician's clinical judgment to optimize therapy. Patients receiving NMBAs should be assessed both clinically and by TOF monitoring with a goal of adjusting the degree of neuromuscular blockade to achieve plane for neurosurgery.

Pattern of nerve stimulation

Single-twitch stimulation

Single-twitch stimulation is the most commonly performed check for adequacy of muscle paralysis during endotracheal intubation.

Stimulus and response: A single supramaximal stimulus of square wave pattern is applied to a peripheral nerve at frequencies ranging from 1.0 Hz (once every second) to 0.1 Hz (once every 10 s). The depression of resultant twitch response depends on the percentage of blockade of postsynaptic nicotinic receptors by NMBA. The level of supramaximal stimulus is first established at the onset of neuromuscular block using a single twitch at 1 Hz (one twitch every second). The onset of neuromuscular block can then be observed, using a single twitch at 0.1 Hz (one twitch every 10 s).

Nondepolarizing and depolarizing neuromuscular blocks: Except for the difference in time factors, no differences in the strength of the evoked responses exist between the two blocks.

Limitation: It is essential to have a control twitch before administering the NMBA. It cannot be used to determine the degree of blockade in a profound neuromuscular blockade

Application time: The most useful time to assess neuromuscular blockade using single-twitch response is at the time of induction.

Train-of-four stimulation

TOF can be used to assess neuromuscular blockade in the anesthetized patient and it does not require control twitch for comparison of evoked responses.

Stimulus and response: Supramaximal twitch stimuli, with a frequency of 2 Hz (four stimuli each separated by 0.5 s), are used to stimulate a peripheral nerve, usually the ulnar nerve. The TOF was then repeated every 10 s (train frequency of 0.1 Hz). TOF ratio is obtained by comparing T4 to T1.

The T4/T1 ratio is important as it is thought to be closely related to T1/T0 (T0—control obtained before neuromuscular block).

Nondepolarizing neuromuscular blockade: When a nondepolarizing agent is given, fade is observed from T1 to T4. There is a decrement in the amplitude of the evoked responses, with T4 affected first, then T3, followed by T2, and finally T1. During a partial nondepolarizing block, the ratio decreases (fades) as the intensity of the block increases. As the nondepolarizing block becomes intense, evoked responses disappear—T4 disappears at about 75% depression of T1, T3 at 80%–85% depression of T1, and T2 at 90% depression of T1. The number of twitches (TOF count) correlates with the degree of neuromuscular block. Twitch suppression of 90% would equate to a TOF count of 1 or less, which is the required maintenance for most neurosurgeries.

Depolarizing neuromuscular blockade: With depolarizing neuromuscular blockade, fade is not observed as all four twitches decrease equally in amplitude (the TOF ratio = 1). This is the same during recovery. However, in cases of phase 2 block produced at larger doses of succinylcholine, which is similar to nondepolarizing block, fade is observed with TOF monitoring.

Application: Disappearance of the TOF count will correspond to optimal intubating conditions. TOF ratio is traditionally used in assessing recovery from neuromuscular block. Achieving a TOF ratio of 0.9 before tracheal extubation has been recently accepted as an indication of adequate reversal rather than the ratio of 0.7, which was previously thought adequate. When the TOF count is 3 or greater, reversal of neuromuscular blockade can be safely achieved.

Advantages: Degree of nondepolarizing blockade can be assessed without control. It is less painful and does not generally affect the degree of neuromuscular blockade, unlike tetanic stimulation.

Limitation: TOF and single-twitch stimulation cannot be used to determine the degree of blockade in a profound neuromuscular blockade.

Tetanic stimulation

Stimulus and response: A frequency of 50–200 Hz with a supramaximal stimulus is used for tetanic stimulation. The stimulus is usually delivered over 5 s. Normal skeletal muscle will show sustained tetanic contraction.

Nondepolarizing neuromuscular blockade: The stimulated muscle shows signs of fade depending on the degree of blockade.

Depolarizing neuromuscular blockade: The response after depolarizing NMBA will be a sustained tetanic contraction, but the amplitude of evoked potential is lower.

Application: This pattern of stimulation is extremely painful but very sensitive to eliciting even minor degrees of neuromuscular block. So, tetanic stimulation is generally used to evaluate residual neuromuscular blockade.

Limitations: It is too painful to use in an unanesthetized patient, which is potentially useful in the postoperative recovery room to look for residual block. However, its use is limited by the fact that tetanic stimulation is extremely painful. Tetanic stimulation is difficult to interpret by either tactile[25,26] or visual evaluation to exclude residual neuromuscular blockade even by experienced observers.

Post-tetanic count

Stimulus and response: PTC refers to the number of responses to single-twitch stimulus, which is obtained after tetanic stimulus. After administration of tetanic stimulus at 50 Hz for 5 s, when no twitch response has been elicited, single twitches at 1 Hz are given 3 s later. There may be a response to this single-twitch stimulation.

Application: PTC can be used to quantify intense neuromuscular blockade.[27] It may be useful in circumstances where there may be no response to TOF or single-twitch stimulation during profound nondepolarizing neuromuscular block. The PTC is more useful when movement or coughing could have devastating effects on surgery, for example, retinal surgery, spinal surgeries, and surgery near the brainstem/motor cortex, in which profound neuromuscular block is required.

Double-burst stimulation

Stimulus and response: In double-burst stimulation (DBS), two short bursts of 50-Hz tetanic stimulation at a supramaximal current separated by 750 ms are applied to a peripheral nerve. The duration of each square wave impulse in the burst is 0.2 ms; each impulse is delivered every 20 ms. A DBS with three impulses in each of the two tetanic bursts ($DBS_{3,3}$) or a DBS with three impulses in one tetanic burst followed by two impulses in the second tetanic burst ($DBS_{3,2}$) is used. Before administration of a neuromuscular blocking drug, the response to DBS is two short muscle contractions of equal strength. The intensity of muscle contraction decreases in the second response in the partially paralyzed muscle, that is fade occurs. DBS ratio refers to the ratio of the amplitude of the second response to the first.

Application: Small degrees of residual neuromuscular block may be detected clinically using DBS.[28] DBS is especially useful during recovery and immediately after surgery.

Advantage: The DBS ratio is very similar to the TOF ratio but tactile evaluation of the $DBS_{3,3}$ response is superior to that of the response to TOF stimulation.[29,30]

Measuring evoked muscle responses

Five methods are available for detecting and measuring evoked responses more accurately. They are as follows:

1 Mechanomyography (MMG): measurement of the evoked mechanical response of the muscle
2 Electromyography (EMG): measurement of the evoked electrical response of the muscle
3 Acceleromyography (AMG): measurement of acceleration of the muscle response
4 Piezoelectric neuromuscular monitor [P_ZEMG]: measurement of the evoked electrical response in a piezoelectric film sensor attached to the muscle
5 Phonomyography (PMG)

Mechanomyography

Mechanomyography is a noninvasive technique that records and quantifies the oscillations generated by evoked muscle tension of the active skeletal muscle fibers. Evoked MMG records changes associated with excitation–contraction coupling and contraction of the muscle as well. Adductor pollicis is most commonly studied using MMG.

Though this technique is considered the gold standard for the assessment of any pattern of nerve stimulation, it has the disadvantage of being cumbersome and impractical for use in the operating theater.

Electromyography

Evoked EMG records the compound action potentials of a peripheral nerve during muscular contraction. Muscles such as adductor pollicis, hypothenar eminence, and first dorsal interosseous can be used to record evoked EMG response. The larynx and diaphragm are the two new sites where recording of EMG response can be done.[31,32] The commonly used nerve is the ulnar or median nerve. Both surface and needle electrodes may be used to transmit or detect electrical signals. The signal picked up by the analyzer is processed by an amplifier, a rectifier, and an electronic integrator. EMG translates these signals into graphs, sounds, or numerical values, and the results are displayed either as a percentage of control or as a TOF ratio.

Advantages of EMG potentials: The equipment needed is easier to assemble. It does not require rigid fixation of arm and hand.

Disadvantages: The readings are affected by diathermy, hand temperature and movements, and improper placement of electrodes. Direct muscle stimulation sometimes occurs. If muscles close to the stimulating electrodes are stimulated directly, the recording electrodes may pick up an electrical signal even though neuromuscular transmission is completely blocked. Another difficulty is that the EMG response often does not return to the control value.

Acceleromyography

Acceleromyography measures the acceleration of the contracting muscle. The principle is based on Newton's second law of motion: force equals mass times acceleration. After nerve stimulation, acceleration of the thumb can be measured using a piezoelectric ceramic wafer with electrodes on both sides. Other muscles preferred for monitoring the acceleration (other than thumb) include orbicularis oculi or the corrugator supercilii in response to facial nerve stimulation.[33]

Advantages: Acceleromyography can be used conveniently in operation theaters and in intensive care units for monitoring evoked responses. AMG is a valuable clinical tool that may eliminate the problem of postoperative residual neuromuscular blockade.[34] TOF and PTC can be monitored using acceleromyography.

Disadvantage: Because of uncertainty of the degree of block with respect to peripheral muscles, it is not recommended for routine monitoring.

Piezoelectric neuromuscular monitors

The technique of piezoelectric monitors is based on the principle that stretching or bending a flexible piezoelectric film generates a voltage that is proportional to the amount of stretching or bending. A piezoelectric film is kept attached to the thumb and the nerve is stimulated. Then, the stretch of the thumb (piezoelectric film) is monitored. Though data indicate that there is a good correlation between AMG and MMG, it is rarely recommended as a valuable clinical tool.

Phonomyography

PMG (acoustic myography) uses special microphones to record intrinsic low-frequency sounds generated from skeletal muscles. It is one of the

methods of monitoring neuromuscular function. PMG can be used to monitor diaphragm, larynx and eye muscles along with adductor pollicis, and also the application is very easy. But the available evidence is scarce for recommendation of PMG in routine anesthesia monitoring.

Opioids

Opioid is the term used in modern pharmacology to describe both natural and synthetic drugs derived from opium. *Opium* is a Greek word, which means "juice" derived from poppy seeds. Opioids play an indispensable role in the field of anesthesiology for preanesthetic medication, systemic and spinal analgesia, supplementation of general anesthetic agents, and as primary anesthetics. Additionally, they are used in critical care and pain management. Opioids are the most commonly used drugs in the treatment of severe acute and chronic pain. They act through opioid receptors expressed in central and peripheral nervous systems. This chapter reviews the clinical uses of opioids with an emphasis on their use in neuroanesthesia.

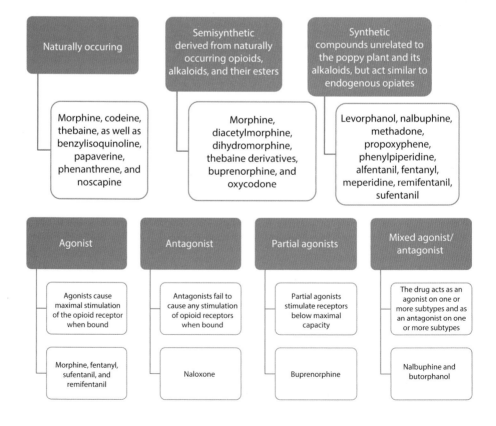

Classification of opioids

There are several ways to classify opioids: by origin, by chemical makeup, by receptor affinity, and by intrinsic receptor activity.

Mechanism of action

Opioids act through three opioid receptors—μ, κ, and δ—that belong to a family of G-protein-coupled receptors.

The binding of opioid agonists with the receptors leads to activation of the G-protein subunits, which leads to inhibition of cAMP production, decreased Ca^{2+} influx, and increased K^+ efflux. This results in hyperpolarization of the membrane and decreased neuronal excitability, producing analgesic effects of opioids.

Metabolism

Most opioids are metabolized by the hepatic microsomal cytochrome P450 (CYP) system, although hepatic conjugation and subsequent excretion by the kidney are important for some drugs.

Therapeutic effects

Primarily, opioids produce significant pain relief by acting at spinal and brain μ receptors. The μ agonists are effective in treating pain sensations carried by unmyelinated C fibers and neuropathic pain. In ambulatory patients, pain relief produced by an opioid does not produce sleep. In addition to analgesia, μ agonists in the brain produce sedation, which is also one of the targeted effects of higher-dose opioids in the perioperative period. Even at higher doses μ agonists do not produce amnesia, so opioids cannot be used as a complete anesthetic agent when used alone. Opioids suppress cough reflex thereby increasing endotracheal tube tolerance.

Opioids in neurosurgery

Premedication and induction

In patients undergoing neurosurgery, especially those with raised ICP, opioids are generally avoided outside the operating room (preoperative room) as they suppress ventilation and increase ICP due to $PaCO_2$ raise. So, it is advisable to give opioids once after the patient is connected to all standard monitors on the operating table. Fentanyl premedication is usually given at doses ranging from 2 to 5 μg/kg to attenuate intubation response and further increase in ICP. Morphine or remifentanil infusions are also used to supplement induction agents and are found useful.[35] The administration of an opioid prior to, rather than after, noxious stimulation attenuates physiologic responses. Opioids significantly reduce the dose of propofol and other agents required for loss of consciousness and during noxious stimulation such as skin incision.[36] Opioids can decrease or abolish responses to an RSI and other noxious stimuli.[37] Studies also have found that opioids are better than esmolol in controlling heart rate during laryngoscopy.[38] Studies have found no difference in alfentanil, fentanyl, and remifentanil in neurosurgery patients in terms of hemodynamic and respiratory variables except for the reduced time of eye opening with remifentanil.[39] An opioid that does not depress cardiac activity at anesthetic doses offers an advantage, especially in patients with cardiac comorbidity.

Pin fixation response in neurosurgery

In addition to inhalational and intravenous anesthetic agents, opioids such as fentanyl or remifentanil are given as intravenous short boluses to cut off the head-pin fixation response.

Scalp block versus opioids: Scalp block is performed by infiltration of local anesthetics in the scalp and forehead to block sensory supply carried by supraorbital nerve, the supratrochlear nerve, the zygomaticotemporal nerve, the auriculotemporal nerve, and the greater and lesser occipital nerves emerging from the skull.[40] This block was used as an adjunct to propofol/remifentanil-based anesthetic during awake craniotomy in an adolescent patient.[41] Besides awake craniotomy, scalp block can be used for all craniotomies under general anesthesia. Scalp block with local anesthetics was shown to prevent the hemodynamic response to skull-pin placement and decrease the need for opioids.[42] The problem associated with the block is infiltration of higher doses of local anesthetics in a highly vascularized area.

Maintenance of anesthesia

Modern anesthesia refers to a balanced technique of using different agents to produce analgesia, amnesia, muscle relaxation, and abolition of autonomic reflexes with maintenance of homeostasis. The analgesic component is maintained by supplementation of opioids. The tight brain checklist includes pain as one of the causes to rule out raised ICP. Opioids do not have a direct effect on increasing or decreasing ICP.[43] Pain in neurosurgery occurs, especially during head-pin fixation, skin incision, craniotomy, dura mater incision, and laminectomy. Intermittent doses of opioids depending on its duration of action to maintain stable hemodynamics may be required. In patients undergoing spine fusion, infusion of fentanyl reduced the infusion rate of propofol necessary to stabilize mean arterial pressure but delayed spontaneous eye opening.[44] Short-acting opioids such as remifentanil can be given as continuous intravenous infusion.

In awake craniotomy and in surgeries in which sensory or motor evoked potential monitoring will be used, anesthesia is preferably maintained with total intravenous anesthesia. Combination of drugs such as propofol and remifentanil/fentanyl or a combination of dexmedetomidine with remifentanil/fentanyl and propofol is widely used to maintain anesthesia. Studies have found that there is no significant difference in emergence time, early postoperative cognitive function, pain, nausea, or vomiting when comparing sevoflurane and fentanyl with propofol and remifentanil.[45] Short-acting opioids and other short-acting anesthetic agents are preferred in neurosurgeries to assess postoperative neurological status of the patients.

Emergence

One of the main goals of extubation in neurosurgery includes smooth extubation to prevent any intracranial bleeding and sequelae. Smooth extubation refers to extubation of a fully conscious patient with good tube tolerance, without any increased fluctuations in hemodynamics and ICP, with good airway reflexes to protect airway after extubation. Intracranial hematoma during emergence is common in patients undergoing neurosurgery due to systemic hypertension.[46] Propofol, fentanyl, remifentanil,[47] Xylocard, esmolol, and lignocaine instillation[48] all have been studied to facilitate smooth extubation. In a study comparing propofol, isoflurane, and fentanyl in craniotomies, the authors found that low-dose fentanyl is more effective in preventing early hypertension at the time of emergence.[49]

Drugs should be given with careful titration according to an individual patient's response, specific condition of the patient, and the expected duration of the operation to avoid postoperative pain or respiratory depression. When the patient's ventilation is supported, there is a wide margin of safety while using opioids. After extubation, postoperative ventilatory depression is the major limitation in using opioids.

References

1. Boonyapisit K, Kaminski HJ, Ruff RL. Disorders of neuromuscular junction ion channels. *Am J Med* 1999;106:97.
2. Naguib M, Flood P, McArdle JJ, Brenner HR. Advances in neurobiology of the neuromuscular junction: Implications for the anesthesiologist. *Anesthesiology* 2002;96:202.
3. Perry J, Lee J, Wells G. Rocuronium versus succinylcholine for rapid sequence induction intubation. *Cochrane Database Syst Rev* 2003;1:CD002788.
4. Stirt JA, Grosslight KR, Bedford RF, Vollmer D. Defasciculation with metocurine prevents succinylcholine-induced increases in intracranial pressure. *Anesthesiology* 1987;67:50–53.
5. Hopkins PM. Malignant hyperthermia: Pharmacology of triggering. *Br J Anaesth* 2011;107(1):48–56.
6. Rosero E, Joshi GP. Total intravenous anesthesia: Present and future. *ASA Monitor.* August 2015; 79(8):10–57.
7. Murray MJ, Coursin DB, Scuderi PE et al. Doubleblind, randomized, multicenter study of doxacurium vs. pancuronium in intensive care unit patients who require neuromuscular-blocking agents. *Crit Care Med* 1995;23:450–458.
8. Lacomis D, Giuliani MJ, Van Cott A, Kramer DJ. Acute myopathy of intensive care: Clinical, electromyographic, and pathological aspects. *Ann Neurol* 1996;40:645–654.
9. Fodale V, Santamaria LB. Laudanosine, an atracurium and cisatracurium metabolite. *Eur J Anaesthesiol* 2002;19(7):466–473.
10. Manthous CA, Chatila W. Atracurium and status epilepticus. *Crit Care Med* 1995;23:1440–1442.

11. Ghoneim AA, El Beltagy MA. Comparative study between sugammadex and neostigmine in neurosurgical anesthesia in pediatric patients. *Saudi J Anaesth* 2015 Jul-Sep;9(3):247–252.

12. Tavernier B, Rannou JJ, Vallet B. Peripheral nerve stimulation and clinical assessment for dosing of neuromuscular blocking agents in critically ill patients. *Crit Care Med* 1998;26:804–805.

13. Rudis MI, Sikora CP, Angus E et al. A prospective, randomized, controlled evaluation of peripheral nerve stimulation versus standard clinical dosing of neuromuscular blocking agents in critically ill patients. *Crit Care Med* 1997;25:575–583.

14. Strange C, Vaughan L, Franklin C, Johnson J. Comparison of train-of-four and best clinical assessment during continuous paralysis. *Am J Resp Crit Care Med* 1997;156:1556–1561.

15. Frankel H, Jeng J, Tilly E, St Andre A, Champion H. The impact of implementation of neuromuscular blockade monitoring standards in a surgical intensive care unit. *Am Surg* 1996;62:503–506.

16. Ford EV. Monitoring neuromuscular blockade in the adult ICU. *Am J Crit Care* 1995;4:122–130.

17. Kleinpell R, Bedrosian C, McCormick L. Use of peripheral nerve stimulators to monitor patients with neuromuscular blockade in the ICU. *Am J Crit Care* 1996;5:449–454.

18. Murray MJ. Monitoring of peripheral nerve stimulation versus standard clinical assessment for dosing of neuromuscular blocking agents. *Crit Care Med* 1997;25:561–562.

19. Tavernier B, Rannou JJ, Vallet B. Peripheral nerve stimulation and clinical assessment for dosing of neuromuscular blocking agents in critically ill patients. *Crit Care Med* 1998;26:804–805.

20. Barnette RE, Fish DJ. Monitoring neuromuscular blockade in the critically ill. *Crit Care Med* 1995;23:1790–1791.

21. Berg H, Roed J, Viby-Mogensen J et al. Residual neuromuscular block is a risk factor for postoperative pulmonary complications. A prospective, randomised, and blinded study of postoperative pulmonary complications after atracurium, vecuronium and pancuronium. *Acta Anaesthesiol Scand* 1997;41:1095–1103.

22. Eriksson LI, Sato M, Severinghaus JW. Effect of a vecuronium-induced partial neuromuscular block on hypoxic ventilatory response. *Anesthesiology* 1993;78:693–699.

23. Eriksson LI, Sundman E, Olsson R, et al. Functional assessment of the pharynx at rest and during swallowing in partially paralysed humans: Simultaneous videomanometry and mechanomyography of awake human volunteers. *Anesthesiology* 1997;87:1035–1043.

24. Viby-Mogensen J. Postoperative residual curarization and evidence-based anaesthesia. *Br J Anaesth* 2000;84:301–303.

25. Dupuis JY, Martin R, Tessonnier JM, Tétrault JP. Clinical assessment of the muscular response to tetanic nerve stimulation. *Can J Anaesth* 1990;37:397.

26. Capron F, Fortier L-P, Racines S, Donati F. Tactile fade detection with hand or wrist stimulation using train-of-four, double-burst stimulation, 50-hertz tetanus, 100-hertz tetanus and acceleromyography. *Anesth Analg* 2006;102:1578.

27. Viby-Mogensen J, Howardy-Hansen P, Chraemmer-Jorgensen B, Ording H, Engbaek J, Nielsen A. Post-tetanic count (PTC). A new method of evaluating an intense nondepolarizing neuromuscular blockade. *Anesthesiology* 1981;55:458.

28. Engbæk J, Østergaard D, Viby-Mogensen J. Double burst stimulation (DBS). A new pattern of nerve stimulation to identify residual curarization. *Br J Anaesth* 1989;62:274.

29. Drenck NE, Olsen NV, Ueda N et al. Clinical assessment of residual curarization. A comparison of train-of-four stimulation and double burst stimulation. *Anesthesiology* 1989;70:578.

30. Saddler JM, Bevan JC, Donati F, Bevan DR, Pinto SR. Comparison of double-burst and train-of-four stimulation to assess neuromuscular blockade in children. *Anesthesiology* 1990;73:401.

31. Hemmerling TM, Schurr C, Walter S, Dern S, Schmidt J, Braun GG. A new method of monitoring the effect of muscle relaxants on laryngeal muscle using surface laryngeal electromyography. *Anesth Analg* 2000;90:494.

32. Hemmerling TM, Schmidt J, Wolf T, Hanusa C, Siebzehnruebl E, Schmitt H. Intramuscular versus surface electromyography of the diaphragm for determining neuromuscular blockade. *Anesth Analg* 2001;92:106.

33. Kirov K, Motamed C, Ndoko S-K, Dhonneur G. TOF count at corrugator supercilii reflects abdominal muscles relaxation better than at adductor pollicis. *Br J Anaesth* 2007;98:611.

34. Mortensen CR, Berg H, El-Mahdy A, Viby-Mogensen J. Perioperative monitoring of neuromuscular transmission using acceleromyography prevents residual neuromuscular block following pancuronium. *Acta Anaesthesiol Scand* 1995;39:797.

35. Gelb AW, Salevsky F, Chung F et al. Remifentanil with morphine transitional analgesia shortens neurological recovery compared to fentanyl for supratentorial craniotomy. *Can J Anaesth* 2003;50(9):946–952.

36. Smith C, McEwan AI, Jhaveri R et al. The interaction of fentanyl on the Cp50 of propofol for loss of consciousness and skin incision. *Anesthesiology* 1994;81:820–828.

37. Van Aken H, Meinshausen E, Prien T, Brüssel T, Heinecke A, Lawin P. The influence of fentanyl and tracheal intubation on the hemodynamic effects of anesthesia induction with propofol/N_2O in humans. *Anesthesiology* 1988;68:157–163.

38. Ebert JP, Pearson JD, Gelman S, Harris C, Bradley EL. Circulatory responses to laryngoscopy: The comparative effects of placebo, fentanyl and esmolol. *Can J Anaesth* 1989;36:301–306.

39. Magni G, Baisi F, La Rosa I et al. No difference in emergence time and early cognitive function between sevoflurane-fentanyl and propofol-remifentanil in patients undergoing craniotomy for supratentorial intracranial surgery. *J Neurosurg Anesthesiol* 2005;17:134–138.

40. Osborn I, Sebeo J. "Scalp Block" during craniotomy: A classic technique revisited. *J Neurosurg Anesthesiol* 2010;22(3):187–194.

41. B. Sung et al. Anesthetic management with scalp nerve block and propofol/remifentanil infusion during awake craniotomy in an adolescent patient—A case report. *Korean J Anesthesiol* 2010;59(Suppl):S179–S182.

42. Pardey G, Grousson S, de Souza EP, Mottolese C, Dailler F, Duflo F. Levobupivacaine scalp nerve block in children. *Pediatr Anesthesia* 2008;18(3):271–272.

43. Guy J, Hindman BJ, Baker KZ et al. Comparison of remifentanil and fentanyl in patients undergoing craniotomy for supratentorial space-occupying lesions. *Anesthesiology* 1997;86(3):514–524.

44. Han T, Kim D, Kil H, Inagaki Y. The effects of plasma fentanyl concentrations on propofol requirement, emergence from anesthesia, and postoperative analgesia in propofol nitrous oxide anesthesia. *Anesth Analg* 2000;90:1365–1371.

45. Coles JP, Leary TS, Monteiro JN et al. Propofol anesthesia for craniotomy: A double blind comparison of remifentanil, alfentanil and fentanyl. *J Neurosurg Anesthesiol* 2000;12:15–20.

46. Basali A, Mascha EJ, Kalfas I, Schubert A. Relation between perioperative hypertension and intracranial haemorrhage after craniotomy. *Anesthesiology* 2000;93:48–54.

47. Lee B, Lee JR, Na S. Targeting smooth emergence: The effect site concentration of remifentanil for preventing cough during emergence during propofol–remifentanil anaesthesia for thyroid surgery. *Br J Anaesth* 2009;102(6):775–778.

48. Chan PBK. On smooth extubation without coughing and bucking. *Can J Anesth* 2002;49(3):324–324.

49. Bhagat H, Dash HH, Bithal PK, Chouhan RS, Pandia MP. Planning for early emergence in neurosurgical patients: A randomized prospective trial of low-dose anesthetics. *Anesth Analg* 2008;107(4):1348–1355.

22

Perioperative steroids

M. V. S. SATYA PRAKASH

Introduction

Steroids are the hormones produced by the adrenal cortex.[1] Among the steroids that are produced by the adrenal cortex, glucocorticoids are used for treatment of a wide range of diseases and in neuroanesthesia applications. The glucocorticoids that are available and in use can be divided into three groups:

Short acting: cortisol, cortisone, prednisone, prednisolone, and methylprednisolone
Intermediate acting: triamcinolone, paramethasone, and fluprednisolone
Long acting: betamethasone and dexamethasone

Pharmacological actions of steroids: Commonly synthetic glucocorticoids are used for most clinical purposes because they have no saltretaining properties and have less affinity for the receptor. The direct actions of steroids are anti-inflammatory, anti-allergy, and immunosuppression. The other actions are hypertension, lipolysis, and broncho-dilation.

Actions of steroids on the central nervous system (CNS): They have both direct and indirect actions. The direct actions are alterations in mood, behavior, and excitability, and the indirect actions are maintaining the blood–brain barrier and electrolyte balance.

On prolonged use, steroids can have side effects such as growth retardation, osteoporosis, myopathy, cataract formation, appearance of moon face, hypertension, peptic ulceration, immunosuppression, delayed and improper wound healing, interaction with non-depolarizing neuromuscular blocking agents, neuropsychiatric disorders, and pancreatitis.

High doses of steroids can cause acutely glucose intolerance, arrhythmia, myocardial infarction, bowel perforation, neuropsychiatric disorders, and rarely pancreatitis.[2]

Hydrocortisone: This is available in oral, topical, intravenous, and rectal administration forms. It is commonly used for treating asthma and shock in oral and intravenous routes. It is topically used for eczema and rectally for ulcerative colitis.

Prednisolone: This is used commonly for treating inflammatory and allergic components of diseases.

Dexamethasone: This is a long-acting drug and does not have salt-retaining properties, so it is commonly used for high-dose therapies and where only less doses can be administered.

Beclomethasone: This is commonly used in topical form to treat skin diseases and is also available in nebulized form for asthma.

Budesonide: This is used for asthma in inhaled form.

Triamcinolone: This is used topically for skin diseases.

Role of steroids in neuroanesthesia

Steroids are used as follows:

1. As perioperative stress dose
2. As replacement therapy during pituitary surgeries
3. For treating intracranial pressure (ICP) during surgery
4. For treating traumatic spinal and brain injuries
5. For treating cerebral edema in cerebral tumors
6. For miscellaneous use such as in carpal tunnel syndrome, Bell's palsy, cranial nerve damage, chronic subdural hematoma (SDH), dexamethasone suppression test, neurodegenerative diseases, and meningitis

Tests

Steroids are generally given when there is alteration in the steroid regulation of synthesis. So there are many tests that are developed for assessment of the hypothalamic–pituitary–adrenal (HPA) axis. They are as follows:

1. Single measurement of serum cortisol and urinary free cortisol
2. Random cortisol estimation
3. Short Synacthen test (SST)
4. Insulin tolerance test (ITT)
5. Corticotropin-releasing hormone (CRH) test
6. Overnight metyrapone test
7. Glucagon stimulation test

Single measurement of serum cortisol and urinary free cortisol

In olden days, single measurement of serum cortisol and urinary free cortisol was used to assess the HPA. As the secretion of the steroids varies depending on the time of the day and working nature of the individuals, many discrepancies were found in this test. So this test is rarely done nowadays.

Random cortisol estimation

When a patient is in severe stress, the endogenous HPA axis function should be at the maximum level. So if we estimate the random serum cortisol level during this situation, it will give an idea about the function of the adrenal gland. Except in this situation, random cortisol estimation may not be useful in patient treatment.

Short synacthen test

Synacthen is a synthetic corticotropin, synthetic polypeptide β. Synacthen (tetracosactrin) is a synthetic analog, comprising amino acids 1–24 of the 39-amino-acid peptide adrenocorticotropic hormone (ACTH). This sequence retains the full biological activity of intact ACTH. Synacthen stimulates the normal adrenal cortex to secrete cortisol, which can then be measured in serum. Prednisolone and hydrocortisone cross-react with cortisol assays, but the SST is suitable for patients who were recently started on steroid replacement or are on low dose steroids. For these patients, the steroid dose should be omitted in the evening before the test (if possible) and on the morning of the test.

Contraindications

Contraindications for this test are pregnancy, allergy to the Synacthen, and use of oral contraceptive pills.

Procedure

No special preparation for the test is required. As the cortisol levels vary throughout the day, it is preferable to perform the test as nearly as possible to 9 A.M. Results can be interpreted to the nearest correct if it is done as nearly as to 9 A.M. First at the start, a sample of blood should be taken to measure basal cortisol level. After which 250 μg Synacthen should be given either IM or IV. Then once again at 30 and 60 min (optional) a blood sample should be taken for measurement of cortisol level for the response to the test. A patient responds normally with the highest peak cortisol level at 30-min interval, and after 60 min the cortisol level starts decreasing and by 4 h reaches normal.

Interpretation

There are many controversies in the interpretation of this test. Interpretation varies depending on the lab and the area where it is performed, as the normal levels vary depending on the ethnicity and area. Hurel et al.[3] assessed 57 healthy volunteers and found that the mean 30-min cortisol value during SST was 390 nmol/L and the 60-min value was 500 nmol/L. Clayton[4] has suggested that by taking a 30-min cortisol value of >600 nmol/L as a pass in the SST, the sensitivity of the test could be increased, the number of false-positive *pass* results reduced to 3.5%, and the number of ITTs undertaken reduced by 25%. But on the whole many investigators agree on 500–600 nmol/L as a cutoff value for interpreting the test as a normal response, so each lab has to determine their value depending on the local area values.

There is a controversy about the amount of Synacthen that should be administered. A few authors propose 1 μg Synacthen and others advise 250 μg Synacthen.[5–8] Some authors consider that the dose of 250 μg Synacthen is supraphysiological and may cause false-positive results in some patients. So using 1 μg Synacthen and measuring cortisol at 30 min will give more sensitivity in at least some patients who are on long-term steroids.

Insulin tolerance test

This is the gold standard test for assessing the function of the HPA axis.[9,10] This test should be performed in an inpatient context under the supervision of trained doctors only.

Indications

This test is used for assessment of growth hormone (GH) and cortisol reserve, and to differentiate between Cushing's syndrome and pseudo-Cushing's syndrome.

Contraindications

1. Age > 60 years.
2. Ischemic heart disease.
3. Epilepsy.
4. Severe panhypopituitarism and hypoadrenalism.
5. Hypothyroidism impairs the GH and cortisol response. Patients should be treated with corticosteroid replacement starting prior to thyroxine as the latter has been reported to precipitate an Addisonian crisis with dual deficiency. If adrenal insufficiency is confirmed, the need for a repeat ITT may need to be reconsidered after 3 months of thyroxine therapy.

Side effects

1. Loss of consciousness
2. Seizures
3. Resistant hypoglycemia
4. Myocardial infarction
5. Unpleasant sensation
6. Sweating
7. Palpitations
8. Severe hypoglycemia

Advantages over other tests

1. As this test provides the stimulus at the level of the hypothalamus, it examines the entire HPA axis.
2. It has more reproducible results than any other test for testing the HPA axis and for detecting cortisol deficiency.
3. Even though there is variability in peak cortisol value in patients with hypopituitarism, repeat testing did not misclassify any patient.

Principle

When insulin is administered neuroglycopenia occurs to less than 2.2 nmol/l, which results in release of both ACTH and GH from the pituitary which in turn leads to release of cortisol from adrenal glands.

Procedure

The patient should be fasting overnight. Once the patient is on the table, he/she should be recumbent until the end of the procedure. A good IV cannula should be secured and 25% dextrose should be ready to combat any untoward incident. Blood sample should be taken for baseline measurements of cortisol and GH, whichever is proper for the patient. Then 0.10–0.15 IU/kg soluble insulin should be given IV to the patient. Blood glucose levels should be checked. A response to hypoglycemia should come to the level of <2.2 mmol/L. Blood samples should be withdrawn at 30, 45, 60, 90, and 120 min after the injection of insulin. At least two samples should be collected once the hypoglycemic response appears. If hypoglycemia is intolerable, the patient should be given 25% glucose or food after 1 h of insulin injection. If hypoglycemia does not appear by 45 min, the test should be repeated.

Interpretation

Peak cortisol level of >500 nmol/L at any time during the test indicates that the HPA axis is working properly to the adequate level.[11] If the peak cortisol level is <500 nmol/L, then it is said to be hypoadrenalism.

Corticotropin-releasing hormone test

The patient should be given 1 μg/kg or 100 μg corticotropin-releasing hormone (CRH) and the maximum cortisol response should be assessed over 2 h. If the maximum cortisol response is >550 nmol/L, then it indicates that the HPA axis is responding normally. This test is useful mainly in differential diagnosis of Cushing's syndrome. But its use is controversial as a routine test to test the HPA axis as its performance in pituitary disease is inferior to estimation of basal cortisol level, and at the same time, it does not provide any further information in the group of patients whose response is intermediate.[12]

Both human and bovine CRH are available for conducting the test. The bovine form has longer duration of action than the human form. So the majority of the labs prefer the bovine form. CRH concentrations should increase during ITT. But many factors (such as CRH binding protein, extrahypothalamic sources of CRH, assay variability in the presence of secretagogues) cause discrepancy in the results. So random/stimulated/suppressed CRH level testing is not useful.

Overnight metyrapone test

In this test, the patient has to be given 30 mg/kg metyrapone at 12 A.M. with food to minimize the gastrointestinal side effects. Plasma cortisol and 11-deoxycortisol has to be measured at 8 A.M. the next day. A 11-dexoycortisol level of >200 nmol/L (7 μg/dL) is a normal response.[13] Measurement of ACTH improves the sensitivity of the test. But until now the cutoff value of ACTH has not been determined to diagnose the normal response. Further trials are needed to use this test as a main test.

Glucagon stimulation test

IM or SC administration of 1 mg glucagon may also stimulate the HPA axis, leading to production of peak cortisol level of >500 nmol/L. As the responses are variable and not reproducible to an adequate level, this test is not used regularly for testing the intactness of the HPA axis.

There is no single test that perfectly determines the adrenal insufficiency. SST is criticized for its lack of uniform pass criteria and also some authors raised doubts about its accuracy. ITT has good accuracy, and an acceptable level of sensitivity and specificity, but it has its own disadvantages. So a battery of tests is required to determine the adequacy of function of the HPA axis. If the basal cortisol level at 8 A.M. is <100 nmol/L or the random cortisol level is >500 nmol/L, then there is no need to proceed for any other testing as they indicate that the patient surely is having adrenal insufficiency or perfect adrenal function. ITT should be reserved for those patients who are showing equivocal results in other tests including SST.

Effect of anesthesia on HPA axis

General anesthesia

Single induction dose of etomidate inhibits cortisol production for 8 h.[14] Midazolam has an imidazole ring in its structure, which also is found to decrease cortisol response.[15,16] Volatile agents are found to have no effect on the HPA axis. Fentanyl with a dose of 50 µg/kg is found to abolish cortisol response to pelvic surgery[17] and with 100 µg/kg in upper abdominal surgery.[18]

Regional anesthesia

If complete afferent and efferent blockade is achieved then the cortisol response to the surgery is abolished. This can be done in limb surgery, eye surgery, and pelvic surgery if the blockade is to the level of T4 to S5.

Perioperative stress-dose steroids

Since the first report of adrenal crisis in a patient on exogenous steroids 65 years ago, there were many postulations, many practices, and many recommendations on perioperative stress-dose steroids. Normally in humans, the adrenal gland secretes cortisol as a response to stress. In olden days, when anesthesia was not developed, this response was supposedly present during surgery. But with the evolution of anesthesia in the present-day scenario, the anesthesia team tries to obtund this response to the maximum level. But anesthesia is not developed to the level that this surgical stress response is prevented at all times in all types of surgeries. During the early period, there used to be a recommendation that supraphysiological doses of steroids are required in patients whose HPA axis is obtunded due to regular treatment with steroids. But during the late 1990s, it was proven that these supraphysiological doses of steroids are unnecessary and not required, and an algorithm was proposed by Kehlet[19], Symreng et al.,[20] and Salem et al.[21] In the twenty-first century and particularly after 2010, there were many articles published contradicting this algorithm also. Kelly and Domajnko[22] opined that this algorithm is also not necessary to follow and it is sufficient to give rescue steroids only when there is unresponsive hemodynamic instability.

But a meta-analysis done by Yong et al.[23] could not refute or support this claim. After considering all these reports, the authors are of the opinion that if it is feasible it is better to establish the intactness of the HPA axis and make a decision. If it is felt that testing the HPA axis is too much for the surgery that is going on, try to follow one of the algorithms advocated by Kehlet[19], Symreng et al.,[20] and Salem et al.[21]

The steroid treatment regimen followed widely is given here.[2] It is assumed that for patients on <10 mg prednisolone per day, the HPA axis is preserved and there is no need of any additional steroid supplementation. If patients are on >10 mg prednisolone per day and if they are undergoing a minor surgery such as herniorrhaphy, they should either take their routine dose of steroids preoperatively or be supplemented with 25 mg hydrocortisone at induction and resume their oral steroid therapy postoperatively. If patients are undergoing a moderate surgery such as total abdominal hysterectomy, they should receive their routine dose of steroids and also 25 mg hydrocortisone at induction and 100 mg hydrocortisone for 24 h as infusion. Patients should start their normal oral steroid supplementation on postoperative day 2. If patients are undergoing a major surgery then they should take their routine dose of steroids and 25 mg hydrocortisone at induction and 100 mg/day hydrocortisone for 48–72 h, and the regular doses of steroids should be started as and when bowel movements return. Patients who were on steroids and had stopped the steroid treatment within less than 3 months should be treated as if they are on steroids, and those patients who have stopped for more than 3 months should be treated as if their HPA axis is working normally. Patients who are on high doses of steroids for immunosuppression have to be given their daily doses of steroid during the perioperative period. Additional doses of steroid are not required as the immunosuppressive doses are more than sufficient to maintain hemodynamic stability.

As replacement therapy during pituitary surgeries

We divide the pituitary tumors into two types for deciding the steroid supplementation during the perioperative period. They are ACTH-secreting and non-ACTH-secreting pituitary adenomas.

Non-ACTH-secreting pituitary adenomas

Before any pituitary surgery, the adequacy of the HPA axis has to be established by a battery of tests. Even though ITT is the gold standard test, many authors are of the opinion that it is an excessive test at this time. Many units consider doing SST at this stage. SST results can be abnormal either because of a nonsecreting tumor or the tumor might be compressing the normal tissue making it temporarily nonfunctional. If the SST result is abnormal, the patient should be started with 15–30 mg hydrocortisone daily depending on the age, sex, ethnicity, and body habitus. Then the patient should be treated with supraphysiological doses of steroid cover during the first 48 h of the perioperative period. The regimens that are suggested are either 50 mg hydrocortisone q 8 h on day 0, 25 mg hydrocortisone q 8 h on day 1, and 25 mg hydrocortisone at 8 A.M. on day 2 or 4 mg dexamethasone at induction, 2 mg dexamethasone at 8 A.M. on day 1, and 0.5 mg dexamethasone at 8 A.M. on day 2. If there are no complications during the surgery and in the postoperative period, the steroid supplementation should be discontinued and plasma cortisol levels collected at 8 A.M. have to be checked on day 3–5 for further management. If the patient had normal SST results preoperatively and the tumor is located in such a way that the surgeon can perform a selective pituitary adenomectomy, then steroid supplementation is not required during the preoperative and intraoperative period. Cortisol level has to be measured at 8 A.M. on day 1–3 for making a decision on steroid supplementation in these patients. If the surgeon is of the opinion that he/she cannot perform a selective adenomectomy or the surgery is extensive, then the patient had to be treated like they have an abnormal SST result.[10]

In the postoperative period, if the 8 A.M. plasma cortisol level (on days 1–3, for the patients who had not received steroid supplementation and on days 3–5, in the patients who had steroid supplementation) is <100 nmol/L then it is confirmed that the patients have HPA axis dysfunction and they should be supplemented with 15–30 mg hydrocortisone daily for further life. If the patient has a cortisol level of >450 nmol/L then the patient is considered to have an absolutely normal HPA axis function and he/she does not require any steroid supplementation. If the patient has an 8 A.M. cortisol level between 100 and 250 nmol/L then the patient has to be supplemented with 10–20 mg hydrocortisone as single morning dose with the instructions that further steroid supplementation has to be done during the periods of stress until the HPA axis is tested at 4–6 weeks into the postoperative period to decide about steroid replacement. If the patient had an 8 A.M. plasma cortisol level between 250 and 450 nmol/L then the patient need not be on routine steroid supplementation, but the patient requires steroid supplementation during the periods of stress and a definitive test needs to be conducted for deciding about steroid supplementation 4–6 weeks into the postoperative period.[10]

ACTH-secreting pituitary adenomas

All the patients with ACTH-secreting pituitary adenomas require steroid supplementation during the perioperative period. After the surgery if the patient has low plasma cortisol level, the patient needs to be supplemented with steroids until the HPA axis function is tested. In this situation, the pituitary gland recovers slowly once the ACTH suppression stops and the steroid had to be supplemented till the HPA axis returns to its normal function. Estimation of 24-h urinary cortisol may help in making a decision and it can be done while receiving physiological replacement with dexamethasone 0.5–0.75 mg daily.

Patients who are hemodynamically unstable and supposedly having pituitary apoplexy have to be supplemented with 100–200 mg hydrocortisone followed up with 2–4 mg continuous infusion or 50–100 mg 6 hourly by IM route after drawing the blood samples for hormone assays.

Steroid supplementation in brain tumors

Use of steroids in brain tumors for reducing edema started more than 60 years ago.[24] Several mechanisms such as inhibition of phospholipase A2, stabilization of lysosomal membranes, and improvement of peritumoral microcirculation have been proposed.[25] But according to recent studies, the corticosteroids reduce the expression of edema-producing factor vascular endothelial growth factor (VEGF) and thereby capillary permeability without causing change in the absorption mechanism.[26] The effect is observed as early as 1 h after administration of the drug. Corticosteroids are effective in reducing the cerebral edema only when the blood–brain barrier is intact. Dexamethasone is the drug of choice in these situations. The dose that is advised is 4 mg/day.[27] Vecht et al.[28] conducted a dose-dependent study in which they gave 4, 8, and 16 mg/day dexamethasone to three different groups and found that the edema-reducing effect was the same in all the three groups but the side effects increased with the increase in the dose. So they concluded that the dose of 4 mg/day dexamethasone is sufficient and effective with minimal side effects. After successful treatment of the tumor by resection, steroids should be tapered gradually within 2–3 weeks. Corticosteroids should be tapered by 50% every 4–5 days if there are no problems and if the surgeon could achieve full tumor resection. But if there are problems and there is partial resection of the tumor, steroids should be tapered at the rate of 25% every 8 days. In some patients, corticosteroid treatment may be continued for a long time at the dose of 1–2 mg/day for acceptable quality of life of the patient. If corticosteroids are tapered too fast, the patient may develop steroid withdrawal syndrome.

Recent studies show promising results for decreasing cerebral edema in brain tumors by administering corticotropin-releasing factor (CRF). But further studies are required to introduce and practice it regularly as a main treatment.

Role in traumatic spinal and head injuries

The National Acute Spinal Cord Injury Studies (NASCIS) II and III in the late 1990s threw some light on the role of corticosteroids in acute spinal cord injury. Even though these studies show some benefit after administration of corticosteroids, now it is level I recommendation to not use corticosteroids for acute spinal cord injuries.[29]

Similarly, even though the Corticosteroid Randomization after Significant Head Injury (CRASH) studies had recommended the use of corticosteroids in head injury, recent Brain Trauma Foundation guidelines published in the *Journal of Neurotrauma* in 2007 provide a level I recommendation that corticosteroids should not be used for moderate and severe traumatic brain injury.

Steroids are also used for treating painful conditions such as low back pain and nerve root pain. They are used in the form of pain blocks and epidural steroids. A recent systematic review states that there is level II evidence for caudal and epidural steroid for 2-year efficacy for low back pain and lower extremity pain for patients with lumbar central spinal stenosis and there is level III evidence for short-term efficacy for transforaminal injections.[30] The drugs that can be used for this purpose are generally mixed with a local anesthetic and then administered. The steroids that are used commonly are 20–40 mg triamcinolone and 40–80 mg methyl prednisolone.

References

1. Abraham R. Steroids in neuroinfection. *Arq Neuropsiquiatr* 2013;71(9B):717–721.
2. Nicholson G, Burrin JM, Hall GM. Peri-operative steroid supplementation. *Anaesthesia* 1998;53:1091–1104.
3. Hurel SJ, Thompson CJ, Watson MJ, Harris MM, Baylis PH, Kendal-Taylor P. The short Synacthen and insulin stress tests in the assessment of the hypothalamic-pituitary-adrenal axis. *Clin Endocrinol* 1996;44:141–146.
4. Clayton RN. Short Synacthen test versus insulin stress test for assessment of the hypothalamo-pituitary-adrenal axis: Controversy revisited. *Clin Endocrinol* 1996;44:147–149.
5. Tordjman K, Jaffe A, Grazas N, Apter C, Stern N. The role of the low dose (1 microgram) adrenocorticotropin test in the evaluation of patients with pituitary diseases. *J Clin Endocrinol Metab* 1995;80:1301–1305.
6. Oelkers W. The role of high- and low-dose corticotropin tests in the diagnosis of secondary adrenal insufficiency. *Eur J Endocrinol* 1998;139:567–570.
7. Thaler LM, Blevins LS Jr. The low dose (1-microg) adrenocorticotropin stimulation test in the evaluation of patients with suspected central adrenal insufficiency. *J Clin Endocrinol Metab* 1998;83:2726–2729.

8. Stewart PM, Clark P. The short Synacthen test: Is less best? *Clin Endocrinol (Oxf)* 1999;51:151–152.

9. Fish HR, Chernow B, O'Brian JT. Endocrine and neurophysiologic responses of the pituitary to insulin-induced hypoglycemia: A review. *Metabolism* 1986;35:763–780.

10. Inder WJ, Hunt PJ. Glucocorticoid replacement in pituitary surgery: Guidelines for perioperative assessment and management. *J Clin Endocrinol Metab* 2002;87(6):2745–2750.

11. Nelson JC, Tindall DJ Jr. A comparison of the adrenal responses to hypoglycemia, metyrapone and ACTH. *Am J Med Sci* 1978;275:165–172.

12. Dullaart RP, Pasterkamp SH, Beentjes JA, Sluiter WJ. Evaluation of adrenal function in patients with hypothalamic and pituitary disorders: Comparison of serum cortisol, urinary free cortisol and the human-corticotrophin releasing hormone test with the insulin tolerance test. *Clin Endocrinol (Oxf)* 1999;50:465–471.

13. Fiad TM, Kirby JM, Cunningham SK, McKenna TJ. The overnight single dose metyrapone test is a simple and reliable index of the hypothalamic-pituitary-adrenal axis. *Clin Endocrinol (Oxf)* 1994;40:603–609.

14. Fragen RJ, Shanks CA, Molteni A, Avram MJ. Effects of etomidate on hormonal responses to surgical stress. *Anesthesiology* 1984;61:652–656.

15. Crozier TA, Beck D, Schlaeger M, Wuttke W, Kettler D. Endocrinological changes following etomidate midazolam, or methohexital for minor surgery. *Anesthesiology* 1987;66:628–635.

16. Desborough JP, Hall GM, Hart GR, Burrin JM. Midazolam modifies pancreatic and anterior pituitary hormone secretion during upper abdominal surgery. *Br J Anaesth* 1991;67:390–396.

17. Hall GM, Young C, Holdcroft A, Alaghband-Zadeh J. Substrate mobilisation during surgery: A comparison between halothane and fentanyl anaesthesia. *Anaesthesia* 1978;33:924–930.

18. Klingstedt C, Giesecke K, Hamberger B, Järnberg PO. High and low dose fentanyl anaesthesia: Circulatory and plasma catecholamine responses during cholecystectomy. *Br J Anaesth* 1987;59:184–188.

19. Kehlet H. A rational approach to dosage and preparation of parenteral glucocorticoid substitution therapy during surgical procedures. A short review. *Acta Anaesthesiol Scand* 1975;19:260–264.

20. Symreng T, Karlberg BE, Kågedal B, Schildt B. Physiological cortisol substitution of long-term steroid-treated patients undergoing major surgery. *Br J Anaesth* 1981;53:949–953.

21. Salem M, Tainsh RE, Bromberg J, Loriaux DL, Chernow B. Perioperative glucocorticoid coverage: A reassessment 42 years after emergence of a problem. *Ann Surg* 1994;219:416–425.

22. Kelly KN, Domajnko B. Perioperative stress-dose steroids. *Clin Colon Rectal Surg* 2013;26:163–167.

23. Yong SL, Marik P, Esposito M, Coulthard P. Supplemental perioperative steroids for surgical patients with adrenal insufficiency. *Cochrane Database Syst Rev* 2009;(4):CD005367.

24. Ruderman NB, Hall TC. Use of glucocorticoids in the palliative treatment of metastatic brain tumors. *Cancer* 1965;18:298–306.

25. Yamada K, Ushio Y, Hayakawa T. Effects of steroids on the blood–brain barrier. In: Neuwelt EA, editor. *Implications of the Blood–Brain Barrier and Its Manipulation.* New York, NY: Plenum Press; 1989, pp. 53–76.

26. Heiss JD, Papavassiliou E, Merrill MJ et al. Mechanism of dexamethasone suppression of brain tumor-associated vascular permeability in rats. Involvement of the glucocorticoid receptor and vascular permeability factor. *J Clin Invest* 1996;98:1400–1408.

27. Kaal EC, Vecht CJ. The management of brain edema in brain tumors. *Curr Opin Oncol* 2004;16:593–600.

28. Vecht CJ, Hovestadt A, Verbiest HB, van Vliet JJ, van Putten WL. Dose–effect relationship of dexamethasone on Karnofsky performance in metastatic brain tumors: A randomized study of doses of 4, 8, and 16 mg per day. *Neurology* 1994;44:675–680.

29. Hurlber RJ, Hadley MN, Walters BC et al. Pharmacological therapy for acute spinal cord injury. *Neurosurgery* 2013;72:93–105.

30. Manchikanti L, Kaye AD, Manchikanti K, Boswell M, Pampati V, Hirsch J. Efficacy of epidural injections in the treatment of lumbar central spinal stenosis: A systematic review. *Anesth Pain Med* 2015;5(1):e23139.

23

Emergence from anesthesia

SONIA KAPIL and HEMANT BHAGAT

Introduction

Emergence from anesthesia is described as the phase whereby the effects of the various general anesthetic agents on amnesia and muscle relaxation are reversed along with the removal of a definitive airway. Emergence from general anesthesia and extubation is a period of physiological stress characterized by sympathetic stimulation leading to hemodynamic and metabolic reactions.[1,2] The phase lasting 5–15 min is associated with increased oxygen consumption, catecholamine secretion, tachycardia, hypertension, changes in arterial blood gases, and hyperglycemia.[3–6] The hemodynamic perturbations are more in the pre-extubation period as compared to the extubation and immediate post-extubation periods.[7] These metabolic and cardiovascular responses may adversely affect the balance between myocardial oxygen supply and demand. The events may increase cerebral blood flow (CBF) and cerebral oxygen consumption, potentially producing elevation of intracranial pressure (ICP), thus favoring cerebral insults.[8,9] This can, however, be tolerated by most of the patients, but the patients with cardiac and cerebrovascular diseases could be prone to complications.

The conduct of emergence from anesthesia should ensure that it is easy, predictable, and smooth. In light of this, this chapter discusses the various aspects of emergence from anesthesia.

Pathophysiological changes during emergence

There can be various pathophysiological changes during emergence from anesthesia. This section deals with the effects of emergence from anesthesia on the systemic physiology (Figure 23.1).

Neurological effects

It is a well-known fact that severe stress increases CBF and cerebral metabolic oxygen requirement ($CMRO_2$), which have been observed during emergence from anesthesia.[4] The mechanisms behind these changes are not fully understood. Sympathetic stimulation acting through

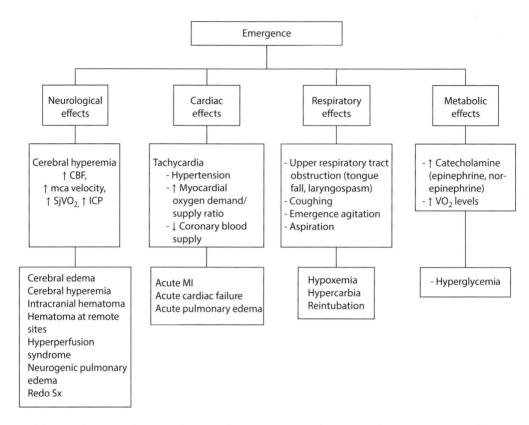

Figure 23.1 A schematic diagram showing the systemic manifestations during emergence from anesthesia. (MI, myocardial infarction; Redo Sx, Redo surgery.)

β-adrenoreceptors may play a role.[10] This adrenergic stimulation may further increase CBF and CMRO$_2$ following neurosurgery in patients with central nervous system (CNS) lesions or disrupted blood–brain barrier (BBB).[11]

Factors related to anesthesia, such as hypocapnia and anesthetic technique, may enhance BBB disruption.[12]

Bruder et al.[8] reported a 60% increase in Vmca above the awake value at extubation while the jugular venous bulb oxygen saturation increased to 81%. They concluded that cerebral hyperemia occurs independently of the anesthesia technique (inhalational or intravenous) and hemodynamic and ventilatory changes. CBF velocity returned gradually toward the baseline values 60 min after extubation.

Endotracheal suctioning also increases ICP and can either increase or decrease cerebral perfusion pressure (CPP).[13–16] The ICP increase usually lasts 2 or 3 min, but can be longer in case of reduced intracranial compliance. This sudden rise in ICP can be anticipated in patients with "tight brain" and thus can have deleterious effects in patients with reduced intracranial compliance.

Cardiovascular effects

Hypertension is frequent during emergence with a reported incidence of 70%–90%. This can cause cerebral hyperemia, leading to the increased incidence of postoperative intracranial edema and hemorrhage.[8,17,18] Hypertension is multifactorial in origin, arising secondary to sympathetic stimulation. If a >20% increase in blood pressure is considered for treatment, 40%–90% of patients require an antihypertensive therapy during emergence.[17–19] The most commonly feared complication after neurosurgery is the development of intracranial hematoma, the incidence of which ranges from 0.8% to 2.2%.[20] Basali et al.[21] described a link between perioperative hypertension and intracranial hemorrhage after craniotomy although a direct causal relationship could not be made.

Arousal from anesthesia, presence of endotracheal tube, and pain could also contribute to emergence hypertension. Neurologic causes of cardiovascular instability include raised ICP, brain stem injury, involvement of T1–T4 sympathetic nerves, spinal shock, and autonomic hyperreflexia after spinal injury. Cardiac dysfunction and neurogenic pulmonary edema may be secondary to significant sympathetic activation after subarachnoid hemorrhage.[22] Postoperative hemodynamic instability is common in patients undergoing carotid endarterectomy. A tight control of blood pressure is mandatory in the patients at risk of "hyperperfusion syndrome."

Respiratory effects

Respiratory complications include local trauma, coughing, desaturation, breath-holding, masseter spasm, laryngospasm, airway obstruction, and aspiration. In the early postoperative period after elective craniotomy, autoregulation is often impaired, with 20% of patients demonstrating raised ICP, and both hypoxemia and hypercarbia can exacerbate the secondary injury in the patients.[23]

Depressed level of consciousness with failure to maintain a patent airway is the most common cause of reintubation in the postoperative period. Respiratory complications specific to neurosurgical patients are related to the disease per se, positioning of the patients in the intraoperative period (prone/sitting), and surgical approach. Decreased or absent gag reflex and diaphragm involvement in high cervical spine injuries may delay extubation. Tongue and upper airway edema should always be considered in prolonged prone and sitting positions. Vocal cord dysfunction is also a possibility in the patients with carotid endarterectomy (CEA) and anterior cervical spine injury. Transsphenoidal surgeries also pose a challenge during emergence because of higher incidence of difficult airway in acromegaly patients, nasal packing, trickling of blood in the oral cavity, and associated comorbidities.

Coughing can be deleterious in neurosurgical patients as it leads to the Valsalva effect and rise in ICP.[24]

Metabolic effects

Increase in oxygen consumption (VO_2), catecholamine levels, and sympathetic activation are the most significant relevant metabolic changes that occur during recovery. Shivering and pain are the most common factors responsible, though a part can be attributed to regaining consciousness and recovery of spontaneous ventilation after a controlled weaning.

Other systemic effects

1. *Nausea/vomiting*: Postoperative nausea and vomiting (PONV) is a common problem, with an overall incidence of 50%–73% in neurosurgical patients. In addition to patient discomfort, there is always a risk of aspiration in patients with altered sensorium and depressed airway reflexes, particularly in the immediate postoperative period. The physical act of vomiting in itself increases ICP. Protracted PONV can cause dehydration and acid–base disturbance.[25]

2. *Pain*: 55%–60% patients have moderate-to-severe pain in the first 24–48 h.[26,27] Adverse effects of analgesics leading to underdosing are commonly observed in neuroanesthesia practices. Inadequate analgesia can complicate emergence, leading to emergence agitation and emergence hypertension. Surgery for posterior fossa tumors and acoustic neuromas is associated with a higher incidence of disabling postoperative headache.[28]

3. *Shivering*: Post-anesthetic shivering affects 5%–65% of the patients after general anesthesia. Abolition of thermoregulation and behavioral mechanisms have been implicated for shivering.[29,30] Hypothermia also prolongs recovery fro neuromuscular antagonists and causes delayed awakening.[30] Mild perioperative hypothermia (33°C –36.4°C) due to long duration of neurosurgeries is a common observation. Shivering leads to increase in VO_2 by 200%–400%.[4,29-33]

4. *Emergence agitation*: Emergence agitation is a state of aggressive agitation that occurs temporarily in the process of emerging from anesthesia and occurs most often during the early stages of emergence. The incidence of

emergence agitation has been found to be less in adults as compared to the pediatric population. However, in adults there may be more possibility of injury as the medical staff may not be able to restrain the patient.

Factors affecting emergence from anesthesia

The factors can be broadly categorized as patient-related factors, surgical factors, and anesthesia-related factors.

Patient-related factors

1. *Age*: Age >65 years has been shown to be associated with the failure of extubation in the immediate postoperative period. Elderly patients may also have increased risk of reintubation.[34]
2. *Sex*: None of the studies, except one where female sex was considered a risk for extubation failure, has shown any difference in reintubation and extubation failure among the two sexes.[35] In our experience, gender does not seem to play any role in emergence.
3. *American Society of Anesthesiologists (ASA) status*: Higher ASA status >II is an independent predictor of failed *On Table* extubation and risk of reintubation.[34,35] Patients with poor ASA status are more likely to remain intubated after major surgery.[36] They also tend to have more surgical and nonsurgical complications after craniotomy.[37]
4. *Glasgow Coma Scale (GCS)/level of consciousness*: Nivatpumin et al.[38] found GCS less than 13 as an independent predictor of delayed extubation while Vidotto et al.[35] and Namen et al.[39] found GCS less than 8 to be significantly associated with extubation failure (i.e., need of reintubation in 24–72 h). This is probably because the patients with low GCS are more likely to get intubated in the preoperative period in view of inability to maintain the airway patency.
5. *Preoperative neurological deficit*: Preoperative involvement of lower cranial nerves in posterior fossa tumors and respiratory muscle weakness in high cervical spine injuries will delay one's decision to extubate the patient in the immediate postoperative period.[37] The integrity of the airway depends predominantly on the proper function on the IX, X, and XI cranial nerves, which can affect swallowing and the cough reflex. Quadriplegia has been found to have a significant high risk of reintubation.[40]

Surgery-related factors

1. *Emergency surgery*: Emergency surgical procedure could be a significant risk factor for delayed extubation as the intracranial pathology is more severe in these patients.[38]
2. *Site of surgery*: It is observed that patients who undergo uneventful supratentorial tumors can be safely extubated in the operating room (OR). The dilemma for early versus delayed emergence persists for the infratentorial surgeries. Tumor location in infratentorial craniectomies depending on brain stem location can lead to delayed extubation.[37]
3. *Size of the tumor*: Patients operated on for large intracranial tumors awaken more slowly than patients after spinal surgery and small brain tumors.[41] In one study, midline shift of more than 5 mm on preoperative imaging has been found to be an independent risk factor for emergence hypertension.
4. *Duration of surgery*: Prolonged duration of surgery also bears a significant relation with delayed emergence.[34,37,42]
5. *Blood loss*: In a retrospective analysis, the group of patients who were not extubated in the OR had a significantly larger intraoperative blood loss and received a larger amount of blood products than those extubated in the OR.
6. *Fluids*: The choice of fluids has not been found to influence emergence. As a general principle, hypoosmolar and dextrose-containing solutions should be avoided in neurosurgical population.[43]
7. *Temperature*: In the past decade, there has been a lot of research regarding the neuroprotective effects of the hypothermia, but it has not been shown to add benefits in current neuroanesthetic practices.[44]

Anesthesia-related factors

1. *Benzodiazepines* (BZDs): Small doses of BZDs and opioids can unmask the preexisting neurological deficits, making it difficult to

distinguish them from the newly developing features of raised ICP and mass effect.[45,46] Midazolam reduces the incidence of emergence agitation in pediatric patients after sevoflurane anesthesia, but had been found to be a risk factor for emergence delirium in adults.[47–49]

2. *Opioids*: Opioids may increase or decrease CBF, $CMRO_2$, and ICP, depending on the use of a background anesthetic agent. They have minimal-to-modest depressive effects on CBF and $CMRO_2$. Rapid intravenous administration of synthetic opioids can cause hypotension with concomitant rise in ICP.[50] Short-acting opioids may decrease the time to emergence and need of hypertensive during emergence as compared to inhalational and intravenous anesthetics.[9]

Morphine and fentanyl: New synthetic opioids have almost replaced morphine, but it is still the most commonly used drug in developing countries. One study compared emergence with use of morphine and fentanyl. The study did not find any difference in time to emergence among the two agents.[51]

a. *Fentanyl and remifentanil*: Some of the studies comparing remifentanil to fentanyl have shown that immediate recovery was faster with remifentanil. Contrarily, the NeuroMorfeo trial on 380 patients concluded that there was no difference in time to reach an Aldrete score ≥9 between remifentanil and fentanyl groups.[52] However, the use of remifentanil has been associated with increased sympathetic tone, postoperative hyperalgesia, arterial hypertension, and tachycardia in the early postoperative period.[19,53]

b. *Remifentanil and sufentanil*: There is no difference in time to extubation with the use of either remifentanil or sufentanil.[19,54]

3. *Hypnotics (inhalational versus intravenous anesthetics)*: The choice of anesthetics, that is, inhalational versus intravenous anesthetic drugs, in neuroanesthesia practices is a topic of debate. The clinicians practicing neuroanesthesia prefer intravenous drugs when there are indications of raised ICP. However, the "ideal" drug in stable patients will vary with the comfort and experience levels of the attending anesthetist. The proponents of intravenous anesthetic drugs advocate their

vasoconstricting and "neuroprotective effects," while those favoring inhalational anesthetics would argue over more predictable recovery profile of these agents. In the past decade, a number of studies have come up comparing the two, but the results have not shown any statistical difference with propofol, sevoflurane, isoflurane, or desflurane in terms of eye opening, time to extubation, and Aldrete score.[18,55–57]

The commonly used inhalational agents are isoflurane, sevoflurane, and desflurane. Though the difference in recovery between the three agents may not be clinically significant, desflurane has shown to be associated with faster emergence.[58–60]

Checklist prior to conduct of emergence in surgical patients

The emergence plan should be laid out at the time of the surgical closure. Check for normotension, normovolemia, normoxia, normocapnia, and normothermia. Ensure surgical hemostasis. Ensure administration of nonopioid analgesics at the time of surgical closure.

Do not completely switch off the anesthetic agents before the surgical dressing has been applied. The reversal for the residual neuromuscular blockade should be done only after ensuring sufficient time lag since the administration of the last dose of the muscle relaxant. Check for facial and tongue edema. Ensure administration of antiemetic prophylaxis. Avoid oral suctioning at the lighter planes of anesthesia. No stimulation should be given except for the verbal commands. Extubation of trachea should be attempted only when the patient has adequate muscle power and respiratory efforts and is responsive to verbal commands.

Monitoring during emergence

1. *Electroencephalogram (EEG)-based monitors*: Use of EEG-based monitors to assess the depth of anesthesia in the intraoperative period, especially with total intravenous anesthesia (TIVA), has considerably increased in the past decade. These monitors decrease the incidence of intraoperative awareness, decrease the total amount of drug used, and also shorten the time to recovery.[61–64]

Their significance is well established in general anesthesia patients, but these effects have not been much studied in neurosurgical patients. The major difficulty in postoperative care in patients after craniotomy is to distinguish the intracranial deficits from the residual effect of general anesthesia. Cerebral state index (CSI) monitoring as described in one study may be a reliable objective method to predict delayed recovery after elective craniotomy.[64]

2. *Neuromuscular monitoring*: In the absence of neuromuscular transmission (NMT) monitoring, the usual practice is to switch off the anesthetic agents, switch over from mechanical ventilation, assist the ventilation manually, and once the adequate respiratory efforts are achieved, administer the anticholinesterase. But these criteria may be associated with inadequate reversal or "decurarization."

If only a single twitch or none at all can be evoked, neostigmine should not be expected to promptly reverse neuromuscular block, and antagonism is best delayed until a train-of-four (TOF) count of 2 is achieved. As little as 0.015–0.025 mg/kg neostigmine is required at a TOF count of 4 with minimal fade whereas 0.04–0.05 mg/kg is needed at a TOF count of 2–3.[65] Previously a TOF ratio, that is, T4:T1 ≥0.7 was thought to be associated with adequate reversal, but it is now believed that a significant residual paralysis may be there with a TOF ratio <0.9; therefore, TOF ratio >0.9 should be achieved before extubation.[65,66]

Early versus delayed emergence

The rationale of rapid and early emergence is more in the context of patients undergoing neurosurgery in order to permit an early neurological evaluation and prevent devastating complications.

The advantages of early extubation are evaluation of the neurological status and re-intervention if needed, earlier assessment of the baseline for further clinical assessment, less hypertension, less catecholamine burst, and if done by an anesthetist familiar with the patient (brain tightness, bleeding, course of the surgery etc.), less cost.

Nevertheless, this fast-tracking has its own pitfalls. The patient may be at the risk of hypoxia, hypothermia, there can be difficulty in monitoring the respiratory status during transfer of the patient to intensive care unit (ICU), and there may be residual hypothermia. However, surgeries lasting for long duration (>6 h), complicated surgeries, massive blood loss during the intraoperative period, hemodynamic instability, preoperative altered level of consciousness, surgeries near the brain stem, a prolonged period of ischemia, involvement of lower cranial nerves in posterior fossa lesions, patients with high cervical spine injuries and trauma, large arteriovenous malformations (AVM) resection, large tumors with midline shift on preoperative scans, intraoperative brain bulge, and patients with severe cardiac and respiratory diseases may warrant delayed emergence and extubation, allowing them to "come out at own."[7,23] The advantages are less chance of hypoxemia and hypercarbia, and a longer period for hemodynamic stabilization.[67]

Delayed emergence can be arbitrarily taken as an emergence time more than 15 min, as was described by Bhagat et al.[9]

In patients with unplanned delayed awakening, one should look for surgical and systemic causes. These can be postoperative intracranial bleed/hemorrhage/thrombosis/infarction, raised ICP, reverse brain herniation (at the time of suction drain opening), antiepileptic drug toxicity, cerebral edema/ischemia, tension pneumocephalus, hypoglycemia, hyponatremia/hypernatremia, hypokalemia, hypothermia, and uncommon causes such as central anticholinergic syndrome, hypothyroidism, and sepsis.[68,69] An urgent CT scan and monitoring of arterial blood gases and electrolytes should be performed in patients with delayed emergence.

Strategies to facilitate smooth emergence

There are a number of pharmacological agents that are used to manage emergence hypertension, coughing, and agitation. Most of them have been described in the context of neurosurgical patients.

1. *Local anesthetics*: Lignocaine is the most common drug used to control emergence hypertension in both neuro and non-neurosurgical patients in our institute. Various routes have been tried for its administration: intravenous, endotracheal cuff inflation, IT instillation, tube lubrication,

and aerosolized form.[70–74] Nontoxic doses of lidocaine produce a dose-related reduction of $CMRO_2$ and CBF. Intravenous (IV) lignocaine in the dose of 1–1.5 mg/kg blunts the hemodynamic responses to extubation, suppresses the cough, and, thus, prevents the secondary rise in ICP.[75]

Intracuff lignocaine (4%) and intratracheal lignocaine (2%) have proved equally efficacious to IV lignocaine in terms of coughing and hemodynamic response attenuation to tracheal extubation.[70,76]

The drawbacks with the use of lignocaine are short duration of action, sedation, and prolonged emergence.[70]

2. *β-Blockers*: Esmolol is a β-receptor antagonist with rapid onset and short duration of action. It has also been found to decrease CBF velocity, heart rate (HR), and mean arterial pressure (MAP) in the neurosurgical patients.[77] The early administration of β-blockers was associated with a 31% reduction in the rate of intracranial hemorrhage in one study.[78]

Labetalol, a longer-acting β-antagonist, is usually given in incremental doses of 0.25–1 mg/kg, to a maximum of 2.5 mg/kg, but it can lead to bradycardia and hypotension in the postoperative period in the absence of any stimulus.[79]

3. *Calcium-channel blockers (CCBs)*: Diltiazem (0.1 mg/kg, IV) and nicardipine (0.03 mg/kg, IV) have been found superior to esmolol (1 and 1.5 mg/kg, respectively) in controlling systolic blood pressure changes.[80–82] Verapamil (0.1 mg/kg) also effectively attenuates the cardiovascular responses to extubation.[83] Combined use of diltiazem (0.1 mg/kg) and verapamil (0.01 mg/kg) has also been reported to effectively treat peroperative hypertensive crisis.[84]

The disadvantage with the use of CCBs is that they may cause cerebral vasodilation and lead to increased CBF.[85]

4. *α2-agonists*: α2-agonists are potent cerebral vasoconstrictors.[86] Dexmedetomidine decreases Vmca in transcranial Doppler (TCD), with maximum reduction at 25% of the hypnotic doses. The $CMRO_2$ and ICP may remain unchanged after dexmedetomidine infusion.[87] The use of dexmedetomidine in a neurosurgical patient has considerably increased in the past decade. It is frequently used for awake craniotomy.

The use of dexmedetomidine as a single bolus dose prior to extubation has been associated with fewer hypertensive episodes with no difference in extubation and recovery time.[88–90]

5. *Scalp block*: Scalp block has emerged as an essential adjuvant along with dexmedetomidine in patients undergoing awake craniotomy.[91] Scalp block decreases the hemodynamic response to pin insertion and skin incision.[92] The wound infiltration with local anesthetics also decreased pain scores on admission to the postanesthesia care unit for up to 1 h.[93] It has also been found to decrease the incidence of chronic postoperative pain.[94]

6. *Supraglottic airway devices*: Use of supraglottic airway devices at the end of the surgery prior to extubation decreased the incidence of coughing, MAP, HR, and regional cerebral oxygenation in one study.[95]

7. *Prone extubation*: Though the evidence is scarce, prone extubation in patients undergoing spine surgery has been shown to have lesser incidence of coughing as compared to supine extubation.[96–98]

Summary

Emergence and extubation in surgical patients is associated with various systemic effects. This can have deleterious effects in patients with reduced cerebrovascular reserve and impaired autoregulation.

An awake patient is the best neurological monitor. Fast-tracking the awakening permits early neurological examination. Apart from early awakening, a smooth "landing" should be the aim. The attending anesthesiologists must plan the emergence well in advance and discuss the various pros and cons. The current evidence does not demonstrate the superiority of either intravenous or inhalational agents for providing early recovery. There are various physiological and pharmacological measures that may help in achieving an early and smooth emergence.

References

1. Ciofolo MJ, Clergue F, Devillier C et al. Changes in ventilation, oxygen uptake, and carbon dioxide output during recovery from isoflurane anesthesia. *Anesthesiology* 1989;70:737–741.

2. Breslow MJ, Parker SD, Franck SM et al. Determinants of catecholamine and cortisol responses to lower extremity revascularization. *Anesthesiology* 1993;79:1202–1209.

3. Udelsman R, Norton JA, Jelenich SE et al. Responses of the hypothalamic–pituitary–adrenal and renin–angiotensin axes and the sympathetic system during controlled surgical and anesthetic stress. *J Clin Endocrinol Metab* 1987;64:986–994.

4. Fàbregas N, Brudera N. Recovery and neurological evaluation. *Bes Pract Res Clin Anaesthesiol* 2007;21:431–447.

5. Hartley M, Vaughan RS. Problems associated with tracheal extubation. *Br J Anaesth* 1993;71:561–568.

6. Miller KA, Harkin CP, Bailey PL. Postoperative tracheal extubation. *Anesth Analg* 1995;80:149–172.

7. Bruder N, Stordeur JM, Ravussin P et al. Metabolic and hemodynamic changes during recovery and tracheal extubation in neurosurgical patients: Immediate versus delayed recovery. *Anesth Analg* 1999;89:674–678.

8. Bruder N, Pellissier D, Grillot P, Gouin F. Cerebral hyperemia during recovery from general anesthesia in neurosurgical patients. *Anesth Analg* 2002;94:650–654.

9. Bhagat H, Dash HH, Bithal PK, Chouhan RS, Pandia MP. Planning for early emergence in neurosurgical patients: A randomized prospective trial of low-dose anesthetics. *Anesth Analg* 2008;107:1348–1355.

10. Bryan RM. Cerebral blood flow and energy metabolism during stress. *Am J Physiol Heart Circ Physiol* 1990;259:H269–H280.

11. Ijima T, Kubota Y, Kuroiwa T, Sankawa H. Blood–brain barrier opening following transient reflex sympathetic hypertension. *Acta Neurochir Suppl* (Wien) 1994;60:142–144.

12. Remsen LG, Pagel MA, McCormick CI et al. The influence of anesthetic choice, $PaCO_2$, and other factors on osmotic blood–brain barrier disruption in rats with brain tumor xenografts. *Anesth Analg* 1999;88:559–567.

13. Brucia J, Rudy E. The effect of suction catheter insertion and tracheal stimulation in adults with severe brain injury. *Heart Lung* 1996;25:295–303.

14. Gemma M, Tommasino C, Cerri M, Giannotti A, Piazzi B, Borghi T. Intracranial effects of endotracheal suctioning in the acute phase of head injury. *J Neurosurg Anesthesiol* 2002;14:50–54.

15. Leone M, Albanese J, Viviand X et al. The effects of remifentanil on endotracheal suctioning-induced increases in intracranial pressure in head-injured patients. *Anesth Analg* 2004;99:1193–1198.

16. White PF, Schlobohm RM, Pitts LH, Lindauer JM. A randomized study of drugs for preventing increases in intracranial pressure during endotracheal suctioning. *Anesthesiology* 1982;57:242–244.

17. Lim SH, Chin NM, Tai HY et al. Prophylactic esmolol infusion for the control of cardiovascular responses to extubation after intracranial surgery. *Ann Acad Med Singapore* 2000;29:447–451.

18. Todd M, Warner D, Sokoll M et al. A prospective, comparative trial of three anesthetics for elective supratentorial craniotomy. *Anesthesiology* 1993;78:1005–1020.

19. Bilotta F, Caramia R, Paoloni FP et al. Early postoperative cognitive recovery after remifentanilpropofol or sufentanil-propofol anaesthesia for supratentorial craniotomy: A randomized trial. *Eur J Anaesthesiol* 2007;24:122–127.

20. Sawaya R, Hammoud M, Schoppa D et al. Neurosurgical outcomes in a modern series of 400 craniotomies for treatment of parenchymal tumors. *Neurosurgery* 1998;42:1044–1055; discussion 1055–1056.

21. Basali A, Mascha EJ, Kalfas I, Schubert A. Relation between perioperative hypertension and intracranial hemorrhage after craniotomy. *Anesthesiology* 2000;93:48–54.

22. Wong DM, Manninen PH. Post anaesthesia care unit. In: Gupta AK, Gelb AW, editors. *Essentials of Neuroanesthesia and Neurointensive Care*, 1st ed. Philadelphia, PA: Elsevier; 2008.

23. Bruder N, Ravussin P. Recovery from anesthesia and postoperative extubation of neurosurgical patients: A review. *J Neurosurg Anesthesiol* 1999;11:282–9316.

24. Prabhakar H, Bithal PK, Suri A, Rath GP, Dash HH. Intracranial pressure changes during Valsalva manoeuvre in patients undergoing a neuroendoscopic procedure. *Minim Invasive Neurosurg* 2007;50:98–101.

25. Wig J, Chandrashekharappa KN, Yaddanapudi LN, Nakra D, Mukherjee KK. Effect of prophylactic ondansetron on postoperative nausea and vomiting in patients on preoperative steroids undergoing craniotomy for supratentorial tumors. *J Neurosurg Anesthesiol* 2007;19:239–242.

26. Mordhorst C, Latz B, Kerz T et al. Prospective assessment of postoperative pain after craniotomy. *J Neurosurg Anesthesiol* 2010;22:202–206.

27. De Benedittis G, Lorenzetti A, Migliore M et al. Postoperative pain in neurosurgery: A pilot study in brain surgery. *Neurosurgery* 1996;38:466–469.

28. Vijayan N. Postoperative headache in acoustic neuroma. *Headache* 1995;2:98–100.

29. Buggy DJ, Crossley AWA. Thermoregulation, mild peri-operative hypothermia, post anaesthetic shivering. *Br J Anaesth* 2000;84(5):614–628.

30. Lenhardt R, Marker A, Goli V et al. Mild intra-oerative hyothermia rolongs ostanaesthetic recovery. *Anaesthesiology* 1997;87:1318–23

31. Alfonsi P. Postanaethetic shivering. Epidemiology, pathophysiology, approaches to prevention and management. *Minerva Anaesth* 2003;69:438–441.

32. Frank SM, Higgins MS, Breslow MJ et al. The catecholamine, cortisol, and hemodynamic responses to mild perioperative hypothermia. A randomized clinical trial. *Anesthesiology* 1995;82:83–93.

33. Motamed S, Klubien K, Edwardes M et al. Metabolic changes during recovery in normothermic versus hypothermic patients undergoing surgery and receiving general anesthesia and epidural local anesthetic agents. *Anesthesiology* 1998;88:1211–1218.

34. Shalev D, Kamel H. Risk of reintubation in neurosurgical patients. *Neurocrit Care* 2015;22:15–19.

35. Vidotto MC, Sogame LCM, Gazzotti MR, Prandini MN, Jardim JR. Analysis of risk factors for extubation failure in subjects submitted to non-emergency elective intracranial surgery. *Respir Care* 2012;57(12):2059–2066.

36. Callaghan CJ, Lynch AG, Amin I et al. Overnight intensive recovery: Elective open aortic surgery without a routine ICU bed. *Eur J Vasc Endovasc Surg* 2005;30:252–258.

37. Cai YH, Zeng HY, Shi ZH et al. Factors influencing delayed extubation after infratentorial craniotomy for tumour resection: A prospective cohort study of 800 patients in a Chinese neurosurgical centre. *J Int Med Res* 2013;41(1):208–217.

38. Nivatpumin P, Srisuriyarungrueng S, Saimuey P, Srirojanakul W. Factors affecting delayed extubation after intracranial surgery in Siriraj Hospital Siriraj. *Med J* 2010;62:119–123.

39. Namen AM, Ely EW, Tatter SB, et al. Predictors of successful extubation in neurosurgical patients. *Am J Respir Crit Care Med* 2001;163(3):658–664.

40. Chen L, Xu M, Li GY, Cai WX, Zhou JX. Incidence, risk factors and consequences of emergence agitation in adult patients after elective craniotomy for brain tumor: A prospective cohort study. *PLoS One* 2014;9(12):e114239.

41. Schubert A, Mascha EJ, Bloomfield EL et al. Effect of cranial surgery and brain tumor size on emergence from anesthesia. *Anesthesiology* 1996;85:513–521.

42. Cata JP, Saager WL, Kurz A, Avitsian R. Successful extubation in the operating room after infratentorial craniotomy: The Cleveland Clinic experience. *J Neurosurg Anesthesiol* 2011;23:25–29.

43. Rusa R, Zornow MH. Fluid management during craniotomy. In: Cottrell JE, Young LY, editors. *Cottrell and Young's Neuroanesthesia*, 5th ed. Philadelphia, PA: Elsevier; 2010.

44. Sandestig A, Romner B, Grande PO. Therapeutic hypothermia in children and adults with severe traumatic brain injury. *Ther Hypothermia Temp Manag* 2014;4(1):10–20.

45. Lazar RM, Fitzsimmons BF, Marshall RS et al. Reemergence of stroke deficits with midazolam challenge. *Stroke* 2002;33:283–285.

46. Thal GD, Szabo MD, Lopez-Bresnahan M, Crosby G. Exacerbation or unmasking of focal neurologic deficits by sedatives. *Anesthesiology* 1996;85:21–51.

47. Lepouse C, Lautner CA, Liu L, Gomis P, Leon A. Emergence delirium in adults in the post-anaesthesia care unit. *Br J Anaesth* 2006;96:747–753.

48. Zhang C, Li J, Zhao D, Wang Y. Prophylactic midazolam and clonidine for emergence from agitation in children after emergence from sevoflurane anesthesia: A meta-analysis. *Clin Ther* 2013;35(10):1622–1631.

49. Kim YH, Yoon SZ, Lim HJ, Yoon SM. Prophylactic use of midazolam or propofol at the end of surgery may reduce the incidence of emergence agitation after sevoflurane anaesthesia. *Anaesth Intensive Care* 2011;39(5):904–908.

50. Sakabe T, Matsumoto M. Effects of anesthetic agents and other drugs. In: Cottrell JE, Young LY, editors. *Cottrell and Young's Neuroanesthesia*, 5th ed. Philadelphia, PA: Elsevier; 2010.

51. Bhagat H, Bhukal I, Bastola P, Bithal P, Dash HH. Does morphine prolong emergence in neurosurgical patients. *Eur J Anaesth* 2012;29:S14.

52. Citerio G, Pesenti A, Latini R et al. A multicentre, randomised, open-label, controlled trial evaluating equivalence of inhalational and intravenous anaesthesia during elective craniotomy. *Eur J Anaesthesiol* 2012;29(8):371–379.

53. Bilotta F, Lam AM, Doronzio A, Cuzzone V, Delfini R, Rosa G. Esmolol blunts postoperative hemodynamic changes after propofol-remifentanil total intravenous fasttrack neuroanesthesia for intracranial surgery. *J Clin Anesth* 2008;20(6):426–430.

54. Djian MC, Blanchet B, Pesce F et al. Comparison of the time to extubation after use of remifentanil or sufentanil in combination with propofol as anesthesia in adults undergoing nonemergency intracranial surgery: A prospective, randomized, double-blind trial. *Clin Ther* 2006;28(4):560–568.

55. Bastola P, Bhagat H, Wig J. Comparative evaluation of propofol, sevoflurane and desflurane for neuroanaesthesia: A prospective randomised study in patients undergoing elective supratentorial craniotomy. *Indian J Anaesth* 2015;59(5):287–294.

56. Talke P, Caldwell JE, Brown R, Dodson B, Howley J, Richardson CA. A comparison of three anesthetic techniques in patients undergoing craniotomy for supratentorial intracranial surgery. *Anesth Analg* 2002;95(2):430–435.

57. Magni G, Baisi F, La Rosa I et al. No difference in emergence time and early cognitive function between sevoflurane fentanyl and propofol–remifentanil in patients undergoing craniotomy for supratentorial intracranial surgery. *J Neurosurg Anesthesiol* 2005;17(3):134–138.

58. Gauthier A, Girard F, Boudreault D, Ruel M, Todorov A. Sevoflurane provides faster recovery and postoperative neurological assessment than isoflurane in long-duration neurosurgical cases. *Anesth Analg* 2002;95(5):1384–1388.

59. Magni G, Rosa IL, Melillo G et al. A comparison between sevoflurane and desflurane anesthesia in patients undergoing craniotomy for supratentorial intracranial surgery. *Anesth Analg* 2009;109:567–571.

60. Bilotta F, Doronzio A, Cuzzone V, Caramia R, Rosa G. Early postoperative cognitive recovery and gas exchange patterns after balanced anesthesia with sevoflurane or desflurane in overweight and obese patients undergoing craniotomy: A prospective randomized trial. *J Neurosurg Anesthesiol* 2009;21(3):207–213.

61. Punjasawadwong Y, Boonjeungmonkol N, Phongchiewboon A. Bispectral index for improving anaesthetic delivery and postoperative recovery. *Cochrane Database Syst Rev* 2007 Oct 17;(4):CD003843.

62. Kreuer S, Biedler A, Larsen R, Altmann S, Wilhelm W. Narcotrend monitoring allows faster emergence and a reduction of drug consumption in propofol–remifentanil anesthesia. *Anesthesiology* 2003;99(1):34–41.

63. Recart A, Gasanova I, White PF et al. The effect of cerebral monitoring on recovery after general anesthesia: A comparison of the auditory evoked potential and bispectral index devices with standard clinical practice. *Anesth Analg* 2003;97(6):1667–1674.

64. Xu M, Lei YL, Zhou JX. Use of cerebral state index to predict long-term unconsciousness in patients after elective craniotomy with delay recovery. *BMC Neurol* 2011;11:15.

65. McGrath CD, Hunter JM. Monitoring of neuromuscular block. *CEAP* 2006;6(1):7–12.

66. Kopman AF, Eikermann M. Antagonism of non-depolarising neuromuscular block: Current practice. *Anaesthesia* 2009;64:22–30.

67. Bruder N, Ravussin P. Anaesthesia for supratentorial tumours. In: *Cottrell and Young's Neuroanesthesia*, 5th ed. Philadelphia, PA: Elsevier; 2010.

68. Prabhakar H, Bithal PK, Garg A. Tension pneumocephalus after craniotomy in supine position. *J Neurosurg Anesthesiol* 2003;15:278–281.

69. Shaikh SI, Lakshmi RR. Delayed awakening after anaesthesia—A challenge for an anaesthesiologist. *Int J Biomed Adv Res* 2014;8:352–354

70. Venkatesan T, Korula G. A comparative study between the effects of 4% endotracheal tube cuff lignocaine and 1.5 mg/kg intravenous lignocaine on coughing and hemodynamics during extubation in neurosurgical patients: A randomized controlled double-blind trial. *J Neurosurg Anesthesiol* 2006;18:230–234.

71. Bidwai AV, Stanley TH, Bidwai VA. Blood pressure and pulse rate responses to extubation with and without prior topical tracheal anaesthesia. *Can Anaesth Soc J* 1978;25:416–418.

72. Gonzalez RM, Bjerke RJ, Drobycki T et al. Prevention of endotracheal tube-induced coughing during emergence from general anesthesia. *Anesth Analg* 1994;79:792–795.

73. Soltani HA, Aghadavoudi O. The effect of different lidocaine application methods on postoperative cough and sore throat. *J Clin Anesth* 2002;14:15–18.

74. Kautto UM, Heinonen J. Attenuation of circulatory response to laryngoscopy and tracheal intubation: A comparison of two methods of topical anaesthesia. *Acta Anaesthesiol Scand* 1982;26:599–602.

75. Sakabe T, Maekawa T, Ishikawa T et al. The effects of lidocaine on canine cerebral metabolism and circulation related to the electroencephalogram. *Anesthesiology* 1974;40:433–441.

76. Jee D, Park SY. Lidocaine sprayed down the endotracheal tube attenuates the airway–circulatory reflexes by local anesthesia during emergence and extubation. *Anesth Analg* 2003;96:293–297.

77. Grillo P, Bruder N, Auquier P, Pellissier D, Gouin F. Esmolol blunts the cerebral blood flow velocity increase during emergence from anesthesia in neurosurgical patients. *Anesth Analg* 2003;96(4):1145–1149.

78. Barron H, Rundle A, Gore J et al. Intracranial hemorrhage rates and effect of immediate beta-blocker use in patients with acute myocardial infarction treated with tissue plasminogen activator. *Am J Cardiol* 2000;85:294–298.

79. Muzzi DA, Cayuman S, Lossaso TJ, Cucchiara RF. Labetolol and Esmolol in the control of hypertension after intracranial surgery. *Anaesth Aanlg* 1990;70(1):68–71.

80. Singh A, Bhosale J, Aphale S. Comparison of diltiazem and esmolol in attenuating the cardiovascular responses to extubation. *Innovative J Med Health Sci* 2015;5:1–5.

81. Kovac AL, Masiongale A. Comparison of nicardipine versus esmolol in attenuating the hemodynamic responses to anesthesia emergence and extubation. *J Cardiothorac Vasc Anesth* 2007;21:45–50.

82. Bebawy JF, Houston CC, Kosky JL et al. Nicardipine is superior to esmolol for the management of postcraniotomy emergence hypertension: A randomized open-label study. *Anesth Analg* 2015;120:186–192.

83. Jajoo SS, Chaudhari AR, Singam A, Chandak A. Attenuation of hemodynamic responses to endotracheal extubation: A prospective randomised controlled study between two different doses of Verapamil. *Int J Biomed Res.* 12/2013; 4(12):663

84. Nakao S, Hirota K, Kurata J et al. Effects of combined intravenous nicardipine and diltiazem administration on the circulatory response to laryngoscopy and tracheal intubation. *J Anesth* 1994;8:163–166.

85. Morimoto Y, Morimoto Y, Kemmotsu O, Gando S, Shibano T, Shikama H. The effect of calcium channel blockers on cerebral oxygenation during tracheal extubation. *Anesth Analg* 2000;91(2):347–352.

86. Zornow MH, Fleischer JE, Scheller MS et al. Dexmedetomidine, an alpha2 adrenergic agonist, decreases cerebral blood flow in the isoflurane-anesthetized dog. *Anesth Analg* 1990;70:624–630.

87. Zornow MH, Maze M, Dyck JB et al: Dexmedetomidine decreases cerebral blood flow velocity in humans. *J Cereb Blood Flow Metab* 1993;13:350–353.

88. Turan G, Ozgultekin A, Turan C, Dincer E, Yuksel G. Advantageous effects of dexmedetomidine on haemodynamic and recovery responses during extubation for intracranial surgery. *Eur J Anaesthesiol* 2008;25(10):816–820.

89. Bekker A, Sturaitis M, Bloom M et al. The effect of dexmedetomidine on perioperative hemodynamics in patients undergoing craniotomy. Anesth Analg 2008;107(4):1340–1347.

90. Kothari D, Tandon N, Singh M, Kumar A. Attenuation of circulatory and airway responses to endotracheal extubation in craniotomies for intracerebral space occupying lesions: Dexmedetomidine versus lignocaine. *Anesth Essays Res* 2014;8(1):78–82.

91. Osborn I, Sebeo J. "Scalp block" during craniotomy: A classic technique revisited. *J Neurosurg Anesthesiol* 2010;22:187–194.

92. Geze S, Yilmaz AA, Tuzuner F. The effect of scalp block and local infiltration on the haemodynamic and stress response to skull-pin placement for craniotomy. *Eur J Anaesthesiol* 2009;26(4):298–303.

93. Bloomfield EL, Schubert A, Secic M et al. The influence of scalp infiltration with bupivacaine on hemodynamics and postoperative pain in adult patients undergoing craniotomy. *Anesth Analg* 1998;87:579–582.

94. Batoz H, Verdonck O, Pellerin C et al. The analgesic properties of scalp infiltrations with ropivacaine after intracranial tumoral resection. *Anesth Analg* 2009;109:240–244.

95. Perelló-Cerdà L, Fàbregas N, López AM et al. ProSeal laryngeal mask airway attenuates systemic and cerebral hemodynamic response during awakening of neurosurgical patients: A randomized clinical trial. *J Neurosurg Anesthesiol* 2015;27(3):194–202.

96. Yörükoğlu D, Alanoğlu Z, Dilek UB, Can OS, Keçik Y. Comparison of different extubation techniques in lumbar surgery: prone extubation versus supine extubation with or without prior injection of intravenous lidocaine. *J Neurosurg Anesthesiol* 2006;18(3):165–169.

97. Olympio MA, Youngblood BL, James RL. Emergence from anesthesia in the prone versus supine position in patients undergoing lumbar surgery. *Anesthesiology* 2000;93:959–963.

98. Kumar S, Sahni N, Bhagat H et al. A randomized clinical trial of prone position extubation reduces the severity of coughing in patients undergoing dorsolumbar spine surgery. *Can J Anaesth* 2016;63:774–775.

PART V

Positioning the neurosurgical patient

24

Positioning of patients

STEFAN JANKOWSKI and JAKE DRINKWATER

Introduction

Although the primary aim of patient positioning is to provide optimum surgical access, there are physiological consequences and risks that need to be considered to avoid complications. Positioning any patient must take into account each of these aspects, be considered as bespoke for that patient, and be tailored accordingly. The surgical team and the anesthetic team share responsibility for the chosen position and its safe execution. An awareness of the risks and benefits associated with each position is essential to inform the decision-making process, counsel, and obtain informed consent.

Some positions, and their potential for severe complications, such as postoperative visual loss (POVL) and venous air embolism (VAE), although rare, are encountered in patients undergoing neurosurgical procedures, and the theater team should have an understanding of the principles outlined in this chapter to mitigate risks, where possible, and to manage complications effectively.

We consider four *principles of positioning* applied to supine, lateral, prone, and sitting positions:

1. Preference: Which position provides optimal surgical access?
2. Practical considerations: What difficulties in positioning might you encounter?
3. Physiological consequences: What are the effects on the patient and how do they influence management?
4. Physical injury: What are the risks to the patient and how are they mitigated?

Preference: Surgical preference and common indications for the position

Head positioning for craniotomies

An optimal surgical approach to an intracranial target requires that the distance from the highest point of the skull, when positioned, to the intracranial target is the shortest possible distance and that the plane of the perimeter of the craniotomy is parallel to the floor.[1]

Types of craniotomies

The five classic surgical approaches for craniotomies are frontal, temporal, occipital, parietal, and posterior fossa. Each provides extensive *regional* exposure of the entire lobes, and they are now only occasionally used when exposure of large areas is required, such as in decompressive craniectomy. In modern neurosurgery, six standard types of craniotomies are used, which are derived from the regional craniotomies by miniaturization and/or combination. They are anterior parasagittal, frontosphenotemporal, subtemporal, posterior sagittal, midline suboccipital, and lateral suboccipital.[1]

Head fixation

Skeletal fixation using either a three- or a four-pin fixation device linked to the operating table by a Mayfield frame has the advantage of ensuring head immobility (essential if stereotactic localization such as BrainLab™ is used) and avoids pressure on the face and eyes. The Mayfield frame consists of an articulating arm that enables movement in all three spatial planes and that can be secured in the locked state once the desired head position has been achieved. It may be used in combination with either a skeletal pin fixation device or a horseshoe headrest. The anesthetist should appreciate that application of skeletal fixation with pins is extremely stimulating, even with the use of local anesthetic, and if left unchecked by appropriate analgesia and depth of anesthesia may result in a dramatic rise in sympathetic outflow with associated arterial hypertension and tachycardia. The potential for this to cause or worsen intracranial pathology should not be underestimated, and continuous arterial blood pressure measurement is recommended. Other potential complications

associated with skeletal fixation are bleeding from pin sites; laceration to the scalp, face, and eyes; air embolus; and even intracranial hemorrhage[2] (Figure 24.1a and b).

Head and neck positioning

Although head and neck rotation, flexion, or extension away from the neutral position may be required to optimize surgical access, each carries attendant risks. Each patient should be assessed with regard to his or her head and neck mobility and this should inform the range of positions that can be safely tolerated. Patients with arthritis, those with osteophytes or rheumatoid conditions affecting the neck, and those with vascular atherosclerosis may be much less tolerant of even modest movements of the head and neck. Some advocate patient self-positioning prior to induction of anesthesia, which may necessitate awake fiber-optic intubation and the application of eye protection prior to final positioning.[3]

- *Neck rotation*: Blood flow in the vertebral arteries, which run through the foramen transversarium of the cervical vertebrae 3–6, is reduced on the ipsilateral side to head and neck rotation with consequent risks of brain and cervical spine ischemia. Extreme rotation may also compromise venous drainage of the head with consequent rises in the intracranial pressure (ICP). The brachial plexus, originating from the anterior spinal nerves C5–T1 and projecting to the ipsilateral arm, is also vulnerable to injury as a result of neck rotation and shoulder depression. Injury occurs as a result of direct stretch and hypoperfusion as a result of the stretch. As a guide, neck rotation in the range 0°–45° is typically well tolerated. A shoulder roll placed beneath the contralateral shoulder to the direction of head rotation helps to achieve the desired position with less rotation of the neck and also prevents internal jugular venous compression (Figure 24.2).
- *Neck flexion*: Hyperflexion of the head and neck may obstruct venous drainage of the head via compression of the internal jugular veins with associated increases in the ICP. Obstructed venous drainage from the tongue can result in macroglossia with consequences for airway

management. Arterial supply of the head may also be compromised if carotid artery compression occurs, with resultant central nervous system (CNS) ischaemia. Chin necrosis may occur if pressed against the manubrium for prolonged periods. Maintaining two to three fingerbreadth thyromental distance is recommended during neck flexion.[4]

- *Neck extension*: Hyperextension of the head carries with it risks of obstructed venous drainage and impaired arterial inflow with the possibility of causing dangerous reductions in cerebral and spinal perfusion pressure.

Practical considerations

For each combination of surgical procedure, patient position, and the individual patient, there are a number of practical considerations. These can be considered in terms of patient factors and anesthetic factors.

Patient factors

The patient's weight, height, and body morphology have particular implications:

- What is the weight limit for the table or frame?
- How many people are needed to safely position the patient?
- Are positioning aids such as slide sheets and IntoProne™ required?
- Should consideration be given to positioning the patient awake prior to induction of anesthesia? Are the dimensions of the frame or table adequate to prevent abdominal compression?

Anesthetic factors

In addition to the practical considerations of placing the patient in the desired position, anesthetic factors include the *geography* of the positioned patient in relation to the anesthetist, anesthetic machine, and surgical trays/equipment.

Airway

- How should the airway be secured?
- Should a throat pack be inserted?
- What length of breathing circuit is required, and how should this be secured?

- What are the risks of intraoperative changes to position, especially to the airway and cervical spine?
- If prone or lateral, what plan is in place if emergent return to supine position (such as airway loss or cardiovascular collapse) is required?

Venous access

- Where should vascular access lines be sited, and will they be visible, especially if using a total intravenous anesthesia (TIVA) technique, once positioned?
- Will additional venous access be possible intraoperatively, if required?

Monitoring

- Will the non-invasive blood pressure (NIBP) cuff give accurate measurements in the position?
- Can arterial lines be accessed, and where should the transducer be leveled?
- If neuromuscular blockade is used, where can the adequacy of paralysis with a peripheral nerve stimulator be monitored?
- If intraoperative monitoring (IOM) is used, what are the implications for neuromuscular blockade?
- Which side should the BIS™/Entropy monitor be placed?
- Should monitoring be disconnected during the act of positioning and if so which?
- Should the ventilator be disconnected from the patient for positioning?
- Should vascular access lines be disconnected during positioning, and what are the implications when using a TIVA technique?

Eye protection

- How should the eyes be protected?

Airway

- A flexometallic tube allows connection of the breathing circuit away from the face, and should not kink, but carries the risk of endobronchial intubation.
- Airway connectors should be accessible during the case.
- Humidity and moisture exchange (HME) filters should not be placed in a dependent loop as they become waterlogged.

- A throat pack may help secure the endotracheal tube and absorb oropharyngeal secretions, but should be used with care, following local guidelines to prevent accidental retention postextubation.
- Glycopyrronium is useful to reduce oral secretions.
- Tube ties may cause venous obstruction at the neck, and adhesive tapes are preferred.
- A bite block should be used if IOM is required.
- The breathing circuit should be preoxygenated and disconnected during positioning to prevent accidental extubation.

Venous access

- Indwelling lines should be disconnected, if possible, during positioning. Valved luer lock connectors (e.g., Bionector™) or extensions (e.g., Octopus™) are recommended for rapid and secure reconnection.
- TIVA lines should be accessible for monitoring throughout the procedure (if a central venous line is used for this purpose, continuous waveform monitoring is recommended).
- TIVA should be interrupted only with great care. Depth of sedation monitoring is recommended.

Monitoring

- Arterial access should be accessible for flushing/sampling, and leveled with the external auditory meatus (EAM) intraoperatively.
- Cardiovascular stability should be ensured prior to positioning; temporary discontinuation of monitoring assists in positioning and prevents inadvertent injury from cables/connectors/transducers, etc.

Eye protection

- Eyelids should be taped shut. Artificial lubricants are not recommended.
- Ideally, the eyes should be visible, using positioning aids such as ProneView™.
- Padding and waterproof dressing is recommended for all cases in which the eyes cannot be visually inspected. Care to prevent pads transmitting pressure to the orbit is required.

Physiological consequences of positioning

Of central importance are cerebral hemodynamics and ICP, which are often related to the cardiorespiratory consequences of the patient position.

Airway

Prolonged prone position is associated with facial and potentially airway edema; the airway should be assessed prior to extubation with consideration of delayed or staged extubation, if necessary.[5]

Respiratory

Although recently challenged,[6] traditional texts describe a ventilation–perfusion relationship that is influenced by gravity (and hence also by changes in position) by its effect on either the intrapleural pressure gradient (ventilation) or the hydrostatic blood column (perfusion), resulting in the readily understood West zones.[7] Changes in functional respiratory capacity might be anticipated following changes in position, but provided abdominal and chest wall movements are not impeded, they should have minimal clinical impact.[8] Clearly, the most detrimental effects on respiratory physiology are found in the head-down position, rarely used in neurosurgery. The sitting position provides the least disruption to normal respiratory physiology as long as lung perfusion is maintained. In the supine position, the dorsal portion of the lung is well perfused, but during anesthesia the dorsal lung compliance is reduced (by the cephalad movement of abdominal content on the diaphragm), so the ventral lung is better ventilated. (In normal breathing, the ventilation–perfusion relationship is maintained in the supine position as the cephalad displacement of the diaphragm places it on an advantageous part of its length–tension curve, and hence supine positioning is often recommended in spontaneously breathing patients with high spinal cord injury.) The prone position improves functional residual capacity (FRC) and oxygenation over the supine position, possibly as a result of reduced cephalad pressure on the diaphragm and reopening of atelectatic segments.[9]

Key points here are to ensure the abdomen is free to allow adequate diaphragmatic excursion by the proper use of chest rolls or specifically designed aids, such as the Wilson frame, the Andrews table, and the Jackson table. The lateral positions will alter the distribution of ventilation and perfusion across the two lungs, but the clinical significance of this is negligible in the absence of unilateral lung pathology.

Cardiovascular

The cardiovascular consequences of positioning are primarily related to venous return. A reduction in sympathetic outflow, and a degree of direct myocardial depression caused by anesthetic agents, frequently results in arterial hypotension relative to the patient's usual blood pressure. The reduction of sympathetic tone causes venodilation of the capacitance vessels and pooling of blood in dependent areas. The magnitude of the capacitance vessels is greater in the territory of the inferior vena cava (IVC) than in the superior vena cava (SVC). Consequently, hypotension due to venous pooling of blood and reduced venous return is more commonly encountered with positions where the lower body and legs are below the level of the heart, such as sitting and deckchair positions.

Conversely, if the head is lower than the level of the heart then venous congestion of the upper body, including the brain, is likely to occur with implications for ICP, cerebral edema, and cerebral perfusion.

Cerebral hemodynamics and intracranial pressure

Key goals of neuroanesthesia are to maintain cerebral perfusion and prevent intracranial hypertension. Cerebral perfusion is a function of cerebral perfusion pressure (CPP) and cerebral autoregulation. Although we have no direct control over the adequacy of cerebral autoregulation, we have considerable control over CPP. CPP is defined as the mean arterial pressure (MAP) at the same vertical height as the brain (usually taken as the level of the foramen of Monro, which correlates with the level of the EAM) minus the higher of either the ICP or the central venous pressure

(CVP). Accepted target values for CPP are in the range of 60–70 mmHg (extrapolated from studies in traumatic brain injury). It follows that CPP can be modified by changing the MAP, the ICP, and/or the CVP.

In the patient lying in the supine position, the MAP at the level of the right atrium (RA) (standard reference point) will equate to the MAP measured at the level of the foramen of Monro. However, if the patient is positioned such that these two points no longer fall on the same horizontal line, there will be a discrepancy in the measured values, which is equal to the vertical difference between the two points in cmH_2O (10.2 cmH_2O = 7.5 mmHg). To illustrate the significance of this, if the patient is in a sitting position where the vertical distance between the two reference points is 30.6 cm, when the transducer placed at the level of the RA registers an MAP of 75 mmHg, the MAP at the foramen of Monro will be 52.5 mmHg. If the ICP in this patient was 10 mmHg, then the CPP would be just 42.5 mmHg, well outside our target range to ensure adequate cerebral perfusion. We recommend placing the transducer at the level of the EAM to facilitate accurate calculation of the CPP, and this is best done by firmly securing it to an adjustable pole or arm that moves with the table.

Impaired cerebral venous drainage causes congestion of the cerebral venous circulation. The implications of this are several fold. It may be that CVP increases above ICP, thus making it a determinant of CPP and tending to reduce CPP. It may reduce the rate at which cerebrospinal fluid (CSF) is absorbed into the dural venous sinuses via the arachnoid granulations. If the skull is closed, the increased CSF pressure may cause a rise in the ICP, or it may lead to interstitial cerebral edema with subsequent rises in ICP. During craniotomy, these factors may also adversely affect operating conditions. A number of simple interventions can help reduce CVP and improve venous drainage of the head. The most relevant to positioning is having the head higher than the level of the heart. A simple head-up tilt of 15°–30° can significantly improve venous drainage from the head and lower ICP, but significantly increases the risk of VAE. Other interventions including the avoidance of obstructed venous drainage due to head/neck position (see 'Head and neck positioning'), endotracheal tube ties, other mechanical compression of the neck (e.g., cervical spine collar), and the avoidance of high ventilation pressures.

Cerebrospinal fluid drainage and the development of pneumocephalus

The CSF pressure decreases with increase in elevation of the head as CSF drains from the cranial compartment. The brain can sag, causing traction on bridging veins to the venous sinuses (which can cause subdural hemorrhage) and allowing air to enter the cranial cavity (which may cause significant postoperative pneumocephalus). Pneumocephalus may delay emergence, or even present a risk to life, and the use of nitrous oxide should be avoided to prevent the development of tension pneumocephalus.

Venous drainage effects on the vertebral venous plexus

Since the vertebral venous plexus is in communication with abdominal and thoracic veins, high pressures transmitted from these cavities will engorge the former, increasing the risk of bleeding (by compression of the thecal sac within the spinal canal) and elevate CSF pressure, increasing the risk of dural injury in spinal surgery and contributing to raised ICP in cranial surgery.

Physical injury

Patients undergoing neurosurgical operations under general anesthesia are at particular risk of physical injury because of the positions that are used, often for extended periods, and it is the responsibility of the theater team to take appropriate preventative measures. Three types of injury are of particular interest: (1) pressure ulceration, (2) perioperative peripheral nerve injury (PPNI), and (3) postoperative visual loss.

Pressure ulceration

If adequate pressure is applied to tissues for long enough, then tissue ischemia leading to necrosis can result. As pressure within the tissues increases

due to the external pressure, the perfusion pressure of the tissue is reduced and the potential for ischemia is increased. Most tissues can withstand short periods of hypoperfusion without significant sequelae, but the longer the hypoperfusion persists, the greater the chance of ischemia and necrosis. Pressure is a function of force divided by area. Thus, by spreading the application of force over a greater area, the pressure increase in the tissues is minimized. Similarly, force being applied to the patient through a small surface area, as may be found with cannula hubs and monitoring wires, should be avoided.

Perioperative peripheral nerve injury

The reported incidence of PPNI is 0.03%–0.14%.[10] Neurosurgery was found to have a hazard ratio of 2.7 (95% CI 1.4–5.1) and was found to be an independent risk factor for PPNI along with orthopedic surgery, general anesthesia, hypertension, diabetes mellitus, and smoking.[11] Other factors associated with PPNI include hypovolemia, dehydration, hypotension, hypoxia, electrolyte disturbance, and induced hypothermia.[12]

Mechanism of PPNI

The etiology of PPNI is multifactorial and involves patient predisposition, and precipitating mechanical and physiological factors.[13] Although direct trauma to peripheral nerves can be the cause of PPNI, it is not the cause in the majority of cases.[13]

One of the most important mechanisms of PPNI is ischemia of the nerve fibers,[14,15] and it has been postulated that ischemia may be the final common pathway of perioperative neuropathy.[16–20] The interdependence between ischemic and mechanical factors (stretch, compression, and inflammation) as a cause of PPNI is well established but incompletely understood.[13]

- *Stretch*: Overstretch of a nerve can result in direct nerve damage due to disruption of axons and vasa vasorum.[13] Stretching a peripheral nerve leads to an increase in the intraneural pressure, thus reducing the perfusion pressure of the nerve fiber with consequent reduction in blood flow and ischemia.[21–23] Injury occurs when the nerve is stretched beyond 5%–15% of its resting length.[21,24,25]

- *Compression*: Compression of a peripheral nerve is another related mechanism of PPNI.[26] It is conceivable that the PPNI results from similar mechanisms to those found with stretch of the peripheral nerve.
- *Inflammation*: Inflammatory mechanisms may play a significant role in PPNI. Biopsy evidence of generalized microneuritis in patients with persistent postoperative ulnar neuropathy and a positive response in these patients to high-dose steroids support this.[27]

It would seem logical then, in addition to the local factors that contribute to PPNI, that more global factors influencing perfusion of peripheral nerves, such as the MAP, cardiac output, peripheral vasomotor tone, and oxygen content of blood, also play an important role in the pathogenesis and prevention of PPNI.

Common sites of PPNI

Ulnar nerve injury

- Most common PPNI[28] (28% of all anesthesia-related nerve injury malpractice claims[29]).
- Commonly presents more than 24 h after procedure (<10% in recovery room).[30]
- Superficial course and vulnerable to external pressure.[20]
- Increases in intramural pressure are not solely due to external pressure.[31]
- More sensitive to ischemia than the median and radial nerves.[17]
- Risk factors include
  - Male gender (70%), the elderly, the very thin, the very obese, and prolonged postoperative immobilization.[30]
  - Induced and prolonged hypotension.[16,32,33]
- Considerations specific to positioning are as follows (Figure 24.3a through d):
  - Forearm position affects pressure over the ulnar nerve at the elbow[20]:
    - Supination (2 mmHg)
    - Neutral (69 mmHg)
    - Pronation (95 mmHg)

Tips to avoid ulnar nerve injury

- Identify high-risk patients (male, extremes of body habitus, prolonged immobilization).
- Avoid direct pressure over the medial humeral condyle (pad with foam or gamgee).
- Aim to have the forearm on the supinated position.
- Aim to flex the elbow to 45°.
- Avoid elbow flexion beyond 90°.
- Avoid shoulder elevation and/or abduction beyond 90°.
- Avoid prolonged wrist dorsiflexion.

- Concomitant shoulder abduction further increases the pressure.[34]
- Elbow flexion
  - Greater than 70°: increased intraneural pressure.[31]
  - Greater than 90°: increased pressure along the ulnar nerve.[34]
  - Greater than 100°: increased extraneural pressure.[31]
- Intraneural and extraneural pressures are lowest with elbow flexion of approximately 45°.[31]
- Increased intraneural pressure with shoulder elevation and wrist dorsiflexion.[35]

Brachial plexus injury

- Second most common PPNI (20% of all anesthesia-related nerve injury malpractice claims).[29]
- Vulnerable to injury resulting from stretch and compression (long course between the vertebrae and the axilla).[12]
- Injury usually involves the upper roots (lower root injuries associated with median sternotomy).[12]
- Positional factors that can stretch the plexus and cause injury are as follows:
  - Shoulder abduction beyond 90°, external rotation of the arm, and posterior shoulder displacement.[12,36]

Tips to avoid brachial plexus injury

- Avoid shoulder abduction beyond 90°.
- Limit lateral neck flexion to avoid stretch of the contralateral plexus.
- Avoid head and neck extension.

- Downward tilting of the head and hyper-abduction of the independent arm in the lateral position.[37]
- Extension and lateral flexion of the head and neck in the supine position (contralateral injury).[12]
- Combinations of the aforementioned components have a cumulative impact.[13]
  - Interpatient variability increases as the number of components leading to stretch on the plexus increases.[38]

Median nerve injury

- Rare (4% of all anesthesia-related nerve injury malpractice claims).[29]
- Elbow extension may overstretch the nerve leading to injury.[39]
- Muscular patients and those with limited elbow extension are at particular risk.[39]
- Reduced range leading to contraction of the nerve is a proposed mechanism making these patients more prone to overstretch.[39]
- Overextension of the elbow to a point which is uncomfortable in the awake patient should be avoided.[40]
- Wrist extension, such as that used to aid placement of radial arterial lines, may stretch the median nerve further, and if prolonged risks injury to the nerve.[41]

Radial nerve injury

- Rare (3% of all anesthesia-related nerve injury malpractice claims).[29]
- Most common mechanism is compression of the nerve as it runs in the spiral groove of the humerus.[13]
- It is associated with
  - Abduction of the dependent arm beyond 90° in the lateral position.[42]
  - Direct compression by the arm board supporting the upper arm when the patient is placed in the lateral position.[13]

Postoperative visual loss

POVL is a rare but devastating complication of positioning and anesthesia for neurosurgical procedures. It is discussed in Chapter 32 of the book.

Tips to avoid median nerve injury

- Identify high-risk patients (muscular patients and those with reduced elbow extension).
- Limit positions to those that are tolerated by the patient when awake.
- Avoid prolonged wrist dorsiflexion.

Tips to avoid radial nerve injury

- Avoid shoulder abduction beyond 90°.
- Avoid direct pressure on the arm in the region of the spiral groove.
- When pressure on the arm is unavoidable, ensure ample padding with foam or gamgee.

General Points

- All positioning should be considered bespoke.
- Surgical drapes/warming blankets, etc., should not be applied until the final position is approved, and all at-risk points are checked.
- At all stages of positioning, the use of continuous capnography and pulse oximetry is recommended.
- Intraoperative adjustments to position risk airway loss and physical injuries (especially when the skull fixation is used) and should be avoided.

Supine (Figures 24.1a and b, 24.2, and 24.3a through d)

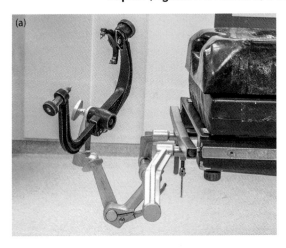

- Anticipate and manage the sympathetic response to skull fixation.
- Fixation devices should be unlocked and the head supported during any repositioning.
- Fixation pins are sharp and should not be left attached to the clamp and Mayfield frame.

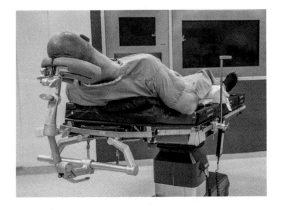

Figure 24.1 (a) Three-pin head clamp. (b) Beware hanging pins!

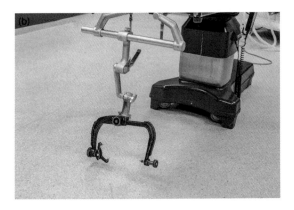

- Head-up tilt of 15° is widely used, but increases the risk of VAE.
- Transducer should be in level with the skull base (approximates to EAM).

Figure 24.2 Supine position with head tilted to the left.

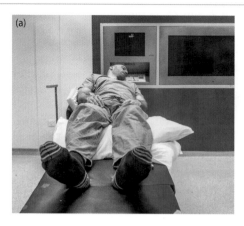

- Use of a sandbag contralateral to the direction of head rotation facilitates surgical positioning without overly rotating the neck.
- Overflexing the neck can lead to tongue and airway edema. Always check for airway edema if marked flexion is used.

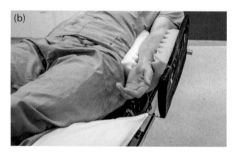

Figure 24.3 **(a)** Supported and well-padded arms and hands. **(b)** Forearm supinated.

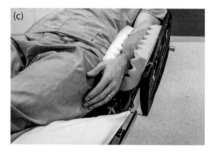

- A pillow behind the knees places the hip in slight flexion, maintaining lumbar lordosis.
- All pressure points should be checked.
- To reduce the risk of peripheral nerve injury, forearms alongside should be padded in neutral/supinated position.

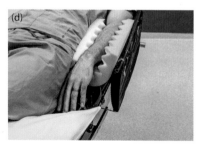

Figure 24.3 **(c)** Forearm neutral. **(d)** Avoid forearm pronated.

Lateral (Figure 24.4a and b, 5a through c]

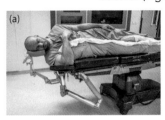

Figure 24.4 (a) Lateral position.

- Vacuum positioning devices assist stability, but negate the pressure-relieving design of modern mattresses.
- Monitoring cables/catheters can be easily trapped between hard surfaces and the patient's skin.

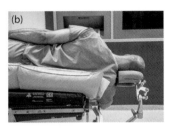

Figure 24.4 (b) Avoid overtraction of upper limb.

- Dependent arm should be supported in a way that relieves traction on the brachial plexus and protects the ulnar nerve.
- Simultaneous upper limb traction and neck abduction can stretch the brachial plexus.

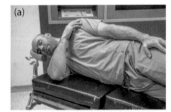

- Brachial plexus injury due to axillary pressure can be avoided by correct placement of the *axillary* roll (not in the axilla).
- Pillows and padding at pressure points and between legs.

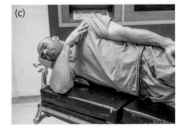

Figure 24.5 (a) Chest weight transferred to dependent axilla. (b) Axillary roll relieving dependent axilla. (c) Axillary roll incorrectly placed in dependent axilla.

Prone (Figure 24.6a through g)

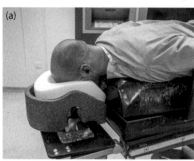

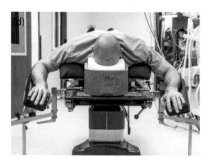

- Montreal mattress is not adjustable, and chest pillows should be used if the abdomen is large.
- Take care to maintain the neck neutral or in flexion when using ProneView™ or similar devices.

Figure 24.6 (a) Prone position: incorrectly supported head. (b) Correctly supported head, eyes visualized in ProneView™ device. (c) Forearms overflexed. (d) Upper arms inadequately supported.

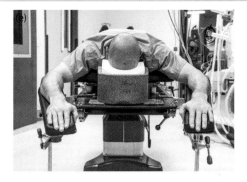

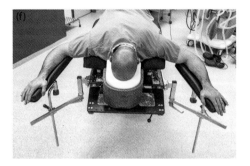

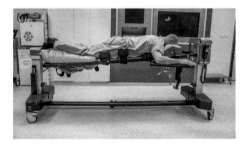

- Wilson frame should be correctly mounted (above the table break), and the width adjusted prior to patient positioning.
- Hips should be lined up to the table break point, but for short patients, the head and neck should be aligned with the top of the frame.
- As the frame is flexed, the head and neck will move and should be supported until positioning is complete.

Figure 24.6 (e) Arms overabducted. (f) Ideal upper limb support. (g) Prone position in alternate type of table.

- The Andrews table (not shown here) is designed to gradually place the patient into a knee–chest position, using the weight of the lower limbs to pull the torso down the table.
- The central portion (chest block and arm supports) of the table can be unlocked to slide freely.
- Chest block and tibial support can be adjusted for optimal final positioning.
- This table facilitates a free hanging abdomen, but the mechanical nature of positioning mandates trained and competent staff to avoid injury.
- The table is not radiolucent.
- The Jackson table (not shown here) is designed to facilitate spinal positioning and can be used to turn the patient in alignment.
- Chest and hip supports are adjustable.
- Free hanging abdomen is facilitated by correct positioning.
- Table design facilitates intraoperative use of X-ray.

Sitting (Figures 24.7a and b)

The sitting position is favored by some surgeons for the superior conditions it affords when accessing the posterior fossa, e.g., pineal surgery. Venous air embolus is a significant risk, and where possible this position should be avoided, although with the correct management it can be safely used.[43]

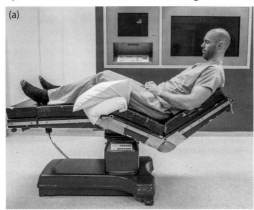

- Proceed in a stepwise manner to ensure cardiovascular stability.
- Pillow under knees reduces sciatic stretch.
- Pressure-relieving mattress or pillows for buttocks.
- Arterial line transducer at level of EAM.
- Apply skull fixation and establish invasive monitoring.
- Use fluid bolus and/or vasoconstrictors to maintain blood pressure.

Figure 24.7   (a) Semi-sitting position.

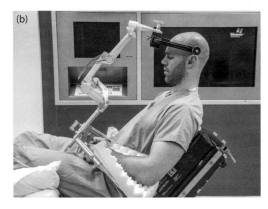

- Arterial line transducer at level of EAM.
- Legs level with the heart.
- Mayfield frame fixed to backrest to allow rapid repositioning in the event of VAE (bringing the head below the level of the heart).
- Avoid extremes of neck flexion.
- Forearms in supination across lap, supported by a pillow.
- All pressure points padded and isolated from contact with metal supports (burn risk from diathermy shorting).
- A pillow to prevent loss of lumbar lordosis; reduces postoperative back pain.

Figure 24.7   (b) Semi-sitting position with Mayfield frame fixed to the table.

References

1. Crowley RW, Dumont AS, McKisic MS, Jane JA. *Positioning for Cranial Surgery*. Amsterdam: Elsevier; 2011, 442–446. doi:10.1016/b978-1-4160-5316-3.00027-7.
2. Lee MJ, Lin EL. The use of the three-pronged Mayfield head clamp resulting in an intracranial epidural hematoma in an adult patient. *Eur Spine J* 2010;19(Suppl. 2):S187–S189. doi:10.1007/s00586-010-1323-z.
3. Malcharek MJ, Rogos B, Watzlawek S. Awake fiberoptic intubation and self-positioning in patients at risk of secondary cervical injury: A pilot study. *J Orthop Res* 2012;24(3):217–221. doi:10.1097/ana.0b013e31824da7e5.

4. Rozet I, Vavilala MS. Risks and benefits of patient positioning during neurosurgical care. *Anesthesiol Clin* 2007;25(3):631–53, x. doi:10.1016/j.anclin.2007.05.009.

5. Ogilvie L. Difficult airway society guidelines for the management of tracheal extubation. *Anaesthesia* 2012;67(11):1277–1278. doi:10.1111/anae.12011.

6. Galvin I, Drummond GB, Nirmalan M. Distribution of blood flow and ventilation in the lung: Gravity is not the only factor. *Br J Anaesth* 2007;98(4):420–428. doi:10.1093/bja/aem036.

7. West JB. Pulmonary blood flow and gas exchange. In: *Respiratory Physiology*. New York, NY: Springer; 1996, 140–169. doi:10.1007/978-1-4614-7520-0_5.

8. Lumb AB, Nunn JF. Respiratory function and ribcage contribution to ventilation in body positions commonly used during anesthesia. *Anesth Analg* 1991;73(4):422–426. doi:10.1213/00000539-199110000-00010.

9. Pelosi P, Croci M, Calappi E et al. The prone positioning during general anesthesia minimally affects respiratory mechanics while improving functional residual capacity and increasing oxygen tension. *Anesth Analg* 1995;80(5):955–960.

10. Lalkhen AG, Bhatia K. Perioperative peripheral nerve injuries. *Contin Educ Anaesth Crit Care Pain* 2012;12(1):38–42. doi:10.1093/bjaceaccp/mkr048.

11. Welch MB, Brummett CM, Welch TD et al. Perioperative peripheral nerve injuries: A retrospective study of 380, 680 cases during a 10-year period at a single institution. *Anesthesiology* 2009;111(3):490–497. doi:10.1097/ALN.0b013e3181af61cb.

12. Sawyer RJ, Richmond MN, Hickey JD, Jarrratt JA. Peripheral nerve injuries associated with anaesthesia. *Anaesthesia* 2000;55(10):980–991. doi:10.1046/j.1365-2044.2001.01870-28.x.

13. Kamel I, Barnette R. Positioning patients for spine surgery: Avoiding uncommon position-related complications. *World J Orthop* 2014;5(4):425–443. doi:10.5312/wjo.v5.i4.425.

14. Myers RR, Yamamoto T, Yaksh TL, Powell HC. The role of focal nerve ischemia and Wallerian degeneration in peripheral nerve injury producing hyperesthesia. *Anesthesiology* 1993;78(2):308–316. doi:10.1097/00000542-199302000-00015.

15. Bonner SM, Pridie AK. Sciatic nerve palsy following uneventful sciatic nerve block. *Anaesthesia* 1997;52(12):1205–1207.

16. Swenson JD, Bull DA. Postoperative ulnar neuropathy associated with prolonged ischemia in the upper extremity during coronary artery bypass surgery. *Anesth Analg* 1997;85(6):1275–1277. doi:10.1097/00000539-199712000-00017.

17. Swenson JD, Hutchinson DT, Bromberg M. Rapid onset of ulnar nerve dysfunction during transient occlusion of the brachial artery. *Anesth Analg* 1998;87(3):677–680. doi:10.1097/00000539-199809000-00035.

18. Yamada T, Muroga T, Kimura J. Tourniquet induced ischemia and somatosensory evoked potentials. *Neurology* 1981;31(12):1524–1524. doi:10.1212/wnl.31.12.1524.

19. Kozu H, Tamura E, Parry GJ. Endoneurial blood supply to peripheral nerves is not uniform. *J Neurol Sci* 1992;111(2):204–208. doi:10.1016/0022-510X(92)90070-2.

20. Prielipp RC, Morell RC, Walker FO, Santos CC, Bennett J, Butterworth J. Ulnar nerve pressure: Influence of arm position and relationship to somatosensory evoked potentials. *Anesthesiology* 1999;91(2):345–354.

21. Ogata K, Naito M. Blood flow of peripheral nerve effects of dissection, stretching and compression. *J Hand Surg: J Br Soc Surg Hand.* 1986;11(1):10–14. doi:10.1016/0266-7681(86)90003-3.

22. Brown R, Pedowitz R, Rydevik BR et al. Effects of acute graded strain on efferent conduction properties in the rabbit tibial nerve. *Clin Orthop Relat Res* 1993 Nov;(296):288–294. doi:10.1097/00003086-199311000-00046.

23. Rydevik BL, Kwan MK, Myers RR. An in vitro mechanical and histological study of acute stretching on rabbit tibial nerve. *J Orthop Res* 1990;8(5):694–701. doi:10.1002/jor.1100080511.

24. Tanoue M, Yamaga M, Ide J. Acute stretching of peripheral nerves inhibits retrograde axonal transport. *J Hand Surg: J Br Soc Surg Hand* 1996;21(3):358–363. doi:10.1016/s0266-7681(05)80203-7.

25. Wall EJ, Massie JB, Kwan MK, Rydevik BL, Myers RR, Garfin SR. Experimental stretch neuropathy. Changes in nerve conduction under tension. *J Bone Joint Surg Br* 1992;74(1):126–129.

26. Winfree CJ, Kline DG. Intraoperative positioning nerve injuries. *Surg Neurol* 2005;63(1):5–18. doi:10.1016/j. surneu.2004.03.024.

27. Staff NP, Engelstad J, Klein CJ et al. Post-surgical inflammatory neuropathy. *Brain* 2010;133(10):2866–2880. doi:10.1093/brain/awq252.

28. Lalonde G. Miller's Anesthesia, Eighth Edition. *Can J Anesth* 2015;62(5):558–559. doi:10.1007/s12630-015-0311-5.

29. Cheney FW, Domino KB, Caplan RA, Posner KL. Nerve injury associated with anesthesia: A closed claims analysis. *Anesthesiology* 1999;90(4):1062–1069.

30. Warner MA, Warner ME, Martin JT. Ulnar neuropathy. Incidence, outcome, and risk factors in sedated or anesthetized patients. *Anesthesiology* 1994;81(6):1332–1340. doi:10.1097/00000542-199412000-00006.

31. Gelberman RH, Yamaguchi K, Hollstien SB et al. Changes in interstitial pressure and cross-sectional area of the cubital tunnel and of the ulnar nerve with flexion of the elbow. An experimental study in human cadavera. *J Bone Joint Surg Am* 1998;80(4):492–501. doi:10.1016/S0072-968X(82)80030-2.

32. Britt BA, Gordon RA. Peripheral nerve injuries associated with anaesthesia. *Can Anaesth Soc J* 1964;11(5):514–536. doi:10.1007/BF03005094.

33. Jones HD. Ulnar nerve damage following general anaesthetic. A case possibly related to diabetes mellitus. *Anaesthesia* 1967;22(3):471–475.

34. Macnicol MF. Extraneural pressures affecting the ulnar nerve at the elbow. *Hand* 1982;14(1):5–11. doi:10.1016/S0072-968X(82)80030-2.

35. Pechan J, Juliš I. The pressure measurement in the ulnar nerve. A contribution to the pathophysiology of the cubital tunnel syndrome. *J Biomech* 1975;8(1):75–79. doi:10.1016/0021-9290(75)90045-7.

36. Dhuner KG. Nerve injuries following operations: Survey of cases occurring during a 6-year period. Anesthesiology 1950; 5:289–293.

37. Ngamprasertwong P, Phupong V, Uerpairojkit K. Brachial plexus injury related to improper positioning during general anesthesia. *J Anesth* 2004;18(2):132–134. doi:10.1007/s00540-003-0220-6.

38. Coppieters MW, Van de Velde M, Stappaerts KH. Positioning in anesthesiology: Toward a better understanding of stretch-induced perioperative neuropathies. *Anesthesiology* 2002;97(1):75–81. doi:10.1097/00000542-200207000-00011.

39. Barash P, Cullen BF, Stoelting RK, Cahalan M, Stock CM, Ortega R. *Clinical Anesthesia, 7e: Print + Ebook with Multimedia*. Philadelphia, PA: Lippincott Williams & Wilkins; 2013. doi:10.1007/s12630-009-9173-z.

40. Jeffrey LA, Richard TC, Robert AC et al. Practice advisory for the prevention of perioperative peripheral neuropathies: A report by the American Society of *Anesthesiologists* Task Force on Prevention of Perioperative Peripheral Neuropathies. Anesthesiology 2000;92(4):1168–1182.

41. Chowet AL, Lopez JR, Brock-Utne JG, Jaffe RA. Wrist hyperextension leads to median nerve conduction block: Implications for intra-arterial catheter placement. *Anesthesiology* 2004;100(2):287–291. doi:10.1097/00000542-200402000-00017.

42. Nicholson MJ, Eversole UH. Nerve injuries incident to anesthesia and operation. *Anesth Analg* 1957;36(4):19–32. doi:10.1213/00000539-195707000-00002.

43. Jadik S, Wissing H, Friedrich K, Beck J, Seifert V, Raabe A. A standardized protocol for the prevention of clinically relevant venous air embolism during neurosurgical interventions in the semisitting position. *Neurosurgery.* 2009;64(3):533–8–discussion538–9. doi:10.1227/01.NEU.0000338432.55235.D3.

PART VI

Fluid management of the neurosurgical patient

25

Perioperative fluids

PETER FARLING and KATIE MEGAW

Introduction

Providing optimal cerebral perfusion pressure, blood flow, and oxygen delivery is of paramount importance in the neurosurgical patient to enhance perioperative outcomes while avoiding the deleterious effects of increased cerebral water content. This is achieved, in part, through ensuring an adequate circulating blood volume and blood composition via the perioperative administration of intravenous fluids. Knowledge of the determinants of intracerebral water content, the pros and cons of available intravenous fluids, and the management of raised cerebral volume and intracranial pressure (ICP) is required by the anesthesiologist for a high standard of care of the neurosurgical patient.

Determinants of fluid movement

Fluid movement between the intravascular compartment and most tissues obeys the Starling equation (Box 25.1).[1] Capillary hydrostatic pressure (P_c) is generated by the *osmolality* of fluid in the capillary (Box 25.2). This generates a potent driving force for fluid flux across a semipermeable membrane from the region of lower osmolality to the region of higher osmolality. *Tonicity* refers to the effective osmolality and is often used when referring to intravenous fluids once they have been infused.

Oncotic pressure describes the osmotic pressure generated by larger solutes, such as plasma proteins, that cannot easily pass through a semipermeable membrane and act to reduce fluid movement. Given that tissue hydrostatic pressure (P_t) in nonedematous tissues is usually negative, from consideration of the Starling equation, the major factor preventing fluid movement from capillary to the interstitial space is plasma oncotic pressure (π_c). This is the case in peripheral tissues.

Fluid movement in the central nervous system (CNS) differs due to the existence of the blood–brain barrier (BBB). Morphologically, it is composed of endothelial cells that form tight junctions in the capillaries supplying the CNS as well as overlapping astrocytes.[2] Tight junctions severely limit the diffusion of both plasma proteins and electrolytes.

Box 25.1 The Starling equation

$$Qf=KfS[(Pc-Pt)-\sigma(\pi c-\pi t)]$$

Q_f is the net quantity of fluid moving between capillary and interstitial space
K_r is the filtration coefficient for the capillary membrane
S is the surface area of the capillary membrane
P_c is the capillary hydrostatic pressure
P_t is the interstitial hydrostatic pressure
σ is the coefficient of reflection— quantitates the "leakiness" of the specific capillary
π_c is the plasma oncotic pressure
π_t is the interstitial oncotic pressure

Box 25.2 Some common terminologies

Osmolality: the number of osmotically active particles per kg of solvent (mOsm/kg)
Osmolarity: the number of osmotically active particles per liter of solution (mOsm/L)
Tonicity: The effective osmolarity. Equal to the sum of the concentrations of solutes that have the capacity to exert an osmotic pressure across a semipermeable membrane

Box 25.3 Fluid movement in the brain and peripheral tissue

- In a healthy brain, the main determinant of fluid movement is the *osmolar gradient* between the intracerebral capillaries and interstitial fluid.
- In peripheral tissues, the main determinant of fluid movement is *plasma oncotic pressure*.

This is in contrast to peripheral tissues in which electrolytes are permitted to move between intravascular and extravascular compartments. For this reason, it is the *osmotic gradient* between capillaries and the CNS and not plasma oncotic pressure that governs cerebral fluid volume (Box 25.3). This is the basis for hyperosmolar therapy in situations of raised ICP or edematous brain and the avoidance of hypoosmolar solutions, which may exacerbate cerebral edema. In injured or diseased areas of brain where there may be disruption of the BBB, the determinants of fluid flux may be altered. The exact nature of this has yet to be clarified.[3,4]

Perioperative fluids for neurosurgical procedures

Types of intravenous fluids available

The properties of maintenance, resuscitative, and hyperosmolar intravenous solutions presently available in the United Kingdom, compared to plasma,

are shown in Table 25.1. Most of the fluids listed are relatively *isoosmolar* with respect to plasma except for 20% mannitol and 3% sodium chloride, which are *hyperosmolar*. Although 5% glucose has a similar osmolarity to plasma, it is *hypotonic*, for example, once infused the glucose is metabolized leaving free water and rendering the solution grossly hypotonic with respect to plasma. Fluids may be described as *balanced*, having a composition resembling plasma, for example, Hartmann's solution and the newer derivatives Plasma-Lyte® and Isolyte® S, or *unbalanced*, for example, 0.9% sodium chloride solution (Table 25.2). Ringer's lactate is a balanced solution similar to, but not identical to, Hartmann's solution. Colloids may be suspended in balanced or unbalanced solutions.

Choice of intravenous fluid for neurosurgical procedures

The choice of fluid for neurosurgical procedures should ideally be determined by high-quality randomized controlled trials. However, there is a paucity of evidence for perioperative fluids in the neurosurgical population. As a result, recommendations have been made based on the evidence available, much of which comes from the critically ill population. Other considerations for the administration of intravenous fluids for neurosurgical patients are summarized in Table 25.3.

Crystalloids

Intraoperative fluid requirement (resuscitative, maintenance, and replacement fluid) for neurosurgical procedures is usually achieved with 0.9% sodium chloride or Hartmann's solution/Ringer's lactate, both solutions having a long history of use. These solutions are relatively isoosmolar with

Table 25.1 The Osmolarity and Oncotic Pressure of Plasma Compared to Common Maintenance, Resuscitative, and Hyperosmolar Intravenous Solutions

Intravenous solutions	Osmolarity (mOsm/L)	Oncotic pressure (mmHg)
Plasma	290	26
Hartmann's solution	278	0
0.9% sodium chloride	308	0
5% glucose	278	0
5% albumin	290	19
6% dextran 70	300	69
4% gelatin (succinylated)	284	34
Tetrastarch	286–308	36
20% mannitol	1098	0
3% sodium chloride	1027	0

Table 25.2 The Composition of Plasma (in Mmol/L) Compared to Common Crystalloid Solutions

	Plasma	Hartmann's solution	Plasma-Lyte®	Isolyte® S	0.9% sodium chloride	5% glucose
Na	140	131	140	141	154	–
Cl	100	111	98	98	154	–
K	5	5	5	5	–	–
Ca	2	2	–	–	–	–
Mg	1	1	1.5	3	–	–
Lactate	0.5	29	–	–	–	–
Acetate	–	–	27	27	–	–
Gluconate	–	–	23	23	–	–
Osmolarity	290	278	294	295	308	278

Table 25.3 Considerations for the Administration of Perioperative Intravenous Fluid for Neurosurgical Procedures

Patient factors	Surgical factors
Preoperative health status	Requirement for brain relaxation
Preoperative fluid deficit	Perioperative fluctuations in ICP
Ongoing fluid losses	Potential for blood loss
Presence of trauma	Potential for diabetes insipidus

respect to plasma and should not exacerbate cerebral edema. The balanced solutions (Hartmann's solution, Plasma-Lyte®, Isolyte® S) more closely resemble plasma in their electrolyte composition and presence of a buffer to maintain the body's acid–base balance. Sodium chloride 0.9% with its high sodium and chloride contents and lower pH is far from "normal" as it is often described; however in some centers, it is used in preference to Hartmann's solution based on its comparative hyperosmolarity, which may have a beneficial effect on cerebral water content.

A recent Cochrane review in perioperative patients has shown that buffered fluids were associated with fewer episodes of hyperchloremia and metabolic acidosis than 0.9% sodium chloride, but with no significant difference in complication rate or mortality; however, there were no neurosurgical patients among the participants and buffered fluids included both crystalloids and colloids.[5] In contrast, balanced crystalloid was associated with a lower rate of postoperative complications compared to 0.9% sodium chloride in a large observational study of over 30,000 patients having open abdominal surgery.[6] In the critically ill population, chloride-rich solutions were associated with increased incidence of renal failure and renal replacement therapy than chloride-restricted solutions.[7] No randomized trial has been conducted comparing 0.9% sodium chloride with balanced crystalloid in neurosurgical patients.

Solutions of glucose alone should not be used as maintenance or resuscitative fluid in adult patients presenting for neurosurgery. Being hypotonic with respect to plasma, they are distributed throughout all body compartments, contributing minimally to intravascular volume. The combination of the syndrome of inappropriate antidiuretic hormone secretion (SIADH) associated with surgery, together with excessive use of hypotonic fluid, can result in hyponatremia and, potentially, cerebral edema. Moreover, hyperglycemia is well known to have deleterious effects on traumatic brain injury (TBI), acute ischemic stroke, and subarachnoid hemorrhage (SAH).[8–10] Glucose solutions do, however, still retain a place in clinical practice in the treatment of hypoglycemia and ketoacidosis and in fasting protocols for diabetic patients.

Colloids

Albumin

Human albumin solution is a by-product of whole-blood fractionation from donor blood and, in the United Kingdom, is available as 4.5%, 5%, and 20% solutions in 0.9% sodium chloride. It is primarily used as a resuscitative fluid following the results of several large randomized studies in critically ill patients demonstrating equal safety compared to crystalloids.[11,12] However, in a subgroup analysis of the Saline versus Albumin Fluid Evaluation (SAFE) study, patients with TBI treated with albumin had significantly higher 28-day mortality than those treated with 0.9% sodium chloride.[11] Until further evidence challenges this, it appears prudent to avoid albumin for resuscitation in neurosurgical patients.

Gelatins

Gelatins are manufactured from thermal degradation of bovine collagen and have a molecular weight range of 30–35 kDa. They are unavailable in the United States and currently succinylated gelatins alone are available in the United Kingdom. Gelatins result in a short duration of plasma expansion (2–3 h) secondary to rapid renal excretion. They have the advantage of minimal effects on coagulation and renal function but show the highest risk of anaphylaxis of the synthetic colloids.[13–15] Recent systematic reviews have shown no mortality benefit in critically ill and perioperative patients who received gelatin compared to crystalloids ± albumin for resuscitation.[16,17] Despite a long history of use, large studies investigating outcomes with gelatins are lacking. In the absence of evidence of benefit, gelatins are not recommended in neurosurgical patients.

Starches

Hydroxyethyl starches (HES) are derived from amylopectin and are classified according to concentration, mean molecular weight in kDa (70–670 kDa), and the average number of hydroxyethyl groups per molecule of glucose. The latter is specified by the molar substitution ranging from 0.4 (tetrastarch) to 0.7 (hetastarch).

Tetrastarch (HES 130/0.4), is the most modern form of HES and is the only formulation presently available in the United Kingdom. Compared to older HES formulations, tetrastarch does not accumulate in plasma and is less likely to cause platelet dysfunction and coagulopathy.[18,19] There have been conflicting results regarding the use of HES in the perioperative setting. A recent meta-analysis found no increase in kidney injury, red cell transfusion, or mortality in surgical patients treated with tetrastarch compared to other fluids.[20] Similar results were reported in a systematic review in surgical patients who received any form of 6% HES.[21] However, a 2013 Cochrane review in different patient populations (critically ill, medical, cardiac, and noncardiac surgery) found that HES solutions were associated with acute kidney injury and renal replacement therapy.[22] In the critically ill population, the use of HES for resuscitation has been found to be significantly associated with a higher risk of acute renal injury and requirement for renal replacement therapy.[16,23] These studies have resulted in a marked decline in the use of HES in all clinical situations, particularly in critical care, and its use is not recommended in neurosurgical patients.

Dextrans

Dextrans are high molecular weight (40–70 kDa) glucopolysaccharides formed by the action of bacteria on sucrose. Although significant volume expanders, they are rarely used as a resuscitative fluid secondary to profound effects on platelet and red blood cell aggregation and anaphylactoid reactions.[24] They have been withdrawn from use by many countries and their use is not advised in neurosurgery.

Blood products

In the operating room, point-of-care hemoglobin (Hb) and hematocrit testing along with measurement of intraoperative blood loss allow for rapid management of intraoperative anemia. Bleeding in neurosurgery depends on the nature of surgery and the clinical situation. Certainly, surgery for intracerebral tumor resection and intracranial surgery in trauma may be associated with significant bleeding and coagulopathy necessitating transfusion of blood products. A balance must be struck between providing adequate Hb for oxygen delivery and an appropriate blood viscosity for optimal microcirculatory flow. Transfusion thresholds will vary according to governing institution; however, a restrictive transfusion strategy aimed at

transfusing at a lower Hb and aiming for a lower target Hb is now an accepted practice.[25,26] In the perioperative setting, transfusion thresholds must be considered along with the presence of active hemorrhage and cardiovascular disease. Plasma may be administered in neurosurgery in massive hemorrhage, trauma, or specific coagulopathies.

How much fluid?

In the perioperative period, patients should first receive resuscitative fluids, if necessary, or fluids to replace a preoperative deficit (the optimized patient for elective surgery). Perioperative intravascular volume depletion may be due to gastrointestinal losses, diuretics, or trauma. The rate of *resuscitative fluid* will depend on the severity of hypovolemia. Insensible fluid losses alone may account for fluid deficit in elective surgery. Losses through skin, respiration, sweat, urine, and feces equate to over 0.5 mL/kg/day and increase by 12% for each degree Celsius above 37°C. Although prolonged fasting is not advised, fasting time up to 10 h has not been shown to contribute to intravascular volume depletion.[27]

The normal maintenance water requirement is 25–30 mL/kg/day. Perioperative *maintenance fluid* should be provided together with replacement of fluid losses from distribution and other surgical losses. Neurosurgical procedures are associated with minimal "third space" fluid loss. Instead, perioperative fluid loss may be attributed to prolonged operating time and mechanical ventilation, sudden hemorrhage, and diabetes insipidus (DI).

There is an unsubstantiated belief that fluid restriction lessens cerebral edema formation.[28] Indeed, it is completely inappropriate to withhold isoosmolar fluids to the point that a patient shows hemodynamic instability due to hypovolemia. Optimal volemic status is imperative to achieve adequate cerebral perfusion while avoiding the deleterious effects of fluid overload, which is associated with increased postoperative complications and increased length of hospital stay.[29]

The physiological response to intravenous fluid according to hemodynamic parameters is used to guide perioperative fluid therapy. Recently, "dynamic" measures of fluid responsiveness in mechanically ventilated patients have been used to guide fluid responsiveness. Methods of dynamic monitoring include systolic pressure variation, pulse pressure variation, stroke volume variation derived from the arterial waveform, plethysmography, or esophageal Doppler. These modalities appear to be superior to standard monitoring, central venous pressure monitoring, and a pulmonary artery catheter used in the assessment of response to a fluid challenge in major surgery or in the hemodynamically unstable patient.[30,31] Although much of the research into the utility of various dynamic monitoring devices has been in elective gastrointestinal surgery, there has been some application in the neurosurgical population.[32-34] Advanced hemodynamic monitoring is an evolving field; however, at present there is a lack of evidence to support the use of one modality over another, and their use in clinical practice is limited by institution availability and user experience.

Hyperosmolar therapy

Hyperosmolar therapy describes the administration of a hyperosmolar solution to reduce cerebral volume. The solutions used are mannitol and hypertonic saline (≥3%). On their administration, the osmotic gradient established between blood and cerebral tissue draws water from the intracellular compartment and interstitial space, resulting in a reduced tissue volume and ICP. Intraoperative administration may be requested to improve surgical access and reduce trauma secondary to surgical retractors, and these solutions are frequently used in an emergency to treat raised ICP secondary to edema or hemorrhage.

Mannitol is a six-carbon sugar with a molecular weight of 182 Da. It is available in 10% or 20% solutions and is given at a dose of 0.25–1 g/kg by rapid intravenous infusion. Traditionally, it has been the "gold standard" treatment for raised ICP via a reduction in brain water content in areas of intact BBB.[35] Before the osmotic effect, mannitol causes immediate plasma expansion and reduction in hematocrit, leading to improved cerebral blood flow and oxygen delivery.[36] However, there are concerns that mannitol may exert a delayed increase in ICP. Mannitol has a reflection coefficient of 0.9 and therefore may cross the BBB, potentially causing a reverse osmotic gradient.[37]

Hypertonic saline (HTS) describes saline solutions of concentrations from 3% to 30%. It appears to be as efficacious as mannitol in equiosmolar concentrations for reducing cerebral volume and ICP.[38-40] Having a reflection coefficient of 1.0 and therefore unable to cross the BBB as well a lack of diuretic effect make HTS an appealing alternative to mannitol, particularly in hemodynamically unstable patients.[41] In a recent review comparing mannitol and HTS for brain relaxation in patients undergoing craniotomy, HTS was found to provide significantly better brain relaxation during craniotomy.[42] Although the methodological quality of included studies ($n = 6$) was not good and only three trials used equiosmolar solutions, subsequent randomized trials comparing equiosmolar solutions obtained the same result.[43,44] There remains, however, a lack of evidence on whether HTS compared to mannitol affects long-term outcomes and mortality. Although both mannitol and HTS may cause electrolyte disturbances, a major disadvantage of HTS is the high sodium load and potential for acute hypernatremia.[44] After administration of any hyperosmolar therapy serum electrolytes should be monitored.

Specific circumstances in neurosurgery

Trauma

Traumatic brain injury is a significant cause of morbidity and mortality worldwide. Maintaining cerebral perfusion is a priority for the anesthesiologist to reduce the impact of secondary brain injury, which occurs in the hours and days after the primary injury. This can be extremely challenging in the face of hypovolemia secondary to bleeding, cardiovascular instability, raised ICP, trauma-induced coagulopathy, other critical injuries, and the requirement for emergency surgery.

The *resuscitative fluid* of choice in head trauma has been a subject of debate. HTS has received particular attention given the potential for significant intravascular expansion using small volumes, in addition to the beneficial effect on cerebral volume and ICP. However, the proposed benefits have not been proven in the literature.[45,46] Resuscitation with any of the available colloids may provide no benefit over crystalloid or may cause harm in TBI.[11,16,17,22–24] Crystalloid solutions, either 0.9% sodium chloride or Hartmann's, therefore remain the leading resuscitative fluids in TBI. The theoretical advantage of the relative hyperosmolarity of 0.9% sodium chloride compared to plasma is weighed against the increased risk of hyperchloremic metabolic acidosis with administration of large volumes. In the case of hypovolemia secondary to hemorrhage, infusion of red cells and coagulation factors should be prioritized and initial resuscitation with crystalloid should be minimized to avoid dilutional coagulopathy.

Regarding the choice of hyperosmolar solution for suspected or confirmed raised ICP, the Brain Trauma Foundation currently advise bolus administration of mannitol as opposed to HTS for ICP reduction in TBI due to a lack of high-quality evidence on the use, concentration, and method of administration of HTS.[36]

Cerebral aneurysms

In the perioperative setting, patients with SAH may present for anesthesia for radiological embolization or surgical clipping of the aneurysm. Hypovolemia after SAH increases the risk of cerebral vasospasm and delayed cerebral ischemia and should be strictly avoided.[47] Such patients should be resuscitated with isoosmolar fluids to achieve normovolemia. Along with the calcium-channel blocker nimodipine, "triple H" therapy or hyperdynamic therapy has been traditionally advised to prevent and treat vasospasm in secured aneurysms. Hyperdynamic therapy comprises modest hemodilution, vasopressor-induced hypertension, and hypervolemia. However, recent systematic reviews have questioned such a therapy in the prophylaxis of vasospasm given the lack of well-designed prospective studies.[48,49]

Diabetes insipidus

Neurogenic DI frequently occurs following pituitary surgery or severe TBI due to damage to the neurons of the supraoptic nuclei of the hypothalamus, resulting in absent or reduced secretion of antidiuretic hormone (ADH). The clinical manifestations include polyuria, polydipsia, a normal or elevated plasma osmolarity, and a rise in serum sodium. In the perioperative period, transient DI begins with an abrupt onset of polyuria within 24–48 h of surgery and resolves over 3–5 days.[50] Left untreated, DI can escalate to hypovolemia and hypotension compromising cerebral perfusion.

Fluid deficit causes a hyperosmotic, hypernatremic state and should be treated with either 0.45% sodium chloride or Hartmann's solution. Administration of 0.9% sodium chloride is inappropriate in this setting due to the hypernatremic state. Concomitant administration of desmopressin, the synthetic analog of ADH, is recommended to treat the underlying cause.

Summary

The major influence on fluid movement in the cerebral circulation is the osmolarity of the intravascular compartment compared to the extravascular compartment. This has an impact on the choice of perioperative fluids for neurosurgical patients. Isoosmolar crystalloids such as 0.9% sodium chloride and Hartmann's solution remain the intravenous fluids of choice in neurosurgical patients for both resuscitation and maintenance fluid requirement. The quantity of fluid administered is guided by hemodynamic monitoring. At present, there appears to be no benefit, if not harm, in administration of any of the available colloids in neurosurgical patients, and consequently, their use is not recommended. Hypotonic fluids such as 5% glucose are not advised in the neurosurgical setting due to their potential to cause cerebral edema. Mannitol and HTS may be requested intraoperatively for brain relaxation or be required in the treatment of acute rises in ICP.

References

1. Starling EH. On the absorption of fluids from the connective tissue spaces. J Physiol 1896;19(4):312–326.
2. Pardridge WM, Oldendorf WH, Cancilla P, Frank HJ. Blood–brain barrier: Interface between internal medicine and the brain. Ann Intern Med 1986;105(1):82–95.

3. Warner DS, Boehland LA. Effects of iso-osmolal intravenous fluid therapy on post-ischemic brain water content in the rat. *Anesthesiology* 1988;68(1):86–91.

4. Drummond J, Patel P, Cole D, Kelly P. The effect of the reduction of colloid oncotic pressure, with and without reduction of osmolality, on post-traumatic cerebral edema. *Anaesthesiology* 1998;88(4):993–1002.

5. Burdett E, Dushianthan A, Bennett-Guerrero E et al. Perioperative buffered versus non-buffered fluid administration for surgery in adults. *Cochrane Database Syst Rev* 2012;12:CD004089.

6. Shaw AD, Bagshaw SM, Goldstein SL et al. Major complications, mortality, and resource utilization after open abdominal surgery: 0.9% saline compared to Plasma-Lyte. *Ann Surg* 2012;255(5):821–829.

7. Yunos NM, Bellomo R, Hegarty C, Story D, Ho L, Bailey M. Association between a chloride-liberal vs chloride-restrictive intravenous fluid administration strategy and kidney injury in critically ill adults. *JAMA* 2012;308(15):1566–1572.

8. Lam AM, Winn HR, Cullen BF, Sundling N. Hyperglycemia and neurological outcome in patients with head injury. *J Neurosurg* 1991;75(4):545–551.

9. Weir CJ, Murray GD, Dyker AG, Lees KR. Is hyperglycaemia an independent predictor of poor outcome after acute stroke? Results of a long-term follow up study. *BMJ* 1997;314(7090):1303–1306.

10. Frontera JA, Fernandez A, Claassen J et al. Hyperglycemia after SAH: Predictors, associated complications, and impact on outcome. *Stroke* 2006;37(1):199–203.

11. Finfer S, Bellomo R, Boyce N et al. A comparison of albumin and saline for fluid resuscitation in the intensive care unit. *N Engl J Med* 2004;350(22):2247–2256.

12. Caironi P, Tognoni G, Masson S et al. Albumin replacement in patients with severe sepsis or septic shock. *N Engl J Med* 2014;370(15):1412–1421.

13. Hussain SF, Drew PJ. Acute renal failure after infusion of gelatins. *BMJ* 1989;299(6708):1137–1138.

14. Laxenaire MC, Charpentier C, Feldman L. Anaphylactoid reactions to colloid plasma substitutes: Incidence, risk factors, mechanisms. A French multicenter prospective study. *Ann Fr Anesth Reanim* 1994;13(3):301–310.

15. de Jonge E, Levi M. Effects of different plasma substitutes on blood coagulation: A comparative review. *Crit Care Med* 2001;29(6):1261–1267.

16. Perel P, Roberts I, Ker K. Colloids versus crystalloids for fluid resuscitation in critically ill patients. *Cochrane Database Syst Rev* 2013;2:CD000567.

17. Thomas-Rueddel DO, Vlasakov V, Reinhart K et al. Safety of gelatin for volume resuscitation—a systematic review and meta-analysis. *Intensive Care Med* 2012;38(7):1134–1142.

18. Treib J, Haass A, Pindur G, Treib W, Wenzel E, Schimrigk K. Influence of intravascular molecular weight of hydroxyethyl starch on platelets. *Eur J Haematol* 1996;56(3):168–172.

19. Treib J, Baron JF, Grauer MT, Strauss RG. An international view of hydroxyethyl starches. *Intensive Care Med* 1999;25(3):258–268.

20. Van Der Linden P, James M, Mythen M, Weiskopf RB. Safety of modern starches used during surgery. *Anesth Analg* 2013;116(1):35–48.

21. Gillies MA, Habicher M, Jhanji S et al. Incidence of postoperative death and acute kidney injury associated with i.v. 6% hydroxyethyl starch use: Systematic review and meta-analysis. *Br J Anaesth* 2014;112(1):25–34.

22. Mutter TC, Ruth CA, Dart AB. Hydroxyethyl starch (HES) versus other fluid therapies: Effects on kidney function. *Cochrane Database Syst Rev* 2013;7:CD007594.

23. Myburgh JA, Finfer S, Bellomo R et al. Hydroxyethyl starch or saline for fluid resuscitation in intensive care. *N Engl J Med* 2012;367(20):1901–1911.

24. Ertmer C, Rehberg S, Van Aken H, Westphal M. Relevance of non-albumin colloids in intensive care medicine. *Best Pract Res Clin Anaesthesiol* 2009;23(2):193–212.

25. Carson JL, Terrin ML, Noveck H et al. Liberal or restrictive transfusion in high-risk patients after hip surgery. *N Engl J Med* 2011;365(26):2453–2462.

26. Carson JL, Carless PA, Hebert PC. Transfusion thresholds and other strategies for guiding allogeneic red blood cell transfusion. *Cochrane Database Syst Rev* 2012;4:CD002042.

27. Jacob M, Chappell D, Conzen P, Finsterer U, Rehm M. Blood volume is normal after pre-operative overnight fasting. *Acta Anaesthesiol Scand* 2008;52(4):522–529.

28. Jelsma LF, McQueen JD. Effect of experimental water restriction on brain water. *J Neurosurg* 1967;26(1):35–40.

29. Brandstrup B, Tonnesen H, Beier-Holgersen R et al. Effects of intravenous fluid restriction on postoperative complications: Comparison of two perioperative fluid regimens: A randomized assessor-blinded multicenter trial. *Ann Surg* 2003;238(5):641–648.

30. Funk DJ, Moretti EW, Gan TJ. Minimally invasive cardiac output monitoring in the perioperative setting. *Anesth Analg* 2009;108(3):887–897.

31. Renner J, Scholz J, Bein B. Monitoring cardiac function: Echocardiography, pulse contour analysis and beyond. *Best Pract Res Clin Anaesthesiol* 2013;27(2):187–200.

32. Berkenstadt H, Margalit N, Hadani M et al. Stroke volume variation as a predictor of fluid responsiveness in patients undergoing brain surgery. *Anesth Analg* 2001;92(4):984–989.

33. Li J, Ji FH, Yang JP. Evaluation of stroke volume variation obtained by the FloTrac/Vigileo system to guide preoperative fluid therapy in patients undergoing brain surgery. *J Int Med Res* 2012;40(3):1175–1181.

34. Byon HJ, Lim CW, Lee JH et al. Prediction of fluid responsiveness in mechanically ventilated children undergoing neurosurgery. *Br J Anaesth* 2013;110(4):586–591.

35. Bell BA, Smith MA, Kean DM et al. Brain water measured by magnetic resonance imaging. Correlation with direct estimation and changes after mannitol and dexamethasone. *Lancet* 1987;1(8524):66–69.

36. Brain Trauma Foundation, American Association of Neurological Surgeons, Congress of Neurological Surgeons et al. Guidelines for the management of severe traumatic brain injury. II. Hyperosmolar therapy. *J Neurotrauma* 2007;24(Suppl. 1):S14–S20.

37. Rudehill A, Gordon E, Ohman G, Lindqvist C, Andersson P. Pharmacokinetics and effects of mannitol on hemodynamics, blood and cerebrospinal fluid electrolytes, and osmolality during intracranial surgery. *J Neurosurg Anesthesiol* 1993;5(1):4–12.

38. Scheller MS, Zornow MH, Seok Y. A comparison of the cerebral and hemodynamic effects of mannitol and hypertonic saline in a rabbit model of acute cryogenic brain injury. *J Neurosurg Anesthesiol* 1991;3(4):291–296.

39. Tseng MY, Al-Rawi PG, Pickard JD, Rasulo FA, Kirkpatrick PJ. Effect of hypertonic saline on cerebral blood flow in poor-grade patients with subarachnoid hemorrhage. *Stroke* 2003;34(6):1389–1396.

40. Vialet R, Albanese J, Thomachot L et al. Isovolume hypertonic solutes (sodium chloride or mannitol) in the treatment of refractory posttraumatic intracranial hypertension: 2 mL/kg 7.5% saline is more effective than 2 mL/kg 20% mannitol. *Crit Care Med* 2003;31(6):1683–1687.

41. Rozet I, Tontisirin N, Muangman S et al. Effect of equiosmolar solutions of mannitol versus hypertonic saline on intraoperative brain relaxation and electrolyte balance. *Anesthesiology* 2007;107(5):697–704.

42. Prabhakar H, Singh GP, Anand V, Kalaivani M. Mannitol versus hypertonic saline for brain relaxation in patients undergoing craniotomy. *Cochrane Database Syst Rev* 2014;7:CD010026.

43. Dostal P, Dostalova V, Schreiberova J et al. A comparison of equivolume, equiosmolar solutions of hypertonic saline and mannitol for brain relaxation in patients undergoing elective intracranial tumor surgery: A randomized clinical trial. *J Neurosurg Anesthesiol* 2015;27(1):51–56.

44. Malik ZA, Mir SA, Naqash IA, Sofi KP, Wani AA. A prospective, randomized, double blind study to compare the effects of equiosmolar solutions of 3% hypertonic saline and 20% mannitol on reduction of brain-bulk during elective craniotomy for supratentorial brain tumor resection. *Anesth Essays Res* 2014;8(3):388–392.

45. Bunn F, Roberts I, Tasker R, Akpa E. Hypertonic versus near isotonic crystalloid for fluid resuscitation in critically ill patients. *Cochrane Database Syst Rev* 2004;(3)(3):CD002045.

46. Bulger EM, May S, Brasel KJ et al. Out-of-hospital hypertonic resuscitation following severe traumatic brain injury: A randomized controlled trial. *JAMA* 2010;304(13):1455–1464.

47. Solomon RA, Post KD, McMurtry JG. 3rd. Depression of circulating blood volume in patients after subarachnoid hemorrhage: Implications for the management of symptomatic vasospasm. *Neurosurgery* 1984;15(3):354–361.

48. Rinkel GJ, Feigin VL, Algra A, van Gijn J. Circulatory volume expansion therapy for aneurysmal subarachnoid haemorrhage. *Cochrane Database Syst Rev* 2004;(4):CD000483.

49. Treggiari MM, Walder B, Suter PM, Romand JA. Systematic review of the prevention of delayed ischemic neurological deficits with hypertension, hypervolemia, and hemodilution therapy following subarachnoid hemorrhage. *J Neurosurg* 2003;98(5):978–984.

50. Schreckinger M, Szerlip N, Mittal S. Diabetes insipidus following resection of pituitary tumors. *Clin Neurol Neurosurg* 2013;115(2):121–126.

26

Hyperosmolar therapy

HEMANSHU PRABHAKAR

Introduction

Hyperosmolar therapy remains the keystone in the management of brain edema and raised intracranial pressure (ICP). It is practiced both in the operation theater and in intensive care units. For achieving brain relaxation in the intraoperative period, hypertonic fluids such as mannitol and hypertonic saline are frequently used. It is by their virtue that water is drawn from intracellular and interstitial compartments into the intravascular compartment, resulting in relaxation of the brain and increased compliance. It is essential that the blood–brain barrier remain intact for the hypertonic fluids to produce their effect on the brain.[1] The transport through the blood–brain barrier is a selective process. The restriction of a particle is expressed as the osmotic *reflection coefficient* (RC), which ranges from 0 to 1.0.

This chapter focuses on the use of two popular hyperosmolar agents, mannitol and hypertonic saline.

Mannitol

- It is a six-carbon sugar alcohol that does not undergo metabolism.
- Its means of clearance is through glomerular filtration.
- Its RC is 0.9.
- Its osmolarity is 1098 mOsm/L.

- It is available as a 20% solution.
- It has a dehydrating effect on the body tissues, including the brain.[2]
- It is a scavenger for oxygen-free radicals, which prevents cellular swelling.
- It produces diuresis with urinary excretion of water, sodium, chloride, and bicarbonate ions.
- It begins to exert effect within 10–15 min. Its peak effect may be seen 15–35 min after infusion. The effect may last up to 2 h.[3,4]
- It transiently increases plasma volume, and decreases hematocrit and blood viscosity, thereby improving blood flow through microvasculature.
- It enhances oxygen delivery to tissues.
- Its loading dose as rapid infusion is 0.25–1 g/kg body weight; this may be repeated after 4–8 h.
- Its recommended maximum dose is 2 g/kg/dose.
- ICP reduction may be observed for 3–8 h.
- It can be administered through a central venous catheter or a peripheral cannula.
- Some of the complications observed with its use are sloughing of skin, hypokalemia, and hyperglycemia in patients with diabetes and in the elderly.[5]
- It is not associated with rebound intracranial hypertension.
- Renal damage may occur with a dose exceeding 200 g.
- The upper limit of serum osmolarity that may be safely attained is 320 mOsm/L.

Hypertonic saline

- It is saline in concentrations ranging from 1.6% to 23.4%.
- 3% hypertonic saline is most commonly used. It is also available in 2% and 7.5%.
- It increases the intravascular compartment by drawing water inside the vessels.
- Its RC is 1.0.
- The osmolarity of 3% hypertonic saline is 1027 mOsm/L.
- Its recommended dose is 1–2 mL/kg/h or 250 mL bolus over 30 min; this may be repeated after 30 min.
- Its recommended maximum dose is 1 mEq/kg/h or 1.9 mL/kg/h.
- It produces hypernatremia, which results in shrinkage of the brain.
- It is a less potent diuretic than mannitol.
- Rebound edema can occur as a result of infusions.
- A central venous catheter is preferred if infusion has to be continued for more than 1 day.
- Congestive cardiac failure may occur in patients with compromised cardiac status.
- Its usage has shown mixed immunomodulatory results.

Mannitol and hypertonic saline remain the fluids of choice for managing raised ICP and achieving brain relaxation during the intraoperative period. Both fluids have similar effects on raised ICP given in equimolar doses. In a recent review comparing mannitol and hypertonic saline for brain relaxation in patients undergoing craniotomy, hypertonic saline was found to provide better brain relaxation during craniotomy.[6] However, there is lack of evidence on whether hypertonic saline compared to mannitol affects long-term outcomes and mortality.

References

1. Tommasino C. Fluids in the neurosurgical patient. *Anesthesiol Clin North America* 2002;20:329–346.
2. Ropper AH. Hyperosmolar therapy for raised intracranial pressure. *N Engl J Med* 2012;367:746–752.
3. Wise BL, Chater N. The value of hypertonic mannitol solution in decreasing brain mass and lowering cerebrospinal fluid pressure. *J Neurosurg* 1962;19:1038–1043.
4. Diuretics. In: Stoelting RK, Hillier SC, editors. *Pharmacology and Physiology in Anesthetic Practice*. 4th ed. Philadelphia, PA: Lippincott Williams and Wilkins; 2006, pp. 486–495.
5. Ropper AH. Management of raised intracranial pressure and hyperosmolar therapy. *Pract Neurol* 2014;14:152–158.
6. Prabhakar H, Singh GP, Anand V, Kalaivani M. Mannitol versus hypertonic saline for brain relaxation in patients undergoing craniotomy. *Cochrane Database Syst Rev* 2014;(7):CD010026.

27

Blood loss and blood transfusion

BHAVNA HOODA

Introduction

Perioperative blood loss in the perioperative period is one of the most common indications of blood transfusion. Approximately 85 million red blood cell (RBC) units are obtained globally. Transfusions account for the most common in-hospital procedures; the magnitude is such that orthopedic surgeries account for 40% of perioperative blood usage approximating to 10% of red cell transfusions. On the one hand, timely resuscitation with blood products can be lifesaving, but on the other hand, blood is a finite source with serious risks of immunomodulation, transfusion reactions, transfusion transmissible infections, and so on. Therefore, a pretransfusion risk–benefit analysis should be done and all efforts made to minimize surgical blood loss and blood transfusion, so to speak implement appropriate comprehensive blood management protocols.

Blood volume

The composition of total body water (TBW) is approximately 60% of the lean body mass, or the equivalent of 42 L in a normal-sized adult man. The blood volume (BV, 5 L) consists of the plasma volume (PV, approximately 55% of BV, i.e., 3 L) and the red cell mass or blood cells (about 45%, i.e., 2 L). Normally, the total blood volume (TBV) amounts to approximately 7% body weight in adults (i.e., 70 mL/kg) and 8% body weight in neonates and children (i.e., 80 and 85 mL/kg, respectively) (Tables 27.1 and 27.2).

Table 27.1 TBV Estimation (mL/kg Body Weight) in Adults Based on Body Composition and Gender (Gilcher's Rule of Five)

	Obese	Thin built	Normal	Muscular built
Males	60	65	70	75
Females	55	60	65	70

Table 27.2 TBV Estimation (mL/kg Body Weight) in Pediatric Age Group

Premature	90
Full-term neonates and infants (up to 9 kg)	85
Young children	75
Older children[a]	70

[a] If 50 kg or more, consider as per adult composition (refer to Table 27.1).

Pathophysiological effects of blood loss

Hemostasis is the process of clot formation at the site of injury to prevent blood loss while under normal conditions to maintain the blood flow within the intact vascular tree. Accordingly a fine balance exists between the coagulation and the fibrinolysis systems (Figure 27.1). Hemorrhage causes hypovolemic shock that leads to hemodynamic instability, coagulopathy, decreased oxygen delivery, decreased tissue perfusion, and cellular hypoxia. There is a resultant oxygen debt between systemic oxygen delivery and oxygen consumption.

Almost 25% of trauma patients develop an endogenous acute trauma–induced coagulopathy (ATC) within minutes of injury due to the combined effects of tissue trauma and hypovolemic shock. It is speculated that similar derangements in coagulation may occur during major surgeries, whereby additional factors such as dilution of clotting factors, hypothermia, anaerobic metabolism-driven lactic acidosis, and systemic inflammatory response may all simulate the lethal trauma triad of hypothermia, coagulopathy, and acidosis. These three factors can result in a downward spiral, leading to physiological exhaustion and multiorgan failure (Figure 27.2).[1]

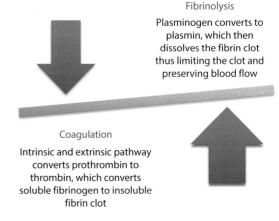

Fibrinolysis
Plasminogen converts to plasmin, which then dissolves the fibrin clot thus limiting the clot and preserving blood flow

Coagulation
Intrinsic and extrinsic pathway converts prothrombin to thrombin, which converts soluble fibrinogen to insoluble fibrin clot

Figure 27.1 Dynamic in vivo relationship of coagulation and fibrinolysis systems

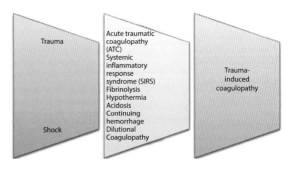

Trauma

Acute traumatic coagulopathy (ATC)
Systemic inflammatory response syndrome (SIRS)
Fibrinolysis
Hypothermia
Acidosis
Continuing hemorrhage
Dilutional Coagulopathy

Shock

Trauma-induced coagulopathy

Figure 27.2 Pathogenesis of trauma-induced coagulopathy. (Adapted from Williams NS et al., *Bailey and Love's Short Practice of Surgery*, Boca Raton, FL, CRC Press, 2013.)

Estimation of blood loss

Accurate and timely assessment of intraoperative blood loss is required for judicious replacement with appropriate amounts of crystalloid/colloid or blood and blood products. Both ends of the spectrum (i.e., underestimation and overestimation) can be detrimental to the patient by compromising on tissue oxygenation on the one hand and exposing the patient to the risks of unwarranted blood transfusion on the other hand. The anesthesiologist is tasked with quantifying blood loss and other surgical losses (evaporative, third spacing, etc.) intraoperatively. Concealed bleeding into the wound or under the surgical drapes complicates these estimates. Further confounding factors such as duration of surgery, rate of blood loss, and the anesthetic technique may also play a role. The estimates may further be flawed by the dependence on the anesthesiologists' expertise in the assessment of the dynamic surgical environment. Apart from these concerns, a major deterrent is nonavailability of a gold standard method that would be appropriate for intraoperative settings whereby one needs to take early and accurate decisions regarding transfusion.

Neurosurgery has special concerns due to difficult visual estimate of lost blood as the surgical field is inaccessible to the anesthesiologist and the operating rooms are poorly lit due to the use of microscopes. Ordinarily, the blood in suction bottles is mixed with irrigation fluid, cerebrospinal fluid (CSF), cavitational ultrasonic surgical aspirator (CUSA), and so on besides the soaked surgical gowns, drapes, sponges, and cotton balls. Also, this is one field that is not amenable to hemorrhage control by applying pressure.

A variety of methods have been described for estimation of blood loss during surgical procedures (e.g., visual estimate, gravimetric test, photometry, radio-tagged RBCs, electrical conductivity, and osmolality), but none has gained wide acceptance due to limitations of poor interobserver reliability, high cost, additional trained personnel, infrastructure, and time constraints. On the one hand, visual estimation, though simplest and easiest to allow repeated assessments, has large interobserver variability and poor correlation with actual blood loss (ABL, 34%). On the other hand, one of the tests, the gravimetric test, shows good correlation with ABL estimation. This basically involves subtracting the dry weighed swabs, sponges, and drapes from the blood-soaked ones and measuring the graduated suction bottles and subtracting the irrigation fluids from it. Though photometry and radiolabeled methods may be the gold standard, their high cost and infrastructure requirements preclude use in clinical practice.

As we emerge into the era of evidence-based medicine, a need has been felt for more objective means of blood loss calculation. A promising entrant into this field is the FDA-approved Triton Fluid Management System (Gauss Surgical, Los Altos, CA) (Figure 27.3), an iPad application that estimates blood loss in surgical sponges using a proprietary algorithm. Photographs of wet sponges are sent to a cloud server by the iPad, which then processes the image and sends back an estimate of the amount of blood in the wet sponges. It is being tested in various settings in clinical trials and shows promising results.

Overall, it is recommended that mathematical models be used for estimation of blood loss. The ABL is calculated by using a modification of the Gross formula[*]:

$$ABL = \frac{TBV[Hct(pre) - Hct(post)]}{Hct(m)}$$

where TBV is total blood volume (calculated from Table 27.1), and Hct (pre), Hct (post), and Hct (m) are pretransfusion, posttransfusion, and mean (of the pre- and posttransfusion values) hematocrits, respectively.

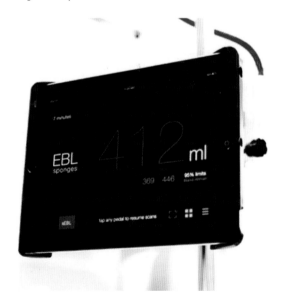

Figure 27.3 Real-time intraoperative monitoring of blood loss with a novel tablet application (Triton Fluid Management System).

---

[*] The Gross formula was actually introduced for the calculation of allowable blood loss intraoperatively. This derivation is based on the premise that the amount of blood loss and response to transfusion is reflected in the changes in hematocrit, assuming normovolemia is maintained.

Monitoring for intravascular volume status

As the intravascular volume is lost to about 10%–15%, compensatory neuroendocrine response causes redistribution of blood from the skin, muscles, and splanchnic circulation to the central compartment, thus preserving flow to the vital organs. Only subtle signs of hypovolemia may be present at this stage. Further losses overwhelm the compensatory mechanisms with decompensation of the cardiorespiratory and renal system. Traditionally, hypovolemia is divided by amount of blood loss (intravascular volume) into four classes:

Class I: Characterized by 15% BV loss
 (<750 mL in adults)
Class II: Characterized by 15%–30% BV loss
 (750–1500 mL)
Class III: Characterized by 30%–40% BV loss
 (1500–2000 mL)
Class IV: Characterized by >40% BV loss
 (>2000 mL)

So although this concept appears simplistic and useful, one needs to bear in mind other confounding factors such as age (children vs. young adults vs. elderly), body composition (athletes, obese), comorbid conditions (cardiorespiratory disease, hypertension, etc.), and concomitant medications such as beta-blockers, pain, and fever.

Therefore, more objective measures of assessing volume status are the need of the hour. Central venous pressure (CVP) monitoring has been a ubiquitous monitor of volume status in patients with normal cardiac and pulmonary functions. However, static CVP readings do not provide an accurate or reliable indication of volume status. Pulmonary artery pressure monitoring has not found favor in clinical practice.

Dynamic noninvasive or minimally invasive methods provide a real-time picture of the volume status and guide goal-directed replacement of surgical losses. These indices predict the volume responsiveness by determining the patient's position on the Frank–Starling curve. Patients on the slope of the curve are said to have preload reserve and are volume or fluid responsive. Critically ill patients or those with underlying cardiovascular disease may have their preload on the plateau of the curve and fluid administration will not improve cardiac output but cause the undue harm of overzealous resuscitation.

The dynamic indices are fast replacing CVP as a measure of volume status and include arterial pulse contour analysis, stroke volume variation estimation (e.g., LiDCO, Vigileo, FloTrac), plethysmography variability index (PVI) estimation, aortic blood flow velocity, the inferior vena cava distensibility index, or the superior vena cava (SVC) collapsibility index.

However in a clinical scenario, the CVP still continues to be used by more than 90% anesthesiologists worldwide. It can be used to make a dynamic assessment of volume status by dynamic fluid challenge testing, that is, change in CVP in response to a fluid challenge of 250–500 mL infused rapidly (more than 5–10 min). Normally, it changes by 2–5 cmH_2O and gradually returns to preinfusion levels in about 20 min. Little or no change may signify exsanguination in a patient, whereas sustained large increases in CVP may be due to circulatory overload (acute left ventricular failure or volume overload) (Figure 27.4).

Replacing blood loss

Ideally, surgical losses (blood loss plus other losses) should be replaced with intravenous fluids, preferably crystalloids, to maintain normovolemia, until the deleterious effects of anemia outweigh the transfusion risks. Usually, a transfusion trigger of hemoglobin concentration below 7 g/dL is considered adequate for optimal oxygen delivery; however, this needs to be individualized in the wake of associated cardiorespiratory diseases, elderly, and neonates. Preferably, the losses are replaced in a ratio of 1:3–4 in the case of crystalloids or 1:1 for colloids until transfusion becomes unavoidable.

The first step in replacing blood loss is estimation of allowable blood loss. This can be done by either of the following methods:

- Percentage method
  - Calculate the patient's BV (see Tables 27.1 and 27.2).
  - Depending on the percentage BV that can be lost without decompensation, while maintaining euvolemia with fluids, i.e., if 20% of BV is appropriate for the individual patient, up to 840 mL (70 kg in adult) could be lost before transfusion becomes essential.
  - Replace the allowable blood loss with crystalloids (3:1) or colloids (1:1) to maintain euvolemia.

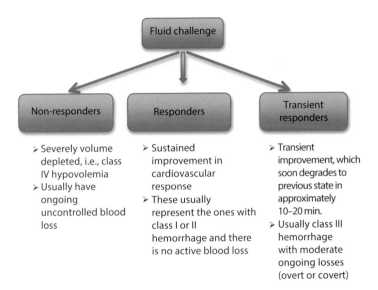

Figure 27.4 Dynamic fluid response.

- If the allowable blood loss volume is surpassed, transfuse blood.
- Hemodilution method
  - Calculate the BV and determine preoperative hemoglobin (or hematocrit), Hb_{pre}.
  - Estimate the lowest acceptable hemoglobin (or hematocrit) that could be safely tolerated by the patient, Hb_{acc}.
  - Allowable blood loss = $BV \times (Hb_{pre} - Hb_{acc})/Hb_m$, where Hb_{pre} is preoperative Hb, Hb_{acc} is lowest acceptable Hb, and Hb_m is average of preoperative and lowest acceptable Hb.
  - Replace blood loss up to the allowable volume with crystalloid or colloid fluids to maintain euvolemia and transfuse once the allowable blood loss volume is surpassed.

Blood transfusion

The history of transfusion of blood dates back to the first canine experiments in 1665. The use of animal-to-human transfusion led to a spate of deaths and then an era of banned transfusions, until the first successful blood transfusion by James Blundell in 1818. Transfusion medicine has come a long way since then, and blood and blood products are much safer and transfusion protocols more stringent; nevertheless, the immune modulation effects and transfusion transmissible infections continue to pose a major threat to well-being.

Furthermore, it is a finite source and therefore judicious use is advocated.

Blood groups

Karl Landsteiner in 1901 described the ABO system of blood grouping, and since then almost 346 red cell antigens and 35 blood group systems have been recognized by the International Society of Blood Transfusion (ISBT). However, the ABO and Rhesus (Rh) systems are the most relevant to clinical practice as incompatibility results in major transfusion reactions. Blood groups show variable frequency depending on ethnicity, geographical distribution, race, natural selection, genetic drift phenomenon, and environment (Table 27.3). In India, there is a preponderance of O (37%) followed by B (32%), A (23%), and AB (8%), whereas 94.6% of the population is Rh-positive. Within each system, individuals mount a strong antibody response (alloantibodies) to the absent allele in their genotype.

The ABO system

Human red cells have the presence of almost 300 different antigens. In the ABO system, there is the presence of one of the three allelic genes A, B, or O antigens, where O is an amorph. The presence or absence of A or B surface antigens therefore determines blood grouping (Table 27.3). Individuals lacking the specific antigen produce alloantibodies to the missing antigen in the first year of life.

Table 27.3 Distribution of ABO and Rh alleles

Phenotype	Genotype	Antigens	Alloantibodies	Frequency in population (%)
O	OO	O	Anti-A, Anti-B	46
A	AO/AA	A	Anti-B	42
B	BO/BB	B	Anti-A	9
AB	AB	A and B	None	3
Rh-positive	D-positive (group of almost 46 antigens)	D	Anti-D	85
Rh-negative	None	None	None (unless sensitized during pregnancy)	15

The Rh system

Individuals with any of the D Rh group of antigens are considered Rh-positive and those lacking this antigen are Rh-negative. This distribution is again affected by ethnicity, race, geographic distribution, and so on. Approximately 85% of the white population is Rh-positive in contrast to 92% in the black population and 94% in the Asian subcontinent. Unlike the ABO groups, naturally occurring antibodies are only expressed in Rh-negative individuals once they receive an Rh-positive transfusion or with pregnancy (Rh-negative mother with an Rh-positive fetus).

Other red blood cell antigen systems

Other systems include MNS, P, Lutheran, Kell, Lewis, Duffy, Ii, Kidd, Diego, Bombay (Oh phenotype), Colton (Null phenotype), Landsteiner-Wiener, Cartwright, Xg, Kx, Sciann, Dombrock, Chido/Rogers (CH/RG), Gerbich, Crome, Knops etc. Except for the MNS ,P, Lewis, kidd, kel, and duffy systems which are tested routinely besides the ABO and Rh systems; other systems are rarely of much clinical concern.

Compatibility testing

Pretransfusion compatibility testing is performed to ensure safe transfusion and basically includes ABO and Rh grouping performed on the donor and recipient samples, antibody screening of the donor and patient sera, and crossmatching.

Blood grouping

ABO incompatibility can result in life-threatening transfusion reactions by causing a fulminant complement-mediated intravascular hemolysis. Therefore, testing patient's erythrocytes with anti-A and anti-B sera determines the ABO typing. Testing the patient's serum against erythrocytes with the same antigen type confirms the blood type. The next step involves testing the patient's red cells against anti-D antibodies to determine Rh status. Rh-negative status is then confirmed by mixing the patient's serum against Rh-positive erythrocytes to determine the presence of anti-D antibody.

Antibody screening

This is the second step in the compatibility screen whereby donor and recipient sera are tested to detect the presence of the antibodies responsible for non-ABO hemolytic reactions. This testing usually requires about 45 min and involves mixing donor serum with commercially prepared RBCs with known antigens. If donor serum contains antibodies to these RBCs, these will coat the red cells and agglutinate when an antiglobulin antibody is added to it. This is called as indirect Coombs test. Antibody screening is performed routinely on donor blood and frequently performed in the likely recipient.

Crossmatching

This is routinely performed as the final step of pretransfusion compatibility testing to serve as a final confirmation of ABO compatibility between donor RBCs and recipient serum as well as to detect antibodies in low titers or antibodies to the other blood group systems missed by the antibody screen. Simplistically, this is the step that mimics actual transfusion and involves mixing small amount of recipient's serum with donor's RBCs; if agglutination occurs, this amounts to incompatible transfusion. Technically, this process has three phases: the first phase (1–5 min) that detects ABO incompatibility and antibodies against the MN, P, and Lewis blood group systems; the second phase (30–45 min in albumin and 10–20 min in low ionic salt solution) detects incomplete antibodies of Rh system (D^u); and the third phase detects low titers of incomplete antibodies of the Rh, Kidd, Kell, and Duffy systems. Thus, it usually takes about 45 min in most laboratories for complete major crossmatching. Units are refrigerated until used. A crossmatched unit is removed from the general blood bank inventory and reserved for the tested patient. Ordinarily, compatibility testing is not required for platelets and plasma components. Only ABO matching is sufficient for fresh frozen plasma (FFP). Platelet concentrates (PCs) and cryoprecipitate need not be tested for compatibility, ABO and Rh typing. Exceptions to this are neonates and alloimmunized individuals in whom use of ABO & Rh-matched platelets might be preferable.

Blood product requisition

Type and screen is the first pedestal of compatibility testing to identify the patient's ABO group and Rh-type and to detect expected and unexpected antibodies in the recipient's serum. The incidence of serious hemolytic reactions after type and screen of blood (ABO- and Rh-compatible transfusion with negative antibody screen and no crossmatch) is less than 1:10,000. Nevertheless crossmatching assures optimal safety in transfusion.

Type and screen

The patient's blood AB and Rh-typing is done and an antibody screen identified for potential alloantibodies. This is requested when it is unlikely that blood will be needed on an emergent basis and therefore no donor units are crossmatched and reserved for a particular patient.

Type and cross

A full gamut of compatibility testing between patient and donor units is conducted and a minimum of two units are crossmatched and reserved specifically for that patient. These units are refrigerated and kept for at least 72 h after which the units are returned back into the inventory. This is requested when it is highly likely that blood will be needed, when the patient's antibody screen is positive, or when the patient is at high risk of alloimmunization.

Emergency transfusions

If the patient's blood type is known, an abbreviated crossmatch can be done in about 1–5 min to confirm ABO compatibility. If the recipient's blood type and Rh status are not known and transfusion cannot be delayed for blood typing, type O (universal donor) red cells (O Rh-negative to women of child-bearing age and O Rh-positive to men) may be used. In more urgent situations, *type-specific* blood (ABO- and Rh-matched) can be issued within 10–15 min.

Blood ordering schedules

It is recommended that blood ordering schedules (BOSs) should be laid down by the hospital transfusion committee on the basis of usual expected blood usage in a particular surgery and accordingly to decide the units of blood to crossmatch or type and screen for a patient undergoing surgical procedures. At the outset, this will prevent unnecessary crossmatching and burdening of the blood bank usage, at the same time preventing injudicious use of blood products. Additionally, there needs to be a system for the perioperative team to overrule the BOS, for example, if a procedure is likely to be more complex than usual or if the patient has a coagulation defect or platelet dysfunction. There should be ready availability in the blood bank of at least two units of group O Rh-negative blood, reserved for use only in an emergency lifesaving situation. A general guide for blood requisition in neurosurgical procedures is given in Table 27.4.

Blood storage

Blood collected from screened donors is typed, screened for antibodies, and tested for hepatitis B, hepatitis C, syphilis, and human immunodeficiency virus (HIV 1 and 2), and stored in a preservative–anticoagulant solution such as CPDA-1

Table 27.4 Rough Guide to Blood Ordering in Neurosurgical Procedures

Craniotomy, craniectomy	T&S
TBI, EDH	T&S
Meningioma and vascular tumors	CM 4 units
Pituitary surgery	T&S
Vascular surgery (aneurysms, A-V malformations)	CM 3–4 units
Spinal fusion procedures, scoliosis	CM 2 units
Disc surgery	T&S

T&S, type and screen; CM, crossmatch; TBI, traumatic brain injury; EDH, epidural/extradural haematoma.

(citrate as an anticoagulant, phosphate as a buffer, dextrose as an energy source for RBCs, and adenosine as a precursor for adenosine triphosphate) or SAG-M solution (saline–adenine–glucose–mannitol) to allow a shelf life to 5 weeks at 2–6°C. Other costly alternative preservative solutions are AS-1 (Adsol) and AS-3 (Nutrice) that extend the shelf life to about 6 weeks. Though fresh whole blood has distinct advantages over components in that it is rich in clotting factors and metabolically active, it is rarely used in civilian practice due to the economically better alternative of component therapy. Also, the effects of storage on whole blood preclude its use in clinical practice: acidosis, progressive rise in plasma potassium concentration, reduced red cell content of 2,3-diphosphoglycerate (2,3-DPG) shifting the oxygen dissociation curve to the right, loss of all platelet function, and reduction in factor VIII levels to 10%–20% of normal within 48 h of donation.

Blood components

The following blood products are commercially available:

1. Blood components:
   a. Components derived from whole blood
      i. Red cell concentrate
      ii. Red cell suspension
      iii. Plasma
      iv. Platelet concentrates
   b. Plasma or platelets collected by apheresis
   c. Cryoprecipitate, prepared from FFP, which is rich in factor VIII and fibrinogen
2. Plasma derivative (human plasma proteins manufactured pharmaceutically):

   a. Albumin
   b. Coagulation factor concentrates
   c. Immunoglobulins

Whole blood is centrifuged to yield approximately 250 mL packed red blood cells (PRBCs) with a hematocrit of 50%–70%. The supernatant is further spun to yield platelets and plasma. Platelet-rich plasma (PRP) contains 50–70 mL plasma and can be stored at 20°C–24°C for 5–7 days. The remaining platelet-poor plasma supernatant is further processed by

- Rapid freezing, which prevents inactivation of labile coagulation factors (V and VIII)
- Slow thawing of FFP, which yields cryoprecipitate rich in factor VIII and fibrinogen

Most platelets are now obtained by apheresis, and a single platelet apheresis (single-donor platelets [SDPs]) unit is equivalent to the amount of platelets derived from 6 to 8 units of whole blood (random-donor platelets [RDPs]) (Figure 27.5).

Packed red blood cells

Each unit of PRBCs is approximately 250 mL with a hematocrit of about 55%–70% and is stored at 2–6°C.[†]

Indications

A restrictive transfusion strategy is recommended over a liberal strategy. It is speculated this would significantly reduce the exposure of patients to transfusions of packed cells by approximately 40%, thereby reducing risks for infectious and noninfectious complications of transfusion. Accordingly it is recommended that

- In adult and pediatric intensive care unit patients, transfusion should be considered at hemoglobin concentrations of 7 g/dL or less.

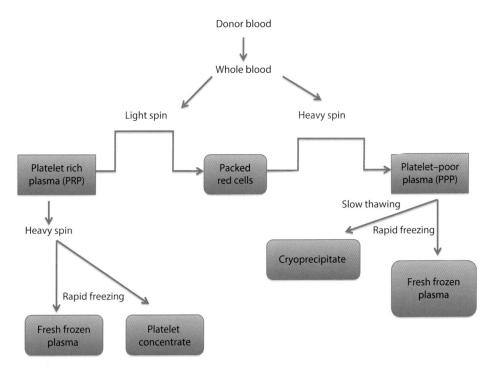

Figure 27.5 A general review of blood component separation by the platelet-rich plasma (PRP) method.

- In postoperative surgical patients, transfusion should be considered at a hemoglobin concentration of 8 g/dL or less or if symptomatic.‡
- In hospitalized, hemodynamically stable patients with preexisting cardiovascular disease, transfusion should be considered at a hemoglobin concentration of 8 g/dL or less or if symptomatic.§

Fresh frozen plasma

Each unit of FFP is about 150–200 mL, stored at −40°C to −50°C, and has a shelf life of 2 years. Each unit of FFP would raise the level of each clotting factor by 2%–3% in adults.**

Indications

1. This is the first-line therapy in the treatment of coagulopathic/microvascular bleeding, that is, if international normalized ratio (INR) > 2.0 in absence of heparin.

2. For correction of excessive bleeding following massive transfusion (MT), usually in a ratio of 1:1:1 or 1:1:2 (FFP/PC/PRBC).
3. For urgent warfarin reversal as an alternative to prothrombin complex concentrate (PCC).
4. For correction of known clotting factor deficiencies due to nonavailability of factor concentrates.

Dose

A dose of 10–15 mL/kg or calculate the transfusion requirement so as to achieve a 30% clotting factor concentration.††

Cryoprecipitate

This is collected as a supernatant precipitate of FFP and stored at −30°C with a 2-year shelf life. Normally, the amount of factor VIII is 80–100 IU/pack and fibrinogen is 150–300 mg/pack. It is rich in factor VIII and fibrinogen. Though the main

† Unless glycerolized frozen red cells in case of rare groups.
‡ Chest pain, orthostatic hypotension or tachycardia unresponsive to fluid resuscitation, or congestive heart failure.
§ Chest pain, orthostatic hypotension or tachycardia unresponsive to fluid resuscitation, or congestive heart failure.
** Use of FFP strongly condemned in the following scenarios:
- Normal prothrombin time (PT) and activated thromboplastin time (aPTT)
- As a means of increasing intravascular volume
-As a source of albumin
†† Normally 4–5 units PC, one unit SDP or one unit fresh whole blood each provide similar level of clotting factors as 1 unit FFP.

indication is low fibrinogen states, use is strictly condemned if levels are >150 mg/dL.

Indications

1. Point-of-care (POC) tests show fibrinolysis.
2. Low fibrinogen states (<80–100 mg/dL), particularly if excessive bleeding.
3. As an adjunct in MT.
4. Congenital hypofibrinogenemia.
5. von Willebrand disease (vWF)/factor VIII deficiency only if no response to desmopressin (DDAVP) or nonavailability of vWF/factor VIII concentrates.

Platelets

Platelets are supplied as a pooled PC and contain about 250×10^9/L and are stored on an agitator at 20–24°C for 5–7 days. Administration of a single unit of platelets may be expected to increase the platelet count by $5000–10,000 \times 10^9$/L, and with administration of a platelet apheresis unit, by $30,000–60,000 \times 10^9$/L.

Indications

1. Thrombocytopenia: Platelet transfusions may be indicated in patients with platelet counts below $10,000 \times 10^9$ per liter due to an increased risk of spontaneous hemorrhage.
2. Invasive procedures are as follows:
   a. Prophylactic platelet transfusion for patients having elective central venous catheter placement if platelet count is $<20,000 \times 10^9$ per liter.
   b. Prophylactic platelet transfusion for patients having elective diagnostic lumbar puncture, epidural anesthesia, liver biopsy, endoscopy with biopsy with a platelet count of $<50 \times 10^9$ cells per liter.
   c. Prophylactic platelet transfusion for patients having major elective non-neuraxial surgery with a platelet count of $<50 \times 10^9$ cells per liter.
   d. It is advisable to have counts $>100,000 \times 10^9$ per liter in patients undergoing neurosurgery and ocular surgery.
3. Known or suspected platelet dysfunction, for example, dual antiplatelet agents, cardiopulmonary bypass, congenital platelet dysfunction, and excessive bleeding.

4. As an adjunct in MT (threshold $< 50,000 \times 10^9$ per liter).

Dose

The dose required to raise the platelet count to a desirable level can be calculated using the following formula:

$$\text{Platelet count } (\times 10^{11}) = \text{PI} \times \text{TBV} \times 1.5/100$$

where PI is desired platelet increment, TBV is total blood volume, and correction factor of 1.5 is for splenic uptake.

Prothrombin complex concentrates

PCCs are highly purified concentrates prepared from pooled plasma. They contain factors II, IX, and X. Factor VII may be included or produced separately.

Indications

It is indicated for the emergency reversal of anticoagulant (warfarin) therapy in uncontrolled hemorrhage. Vitamin K should also be administered simultaneously.

Dose

Dosing is based on the pretreatment INR:

- INR 2–4: 25 units/kg; not to exceed 2500 units
- INR 4–6: 35 units/kg; not to exceed 3500 units
- INR > 6: 50 units/kg; not to exceed 5000 units

Infusion rate of 0.12 mL/kg/min (~3 units/kg/min), up to a maximum rate of 210 units/min.

Perioperative blood management

The World Health Organization (WHO) recognized patient blood management in 2010 as the new standard of care.[2] These protocols are being recommended for the perioperative management of blood products and adjuvant therapies to optimize patient outcome and minimize transfusion. Patient blood management is currently defined by the Society for the Advancement of Blood Management (available at http://www.sabm.org) as "the timely application of evidence based medical and surgical concepts designed to maintain haemoglobin, optimize

‡‡ Anemia (defined as <13 g/dL in males and <12 g/dL in females) increases the risk of mortality by two- to fivefold, increases postoperative infections, and increases hospital length of stay.

haemostasis and minimise blood loss in an effort to improve patient outcome." There is a paradigm shift from the previous transfusion-centric approach to a patient-centric approach, that is, primarily relying on the patient's blood rather than donor blood. This change has occurred due to an increasing gap between blood supply-to-demand ratio, escalating costs, concerns about product safety, adverse outcomes with transfusion, and questionable efficacy of transfusion. It is suggested to address the following three pillars of patient blood management (PBM)[3] to minimize blood usage so that the risks of blood transfusion can be minimized while maximizing clinical outcome:

First pillar: Optimize hematopoiesis
Second pillar: Minimize blood loss and bleeding
Third pillar: Optimize tolerance of anemia

Keeping in mind these objectives, the following are recommended in all surgical patients:

1. *First pillar*: This is the foundation of PBM, an important link in the chain and should preferably be done well in advance (≈3–4 weeks) of the scheduled procedure to allow for *optimal patient preparation*.
   a. Order and review laboratory test results, including hemoglobin, hematocrit, and coagulation profiles to elicit any coagulopathy or anemia.
   b. Screen and diagnose anemia (iron deficiency, anemia of chronic disease, nutritional anemia).[‡‡]
   c. Treat anemia.[§§]
   d. Anemia is an absolute contraindication for elective surgery.
2. *Second pillar*:
   a. *Preoperative*:
      i. Patient history and physical examination: The patient should be interviewed

for any previous transfusion, intake of drugs interfering with coagulation (warfarin, antiplatelet agents, herbal supplements, etc.), any congenital bleeding diathesis/coagulopathy, thrombotic events, cardiopulmonary diseases, and so on. Any signs of pallor, abnormal bruising, or ecchymosis should also be evaluated.
      ii. Explain the risk versus benefits of blood transfusion and discuss patient preferences on transfusion.
      iii. Decide on the need to continue warfarin or thienopyridines[***] in consultation with concerned specialist.
      iv. Consider risk of bleeding versus thrombosis while altering anticoagulant/antiplatelet therapy.
      v. If patient agrees to preoperative autologous blood donation (PABD), institute the protocol to allow collection of 3–5 units of packed cells with supplemented ESA therapy.[†††]
   b. *Intraoperative*:
      i. Meticulous surgical technique: Diathermy, tourniquets, vasoconstrictors, etc.
      ii. Blood-conserving strategies: Damage control surgery, preoperative embolization.
      iii. Anesthetic techniques: Consider neuraxial block over general anesthesia (GA) and total intravenous anesthesia (TIVA) over inhalation anesthesia; avoid sympathetic discharge.
      iv. Consider acute normovolemic hemodilution (ANH)/cell salvage.
      v. Reversal of anticoagulants:
         – Administer PCC for urgent reversal of warfarin along with vitamin K.
         – If PCC not available, administer FFP.

§§ Give iron and vitamin B12 supplementation to patients with nutritional anemia. Consider erythropoiesis-stimulating agents (ESA; erythropoietin 600 U/kg weekly at least 3 weeks prior to surgery) if time and cost is not a deterrent, particularly in chronic kidney disease, anemia of chronic disease, or patient refusal for transfusion.
*** Though aspirin can be continued for all elective surgery, thienopyridines need to be discontinued for a minimum of 5 days prior to the scheduled procedure. In patients who need to be continued on dual antiplatelets, consider postponing surgery for 14 days following balloon angioplasty, 6 weeks following bare-metal stents (BMSs), and 365 days following drug-eluting stents (DESs). Consider bridging therapy, if emergent procedure on dual-antiplatelet therapy (DAPT) is within the vulnerable period and excessive bleeding is anticipated. Warfarin anticoagulation needs to be bridged with heparin in consultation with cardiologist and target INR < 2.0 preoperatively and heparin stopped 6 h prior.
††† The last unit of autologous blood should be collected not less than 72 h prior to surgery.

vi. For elective surgery where warfarin is discontinued, give vitamin K to get INR < 2.

vii. Antifibrinolytics:
  – Consider intraoperative use of epsilon aminocaproic acid (EACA) in cardiac surgery (cardiopulmonary bypass [CPB]).
  – Consider tranexamic acid in liver, orthopedic, and spinal surgery.

viii. Consider ANH in major cardiac, vascular, liver, and orthopedic surgery.

ix. Liberal use of topical hemostatic agents (e.g., fibrin glue, Surgicel, and Abgel etc.).

x. Optimal management of hemostasis by relying on rapid turnaround POC tests of coagulation (e.g., thromboelastography [TEG] and rotational thromboelastometry [ROTEM]).

c. *Postoperative*:
  i. Vigilantly monitor and manage postoperative bleeding/secondary hemorrhage.
  ii. Minimize iatrogenic blood loss.
  iii. Maintain normothermia.
  iv. Postoperative blood salvage.
  v. Treat infections promptly.

3. *Third pillar*: This arm of the PBM protocol emphasizes improving the patient tolerance for anemia and setting up a transfusion trigger.

a. *Preoperative*:
  i. Assess patient's cardiopulmonary reserve.
  ii. Calculate estimated blood loss for the surgery and calculate patient-specific allowable blood loss.
  iii. Make a patient-focused transfusion trigger. A restrictive RBC transfusion strategy is advised (transfuse if Hb falls below 7 g/dL).
  iv. Consider transfusion based on ongoing bleeding and cardiopulmonary reserve.

v. Institutional transfusion committee should have a maximal surgical BOS in place.

b. *Intraoperative*:
  i. Optimize cardiac output.
  ii. Optimize oxygenation.
  iii. Transfuse based on a restrictive trigger.

c. *Postoperative*:
  i. Optimize and treat anemia.
  ii. Optimize oxygen supply and demand.
  iii. Treat infections promptly.
  iv. Maintain a restrictive transfusion trigger.

Complications of blood transfusion

Acute Complications (Table 27.5):

These occur usually within 24 h of transfusion. According to the severity, these can be classified as follows:

1. Hypersensitivity reactions, such as allergic, urticarial reactions, and anaphylaxis
2. Febrile nonhemolytic reactions (due to antibody to leukocytes, platelets, plasma proteins, IgA)
3. Possible bacterial contamination and pyrogens, which can present as septic shock
4. Acute hemolytic reactions
5. Fluid overload
6. Transfusion-related acute lung injury (TRALI)

Delayed complications

These are usually delayed for days or even months after the transfusion.

Transfusion-transmitted infections

- HIV-1 and HIV-2
- Human T-lymphotropic virus (HTLV-I and II)
- Viral hepatitis B and C
- Syphilis
- Chagas disease
- Malaria
- Cytomegalovirus
- Other rare infections (e.g., human parvovirus B19 and hepatitis A)

‡‡‡ This set of criteria for MT, however, do not apply to the pediatric population and the following is a suggested definition by Diab, Woong, and Luban:[4]
Transfusion of >100% TBV within 24 h
Transfusion of >40 ml/kg body weight
- Transfusion rate of >10% TBV/min
- Replacement of >50% TBV with blood products within 3 h

Table 27.5 Guide to Clinical Presentation and Management of Acute Transfusion Reactions

Category	Signs and symptoms	Likely cause	Management
Mild	Urticaria, rash, pruritus	Mild hypersensitivity	Slow the transfusion Administer antihistamine (chlorpheniramine 0.1 mg/kg or equivalent IM) If no clinical improvement within 30 min or if signs and symptoms worsen, treat as Category 2
Moderately severe	Flushing, headache, urticarial rash, rigors, fever, restlessness, tachycardia, anxiety, palpitations, mild dyspnea	Moderate-to-severe hypersensitivity, febrile nonhemolytic reactions, possible contamination with bacteria/pyrogens	Stop the transfusion. Replace the infusion set and keep IV line open with normal saline Notify the blood bank immediately Send blood unit with infusion set, freshly collected urine, and new blood samples (one clotted and one anticoagulated) from vein opposite infusion site with appropriate request form to blood bank and laboratory for investigations Administer antihistamine IM (e.g., chlorpheniramine 0.1 mg/kg or equivalent) and oral or rectal antipyretic (e.g., paracetamol 15 mg/kg) Give IV corticosteroids and bronchodilators if bronchospasm, stridor Collect urine for next 24 h for evidence of hemolysis and send to laboratory If clinical improvement, restart transfusion slowly with new blood unit and observe carefully If no clinical improvement within 15 min or if signs and symptoms worsen, treat as Category 3

(Continued)

Table 27.5 Guide to Clinical Presentation and Management of Acute Transfusion Reactions (Continued)

Category	Signs and symptoms	Likely cause	Management
Life threatening	Rigors, fever, restlessness, anxiety, chest pain, pain near infusion site, loin/back pain, headache, hypotension (fall of ≥20% in systolic blood pressure [SBP]), tachycardia (rise of ≥20% in heart rate), hemoglobinuria (red urine), unexplained bleeding (disseminated intravascular coagulation [DIC]), respiratory distress	Acute intravascular hemolysis, bacterial contamination and septic shock, fluid overload, anaphylaxis, TRALI	Stop the transfusion. Replace the infusion set and keep IV line open with normal saline Infuse crystalloid bolus (initially 20–30 mL/kg) to maintain SBP Maintain airway and give high flow oxygen by mask Administer adrenaline 0.01 mg/kg by slow IM injection Give IV corticosteroids and bronchodilators if bronchospasm, stridor Give frusemide 1 mg/kg IV or equivalent Notify the blood bank immediately Send blood unit with infusion set, fresh urine sample, and new blood samples (one clotted and one anticoagulated) from vein opposite infusion site with appropriate request form to blood bank and laboratory for investigations Check a fresh urine specimen visually for signs of hemoglobinuria (red or pink urine) Assess for bleeding from puncture sites or wounds. If there is clinical or laboratory evidence of DIC, give platelets (adult: 5–6 units) and either cryoprecipitate (adult: 12 units) or FFP (adult: 3 units). Use viral-inactivated plasma coagulation products, wherever possible Reassess If hypotensive, give further saline bolus Administer inotrope If urine output falling or laboratory evidence of acute renal failure, consider renal replacement therapy If bacteremia is suspected, start broad-spectrum antibiotics IV, to cover pseudomonas and gram positives

Other delayed complications of transfusion

- Delayed hemolytic reaction
- Posttransfusion purpura
- Graft-versus-host disease
- Iron overload (after repeated transfusions)

Massive blood transfusion

In general terms, MT is defined by infusion of large amounts of blood products over a short period in patients with severe uncontrolled or ongoing bleeding. This could be in the settings of trauma, obstetric hemorrhage, cardiopulmonary bypass, major surgery, and so on. About 40% trauma-related mortality is due to ongoing uncontrollable bleeding and approximately 10% war casualties and 5% civilian patients requiring MT.

Traditionally, it has been defined as replacement of one entire BV within 24 h; however, this definition lacks the basic premise of early recognition to reduce the mortality in these patients. Therefore, the following more definitive criteria have been designed:

- Transfusion of >= 10 units of PRBCs in 24 h
- Transfusion of >= 20 units of PRBCs in 24 h
- Transfusion of >= 6 units PRBCs in 12 h
- Transfusion of >=4 units of PRBCs in 1 h when ongoing need is anticipated
- Bleeding in excess of 150 ml/min with hemodynamic instability and ongoing need for transfusion
- Replacement of 50% TBV within 3 h[‡‡‡]

Complications of massive transfusion

Besides the hemolytic and immune-mediated reactions, there are certain adverse effects specific to MT.

Problems secondary to volume resuscitation

Inadequate resuscitation

Hypovolemia secondary to massive blood loss may cause hypoperfusion causing lactic acidosis, which added onto the systemic inflammatory response syndrome (SIRS) initiated by the injury may cause DIC and multiorgan dysfunction.

Overzealous resuscitation

Transfusion-associated circulatory overload (TACO): In neonates, elderly, and those with compromised left ventricular function, rapid infusion of IV fluids and blood products may result in a volume overload state. This needs to be differentiated from transfusion-related acute lung injury (TRALI).

Transfusion-related acute lung injury: As per the Serious Hazards of Transfusion (SHOT) hemovigilance data, TRALI risk per component was 6.9 times higher for FFP than for red cells. Data from the American Red Cross and the SHOT demonstrated a TRALI incidence of 1:51,000–65,000 plasma units. It typically presents as acute onset hypoxemia, acute respiratory distress, and increased peak pressure (within 6 h of transfusion), that is, noncardiogenic pulmonary edema due to transfusion of anti-human leukocyte antigen (HLA) antibodies or granulocyte-specific antibodies, which cause complement-mediated damage to the alveolar–capillary membrane.

Coagulopathy

Following MT, the most common coagulopathic defect is dilutional thrombocytopenia, though significant reductions in clotting factor levels are also noted. Although the standard coagulation tests (PT, aPTT, fibrinogen levels, platelet count, etc.) should guide the transfusions, these are time-consuming. MT may therefore be an appropriate setting for the POC viscoelastic tests of coagulation, that is, TEG, ROTEM, or Sonoclot.

Citrate toxicity

About 80 mL of CPDA solution present in each blood bag contains approximately 3 g citrate that gets metabolized in the liver in less than 5 min in healthy adults. However, hypoperfusion or hypothermia associated with massive blood loss reduces this rate of metabolism, leading to citrate toxicity. Ionized calcium and magnesium gets bound to unmetabolized citrate following large volumes of preserved blood transfusions causing hypocalcemia and hypomagnesemia with myocardial depression, bradycardia, dysrhythmias, and so on. Calcium supplementation may be required, particularly if hypotension is noted.

Hypothermia

Rapid infusion of cold IV fluids and blood products, opening of body cavities, cold ambient OR temperature, cold anesthetic gases, decrease in heat production, and impaired thermal control may all contribute to significant hypothermia. Besides slowing drug and citrate metabolism, slowing of enzyme activity and decreased platelet function also contribute to hypothermic coagulopathy at core temperatures below 34°C. Therefore, all blood products and IV fluids should be warmed to body temperature. Also, use of rapid infusion devices with efficient heat transfer capability should be used.

Acid–base balance

After 2 weeks of storage, the acid load of packed cells is about 6 mEq/L per unit due to glycolysis and buffering of citrate, so that the pH is below 7.0. Both extrinsic and intrinsic pathways of clotting are reduced by acidosis, that is, decrease in pH from 7.4 to 7.0 reduces the activity of factor VIIa and factor VIIa/tissue factor by more than 90% and 60%, respectively. Under normal circumstances, metabolic acidosis does not occur due to rapid metabolism of citric acid and lactate to bicarbonate by the liver. However in the setting of exsanguinating hemorrhage, there is hypoperfusion, liver dysfunction, and citrate overload, all of which result in metabolic acidosis. As the perfusion is restored, metabolic alkalosis develops as the citrate and lactate are converted to bicarbonate by the liver.

Potassium imbalance

Potassium concentrations in PRBCs may range from 7 to 77 mEq/L depending on the age of stored blood. It is estimated that approximately 4 mEq/L of extracellular potassium is transfused with each unit because of hemolysis of RBC from storage, irradiation, or both, irrespective of the age of blood. Therefore, hyperkalemia can develop if transfusion rates exceed 100–150 mL/min. Neonates and patients with preexisting cardiac and renal diseases are at particular risk for hyperkalemia. Concomitant hypocalcemia and acidosis further exaggerate the cardiac adverse effects of hyperkalemia. The risk can be reduced by using Fresh RBCs (5–10 day old), pre transfusion washing of irradiated packed cells, avoiding transfusion of recently irradiated RBCs (within 24 hours of irradiation), and use of in-line potassium filters. Potassium reentry into transfused RBCs, stress hormone–induced hyperglycemia, or metabolic alkalosis may all result in hypokalemia. Therefore,

monitoring and correction of potassium concentration is recommended.

Massive transfusion protocols

Timely interruption of the lethal triad of acidosis, hypothermia, and coagulopathy of MT determines the outcomes of MT. It is therefore suggested to have in place proactive standardized protocols, called massive transfusion protocols (MTPs), in patients with massive bleeding. The basic premise of an MTP is reduced dependence on laboratory testing during the acute resuscitation phase of hemorrhagic patient, and obviate the need for regular communication between the blood bank, laboratory, and physician. These are designed to be activated by the treating clinician in response to exsanguination in quick communication with the blood bank. A validated score for Trauma MTP activation is the Assessment of Blood Consumption score (ABC) to evaluate bedside exsanguinating trauma patients. Four point score based on presence of penetrating mechanism, ED systolic BP <=90 mmHg, ED heart rate >=120/ minute, and positive FAST (Focussed assessment with sonography in trauma) whereby score of 2 or more entails MTP activation. Ordinarily, MTP is activated after transfusion of 4–10 units. MTPs have a predefined ratio of RBCs, FFP/cryoprecipitate, and platelet units (RDPs) in each pack (e.g., 1:1:1 or 2:1:1 ratio) for transfusion. Once the patient is recruited in the protocol, the blood bank ensures rapid and timely supply of all blood components in fixed ratio to facilitate resuscitation.

Trauma and blood transfusion

Approximately 20%–40% deaths due to trauma after hospital admission involve massive hemorrhage and are potentially preventable with rapid hemorrhage control and resuscitation. The pathophysiology of the trauma-induced coagulopathy–hypothermia–acidosis triad mandates early institution of damage control resuscitation (DCR) (Figure 27.2).

The Prospective Observational Multicenter Major Trauma Transfusion (PROMMTT) study demonstrated that clinicians generally were transfusing patients with a blood product ratio of 1:1:1 or 1:1:2 and that early transfusion of plasma (within minutes of arrival to a trauma center) was associated with improved 6-h survival after admission.

The Pragmatic, Randomized Optimal Platelet and Plasma Ratios (PROPPR) trial is the first multicenter randomized trial using approved blood products to compare two transfusion ratios with mortality as the primary end point. The patients predicted to be massively transfused were randomized to two groups of plasma: platelets—PRBCs ratio of 1:1:1 versus 1:1:2, no significant differences in overall mortality at 24 h or 30 days were detected. Also more patients achieved hemostasis in the 1:1:1 group, fewer patients died of bleeding, and there was no significant difference between the groups in terms of inflammation-mediated complications such as acute respiratory distress syndrome, multiple organ failure, infection, venous thromboembolism, and sepsis.

Damage control resuscitation

The concepts from the PROMMTT study and the PROPPR trial have been translated into a new paradigm for the management of trauma patients with active bleeding called DCR. It is therefore defined as rapid hemorrhage control through early administration of blood products in a balanced ratio (1:1:1 for units of plasma to platelets to RBCs, a ratio that is the closest approximation to reconstituted whole blood), prevention and immediate correction of coagulopathy, and minimization of crystalloid fluids. This strategy was extended from battlefield resuscitation into civilian trauma patients with an aim to treat intravascular volume deficits, treat acute coagulopathy of trauma (ATC), preserve oxygen-carrying capacity, repair the endothelium, prevent dilutional coagulopathy, and treat hypothermia that develops due to infusion of large quantities of cold IV fluids. DCR principles have been associated with improved outcomes compared with more traditional transfusion practices.

Conclusion

Blood is a precious resource with scarce availability and transfusion carries significant health risks. There is a need for institutional transfusion committees that can implement patient blood management protocols in the perioperative period to minimize blood loss and optimize judicious use of blood products so that transfusion risks are negligible.

References

1. Williams NS, Bulstrode CJK, O'Connell PR. *Bailey and Love's Short Practice of Surgery*, 26th ed. Boca Raton, FL: CRC Press; 2013. ISBN 13: 978-1-4665-8514-0.
2. World Health Organization (WHO). The Clinical Use of Blood in Medicine, Obstetrics, Paediatrics, Surgery and Anaesthesia, Trauma and Burns. Geneva: World Health Organization, Blood Transfusion Safety (WHO/BTS), 2010; pp. 255–292.
3. American Society of Anesthesiologists. Practice guidelines for perioperative blood management. An updated report by the American Society of Anesthesiologists task force on perioperative blood management. *Anesthesiology* 2015;122:241–275.
4. Diab YA, Wong EC, Luban NL. Massive transfusion in children and neonates. *Br J Haematol* 2013;161:15–26.

Suggested reading

1. Roback JD, Caldwell S, Carson J. Evidence-based practice guidelines for plasma transfusion. *Transfusion* 2010;50:1227–1239.
2. Kaufman RM, Djulbegovic B, Gernsheimer T. Platelet transfusion: A clinical practice guideline from the American Association of Blood Banks (AABB). *Ann Intern Med* 2015;162(3):205–213.
3. Kozek-Langenecker SA, Afshari A, Albaladejo P. Management of severe perioperative bleeding: Guidelines from the European Society of Anaesthesiology. *Eur J Anaesthesiol* 2013;30:270–382.
4. Goodnough LT, Shander A. Patient blood management. *Anesthesiology* 2012;116:1367–1376.
5. Vamvakas EC. Reasons for moving toward a patient-centric paradigm of clinical transfusion medicine practice. *Transfusion* 2013;53:888–901.
6. Pham HP, Shaz BH. Update on massive transfusion. *Br J Anaesth* 2013;111(Suppl. 1):i71–i82.
7. Clevenger B, Kelleher A. Hazards of blood transfusion in adults and children. *Contin Educ Anaesth Crit Care Pain* 2014;14:112–118.

PART VII

Case-specific management

Aqueductal stenosis

SAMUEL Y. LEE and ALAA ABD-ELSAYED

1. *Goals of anesthesia*
   a. To avoid increase in intracranial pressure (ICP) secondary to awake tracheal intubation, crying, struggling, or straining.
   b. To provide intraoperative immobilization during the delicate intraventricular surgical movements.
   c. Rapid emergence to expedite a neurological examination in the operating room by surgical team.
   d. To maintain adequate cerebral perfusion pressure (CPP).
2. *Investigations*
   a. Preoperative evaluation is focused on the current neurological status, including signs of increased ICP, hydration status, vomiting, and the underlying primary disease process.
   b. Associated medical illnesses, in particular cervical spine abnormalities, syndromes, and current medication regimen, might influence the perioperative anesthesia planning.
3. *Premedication*
   a. May not be required or desired because of associated problems such as intracranial hypertension and/or altered mental status.
   b. Prolonged postoperative sedation is preferably avoided. Careful titration of premedication with anxiolytic or narcotics, as procedures are usually very short and fast postoperative neurological assessment is desirable.
4. *Intravenous access*: One or two IV access lines; most authors recommend invasive blood pressure monitoring with an indwelling arterial catheter in all patients.
5. *Monitors*
   a. Standard monitors (electrocardiogram, capnography).
   b. Invasive blood pressure monitoring via arterial line.
   c. Continuous measurement of ICP and CPP is strongly suggested. Increased ICP can be caused by high-flow rinsing and obstruction of outflow channel by blood clots, tissue debris, or kinking of outflow tubes; it is imperative to detect these increases in ICP as soon as possible to avoid severe complications such as cardiovascular instability, retinal bleeding, excessive fluid resorption, and herniation syndromes.
6. *Induction*
   a. Smooth controlled induction and being ready to treat any hemodynamic changes that might occur with intubation.
   b. Avoid increases in ICP during intubation.
7. *Maintenance*
   a. Remifentanil + IV or volatile hypnotic.
   b. Nitric oxide should not be used to avoid elevations in ICP, due to additional risk of venous air embolism and the risk of diffusion into ventricular air bubbles.

8. *Positioning*
   a. Patient is in the supine or semi-sitting position with the head flexed, so that the burr hole is located at the apex.
   b. Anesthesia team and equipment are usually situated on the left side of the patient.
   c. Surgical team is positioned directly around the head of the patient, with video monitors at the foot of the patient to navigate the endoscope.
9. *Intravenous fluids*
   a. Crystalloids, administered at body temperature; cold fluids may cause bradycardia. Ringer's lactate solution is to be avoided as it is hyposmolar and can cause cerebral edema.
   b. Blood and blood products, if required.
10. *Other drugs*
    a. Mannitol (0.5–1 g/kg), 3% hypertonic saline (3–5 mL/kg over 10–20 min), furosemide for brain relaxation.
    b. Phenylephrine (50–100 µg bolus every 10–15 min or 0.5 µg/kg/min, titrated to desired response) for maintaining blood pressure.
11. *Intraoperative concerns*
    a. Adequate care for thermoregulation must be taken. Patients (particularly small children) are at risk for hypothermia during neuroendoscopy due to large exchanges of irrigating fluid and ventricular cerebrospinal fluid (CSF).

   b. Injury of basilar artery complex, leading to massive intraventricular and subarachnoid hemorrhage, hemiparesis, and midbrain damage.
   c. Meningeal irritation, headache, and high fever secondary to inflammatory response to irrigation fluids.
   d. Uncontrolled ICP can cause retinal hemorrhage, leading to Terson syndrome.
12. *Postoperative analgesia*
    a. A combination of a low dose of opiates (such as morphine 0.03 mg/kg) and paracetamol usually provides adequate analgesic effect without compromising neurological evaluation.
    b. Nonsteroidal anti-inflammatory drugs (NSAIDs) should be discouraged due to hemostatic concerns.
13. *Postoperative concerns*
    Transient neurological deficits (e.g., delayed emergence, confusion, memory loss, transient papillary dysfunction, and transient hemiplegia), central nervous system (CNS) infections, postoperative hemorrhagic complications (e.g., subdural hematoma, intracerebral hematoma [ICH], and epidural hematoma), and systemic complications (e.g., hyponatremia, infections, and deep vein thrombosis [DVT]).

b

Arnold–Chiari malformation

SAMUEL Y. LEE and ALAA ABD-ELSAYED

1. *Goals of anesthesia*
   a. To facilitate surgical access.
   b. To maintain respiratory and cardiovascular stability.
   c. To anticipate and deal with possible airway difficulties.
   d. To maintain adequate cerebral perfusion pressure (CPP) (mean arterial pressure [MAP]—intracranial pressure [ICP] or central venous pressure [CVP], whichever is greater).
2. *Investigations*
   a. Complete medical history, including cardiac and pulmonary function, to decrease perioperative morbidity and mortality.
   b. Magnetic resonance imaging (MRI) for visualization of posterior fossa anatomical structures.
   c. Careful physical examination for signs of increased ICP and trophic lesions in skin that may limit venous access.
   d. Routine investigations, including completed blood count (CBC), blood chemistry, coagulation profile, electrocardiogram (ECG), and chest X-ray (CXR).
3. *Premedication*
   a. For example, 2 mg midazolam for anxiety; 4 mg ondansetron or 50 mg ranitidine for aspiration prophylaxis.

   b. Oral benzodiazepines 60 min prior are effective in reducing anxiety and do not have significant effect on ICP.
4. *Intravenous access*
   Two IV access lines (16 G and 18 G); central line (optional).
5. *Monitors*
   Heart rate (HR), ECG, noninvasive blood pressure (NIBP), invasive blood pressure (IBP), pulse oximetry (SpO$_2$), CVP, urine output, end-tidal carbon dioxide (EtCO$_2$), precordial Doppler, or transesophageal echocardiogram (TEE).
6. *Induction*
   Standard induction. Various agents may be used; smooth and gentle induction is more important:
   a. Propofol 2 mg/kg IV + vecuronium 0.1 mg/kg IV + lidocaine 1.5 mg/kg IV.
   b. Fentanyl can be used to decrease stimulation during intubation, which may increase ICP.
7. *Maintenance*
   Narcotics-based technique with inhalational agents such as sevoflurane and desflurane. Total IV anesthetic technique can be used as well.
8. *Positioning*
   a. Sitting, prone, or lateral/park-bench position.

b. Careful positioning is required, as patients may have disorganized joints and fixed flexion deformities.

9. *Intravenous fluids*
Crystalloids; blood and blood products, if necessary.

10. *Other drugs*
    a. Vecuronium bromide 5 mg for muscle relaxation.
    b. Neostigmine 2.5 mg and glycopyrrolate 0.5 mg for reversal of neuromuscular blockade.
    c. Sufentanil 0.5–1 µg/kg loading dose, followed by either incremental bolus or IV infusion of 0.25–0.5 µg/kg/h may be used as an alternative to fentanyl.

11. *Intraoperative concerns*
Brain stem and cranial nerve (CN) stimulation (hypertension, bradycardia, hypotension, ventricular/supraventricular arrhythmias), cerebral ischemia, and venous air embolism.

12. *Reversal or elective mechanical ventilation*
Neostigmine and glycopyrrolate to reverse the effect of neuromuscular blockade before extubation.

13. *Postoperative analgesia*
Fentanyl 25–50 µg IV per dose, up to 250 µg and/or hydromorphone IV 0.2 mg/dose for a total of 2 mg as tolerated, with watching for any respiratory depression.

14. *Postoperative concerns*
Pneumocephalus, macroglossia, quadriplegia, and hypertension.

Awake craniotomy

FILIZ UZUMCUGIL and ALTAN SAHIN

1. *Goals of anesthesia*
   a. To provide *conscious sedation* throughout the procedure or to provide *asleep–awake–asleep* periods with respect to painful stimulus during the procedure.
   b. To provide comfort, sedation, and analgesia during head frame placement and drilling of burr holes. Scalp block combined with conscious sedation is one of the techniques of choice.
   c. To maintain the most comfortable position during a potentially long procedure with an actual limitation to movement. To provide a semi-sitting position and consider the potential risk of venous air embolism during spontaneous breathing if a sitting position is preferred for the procedure.
   d. To anticipate and be prepared for a possible respiratory compromise in a patient with a head frame in place.
   e. To keep hemodynamic parameters stable and to avoid hypertension and fluctuations in blood pressure to minimize intracranial bleeding.
   f. To avoid agents that interfere with microelectrode recording (MER) in deep brain stimulation (DBS) and spontaneous seizure activity in seizure surgery.
   g. To preserve patient's ability to respond to assessments of speech, memory, and motor/sensory responses to cortical stimulation during seizure surgery.

2. *Investigations*
   Hemogram, serum electrolytes, renal and liver function tests, coagulation parameters, electrocardiography (ECG), and chest X-ray (CXR). Echocardiography should be considered to detect any existing patent foramen ovale for patients scheduled for craniotomy in sitting position.

3. *Premedication*
   Preoperative evaluation should include informing the patient about the nature of the procedure, in terms of duration and restriction of movement. For seizure surgery, discontinue or lower the doses of anticonvulsants if electrocorticography is to be used and avoid any drug exerting anticonvulsing effect, which eventually interfere with electroencephalography (EEG) localization. Avoid benzodiazepines. For stereotactically guided procedures, such as biopsy or DBS, antiplatelet agents (including herbal medicine) should be discontinued as appropriate.

4. *Intravenous access*
   Two intravenous catheters and a radial arterial line should be in place. A large-bore multiorifice central venous catheter placement should be considered with its tip above the superior vena caval–right atrium (RA) junction to attempt aspiration of air from the RA.

5. *Monitors*
   ECG, pulse oximetry (SpO_2), noninvasive blood pressure (NIBP) and invasive

blood pressure (IBP), central venous pressure (CVP), end-tidal carbon dioxide (EtCO$_2$), precordial Doppler ultrasonography (USG), and temperature. A nasal cannula with EtCO$_2$ monitoring should be used.

6. *Induction-anesthetic management*
In *asleep–awake–asleep* technique, IV propofol (100 µg/kg/min) and dexmedetomidine (0.3–0.6 µg/kg/h) infusions can be used to eliminate the reaction to local anesthetic infiltration for the scalp block to provide pin insertion and head frame placement. Scalp block can be performed by injection of 3–5 mL of 0.25%–0.5% bupivacaine to each site of supraorbital, supratrochlear, lesser and greater occipital, and zygomaticotemporal and auriculotemporal nerves. Pin site local anesthetic infiltration may be considered as well.
Benzodiazepines are to be avoided due to their interference with MER during DBS; and due to their anti-convulsing effects during seizure surgery.

7. *Maintenance*
Discontinue propofol infusion before MER in DBS. Dexmedetomidine can be used within an infusion rate of 0.1–0.2 µg/kg/h without interfering with recordings and without suppressing the symptoms of the patient (e.g., parkinsonian tremor). After MER is completed, restart propofol infusion to supplement dexmedetomidine to provide comfortable closure of surgical sites and removal of head frame and pins.

8. *Positioning*
If sitting position is preferred for the procedure, the modified semi-sitting position, to decrease the gradient between the operation site and the RA, should be preferred. The most comfortable position should be maintained throughout the procedure, especially due to prolonged restriction of movement.

9. *Intravenous fluids*
Crystalloids; blood products if necessary.

10. *Other drugs*
Mannitol 0.5–1 g/kg for brain relaxation.

11. *Intraoperative concerns*
    a. Respiratory compromise, increased blood pressure, seizure, shivering, brain bulge.
    b. The head frame system prevents appropriate airway management, including mask ventilation, laryngoscopy, neck extension, and endotracheal intubation.
    c. Intracerebral hematoma may develop during stereotactic procedures.
    d. Venous air embolism event has a higher risk in those patients due to spontaneous breathing.

12. *Postoperative analgesia*
Paracetamol 1 g every 8 h after the effect of local anesthetic wears off. Rarely nonsteroidal anti-inflammatory drugs (NSAIDs) and opioids are necessary.

13. *Postoperative concerns*
No special requirements from the anesthetic technique itself. After the procedure, the patients are fully alert in the immediate postoperative period, and a prolonged stay in the high-dependency area is usually unnecessary.

Brachial plexus injury

FILIZ UZUMCUGIL and ALTAN SAHIN

1. *Goals of anesthesia*
   a. To avoid aspiration of gastric contents in an emergency surgery. Rapid sequence induction may be required.
   b. To maintain hemodynamic parameters and avoid fluctuations in these parameters during anesthetic induction.
   c. To avoid agents interfering with electrophysiological monitoring.
   d. To be prepared with blood products in case of massive bleeding due to vascular injury.
   e. To avoid a venous air embolism (VAE) event and to detect it early in case of development during exposure of vascular structure at the injury site.

2. *Investigations*
   Hemogram, serum electrolytes, coagulation parameters, electrocardiography (ECG), and chest X-ray (CXR). Echocardiography and ultrasonography (USG) can be used to detect any adverse signs pertaining to injuries to organs both in the abdomen and in the thorax.

3. *Premedication*
   Midazolam (0.02–0.04 mg/kg IV; titrated to desired effect with repeated doses every 5 min up to 0.1–0.2 mg/kg) for sedation; fentanyl (0.5–1 µg/kg IV [50–100 µg/dose]; titrated to desired effect) for analgesia.

4. *Intravenous access*
   In addition to two large-bore IV catheters, a large-bore multiorifice central venous catheter placement at the contralateral subclavian vein can be considered. A radial arterial line can be used for real-time monitoring and frequent blood sampling.

5. *Monitors*
   ECG, pulse oximetry (SpO_2), non-invasive blood pressure (NIBP) and invasive blood pressure (IBP), central venous pressure (CVP), end-tidal carbon dioxide ($EtCO_2$), precordial Doppler USG, urine output, and temperature.

6. *Induction-anesthetic management*
   Propofol (2–3 mg/kg), etomidate (0.3 mg/kg), or thiopental (5–7 mg/kg) in combination with fentanyl (1–2 µg/kg) can be used for induction. In major vascular injury, ketamine (1–2 mg/kg) can be used in case of hemorrhagic shock. Rocuronium (0.6 mg/kg) or vecuronium (0.1 mg/kg) can be used for neuromuscular blockade (avoid repeated doses if motor evoked potential [MEP] monitoring is used).

7. *Maintenance*
   Sevoflurane and desflurane in oxygen–air mixture can be used. Total intravenous anesthesia (TIVA) can be preferred if electrophysiological monitoring is used. In major vascular surgery, nitrous oxide (N_2O) should be avoided due to the potential risk of VAE. Remifentanil (0.05–2 µg/kg/min) can be the analgesic of choice during the surgery. Intermittent bolus doses of any IV anesthetic agent should be used with caution if electrophysiological monitoring is used.

8. *Positioning*

   Supine position is the most commonly preferred position. However, the position is to be discussed with the surgical team.

9. *Intravenous fluids*

   Crystalloids; blood products in case of vascular injury.

10. *Other drugs*

    Vasopressors and inotropes may be required, in addition to sufficient volume replacement with crystalloids and blood products, to avoid fluctuations in hemodynamic parameters.

11. *Intraoperative concerns*

    a. Massive bleeding may result in hemodynamic derangement.

    b. Major vascular injury exposed in the operation site for surgical repair, may cause VAE.

    c. Bolus administration of any IV anesthetic agent or change in the depth of anesthesia by using inhalational agents may interfere with the quality of electrophysiological recordings; hence, it should be avoided.

12. *Postoperative analgesia*

    Patient-controlled analgesia with fentanyl; concentration, 10 μg/mL; demand dose, 0.5–1 μg/kg/dose; lockout interval, 6–8 min; basal rate, 0–0.5 μg/kg/h.

13. *Postoperative concerns*

    Patients with complex regional pain syndrome-2 (CRPS-2) (previously called causalgia) may need repeated sympathetic blocks. However, they may eventually require cervical sympathectomy or radiofrequency (RF) lesioning for permanent pain relief. Other distinct patterns of pain may also develop, such as neurostenalgia, posttraumatic neuralgia, and central pain.

Brain abscess

INDU KAPOOR

1. *Goals of anesthesia*
   a. To facilitate smooth and rapid induction of anesthesia.
   b. To prevent rise in intracranial pressure or brain edema.
   c. To maintain adequate cerebral perfusion pressure.
   d. To maintain hemodynamic stability.
   e. To facilitate smooth and rapid emergence from anesthesia.

2. *Investigations*
   Complete blood count, serum creatinine, serum electrolytes, blood sugar, coagulation profile, electrocardiography (ECG), chest X-ray CXR (if indicated).

3. *Premedication*
   a. Avoid preoperative sedation.
   b. Continue anticonvulsants until the morning of surgery.
   c. Continue antacid prophylaxis (ranitidine/perinorm).

4. *Intravenous access*
   a. Minimum two IV access lines.
   b. Arterial line (radial artery or dorsalis pedis artery) if hemodynamically unstable.

5. *Monitors*
   a. ECG, noninvasive blood pressure (NIBP), pulse oximetry (SpO_2), end-tidal carbon dioxide ($EtCO_2$), invasive blood pressure (IBP), core temperature (nasopharyngeal).
   b. Urinary catheter.

6. *Induction*
   a. Induce fentanyl/ketamine/propofol/thiopentone/rocuronium or atracurium.
   b. Attenuate intubation response with lignocaine 2%, propofol, and opioid.
   c. Secure airway with endotracheal tube (ETT) and fix it with tape or thread.
   d. Tape eyes to avoid exposure keratitis.
   e. Insert nasopharyngeal temperature probe.

7. *Maintenance*
   a. Oxygen/nitrous oxide/air combination (50:50) with sevoflurane (0.8–1 minimum alveolar concentration [MAC]) or total intravenous anesthesia (TIVA) propofol @ 100–150 µg/kg/min.
   b. Intermittent boluses or infusion of fentanyl and muscle relaxant.

8. *Positioning*
   Supine position.

9. *Intravenous fluids*
   a. Crystalloids (normal saline).
   b. Avoid hypotonic and dextrose-containing solutions.

10. *Other drugs*
    a. Mannitol (0.5–1 g/kg) over 20–30 min or hypertonic saline (3% @ 3 mL/kg) for brain relaxation.
    b. Phenytoin (15 mg/kg) over 30–45 min.
    c. Vasopressors (noradrenaline/dopamine) if required.

11. *Intraoperative concerns*
    a. Tense brain.
    b. Seizures.
    c. Cardiac arrhythmias.
    d. Hemodynamic instability.
12. *Reversal or elective mechanical ventilation*
    a. Patients can be extubated with controlled intraoperative management.
    b. Patients with preoperative impaired level of consciousness, unprotected airway, and hemodynamic instability may require mechanical ventilation.
13. *Postoperative analgesia*
    a. Paracetamol or fentanyl.
    b. Scalp block.
14. *Postoperative concerns*
    a. Pain and postoperative nausea and vomiting (PONV).
    b. Hemodynamic instability.
    c. Pneumocephalus.
    d. Seizures.

Carotid angioplasty

INDU KAPOOR

1. *Goals of anesthesia*
   a. To facilitate rapid and smooth induction of anesthesia.
   b. To maintain hemodynamic stability to protect the heart and brain from ischemic events.
   c. To maintain normocarbia, normal sugar levels, and normal temperature.
   d. To maintain depth of anesthesia.
   e. To maintain adequate analgesia.
   f. To avoid coughing and straining at emergence from anesthesia.
2. *Investigations*
   Hemoglobin, blood urea and serum creatinine, serum electrolytes, blood sugar, coagulation profile, electrocardiogram (ECG), chest X-ray (CXR) (if indicated).
3. *Premedication*
   a. Antiplatelet therapy (aspirin/clopidogrel) to be continued until the morning of surgery.
   b. Antacid prophylaxis (ranitidine/perinorm).
   c. Short-acting anxiolytic drug, if required.
4. *Intravenous access*
   a. Minimum two IV access lines.
   b. Arterial line (radial artery or dorsalis pedis artery).
5. *Monitors*
   a. ECG, noninvasive blood pressure (NIBP), pulse oximetry (SpO$_2$), end-tidal carbon dioxide (EtCO$_2$), invasive blood pressure (IBP), temperature, and bispectral index (BIS).
   b. Optional: electroencephalogram (EEG), somatosensory evoked potential (SSEP), transcranial Doppler (TCD), cerebral oximetry.
   c. Urinary catheter.
6. *Induction*
   a. General anesthesia

      Fentanyl/propofol/rocuronium or atracurium

      Attenuate intubation response with lignocaine 2%, propofol, opioid

      Secure airway with endotracheal tube (ETT) and fix it

      Tape eyes to avoid exposure keratitis

      Insert nasopharyngeal temperature probe or skin probe

      Apply BIS sensors on patient's forehead

      OR

   b. Regional with sedation

      Superficial cervical block: Infiltrate with local anesthetic along the posterior border of sternocleidomastoid muscle

      Deep cervical plexus block: Injection of local anesthetic sat the transverse process of C2, C3, and C4

      Propofol infusion @ 50–100 μg/kg/min or dexmedetomidine @ 0.5–0.7 μg/kg/min or fentanyl @ 1–2 μg/kg/h

277

7. *Maintenance*
   a. Oxygen/nitrous oxide/air combination (50:50) with sevoflurane (0.8–1 minimum alveolar concentration [MAC]).
   b. Intermittent boluses of fentanyl or remifentanil infusion.
   c. Maintain blood pressure at mid to high normal during cross clamping and mid to normal at the end of the procedure.
8. *Positioning*
   Supine position.
9. *Intravenous fluids*
   a. Crystalloids (normal saline).
   b. Blood and blood products if required.
10. *Other drugs*
    a. Aspirin/clopidogrel/dipyridamole.
    b. Heparin (5000–7500 units) 3–5 min before arterial occlusion to increase the activated clotting time to 250–300 s.
    c. Lidocaine 1% to blunt baroreceptor reflex.
    d. Vasopressors (noradrenaline/dopamine), if required.

e. IV paracetamol for pain relief.
   f. Antiemetics to avoid postoperative nausea and vomiting (PONV).
11. *Intraoperative concerns*
    a. Bradycardia, hypotension, or hypertension.
    b. Risk of massive blood loss.
    c. Stroke or myocardial infarction.
12. *Reversal or elective mechanical ventilation*
    a. Patients can be extubated with controlled intraoperative management.
    b. Patients with massive intraoperative blood loss and hemodynamic instability may require mechanical ventilation.
13. *Postoperative analgesia*
    Paracetamol or fentanyl.
14. *Postoperative concerns*
    a. Stroke or myocardial infarction.
    b. Hypotension or hypertension.
    c. Cerebral hyperperfusion syndrome.
    d. Cranial nerve injury and dysfunction.
    e. Pain and PONV.
    f. Abnormal coagulation profile following major blood loss.

Cerebellopontine angle tumor

JUDITH DINSMORE

1. *Goals of anesthesia*
   a. To prevent increases in intracranial pressure (ICP).
   b. To maintain hemodynamic stability and adequate cerebral perfusion pressure (CPP).
   c. To facilitate intraoperative neurophysiological monitoring.
   d. To facilitate rapid and smooth induction and emergence from anesthesia.

2. *Investigations*
   Hemoglobin, urea and electrolytes, blood sugar (if on dexamethasone), electrocardiography (ECG), chest X-ray (CXR) (if indicated), bubble-contrast echocardiogram (ECHO) (if sitting position planned).

3. *Premedication*
   a. Continue preoperative medications such as antihypertensives.
   b. Consider antacid prophylaxis.
   c. Consider prophylactic antiemetics such as hyoscine patch.

4. *Intravenous access*
   Two intravenous access lines (at least one, 16 G); central line (optional).

5. *Monitors*
   a. ECG, pulse oximetry (SpO_2), end-tidal carbon dioxide ($EtCO_2$), noninvasive blood pressure (NIBP), invasive arterial pressure (IAP), central venous pressure (CVP), urinary catheter, temperature, neuromuscular transmission (NMT), and bispectral index (BIS) or entropy (if required).
   b. Facial nerve monitoring (if required).
   c. Lumbar drain (if required).
   d. Precordial Doppler or transesophageal echocardiogram (TOE), if in sitting position.

6. *Induction*
   a. Induce propofol/non-depolarizing muscle relaxant, for example, rocuronium or atracurium. Attenuate pressor response with opiate, for example, fentanyl or remifentanil infusion. Use nerve stimulator and intubate when twitches have disappeared. Avoid dropping arterial pressure and maintain CPP with fluids or vasopressors, if needed.
   b. Tape rather than tie armored endotracheal tube (ETT), to avoid venous congestion. Tape and pad eyes.
   c. Use nasogastric (NG) tube, if bulbar dysfunction.

7. *Maintenance*
   Maintain anesthesia with sevoflurane (0.8–1 minimum alveolar concentration [MAC]) and remifentanil target-controlled infusion (TCI) (4–6 ng/mL) or sevoflurane (1 MAC) and fentanyl boluses) or total intravenous anaesthesia (TIVA) (propofol TCI 3–6 µg/mL and remifentanil TCI 4–6 ng/mL). Avoid nitrous oxide (N_2O).

8. *Positioning*
   Lateral, park-bench, or sitting position.

9. *Intravenous fluids*
Crystalloids; avoid glucose-containing fluids; blood if required.
10. *Other drugs*
    a. Mannitol (0.5–1 g/kg) or 3% hypertonic saline (3–5 mL/kg over 10–20 min) for brain relaxation.
    b. Vasopressors as needed to maintain MAP, for example, phenylephrine (50–100 μg boluses or 0.5 μg/kg/min titrated to effect).
    c. Antiemetic prophylaxis as high risk of postoperative nausea and vomiting (PONV).
    d. Morphine or fentanyl bolus about 45 min before the end of surgery, if remifentanil used.
11. *Intraoperative concerns*
    a. Tight brain.
    b. Avoid muscle relaxants if using facial nerve stimulator.

c. Risk of postural hypotension in sitting position.
d. Risk of venous air embolism (VAE) in sitting position.
12. *Reversal or elective mechanical ventilation*
    a. The majority of patients can be extubated at end of procedure.
    b. Patients with preexisting bulbar dysfunction may need mechanical ventilation and/or tracheostomy.
13. *Postoperative analgesia*
    a. Regular paracetamol.
    b. Intermittent morphine or fentanyl as required. Infusions if ventilated.
14. *Postoperative concerns*
    a. Pain and PONV.
    b. Bulbar dysfunction.

Cerebral aneurysm

CHARU MAHAJAN

1. *Goals of anesthesia*
   a. To strictly control hemodynamic parameters and to maintain adequate cerebral perfusion pressure.
   b. To avoid fluctuations in intracranial pressure (ICP) to avoid aneurysm rupture.
   c. To facilitate surgical exposure by reducing brain bulk.
   d. To provide neuroprotection when required.
   e. To ensure smooth emergence.
2. *Investigations*
   Hemogram, serum electrolytes, renal function test, electrocardiograph (ECG), chest X-ray (CXR). Optional: echocardiograph (ECHO), if required.
3. *Premedication*
   a. Preoperative medications such as nimodipine and any antihypertensive to be continued.
   b. Antacid prophylaxis.
   c. A short-acting anxiolytic such as alprazolam in patients with grade I and II subarachnoid hemorrhage (SAH) is optional.
4. *Intravenous access*
   Two intravenous access lines (18 G and 16 G); central line (optional).
5. *Monitors*
   ECG/noninvasive blood pressure (NIBP)/invasive blood pressure (IBP)/pulse oximetry (SpO_2)/end-tidal carbon dioxide ($EtCO_2$)/central venous pressure (CVP)/urine output (UOP)/temperature/neuromuscular

transmission (NMT). Bispectral index (BIS)/entropy optional (if neuroprotectant drug administration is planned). Noninvasive cardiac output monitor, if neurogenic stunned myocardium (NSM) present. Evoked potential monitoring, where available.

6. *Induction*
   Oxygen + fentanyl (2 µg/kg) + thiopentone (5–7 mg/kg)/propofol (2 mg/kg)/etomidate (0.3 mg/kg) + rocuronium (0.6 mg/kg)/vecuronium (0.1 mg/kg).
7. *Maintenance*
   Oxygen with air or nitrous oxide + isoflurane/sevoflurane/desflurane (<1 minimum alveolar concentration [MAC]) or propofol 100–200 µg/kg/min/infusion + fentanyl 0.5 µg/kg/h/remifentanil infusion 0.25–0.05 µg/kg/min + rocuronium 0.4–0.5 mg/kg/h/vecuronium 1 µg/kg/min.
8. *Positioning*
   Supine position for anterior circulation and upper posterior circulation aneurysms. Lateral position for lower basilar trunk and vertebral artery aneurysms.
9. *Intravenous fluids*
   Crystalloids; blood and blood products (if required).
10. *Other drugs*
    a. Mannitol (0.5–1 g/kg) or 3% hypertonic saline (3–5 mL/kg over 10–20 min) for brain relaxation.
    b. Thiopentone for neuroprotection: loading dose of 5 mg/kg followed by 5 mg/kg/h.

   c. Propofol or isoflurane/sevoflurane titrated to burst suppression may also be used.

   d. Phenylephrine (50–100 μg bolus every 10–15 min or 0.5 μg/kg/min, titrated to desired response) for maintaining blood pressure.

   e. Adenosine 0.3–0.4 mg/kg; ideal body weight (IBW) for inducing flow arrest.

11. *Intraoperative concerns*
Brain bulge, aneurysm rupture, prolonged temporary clipping time.

12. *Extubation or elective mechanical ventilation*
Good grade SAH patients with uneventful intraoperative course can be reversed and tracheally extubated. Poor grade SAH patients, prolonged temporary clipping time, aneurysm rupture, cardiopulmonary problems—favor elective mechanical ventilation.

13. *Postoperative analgesia*
Paracetamol 1 g every 8 h. Fentanyl infusion (0.5–1 μg/kg/h) in patients on mechanical ventilation.

14. *Postoperative concerns*
Vasospasm, electrolyte disturbances, hydrocephalous, rebleeding from residual aneurysm.

Cerebral arteriovenous malformation

JAMIE UEJIMA and LAURA B. HEMMER

1. *Goals of anesthesia*
   a. To maintain hemodynamic stability and cerebral perfusion pressure.
      i. Although less common in elective arteriovenous malformation (AVM) resections, it is possible that the patient may have some degree of intracranial hypertension.
      ii. In approximately 10% of patients, a coexisting intracranial aneurysm is present.
   b. To avoid increases in intracranial pressure (ICP) (if mass effect present from size of AVM or from intracranial hemorrhage).
   c. To provide brain relaxation.
   d. To facilitate smooth and rapid emergence.
2. *Investigations*
   Complete metabolic profile (CMP), complete blood count (CBC), coagulation profile, type and cross, electrocardiogram (ECG); for elective resections, optimize patient comorbidities before surgery.
3. *Premedication*
   a. Administer short-acting anxiolytics (e.g., midazolam) prn (*pro re nata*) and with consideration to neurological status.
   b. Administer aspiration prophylaxis prn.
   c. Continue antiepileptic medications.
4. *Intravenous access*
   Prepare for possible rapid, massive blood loss. If AVM successfully embolized, place at least two large-bore peripheral IV lines. If AVM has not been embolized or is especially large, consider central venous access.
5. *Monitors*
   ECG, noninvasive blood pressure (NIBP), pulse oximetry, end-tidal CO_2, invasive blood pressure, urine output, temperature, and neuromuscular blockade monitor. Additional monitor for anesthetic depth at anesthesiologist's discretion. Central venous pressure (CVP) as indicated. Evoked potential monitoring, where available, including somatosensory evoked potentials (SSEPs), motor evoked potentials (MEPs), and electroencephalography (EEG). If operative site is above the level of the heart, consider a precordial Doppler to monitor for air entrapment and placement of multiorifice catheter for air aspiration.
6. *Induction*
   a. Oxygen (O_2) + fentanyl (2–5 µg/kg) + propofol (2 mg/kg)/etomidate (0.3 mg/kg) + succinylcholine (1 mg/kg)/rocuronium (0.6 mg/kg)/vecuronium (0.1 mg/kg)
   b. If evoked potential monitoring is to be used, anticipate the need to avoid or tightly control neuromuscular blockade during surgery. Use of intermediate-acting neuromuscular blockade is acceptable to facilitate intubation.
7. *Maintenance*
   Consider using anesthetics that decrease cerebral metabolic rate and do not promote

significant cerebral vasodilation. If evoked potential monitoring is to be used, limiting volatile agents may be necessary (especially if MEP monitoring). Consider O_2 with air + ≤0.5 minimum alveolar concentration (MAC) sevoflurane/desflurane + propofol 25–50 µg/kg/min infusion + remifentanil (≥0.1 µg/kg/min infusion while in head fixation device); alternatively, a total IV anesthetic technique can be used.

8. *Positioning*
   Depends on AVM; ensure head position allows for adequate cerebral venous drainage.

9. *Intravenous fluids*
   Use isotonic fluids to minimize brain swelling; blood and blood products (if required); maintain euvolemia.

10. *Other drugs*
    a. Diuretic therapy for brain relaxation (e.g., mannitol, ±3% hypertonic saline, ±loop diuretic).
    b. Indocyanine green for video angiography (if required).
    c. Phenylephrine boluses or infusion for maintenance of blood pressure.
    d. Antihypertensive medications (e.g., nicardipine) to avoid hypertensive episodes (especially during emergence), or if periods of induced hypotension required for control of surgical bleeding intraoperatively.
    e. Induction of burst suppression (usually with propofol) for theoretical brain protection if desired by neurosurgeon.

11. *Intraoperative concerns*
    Rapid blood loss, hemodynamic instability, brain bulge; avoid hyperglycemia and hyperthermia.

12. *Reversal or elective mechanical ventilation*
    If the patient had an uncomplicated surgical and anesthetic course, then the patient can be emerged and extubated in the operating room.

13. *Postoperative analgesia*
    If the patient is awake with a stable neurological examination, consider the careful titration of opioids (e.g., IV boluses of fentanyl or hydromorphone) along with nonopioid medications (e.g., acetaminophen). The ventilated patient may require an opioid infusion.

14. *Postoperative concerns*
    Need for neurological examination, hyperemic complications, including cerebral hemorrhage and edema (possibly normal perfusion pressure breakthrough), electrolyte disturbances, anemia, seizures, and infarct.

Cervical spine surgery

JAMIE UEJIMA and LAURA B. HEMMER

1. *Goals of anesthesia*
   a. To take precautions to prevent cervical spine injury during airway management and positioning.
   b. To maintain mean arterial pressures (MAPs) in the high–normal range, may require MAPs >85–90 mmHg; discuss blood pressure (BP) goals with spine surgeon.
   c. To facilitate smooth intubation and emergence.
2. *Investigations*
   Depend on the patient's comorbidities and the complexity of the surgery, but would include basic metabolic profile (BMP), complete blood count (CBC), coagulation profile, type and screen (cross match pending extent of expected blood loss); for acute cervical spinal cord injuries also include electrocardiogram (ECG), chest X-ray, serial vital capacity measurements, and arterial blood gases.
3. *Premedication*
   a. Anxiolytic (e.g., midazolam) prn (*pro re nata*).
   b. Aspiration prophylaxis prn.
   c. Antisialagogue if fiberoptic intubation planned.
4. *Intravenous access*
   At least two intravenous access lines, with need based on expected blood loss and since access to IV lines would be limited with arms likely tucked during surgery; with

anticipation of need for vasoactive drug administration in acute spinal cord injury, central access desirable.
5. *Monitors*
   ECG, noninvasive blood pressure (NIBP), pulse oximetry, end-tidal CO_2, urine output, temperature, and neuromuscular blockade monitor. Based on the patient's comorbidities and complexity of the surgery, consider invasive blood pressure (IBP); IBP indicated in acute cervical spine injury. Additional monitor for anesthetic depth at anesthesiologist's discretion. Discuss with spine surgeon about the use of neuromonitoring (somatosensory and motor evoked potentials and electromyography) where available.
6. *Induction*
   Cervical spine immobilization should be strictly maintained for an unstable cervical spine. There is insufficient data to support one intubation technique over another (authors' preference is awake fiber-optic intubation after local anesthetic topicalization and cautious sedation with midazolam and fentanyl for an unstable cervical spine if intubation is not emergently necessary).
   a. Oxygen (O_2) + fentanyl (2 µg/kg) + propofol (2 mg/kg)/etomidate (0.3 mg/kg) + succinylcholine (1 mg/kg)/rocuronium (0.6 mg/kg)/vecuronium (0.1 mg/kg).
   b. Anticipate need to avoid muscle relaxation for neuromonitoring. Avoid

succinylcholine if denervation state >24 h in spinal cord injury.

7. *Maintenance*
O_2 with air + balanced anesthetic with volatile inhalation agent and opioid titration.
   a. If evoked potential monitoring is to be used, limiting volatile agents may be necessary. Consider O_2 with air + sevoflurane/desflurane (≤0.5 minimum alveolar concentration [MAC]) + propofol 25–50 µg/kg/min infusion + an opioid infusion such as remifentanil 0.05–0.1 µg/kg/min.
   b. For more extensive surgery, sufentanil infusion can substitute for remifentanil infusion. Total intravenous anesthesia (TIVA) is recommended to facilitate neuromonitoring in patients with neurologic deficit. (See point 6 for possible need to avoid muscle relaxation with neuromonitoring.)

8. *Positioning*
Supine position for anterior surgical approach; prone position for posterior surgical approach. Arms are usually tucked.

9. *Intravenous fluids*
Crystalloids, colloids, and blood and blood products (as required).

10. *Other drugs*
Vasopressor (e.g., phenylephrine) and/or inotropes may be necessary to maintain BP goals.

11. *Intraoperative concerns*
Maintenance of high-normal MAPs; caution with excessive fluid administration if in prone position to minimize laryngeal edema.

12. *Reversal or elective mechanical ventilation*
Patients with an uneventful intraoperative course can be reversed (if neuromuscular blockade was used during the case) and extubated in the operating room (OR). For patients in the prone position for a prolonged period or if patient required large-volume fluid resuscitation during the case, a cuff leak test should be performed prior to extubation. If there is no cuff leak and/or the patient has significant facial edema, consider keeping patient intubated and allowing edema to diminish prior to extubation.

13. *Postoperative analgesia*
Multimodal analgesia including opioids such as fentanyl or hydromorphone.

14. *Postoperative concerns*
Venous thromboembolism, skin breakdown, anemia, and postoperative visual loss after prone surgery (rare).

Craniosynostosis

INDU KAPOOR

1. *Goals of anesthesia*
   a. To facilitate rapid and smooth induction of anesthesia.
   b. To prevent rise in intracranial pressure.
   c. To maintain adequate cerebral perfusion pressure.
   d. To maintain hemodynamic stability.
   e. To maintain depth of anesthesia.
   f. To avoid venous air embolism.
   g. To maintain adequate analgesia.
   h. To facilitate smooth emergence from anesthesia.
2. *Investigations*
   Hemoglobin, blood urea and serum creatinine, serum electrolytes, blood sugar, coagulation profile, electrocardiography (ECG), and chest X-ray (CXR) (if indicated).
3. *Premedication*
   a. Continue anticonvulsants till the morning of surgery.
   b. Administer antacid prophylaxis (ranitidine/perinorm).
4. *Intravenous access*
   a. Minimum two intravenous access lines.
   b. Central venous pressure (CVP) line (size in French: depending on the patient's age).
   c. Arterial line (radial artery or dorsalis pedis artery).
5. *Monitors*
   a. ECG, noninvasive blood pressure (NIBP), pulse oximetry (SpO_2), end-tidal carbon dioxide ($EtCO_2$), invasive blood pressure (IBP), CVP, temperature, and bispectral index (BIS).
   b. Urinary catheter.
   c. Lumbar drain (if required).
6. *Induction*
   a. Induce fentanyl/propofol/rocuronium or atracurium.
   b. Attenuate intubation response with lignocaine 2%, propofol, opioid.
   c. Secure airway with endotracheal tube (ETT) and fix securely.
   d. Tape eyes to avoid exposure keratitis.
   e. Insert nasopharyngeal temperature probe or skin probe, if difficulty encountered with nasopharyngeal site.
   f. Apply BIS sensors on patient's forehead.
7. *Maintenance*
   a. Oxygen/nitrous oxide combination (50:50) with sevoflurane (0.8–1 minimum alveolar concentration [MAC]).
   b. Intermittent boluses of fentanyl.
8. *Positioning*
   Supine/semi-sitting position.
9. *Intravenous fluids*
   a. Crystalloids (normal saline).
   b. Blood and blood products if required.
10. *Other drugs*
    a. Mannitol (0.5–1 g/kg) over 20–30 min for brain relaxation.
    b. Vasopressors (noradrenaline/dopamine), if required.

    c. IV paracetamol for pain relief.

    d. Antiemetics to avoid postoperative nausea and vomiting (PONV).

11. *Intraoperative concerns*

    a. Tense brain.

    b. Risk of massive blood loss.

    c. Risk of venous air embolism in semi-sitting position.

    d. Risk of postural hypotension in semi-sitting position.

12. *Reversal or elective mechanical ventilation*

    a. Most patients can be extubated with controlled intraoperative management.

    b. Patients with massive intraoperative blood loss and hemodynamic instability may require mechanical ventilation.

13. *Postoperative analgesia*

    a. Paracetamol or fentanyl.

    b. Scalp block.

14. *Postoperative concerns*

    a. Pain and PONV.

    b. Abnormal coagulation profile following major blood loss.

Epilepsy surgery

INDU KAPOOR

1. *Goals of anesthesia*
   a. To facilitate rapid and smooth induction of anesthesia.
   b. To prevent rise in intracranial pressure (ICP).
   c. To maintain adequate cerebral perfusion pressure (CPP) and hemodynamic stability.
   d. To maintain adequate depth of anesthesia.
   e. To avoid intraoperative seizure.
   f. To avoid venous air embolism (VAE).
   g. To facilitate intraoperative neuromuscular and depth of anesthesia monitoring.
   h. To facilitate smooth emergence from anesthesia.
2. *Investigations*
   Complete blood count, blood urea and serum creatinine, serum electrolytes, blood sugar, liver function test, coagulation profile, electrocardiography (ECG), chest X-ray (CXR) (if indicated), blood group.
3. *Premedication*
   a. All antiepileptics to be continued until the morning of surgery.
   b. Antisialagogue (intramuscular glycopyrrolate @ 0.01 mg/kg [adults] and oral atropine @ 0.02 mg/kg [children]).
   c. Administer antacid prophylaxis (ranitidine/perinorm).
   d. Avoid sedative premedication.
4. *Intravenous access*
   a. Minimum two intravenous access lines.
   b. Central venous pressure (CVP) line (internal jugular vein or subclavian vein).
   c. Arterial line (radial artery or dorsalis pedis artery).
5. *Monitors*
   a. Electrocardiography (ECG), noninvasive blood pressure (NIBP), invasive blood pressure (IBP), pulse oximetry (SpO_2), end-tidal carbon dioxide ($EtCO_2$), CVP, temperature.
   b. Bispectral index (BIS), neuromuscular monitoring (NMT), neurophysiological monitoring (electroencephalogram [EEG] and electrocorticogram [ECOG]).
   c. Urinary catheter.
6. *Induction*
   a. Induce fentanyl (2–5 µg/kg)/propofol (2–3 mg/kg)/thiopental sodium (3–5 mg/kg)/sevoflurane (7%–8%)/rocuronium (1 mg/kg) or atracurium (0.5 mg/kg).
   b. Perform rapid sequence induction (if risk of aspiration from vomiting due to raised ICP).
   c. Attenuate intubation response with lignocaine 2%, propofol, or opioids.
   d. Secure airway with endotracheal tube (ETT) and fix it securely.
   e. Tape eyes to avoid exposure keratitis.

f. Insert nasopharyngeal temperature probe or skin probe (if difficulty encountered with nasopharyngeal site).

g. Apply BIS sensors on patient's forehead.

h. Apply NMT on adductor pollicis muscle on hand.

7. *Maintenance*

a. Oxygen/nitrous oxide combination (50:50) with sevoflurane (0.8–1 minimum alveolar concentration [MAC]) or total intravenous anesthesia (TIVA) (propofol 100–150 µg/kg/min).

b. Intermittent boluses of fentanyl.

8. *Positioning*

Supine/semi-sitting position (depending on location of the seizure focus).

9. *Intravenous fluids*

a. Crystalloids (normal saline).

b. Blood and blood products if required.

10. *Other drugs*

a. Mannitol (0.5–1 g/kg) over 20–30 min for brain relaxation.

b. Anticonvulsant:

  i. Eptoin loading dose @ 15–20 mg/kg IV over 20–30 min followed by maintenance dose of 100 mg tds (i.e., three times a day) IV.

  ii. Methylprednisolone @ 30 mg/kg IV over 20–30 min followed by 5.4 mg/kg/h.

c. Vasopressors (noradrenaline/dopamine) if required.

d. IV paracetamol for pain relief.

e. Antiemetics to avoid postoperative nausea and vomiting (PONV).

11. *Intraoperative concerns*

a. Tense brain, seizure.

b. Risk of venous air embolism in semi-sitting position.

c. Risk of postural hypotension in semi-sitting position.

d. Risk of massive blood loss.

12. *Reversal or elective mechanical ventilation*

a. Most patients can be extubated with controlled intraoperative management.

b. Patients with massive intraoperative blood loss, seizures, and hemodynamic instability may require mechanical ventilation.

13. *Postoperative analgesia*

a. Paracetamol or fentanyl.

b. Scalp block.

14. *Postoperative concerns*

a. Seizures.

b. Pain and PONV.

c. Abnormal coagulation profile following major blood loss.

Extradural hematoma

INDU KAPOOR

1. *Goals of anesthesia*
   a. To facilitate rapid and smooth induction of anesthesia.
   b. To prevent rise in intracranial pressure (ICP).
   c. To maintain adequate cerebral perfusion pressure (CPP) and oxygenation.
   d. To maintain hemodynamic stability.
   e. To maintain adequate depth of anesthesia.
   f. To avoid secondary damage to brain.
   g. To avoid venous air embolism (VAE).
   h. To facilitate smooth emergence from anesthesia.
2. *Investigations*
   Complete blood count, blood urea and serum creatinine, serum electrolytes, blood sugar, coagulation profile, electrocardiography (ECG), chest X-ray (CXR) (if indicated), blood group.
3. *Premedication*
   Antisialagogue (IM glycopyrrolate @ 0.01 mg/kg [adults] and oral atropine @ 0.02 mg/kg [children]).
   a. Administer antacid prophylaxis (ranitidine/perinorm).
   b. Avoid sedative premedication.
4. *Intravenous access*
   a. Minimum two IV access lines (18 G or 16 G).
   b. Arterial line (radial artery or dorsalis pedis artery).

5. *Monitors*
   a. ECG, noninvasive blood pressure (NIBP), invasive blood pressure (IBP), pulse oximetry (SpO$_2$), end-tidal carbon dioxide (EtCO$_2$), temperature, central venous pressure (CVP) (If indicated).
   b. Urinary catheter.
6. *Induction*
   a. Induce fentanyl (2 µg/kg)/propofol (2–3 mg/kg)/thiopental sodium (3–5 mg/kg)/sevoflurane (7%–8%)/ rocuronium (1 mg/kg)/atracurium (0.5 mg/kg).
   b. Perform rapid sequence induction (if full stomach/risk of aspiration from vomiting due to raised ICP).
   c. Attenuate intubation response with lignocaine 2%, propofol, or opioids.
   d. Secure airway with endotracheal tube (ETT) and fix it securely.
   e. Tape eyes to avoid exposure keratitis.
   f. Insert nasopharyngeal temperature probe or skin probe (if difficulty encountered with nasopharyngeal site).
7. *Maintenance*
   a. Oxygen/nitrous oxide or air combination (50:50) with sevoflurane (0.8–1 minimum alveolar concentration [MAC]) or total intravenous anesthesia (TIVA) (propofol 100–150 µg/kg/min).
   b. Intermittent boluses of fentanyl.

8. *Positioning*
   Supine/lateral decubitus/semi-sitting position (depending on location of extradural hematoma [EDH]).
9. *Intravenous fluids*
   a. Crystalloids (normal saline).
   b. Blood and blood products, if required.
10. *Other drugs*
    a. Mannitol (0.5–1 g/kg) over 20–30 min for brain relaxation, but avoid before evacuation of hematoma.
    b. Anticonvulsant:
       i. Eptoin loading dose @ 15–20 mg/kg IV over 20–30 min followed by maintenance dose of 100 mg tds (three times a day) IV.
       ii. Methylprednisolone @ 30 mg/kg IV over 20–30 min followed by 5.4 mg/kg/h.
    c. Vasopressors (noradrenaline/dopamine), if required.
    d. IV paracetamol for pain relief.
    e. Antiemetics to avoid postoperative nausea and vomiting (PONV).
11. *Intraoperative concerns*
    a. Tense brain, seizure.
    b. Risk of VAE in semi-sitting position.
    c. Risk of postural hypotension in semi-sitting position.
    d. Risk of blood loss.
12. *Reversal or elective mechanical ventilation*
    a. Most of patients can be extubated with controlled intraoperative management.
    b. Patients with poor preoperative Glasgow Coma Scale (GCS) score, massive intraoperative blood loss, seizures, and hemodynamic instability may require mechanical ventilation.
13. *Postoperative analgesia*
    a. Paracetamol or fentanyl.
    b. Scalp block.
14. *Postoperative concerns*
    a. Seizures.
    b. Pain and PONV.
    c. Abnormal coagulation profile following blood loss.

Lumbar meningomyelocele

INDU KAPOOR

1. *Goals of anesthesia*
   a. To facilitate rapid and smooth induction of anesthesia.
   b. To maintain adequate spinal cord blood flow.
   c. To position properly to maintain patent airway.
   d. To avoid injury to eyes and peripheral nerves.
   e. To maintain hemodynamic stability.
   f. To maintain adequate body temperature.
   g. To monitor closely fluid balance.
   h. To maintain latex precautions.
   i. To maintain adequate analgesia.
   j. To facilitate smooth emergence from anesthesia.
2. *Investigations*
   Hemoglobin, total leukocyte count, serum electrolytes, blood sugar, electrocardiography (ECG) and chest X-ray (CXR) (if indicated).
3. *Premedication*
   Oral atropine @ 0.02 mg/kg 30 min prior to surgery.
4. *Intravenous access*
   Minimum two IV access lines.
5. *Monitors*
   a. ECG, noninvasive blood pressure (NIBP), pulse oximetry (SpO$_2$), end-tidal carbon dioxide (EtCO$_2$), temperature, and invasive blood pressure (IBP) (if indicated).
   b. Urinary catheter.

6. *Induction*
   a. Induce sevoflurane 8% or fentanyl/propofol/thiopental sodium/rocuronium or atracurium.
   b. Secure airway with endotracheal tube (ETT) and fix it securely.
   c. Tape eyes to avoid exposure keratitis.
   d. Use proper padding to avoid pressure sore or compression on the defect.
   e. Insert nasopharyngeal temperature probe or skin probe, if difficulty encountered with nasopharyngeal site.
7. *Maintenance*
   a. Oxygen/nitrous oxide or air combination (50:50) with sevoflurane (0.8–1 minimum alveolar concentration [MAC]).
   b. Intermittent boluses of fentanyl.
8. *Positioning*
   Lateral decubitus/prone position.
9. *Intravenous fluids*
   a. Crystalloids (normal saline).
   b. Blood and blood products, if required.
10. *Other drugs*
    a. Paracetamol (IV/suppository) for pain relief.
    b. Antiemetics to avoid postoperative nausea and vomiting (PONV).
11. *Intraoperative concerns*
    a. Risk of hypothermia.
    b. Risk of exposure keratitis.
    c. Risk of pressure sores.
    d. Risk of postural hypotension in prone position.

12. *Reversal or elective mechanical ventilation*
    Most of patients can be extubated with
    controlled intraoperative management.
13. *Postoperative analgesia*
    a. Paracetamol (IV/suppository).
    b. Fentanyl.
14. *Postoperative concerns*
    a. Apnea (preterm infant).
    b. Hypothermia.
    c. Cerebrospinal fluid (CSF) leak with
       infection.
    d. Poor wound healing.
    e. Hydrocephalus.

Moyamoya disease

HELENA OECHSNER

1. *Goals of anesthesia*
   a. To avoid brain ischemia!
   b. To understand the effect of hyperventilation: moyamoya vessels overreact from hyperventilation.
   c. To understand the detrimental effect of *hypocapnia*. It can occur from crying, pain, or mechanical hyperventilation and is the main risk factor for ischemic complications. However, short periods of modest hypocapnia were not associated with neurological deterioration in children with moyamoya disease (MMD) anesthetized with potent inhalation agents.
   d. To understand the detrimental effect of *hypercapnia*. It causes reactive dilatation of normal cerebral vessels and results in steal phenomenon, causing ischemia in patients with MMD.
   e. To avoid abrupt normalization of a hypocapnic state, which can result in cerebral swelling.
   f. To maintain appropriate levels of end-tidal carbon dioxide ($ETCO_2$). Values over lower than 31 mmHg and higher than 35 mmHg were associated with statistically significant prolongation of hospital stay.
   g. To maintain perfusion of stenotic brain vessels by maintaining *normovolemia*.
   h. To balance cerebral oxygen demand and supply. An appropriate depth of anesthesia minimizes increases in cerebral oxygen consumption (cerebral metabolic rate of oxygen [$CMRO_2$]) during laryngoscopy or surgical stimulation.

2. *Preoperative assessment*
   a. Carefully assess patient's neurological status, frequency of ischemic attacks, and review the computed tomography (CT)/ magnetic resonance imaging (MRI) for evidence of infarction.
   b. Frequent ischemic attacks signal a high risk for ischemic complications.
   c. Avoid decreased cerebral blood flow (CBF) due to dehydration by maintaining clear liquids intake up to 2 h before scheduled procedure and/or IV hydration if possible.
   d. Continue antiseizure medication, calcium channel blockers, and anticoagulation.

3. *Premedication*
   A short-acting benzodiazepine such as midazolam may be beneficial to avoid hyperventilation from crying and anxiety. Be vigilant for signs of oversedation and hypoventilation as well.

4. *Monitors*
   Standard anesthesia monitors include electrocardiogram (ECG), noninvasive blood pressure (NIBP), pulse oximetry (SpO_2), $ETCO_2$, arterial line for continuous blood pressure monitoring (typically placed after induction), urine output, and core temperature. Also consider the use

of cerebral oximetry or bispectral index (BIS), if evoked potential monitoring is not available.

5. *Intravenous access*

   Two peripheral IV (PIV) lines for medications, continuous drips, and volume replacement. A central line is recommended if PIV access is insufficient or other underlying medical conditions warrant its use.

6. *Induction*

   a. If no IV access is present, a careful inhalation induction with sevoflurane in 100% oxygen and gentle assistance of respiration is reasonable.

   b. After inserting the PIV, assume full control of respiration to maintain normocarbia; administer 1–2 μg/kg fentanyl, muscle relaxants, possibly lidocaine, to assure adequate level of anesthesia and analgesia prior to laryngoscopy and intubation.

7. *Maintenance*

   Some studies have suggested improved regional blood flow with total intravenous anesthesia (TIVA) using propofol compared to inhalation anesthesia. If volatile anesthetics are used, CBF autoregulation may be better preserved with sevoflurane compared to isoflurane.

However, no studies demonstrated superiority of any particular anesthetic technique on the postoperative neurological outcomes.

8. *Hemodynamic control*

   Maintain normovolemia and blood pressure within 10%–20% of patient's baseline. Treat hypotension with ephedrine or phenylephrine; and hypertension with esmolol, labetalol, or hydralazine.

9. *Intravenous fluids*

   Crystalloids and blood and blood products are used as required for maintenance and blood loss replacement.

10. *Temperature monitoring*

    Normal body temperature should be maintained perioperatively. Hyperthermia increases $CMRO_2$ and should be prevented.

11. *Other considerations*

    If cerebral function monitoring with motor evoked potentials (MEP) is used during the surgery, reversal of any residual muscle paralysis is required after positioning of the patient. To obtain good evoked potentials, anesthesia must be maintained to lower minimum alveolar concentration (MAC) of inhalation agent while providing steady-state anesthesia and analgesia. Typically, 0.5 MAC of inhalation agent combined with infusion of remifentanil and occasionally propofol is used.

Neuroendoscopy

HELENA OECHSNER

1. *Goals*
   To provide a short anesthetic with early emergence to facilitate early neurologic evaluation.
2. *Preoperative data*
   Make sure to assess the current neurological state with possible signs of increased intracranial pressure (ICP) and underlying pathology such as intraventricular hemorrhage (IVH), tumor, cyst, and evaluation of other comorbidities.
3. *Premedication*
   May not be required or desired because of age, altered mental status, or need for fast awakening at the conclusion of surgery.
4. *Monitors*
   a. Anesthesia monitoring includes standard monitors: electrocardiogram (ECG), noninvasive blood pressure (NIBP), pulse oximetry (SpO2), capnography, and core temperature.
   b. An arterial line is not usually required unless there are concerns about serious comorbidities.
   c. If there is a concern about venous air embolism, a precordial Doppler monitor can be used.
5. *Intravenous access*
   Single peripheral IV line is usually sufficient for endoscopic third ventriculostomy (ETV); two lines may be considered for endoscopic strip craniectomy (ESC) where blood loss may be potentially higher.

6. *Induction*
   Either IV or inhalation induction represent equally good options. Endotracheal intubation is required and careful positioning (beware of the flexed head position!) and securing of the endotracheal tube are prudent.
7. *Maintenance*
   a. Maintenance of anesthesia is best achieved by using a short-acting inhalation anesthetic without nitrous oxide, a minimal amount of short-acting opioids, and a muscle relaxant with full reversal at the end of surgery.
   b. Local anesthetic for field infiltration by the surgeon helps to decrease opioid use as does preoperative acetaminophen and postoperative ketorolac. Consider reducing the maximum dose because of concern for rapid absorption from the scalp.
8. *Positioning*
   Supine position for ETV and metopic and coronal ESC; prone position for sagittal and lambdoid ESC.
9. *Intravenous fluids*
   With uneventful ETV procedures, only maintenance fluids plus NPO (*nil per os*) deficit are required because of low blood loss. All patients undergoing ESC must have typed and crossed blood products available, and vigilant replacement of ongoing blood loss is vital.

10. *Postoperative*
    a. Bradycardia and apnea (may be a sign of continued increased ICP).
    b. Any new cranial nerve deficits.
11. *Other considerations and complications*
    a. *Hypothermia* is common secondary to relatively large surface area of the infant's cranium: active warming during induction, surgical preparation, and also during the procedure is necessary for maintaining normothermia. A carefully planned setup of anesthesia equipment and extended breathing circuit is required for procedures where the operating table is turned 180° after induction.
    b. Intraventricular procedures: Cold irrigation used for the endoscope can cause bradycardia, hypothermia, or toxic reactions such as fever, meningitis, headache, and increased cell count.
    c. Dilatations of ventricles (a common occurrence during the ventricular endoscopy) may cause a Cushing-type response with hypertension, bradycardia/tachycardia from impaired perfusion, and/or stimulation of preoptic area.
    d. Mastery of the technique and anatomy by the surgeon is important to minimize tissue trauma. While navigating the endoscope through the foramen of Monro, potential injury to the fornix can lead to transient memory loss, personality changes, and injury to cranial nerves III and VI.
    e. ESC is usually performed on infants less than 3 months of age weighing just over 5 kg. It is associated with a small amount of blood loss, low incidence of blood transfusion, and short hospital stay as compared to the typical open craniosynostosis repair.
    f. The risk of venous air embolism is lower in the endoscopic procedure but remains a concern, especially in the sagittal ESC due to higher risk of bleeding from emissary veins.

Occipital encephalocele

CHARU MAHAJAN

1. *Goals of anesthesia*
   a. To safely secure the airway (difficult airway cart should be ready).
   b. To position carefully.
   c. To maintain hemodynamic stability and normothermia.
   d. To take care of other congenital anomalies, if any.
   e. To facilitate rapid and smooth emergence from anesthesia.
2. *Investigations*
   Hemoglobin, renal function tests, coagulation profile, serum electrolytes, electrocardiography (ECG), chest X-ray (CXR) (if indicated). Special investigation according to the presence of other congenital anomaly.
3. *Premedication*
   Oral atropine 20 µg/kg, 1 h before induction (will help to keep airway dry when fiber-optic bronchoscopy (FOB) is planned).
4. *Invasive lines*
   a. Two peripheral IV access lines.
   b. A radial arterial catheter for invasive blood pressure (IBP) if encephalocele is large in size.
5. *Monitors*
   ECG, pulse oximetry (SpO_2), end-tidal carbon dioxide ($EtCO_2$), noninvasive blood pressure (NIBP), intra-arterial pressure (IAP), urinary catheter, temperature.
6. *Intubating position*
   Right lateral position (alternative positions may be supine with head held beyond the edge of table or swelling supported by foam cushions or doughnut ring).
7. *Induction*
   Anticipated difficult intubation: plan according to the available airway gadgets and expertise. Induce fentanyl (2 µg/kg)/thiopentone (3–5 mg/kg) or propofol (1.5–2 mg/kg), if able to ventilate then succinylcholine (1 mg/kg) or rocuronium (0.6 mg/kg), intubate with cuffed endotracheal tube (ETT).
8. *Maintenance*
   Maintain anesthesia with sevoflurane (1 minimum alveolar concentration [MAC])/intermittent fentanyl boluses 1 µg/kg/atracurium 0.5 mg/kg bolus.
9. *Positioning*
   Prone position.
10. *Intravenous fluids*
    Crystalloids; avoid glucose-containing fluids; blood if required.
11. *Other drugs*
    a. Rectal paracetamol suppository 40 mg/kg (in children); IV paracetamol.
    b. Perioperative antibiotic.
    c. Antiemetic prophylaxis 30 min before end of surgery.
12. *Intraoperative concerns*
    a. Hemodynamic instability—bradycardia may be noted commonly.
    b. Hypothermia.
    c. Respiratory complications.
    d. Dislodgement of ETT, invasive lines.
    e. Complications related to positioning.

13. *Reversal or elective mechanical ventilation*
    a. The majority of patients can be extubated at the end of the procedure.
    b. Reasons of ventilation include hemodynamic instability, inadequate recovery, hypothermia, or other intraoperative complications.

14. *Postoperative analgesia*
    Paracetamol intravenously.

15. *Postoperative concerns*
    a. Respiratory complications (apnea may even occur).
    b. Hemodynamic instability.
    c. Seizures.
    d. Hydrocephalus.

Pituitary surgery

JOHN ANDRZEJOWSKI

1. *Goals of anesthesia*
   a. To understand possible presentation/comorbidities of pituitary disease:
      i. Hormone hypersecretion: acromegaly, Cushing's, prolactinoma.
      ii. Hormone hyposecretion: diabetes insipidus, hypothyroidism.
   b. To optimize endocrine function/review by endocrinology preoperatively.
   c. To avoid any hemodynamic instability:
      i. Hypertension can make surgery more difficult and increases the risk of post operative hemorrhage.
      ii. Hypotension may affect cerebral perfusion.
   d. To protect airway from soiling intraoperatively and postoperatively.
2. *Investigations*
   a. Full blood count, urea and electrolytes, glucose levels, electrocardiography (ECG), echocardiograph (ECHO) particularly if cardiac complications are suspected.
   b. Endocrine assays as indicated.
   c. Sleep studies, if sleep apnea is suspected (e.g., acromegalics).
   d. Computed tomography (CT) or magnetic resonance imaging (MRI) to exclude hydrocephalus; document visual fields preoperatively.
3. *Premedication*
   a. Continue preoperative medications such as cortisol and antihypertensives.
   b. Use antacid prophylaxis and anxiolytic according to local preferences.
   c. Warn patient regarding surgical use of nasal packs postoperatively.
4. *Intravenous access*
   a. Two IV access lines.
   b. Arterial line on side nearest to anesthetic machine (ideally placed preinduction to facilitate smooth induction); central line only if patient's comorbidity warrants this.
5. *Monitors*
   a. ECG/noninvasive blood pressure (NIBP)/invasive blood pressure (IBP)/pulse oximetry (SpO_2)/end-tidal carbon dioxide ($EtCO_2$)/core temperature/neuromuscular transmission (NMT).
   b. Urinary catheter usually not required.
   c. Bispectral index (BIS)/entropy, especially if total intravenous anesthesia (TIVA) with muscle relaxation to be used.
6. *Induction*
   a. Opiate coinduction decreases stress response (e.g., fentanyl 2 µg/kg or TCI remifentanil @ 4–6 ng/mL).
   b. Thiopentone 5–7 mg/kg or propofol 2 mg/kg. These should be titrated slowly to avoid BP changes. Further small dose of induction agent after confirmation of relaxation with NMT is recommended (BIS is usually around 35–40 at this point).

c. Muscle relaxant as per local practice (e.g., rocuronium 0.6 mg/kg).

d. Acromegalics may have difficult airways; consider fiber-optic intubation.

7. *Maintenance*

a. Propofol maintenance (TIVA) minimizes postoperative nausea and helps with smooth emergence. (depth monitor then required) or use a volatile (e.g., sevoflurane) at 0.7–1 minimum alveolar concentration (MAC).

b. Remifentanil infusion useful for intraoperative BP control.

c. Muscle relaxant (e.g., rocuronium) infusion useful although not required if higher doses of remifentanil are used, for example 5–6 ng/mL effect-site concentration (0.2 µg/kg/min).

8. *Positioning*

a. Supine with head in horseshoe headrest.

b. Endotracheal tube (ETT) should be kept out of the way of surgical field (e.g., armored tube or south facing RAE coming out of left side of mouth for right-handed surgeon).

c. Careful deep vein thrombosis (DVT) prophylaxis (e.g., flowtron boots) required.

d. Use intraoperative warming to avoid hypothermia.

9. *Intravenous fluids*
Crystalloids; blood and blood products (if required).

10. *Other drugs*

a. Nasal decongestants (e.g., Moffat's solution).

b. Hydrocortisone (reducing regime is standard and started in the operating theater [OT])

c. Antiemetics (e.g., ondansetron and dexamethasone).

d. Antibiotics according to local protocol.

e. Vasopressor (e.g., metaraminol infusion) useful if high-dose remifentanil is used.

11. *Intraoperative concerns*

a. Surgical infiltration using local anesthetic containing adrenaline at the start can result in profound hypotension, which should not be treated as it is due to transient vasodilatation from beta 2 adrenoceptor activation.

b. Bleeding is rare. Tranexamic acid useful if very vascular. A throat pack is recommended and should be included in the swab count to ensure removal prior to extubation.

c. Lumbar drain may be requested to facilitate surgery and help prevent postoperative CSF leak.

12. *Extubation or elective mechanical ventilation*
Patients should be extubated in lateral position to prevent airway soiling or awake in the sitting position to minimise further bleeding and maximize post operative oxygen exchange.

13. *Postoperative analgesia*

a. Paracetamol 1 g every 6 hours started in OT.

b. Nonsteroidal anti-inflammatory drugs (NSAIDs) controversial; ask the surgeon before giving.

c. Longer acting opiates: e.g., IV Morphine titrated to effect, then oral doses as required.

14. *Postoperative concerns*

a. Patients usually kept in a high dependency unit after operation:

i. Monitor sodium and glucose levels closely: Desmopressin may be needed for persistent diabetes insipidus (DI). Syndrome of inappropriate anti diuretic hormone (SIADH) will require fluid restriction +/– demeclocycline.

ii. Hormone replacement (e.g., cortisol, TSH as directed by endocrine review.

iii. CPAP is contraindicated in these patients.

iv. Care with lumbar drain to avoid overdrainage of cerebrospinal fluid (CSF).

Posterior fossa tumor

PRASANNA U. BIDKAR

1. *Goals of anesthesia*
   a. To facilitate smooth induction and avoidance of increases in intracranial pressure (ICP) during laryngoscopy and intubation.
   b. To position properly the patients requiring surgery.
   c. To maintain hemodynamic stability during the intraoperative period.
   d. To facilitate cranial nerve monitoring.
   e. To plan emergence from anesthesia in the postoperative period.
2. *Investigations*
   a. Routine investigations: hemoglobin, complete blood count, serum electrolytes, chest X-ray (CXR).
   b. Specific investigations: computed tomography (CT) scan and magnetic resonance imaging (MRI).
3. *Premedication*
   Routine sedative premedications are generally avoided in these patients due to risk of hypercapnia, induced increases in ICP, and risk of pulmonary aspiration in patients with lower cranial nerve involvement.
4. *Intravenous access*
   A large-bore IV cannula (16 G) with a central venous catheter or two large-bore IV cannulas.
5. *Monitors*
   a. Routine monitoring: heart rate (HR), electrocardiography (ECG), noninvasive

blood pressure (NIBP), pulse oximetry (SpO_2), end-tidal carbon dioxide ($EtCO_2$), temperature.
   b. Specific monitoring: invasive blood pressure (IBP), central venous pressure (CVP), cranial nerve monitoring (electromyography [EMG]), brain stem auditory evoked responses (BAERs), transesophageal echocardiography (TEE)/ precordial Doppler (if sitting position).
   c. Bispectral index (BIS) monitoring for depth of anesthesia (in patients in whom no neuromuscular blockers are used).
6. *Induction*
   Oxygen + fentanyl (2 µg/kg) + thiopentone (5–7 mg/kg)/propofol (2 mg/kg)/etomidate (0.3 mg/kg) + rocuronium (0.6 mg/kg)/ vecuronium (0.1 mg/kg).
7. *Maintenance*
   a. Oxygen (O_2) with air or nitrous oxide + isoflurane/sevoflurane/desflurane (<1 minimum alveolar concentration [MAC]) or propofol (100–200 µg/kg/ min) infusion + fentanyl (0.5 µg/kg/h)/ remifentanil infusion (0.25–0.05 µg/kg// min) + rocuronium (0.4–0.5 mg/kg/h)/ vecuronium (1 µg/kg/min).
   b. In patients planned for EMG for facial nerve/lower cranial nerves: avoid muscle relaxants. A combination of infusions of propofol (75–150 µg/kg) with isoflurane/ sevoflurane/desflurane (0.8–1 MAC).

8. *Positioning*
   a. Lateral position: for CP angle tumors.
   b. Prone position: for midline posterior fossa tumors.
   c. Sitting position: for brain stem tumors and pineal gland tumors.
9. *Intravenous fluids*
   Crystalloids, colloids; and blood products (if required).
10. *Other drugs*
    a. Mannitol (0.5–1 g/kg) or 3% hypertonic saline (3–5 mL/kg over 10–20 min) for brain relaxation.
    b. Phenytoin sodium 300–500 mg loading for prevention of postoperative seizures.
    c. Phenylephrine (50–100 µg bolus every 10–15 min or 0.5 µg/kg/min, titrated to desired response) for maintaining blood pressure.
11. *Intraoperative concerns*
    a. Intraoperative blood loss.
    b. Venous air embolism (in sitting position).
    c. Hemodynamic disturbances.
    d. Bradycardia and hypertension during cranial nerve handling.
12. *Reversal or elective mechanical ventilation*
    a. Extubation: in patients with stable hemodynamics and preserved cranial nerve functions.
    b. Elective ventilation: in patients with lower cranial nerve palsy, prolonged surgery, massive blood loss, and hypothermia.
13. *Postoperative analgesia*
    Injection paracetamol 1 g IV every 8h, with intermittent boluses of fentanyl 1 µg/kg or morphine 0.1 mg/kg.
14. *Postoperative concerns*
    Mechanical ventilation, lower cranial nerve dysfunction leading to aspiration, exposure keratitis (if facial nerve injury).

t

Status epilepticus

SALLY H. VITALI

1. *Goals of medical management*
   a. To facilitate seizure cessation to prevent brain injury.
   b. To prevent respiratory failure (hypoxemia, hypercarbia).
   c. To prevent aspiration.
   d. To prevent further seizures.
2. *Investigations*
   a. Antiepileptic drug (AED) levels.
   b. Serum chemistry (sodium, calcium, magnesium) and glucose.
   c. Toxicology panel (ethanol, tricyclic antidepressants, urine, and blood toxicology screen).
   d. Neuroimaging (computed-tomography [CT] scanning vs. magnetic resonance imaging [MRI]).
   e. Lumbar puncture after imaging to ensure there are no concerns for raised intracranial pressure (ICP) = potential for herniation (opening pressure, cell count, differential, gram stain, culture, glucose, and protein).
3. *Intravenous access*
   a. Peripheral venous access.
   b. Central venous access for refractory status epilepticus (RSE) requiring concentrated midazolam infusion or pentobarbital coma.
   c. Peripheral arterial access for invasive blood pressure monitoring during high-dose midazolam infusion or pentobarbital coma.
4. *Monitors*
   a. Heart rate and noninvasive blood pressure monitoring to assess for evidence of seizure (tachycardia, hypertension) in the setting of nonconvulsive status epilepticus (NCSE) or after chemical paralysis. Blood pressure monitoring also to assess for malignant hypertension as a treatable cause of status epilepticus (SE) or hypotension as a result of AED therapy.
   b. Pulse oximetry to assess for hypoxemia.
   c. Continuous electroencephalography (cEEG) for RSE.
   d. Arterial blood pressure monitoring for high-dose midazolam infusion or pentobarbital coma.
5. *Medications*
   a. First line: benzodiazepines
      i. IV: lorazepam or diazepam.
      ii. If no IV established: diazepam PR, midazolam IM, IN, or buccal.
   b. Second line: fosphenytoin.
   c. Alternate/subsequent second line: phenytoin (if fosphenytoin not available), levetiracetam, phenobarbital, valproate, lacosamide.
   d. Third line (anesthetics delivered by continuous infusion): high-dose midazolam, pentobarbital.
6. *Maintenance*
   a. Neurology/epileptology consultation important.

b. Restarting or continuation ± adjustment of patient's usual maintenance AEDs.

c. For those with no history of seizure but likelihood of future seizures, consider maintenance levetiracetam or fosphenytoin for seizure prophylaxis.

7. *Positioning*

a. Protect the patient from injuring the head or extremities by falling or hitting against the bedrails. Monitor potential for injury in the neurosurgical patient immobilized by pins.

b. Recovery position will help maintain airway but transition to positioning for effective bag-mask ventilation may be required.

8. *Intravenous fluids*

Isotonic maintenance fluids with dextrose (e.g., dextrose 5% normal saline [D5 NS]) to avoid hyponatremia and hypoglycemia.

9. *Other drugs*

a. Antipyretics if the patient is febrile.

b. Empiric meningitic dosing of antibiotics if meningitis is suspected. Can consider lumbar puncture (LP) first if seizures are controlled, imaging has ruled out concern for elevated ICP, and the patient is otherwise stable.

c. Thiamine concurrently for hypoglycemia in adults to prevent Wernicke–Korsakoff syndrome in the situation of chronic alcohol intoxication.

d. Pyridoxine empirically for SE in children under 2 to rule out pyridoxine-dependent seizures.

10. *Airway management, intubation, and mechanical ventilation*

a. Most patients will breathe effectively during a short seizure, but prolonged seizures and/or AED medications may cause apnea, hypopnea, airway obstruction, and/or blunting of airway reflexes and necessitate assisted ventilation and possibly endotracheal intubation.

b. Consider an induction medication with antiepileptic properties (benzodiazepine, barbiturate, or propofol); etomidate may cause myoclonus; avoid ketamine if there are concerns of raised ICP or hypertension.

c. Consider a short-acting muscle relaxant for intubation as clinical seizures will be masked during chemical paralysis. cEEG is helpful during this time but close attention to heart rate, blood pressure, and rapid, unexplained increases in $EtCO_2$ are helpful indicators of seizure as well.

d. Once seizures and their underlying causes have been controlled the patient may be allowed to wake up and extubate.

Subdural hematoma

INDU KAPOOR

1. *Goals of anesthesia*
   a. To facilitate fast and smooth induction of anesthesia.
   b. To prevent rise in intracranial pressure.
   c. To maintain adequate cerebral perfusion pressure.
   d. To prevent secondary brain injury.
   e. To maintain hemodynamic stability.
   f. To maintain depth of anesthesia.
   g. To facilitate smooth emergence from anesthesia.

2. *Investigations*
   Hemoglobin, blood urea and serum creatinine, serum electrolytes, blood sugar, coagulation profile, electrocardiography (ECG), and chest X-ray (CXR) (if indicated).

3. *Premedication*
   a. Continue anticonvulsants.
   b. Administer antacid prophylaxis (ranitidine/perinorm).

4. *Intravenous access*
   a. Minimum two IV access lines.
   b. Central venous pressure (CVP) line (size in French: depending on the age of the patient).
   c. Arterial line (radial artery or dorsalis pedis artery).

5. *Monitors*
   a. ECG, noninvasive blood pressure (NIBP), pulse oximetry (SpO_2), end-tidal carbon dioxide ($EtCO_2$), invasive blood pressure (IBP), CVP, temperature.
   b. Urinary catheter.

6. *Induction*
   a. Induce fentanyl/propofol/rocuronium or atracurium or rapid sequence induction with succinyl choline (full stomach).
   b. Attenuate intubation response with lignocaine 2%, propofol, or opioid.
   c. Secure airway with endotracheal tube (ETT).
   d. Maintain manual inline stabilization in case of unstable cervical spine.
   e. Tape eyes to avoid exposure keratitis.
   f. Insert nasopharyngeal or esophageal temperature probe.

7. *Maintenance*
   a. Oxygen/nitrous oxide or air combination (50:50) with sevoflurane (0.8–1 minimum alveolar concentration [MAC]).
   b. Intermittent boluses of fentanyl or remifentanil infusion.

8. *Positioning*
   Supine position.

9. *Intravenous fluids*
   a. Crystalloids (normal saline).
   b. Avoid hypotonic or dextrose-containing fluids.
   c. Blood and blood products, if required.

10. *Other drugs*
    a. Mannitol (0.5–1 g/kg) over 20–30 min or 3% hypertonic saline @ 3 mL/kg over 20–30 min for brain relaxation.
    b. Furosemide (10–20 mg).
    c. Vasopressors (noradrenaline/dopamine) if required.

d. IV paracetamol for pain relief.
e. Antiemetics to avoid postoperative nausea and vomiting (PONV).

11. *Intraoperative concerns*
    a. Tight brain.
    b. Risk of massive blood loss.
    c. Risk of hemodynamic instability.

12. *Reversal or elective mechanical ventilation*
    a. Most patients can be extubated with controlled intraoperative management.
    b. Patients with massive intraoperative blood loss and hemodynamic instability may require mechanical ventilation.

13. *Postoperative analgesia*
    a. Paracetamol and fentanyl.
    b. Scalp block.

14. *Postoperative concerns*
    a. Hemodynamic instability.
    b. Seizure.
    c. Coagulopathy.
    d. Pain and PONV.

Supratentorial tumor

INDU KAPOOR

1. *Goals of anesthesia*
   a. To facilitate smooth and rapid induction of anesthesia.
   b. To prevent rise in intracranial pressure or brain edema.
   c. To maintain cerebral homeostasis with adequate cerebral perfusion pressure.
   d. To maintain hemodynamic stability.
   e. To maintain depth of anesthesia.
   f. To facilitate smooth and rapid emergence from anesthesia to enable early neurological assessment.

2. *Investigations*
   a. Complete blood count, serum creatinine, serum electrolytes, blood sugar, coagulation profile, electrocardiography (ECG), chest X-ray (CXR).
   b. Crossmatched blood (2–4 units).

3. *Premedication*
   a. Avoid preoperative sedation.
   b. Continue anticonvulsants until the morning of surgery.
   c. Administer antacid prophylaxis (ranitidine/perinorm).

4. *Intravenous access*
   a. Minimum two large-bore IV access lines (16 G or 18 G).
   b. Central venous pressure (CVP) line (optional) (size in French: depending on the age of the patient).
   c. Arterial line (radial artery or dorsalis pedis artery).

5. *Monitors*
   a. ECG, noninvasive blood pressure (NIBP), pulse oximetry (SPO_2), end-tidal carbon dioxide ($EtCO_2$), invasive blood pressure (IBP), CVP, core temperature (nasopharyngeal or esophageal), bispectral index (BIS), urinary catheter.
   b. Others (optional): neurophysiological monitoring, jugular venous bulb oxygen saturation.

6. *Induction*
   a. Induce fentanyl/propofol/thiopentone/rocuronium or atracurium.
   b. Attenuate intubation response with lignocaine 2%, propofol, opioid.
   c. Secure airway with endotracheal tube (ETT) and fix it with tape or thread.
   d. Tape eyes to avoid exposure keratitis.
   e. Insert nasopharyngeal or esophageal temperature probe.

7. *Maintenance*
   a. Oxygen/nitrous oxide or air combination (50:50) with sevoflurane (0.8–1 minimum alveolar concentration [MAC]) or total intravenous anesthesia (TIVA): propofol @ 100–150 µg/kg/min.
   b. Intermittent boluses or infusion of fentanyl/remifentanil and/or muscle relaxant.

8. *Positioning*
   Supine position.

9. *Intravenous fluids*
   a. Crystalloids (normal saline).
   b. Avoid hypotonic and dextrose-containing solutions.
   c. Blood and blood products.
10. *Other drugs*
    a. Mannitol (0.5–1 g/kg) over 20–30 min or hypertonic saline (3% @ 3 mL/kg) for brain relaxation.
    b. Phenytoin (15 mg/kg) over 30–45 min.
    c. Furosemide (10–20 mg).
    d. Vasopressors (noradrenaline/dopamine), if required.
    e. Antiemetics to avoid postoperative nausea and vomiting (PONV).
11. *Intraoperative concerns*
    a. Intraoperative tense brain.
    b. Risk of massive blood loss leading to coagulopathy.
    c. Risk of hemodynamic instability following large fluid shift and blood loss.
    d. Risk of venous air embolism.
12. *Reversal or elective mechanical ventilation*
    a. Most patients can be extubated with controlled intraoperative management.
    b. Patients with massive intraoperative blood loss and hemodynamic instability may require mechanical ventilation.
13. *Postoperative analgesia*
    a. Paracetamol and fentanyl.
    b. Scalp block.
14. *Postoperative concerns*
    a. Pain and PONV.
    b. Abnormal coagulation profile following major blood loss.
    c. Hemodynamic instability.
    d. Pneumocephalus.
    e. Seizures.

Ventriculoperitoneal shunt

MARC-ALAIN BABI and SALMAN AL JERDI

1. *Goals of anesthesia*
   a. To permit control of hemodynamic parameters in a controlled environment.
   b. To ensure adequate cerebral perfusion pressure.
   c. To avoid fluctuations in cerebral perfusion pressure that may lead to permanent brain injury.
   d. To provide smooth emergence from sedation.
2. *Investigations*
   Hemogram with differential, arterial blood gas, serum electrolyte including magnesium, calcium, and phosphorus, baseline renal function, baseline liver function, coagulation, electrocardiography (ECG), chest X-ray (CXR), echocardiogram recommended if underlying cardiac history or high-risk patient.
3. *Premedication*
   a. Preoperative medications prescribed prior to surgery, such as carbonic acid anhydrase or other medications that are typically used to treat intracranial hypertension, may be continued at the discretion of the treating physician.
   b. Anticonvulsant (antiepileptic) medications prescribed to treat underlying epilepsy disorder need to be continued. Anticonvulsants may also be prescribed prophylactically, at the discretion of the treating physician.
   c. Gastric ulcer prophylaxis: H_2-blockers or proton pump inhibitors (PPIs) are recommended in patients undergoing general anesthesia and who are made NPO (*nil per os*).
   d. In anxious patients, small doses of midazolam may be given prior to entering the operation room (OR) but not necessarily.
4. *Intravenous access*
   a. One large-bore IV access line (18 G or 16 G) is recommended.
   b. Arterial line placement in the radial artery for hemodynamic monitoring. The arterial line is placed before induction under local anesthesia or light IV sedation in cardiac and unstable patients.
5. *Monitoring*
   Continuous ECG; continuous invasive and noninvasive blood pressure (NIBP) monitoring; continuous pulse oximetry, end-tidal carbon dioxide ($EtCO_2$) gases. Strict intake/output monitoring, temperature.
6. *Induction*
   a. Continuous oxygen.
   b. Fentanyl (1–2 µg/kg).
   c. Propofol (2 mg/kg) or thiopental (4–5 mg/kg).
   d. Etomidate (0.3 mg/kg), rocuronium (0.6 mg/kg), or vecuronium (0.1 mg/kg) until loss of eyelid reflex.
   e. Facilitation of intubation: rocuronium (0.6 mg/kg).

f.   Once intubated, the endotracheal tube is fixed and eyes should be taped to avoid inadvertent corneal abrasions intraprocedurally.

7. *Maintenance*

a.   Oxygenation: The patient is ventilated with oxygen at different fraction of inspired oxygen (FiO_2) (at the discretion of the anesthetist) to provide normoventilation or mild hyperventilation and normal oxygenation. A potent inhalatory agent, sevoflurane or isoflurane, is added at less than 1 minimum alveolar concentration (MAC).

b.   Analgesia: fentanyl increments.

c.   Muscle relaxation/paralysis: generally atracurium (0.5 mg/kg/h) or rocuronium (0.4–0.5 mg/kg/h) or vecuronium (1 µg/kg/min).

8. *Positioning*
Supine position.

9. *Intravenous fluids*
Crystalloid fluids, typically normal saline.

10. *Other drugs*

a.   Perioperative antibiotic: Typically 1 g IV cefazolin is administered. In patients allergic to penicillin, 600 mg IV clindamycin is administered.

b.   Seizure prophylaxis: This is not routinely administered, but remains at the discretion of the treating physician. Different anticonvulsants such as valproate, levetiracetam, phenytoin, or lacosamide may be used.

11. *Intraoperative concerns*

a.   Hypertension and tachycardia during the tunneling phase of the surgery.

b.   Venous air embolism (VAE): not that common, but can occur at any stage of surgery.

c.   Cardiac complications: due to sudden and drainage of large amount of CSF.

12. *Extubation or elective mechanical ventilation*

a.   There is no clear reason to keep the patients electively intubated/ventilated unless intraoperative complications or concerns have arisen.

b.   For the extubation procedure, we suggest the following approach:

i.   Stop neuromuscular blockade at least 30 min before the end of procedure.

ii.   May need (but not necessarily) to administer either fentanyl (1.0–1.5 µg/kg) or ondansetron (4–8 mg) for postoperative nausea/vomiting prevention as retching may further cause secondary complications.

iii. May need to reverse any residual curarization with atropine/neostigmine.

iv.   The patient should awaken in about 10–15 min. If hypertension occurs, this should be treated with titratable blood pressure (BP) medication (e.g., labetalol or nicardipine).

13. *Postoperative analgesia*

a.   For mild-to-moderate analgesia, one can administer acetaminophen 650 mg every 6 h, but not to exceed 4000 mg every 24 h. This should be avoided in patients with underlying liver disorder.

b.   For moderate-to-severe analgesia, one can use fentanyl 25–100 µg depending on the pain severity. If repeated doses of fentanyl are used, one will need to monitor mental status and airway.

14. *Postoperative concerns*
Hemorrhage, postoperative wound dehiscence, electrolytes disturbance, seizure, shunt infection, shunt malfunction, and shunt failure/migration.

PART VIII

Perioperative complications in neurosurgical patients

28

Venous air embolism

FILIZ UZUMCUGIL and ALTAN SAHIN

Introduction

Venous air embolism (VAE) is one of the major complications of neurosurgical procedures. The studies addressing VAE have reported different incidences within a wide range of 7%–76%.[1] This range has been most commonly attributed to differences between surgical techniques, anesthesia practices, patient positioning, detection method, or definition of VAE. The overall incidence in the sitting position is about 39% in posterior fossa surgery and 11% in cervical procedures[2] whereas the incidence is about 1%–9% in awake patients undergoing deep brain stimulation (DBS) surgery. Although it was reported to occur more commonly in sitting positions, air embolism may occur in any surgical position, including prone, as long as a gradient develops between the operation site and the heart.[3,4] In awake patients undergoing surgery in the sitting position, the negative intrathoracic pressure generated with each breath during spontaneous breathing increases the pressure gradient between the operative site and the right atrium (RA), leading to an increased risk of VAE, which may cause significant morbidity and mortality if not recognized and treated early.[1]

How does VAE occur?

The major air emboli often originates from noncollapsible cerebral venous sinuses, mostly the transverse, sigmoid, and the posterior half of sagittal sinus, via venous channels in the diploic space within the cancellous bone of skull (which may occur during craniotomy and also pin fixation). The diploic space is not actually a bleeding site and provides a one-way passage for air to enter the circulation.[1] However, any vein opened during a surgical procedure, such as those veins transected during scalp incision, may become a source for air entrance. Air may enter via *emissary veins*, which can be opened to atmosphere at their point of entry to the occipital bone, during procedures requiring dissection of suboccipital muscle.[4,5] The veins within or below the dura may also become an entrance site. The *intradural venous channels* are frequently opened, but may not be coagulated effectively due to the confined space of burr holes.[1] Air under pressure in the ventricles or subdural space may also enter the venous system, probably through the egress route of cerebrospinal fluid via arachnoid granulations.[5]

VAE may cause significant morbidity including lung injury, neurologic injury, cardiovascular compromise, and mortality due to cardiovascular collapse caused by obstruction to blood flow from the right heart.[4,6,7] The LD_{50} of bolus air is estimated to be 200–300 mL in humans. When a *large volume of air* is entrained in the venous system, it moves to the RA and ventricle and interferes with the tricuspid and pulmonary valves, which results in "air lock" of the right heart, reducing the stroke volume.[6,7] The decrease in cardiac output eventually causes hypotension, tachycardia or bradycardia, reduction in pulmonary arterial pressure, and a rise in central venous pressure (CVP). VAE may also occur as *slow passage of air* to the venous system in a longer period of time, such as an "air infusion." VAE during sitting craniotomy occurs more via this way. The pathophysiologic consequence of slow air infusion is different from that of large air emboli, because small air bubbles pass through the right heart to lodge in the pulmonary vasculature, resulting in mechanical obstruction to pulmonary blood flow. This obstruction causes a progressive right ventricular (RV) overload that eventually leads to cardiovascular decompensation. In contrast to large volume of air emboli, the pulmonary arterial pressure and CVP gradually rise, while cardiac output gradually decreases. The consequences of the effects of air emboli most commonly depend on volume and rate of accumulation.[2,6] In a study addressing the hemodynamic effects of volume of air emboli in dogs, it was reported that the effects begin at an infusion rate of 0.5 mL/kg/min and severe cardiovascular impairment occurs at >1.5 mL/kg/min.[6]

VAE has been classified by using different grading scales according to its severity. Most of the detected VAE events were reported to reveal minor or no clinical alterations.[8–10]

			Grading Scales for VAE		
Scale	Grade 1	Grade 2	Grade 3	Grade 4	Grade 5
Girard Scale (Girard)	PcDoppler signal positive No hemodynamic alteration	PcDoppler signal positive and increase in SPAP by >5 mmHg and/or decrease in $etCO_2$ >3 mmHg	PcDoppler signal positive and decrease in ABP by >20% or increase in HR by >20% and at least one positive Grade 2 criterion	Abrupt decrease in ABP by ≥40% or an increase in HR by 40% and at least one positive Grade 2 criterion	Cardiocirculatory collapse with at least one positive Grade 2 criterion
Tubingen Scale (Feigl)	TEE: Air bubbles	TEE: Air bubbles and decrease in $etCO_2$ by ≤3 mmHg	TEE: Air bubbles and decrease in $etCO_2$ by >3 mmHg	TEE: Air bubbles and decrease in $etCO_2$ by >3 mmHg and decrease in MAP by ≥20% and/or increase in HR by ≥40%	Arrhythmia with hemodynamic instability requiring CPR

Scale	Grade 1	Grade 2	Grade 3	Grade 4	Grade 5
		Grading Scales for VAE			
Jadik Scale (Jadik)	Minor clinical alteration: TEE positive and etCO$_2$ decreased by >3 mmHg	Moderate clinical alteration: TEE positive and ABP decreased or HR increased	Several clinical alterations: TEE positive and ABP decreased by >40% or HR increased by >40%, including CPR	–	–

Source: Girard F et al., Neurosurgery 53, 316-320, 2003; Feigl GC et al., World Neurosurg 81, 159-164, 2014; Jadik S et al., Neurosurgery 64, 533-539, 2009.
ABP, arterial blood pressure; CPR, cardiovascular resuscitation; etCO$_2$, end-tidal carbon dioxide; HR, heart rate; MAP, mean arterial pressure; PcDoppler, precordial Doppler; TEE, transesophageal echocardiography; SPAP, systolic pulmonary artery pressure

Transpulmonary passage of air

Air can pass from the pulmonary vascular bed and reach systemic circulation. This passage is more likely to occur in the presence of large volumes of air in the pulmonary vascular filter. Pulmonary vasodilators and inhalational anesthetic agents may decrease the threshold for the air passage. Despite this probable effect of volatile anesthetics, it does not mandate a specific plan for the anesthetic technique. However, N$_2$O should be immediately discontinued irrespective of the volume of detected VAE, because air may pass via a patent foramen ovale (PFO) or pulmonary vascular bed to left-sided circulation.[5]

Paradox air embolism

A patent foramen ovale, which is known to be present in 25% of adults, may cause major cerebral and coronary morbidity in the presence of an air embolic event.[5] The incidence of paradoxical air embolism (PAE) in patients undergoing neurosurgical procedures has been reported to be quiet low (0%–14%). The cause of this low incidence is most probably due to lower use of the sitting position in patients diagnosed to have PFO and using inaccurate or insufficient methods for detection. Whatever the incidence is, and however rare it is, PAE results in severe brain ischemia and causes damage to other organs.[2] In the study by Feigl et al.,[9] patients known to have PFO were addressed in terms of the incidence of PAE during the semi-sitting position. This study suggested that patients with PFO can be operated on safely in a semi-sitting position provided that modified sitting position and highly sensitive monitoring techniques are used for VAE.[9] As the actual incidence differs in studies, some clinicians prefer to accept the presence of PFO as a contraindication for the sitting position whereas others do not.[11] In the review by Fathi et al.[2] addressing the use of the sitting position during neurosurgery in the presence of PFO, it was recommended to perform transesophageal echocardiography (TEE) to identify PFO in patients scheduled for operation in a sitting position. Since percutaneous PFO closure has been shown to be both safe and effective, preoperative closure should be considered in the case of a surgical procedure indicating a sitting position. If the surgical procedure has a higher risk when performed in a horizontal position, closure of PFO should be considered 2–4 weeks before surgery. Preoperative closure of PFO can either be declined by the patient or may fail, hence under these circumstances, a horizontal position may be considered despite a higher surgical risk.[2] Either way, it is recommended to perform surgeries in such patients under strict protocols, including a modified semi-sitting position, and monitor the patient by applying highly sensitive techniques.[2,11]

As PAE causes an obstruction in the cerebral blood flow, symptoms pertaining to a transient ischemic attack often occur.[1] A major contributing factor to the development of PAE is the pressure in RA, which may also rise in a major VAE. The gradient between right and left atria may be influenced by many factors. The use of positive end-expiratory pressure (PEEP) increases the incidence of a positive RAP-PCWP gradient whereas fluid administration reduces it. Hence, the use of PEEP to prevent air entrainment was abandoned while generous fluid administration during posterior-fossa procedures evolved. However, during each cardiac cycle, the interatrial pressure gradient may transiently reverse and may still result in PAE.

Even after successful acute treatment, PAE may still occur, leading to long-term sequelae. Hyperbaric O_2 therapy may be of benefit in this situation by reducing the bubble size.[6]

Nitrous oxide (N_2O)

N_2O is well known to diffuse into air bubbles in vasculature and should be discontinued and eliminated when a clinically relevant VAE event is detected, in order to avoid catastrophic cardiovascular effect. N_2O may also increase the risk of PAE, and avoidance of its use or elimination of it immediately after the detection of VAE gains more importance when it comes to the presence of PFO. However, the gradient between the RA and left atrium (LA) is managed throughout surgery when a major VAE occurs; the RAP rises abruptly and causes PAE. The use of N_2O can simply be avoided in procedures with a significant risk of VAE or can be used provided that it is immediately eliminated when VAE is detected.

How to prevent VAE

The sitting position is the preferred position for 45% of posterior fossa surgeries and 39% of cervical spinal surgeries.[4] This position reduces bleeding and intracranial pressure by gravity-assisted blood drainage and cerebellar retraction. These effects result in a clear surgical exposure. Aside from the beneficial effects, this position has some major risks including hemodynamic instability, VAE, and pneumocephalus. It was previously suggested by Jadik et al.[10] that these risks of the sitting position can be reduced by some modifications, and these modifications were used in most of the recent prospective trials addressing the issue. The aim of this

Modified Semi-Sitting Position[10,11]

- Elevate the upper body and legs by adjusting the operating table to flex the hip to a maximum of 90°.
- Flex the knees to 30° to avoid overstretching of tendons and nerves.
- Limit the head flexion to maintain a two-finger distance between the sternal notch and chin, to preserve venous drainage.
- Stabilize all extremities with pads to avoid pressure sores.
- Set the operating table to lower the head providing that the legs are at the level of the vertex.

modification is simply to provide a positive venous pressure at the operation site to decrease the gradient between this site and the RA. Despite this modified semi-sitting position, these patients require specific monitoring to provide a safer surgery.[11]

The potential risk of VAE can also be reduced during microelectrode recording and positioning the leads in DBS in awake patients.

Risk Reduction for VAE during DBS in Awake Patients

- Waxing burr hole edges
- Filling the burr hole with Gelfoam
- Sealing with fibrin glue
- Positioning the operating table horizontally
- Using a small-bore twist drill

A central venous catheter (CVC) with its tip localized in the superior vena caval–RA junction is recommended to be placed in all patients scheduled for an operation in the sitting position. Hence, the air in the RA can be aspirated in case of major embolic events.[8] The Trendelenburg position should be used when placing or removing CVCs.[6] A controlled fluid load before positioning the patient according to the intravascular volume status may be considered for these procedures.[2] In addition, if a pressurized infusion system is used, all air should be removed from IV fluid bags before use.

In nonsitting positions, it may be acceptable to omit right heart catheterization with documented discussion with the surgical team. The degree of the head-up position according to the surgical procedure should be the most important factor for the decision to omit or go for a right heart catheter. It was suggested that a multi-orifice catheter should be advanced up to 2 cm below the superior vena caval–RA junction and a single-orifice catheter with its tip 3 cm above the superior vena caval–RA junction. These locations may well serve for optimal recovery from small volumes of air emboli when cardiac output is well maintained. However, any location in the RA will be sufficient for massive air emboli, resulting in cardiovascular collapse. The right heart placement can be verified by either radiography or intravascular electrocardiography. The catheter, via the right internal jugular vein, may be advanced up to a distance to the second or third right intercostal space to have a sufficient placement in the RA, which can easily be confirmed radiographically. The electrocardiogram (ECG) electrode placed in the RA will initially reflect an increasing positivity as the P-wave vector approaches it, then an increasing negativity as the depolarization wave passes and moves away from the electrode, resulting in the typical biphasic P wave reflected by the electrode placed in the atrium. The catheter should be withdrawn until P waves become inverted.[5,6]

How to detect VAE

Mild VAE may not be detected easily; however, it is generally tolerated well and simple measures like waxing the bone edges often prevent further air entrance, solving the problem. Hence, minor events revealing no clinical signs or symptoms may not be detected by using routine monitoring techniques and may remain unnoticed in routine practice.[12] VAE associated with significant hemodynamic compromise occurs in 1.9%–3.3% of patients.[9,13]

The monitors used to detect the VAE should respond rapidly with high sensitivity and specificity. In addition, the volume of air should also be detected to anticipate the prognosis. Monitors for VAE can be put in order, from most sensitive to least sensitive: TEE > precordial Doppler ultrasonography (pcDoppler) > increased pulmonary artery pressure (PAP) > decreased end-tidal carbon

dioxide ($EtCO_2$) > increased end-tidal nitrogen (etN_2).[6] TEE is the most sensitive as it can actually detect small volumes of air like 0.02 mL/kg and also offers information about right-to-left shunting of air. However, enough data are not available about the safety of its prolonged use. Moreover, the gradual rise in continuous use of TEE increases the incidence of false-positive results.[11] TTE, which is accepted to be the noninvasive alternative to invasive TEE, can detect 0.25 mL/kg of air when performed by experienced clinicians. pcDoppler is also not invasive, and its combination with an $etCO_2$ monitor is the accepted current practice in neurosurgery to detect VAE. The combination of these two techniques can detect VAE before physiological alterations begin. A "washing machine" or "drum-like" sound can be used as an early sign to detect air embolus; however, it requires an experienced, dedicated technician and may show false-positive results during electrocautery.[1,14] The detection of VAE by Doppler is higher when the location of the probe is between the second and third or third and fourth ribs in either the left or right parasternal site. The quality of heart tones verifies adequate placement.

The wide range of monitoring also includes invasive techniques such as the pulmonary artery catheter (PAC). The PAC can be used to detect VAE; however, the rise in PAP cannot directly reveal VAE and must be used in combination with clinical signs and symptoms.[1] Nitrogen analysis in expired air can be used to detect VAE; however, its concentration is very small in any circumstance less than major catastrophic VAE.

Air embolism cannot be confirmed or excluded with any clinical or laboratory finding, hence application of multiple monitoring techniques is recommended.[3] If the sensitive monitors to be used cannot provide data continuously, then there should be parameters to describe the relationship between the clinical signs or symptoms and air embolism. In a study conducted by Spektor et al.,[3] the authors defined these parameters to calculate the probability of the event to be related with VAE. They described that if there is a sustained (1) decrease in $etCO_2$ by >5 mmHg, (2) increase in heart rate >15%, and (3) decrease in systolic blood pressure >20% for ≥5 min, then it should be accepted to indicate a high probability. And if parameters (1) and (2) sustain for ≥5 min, it should be accepted to indicate a possibility for VAE.

The detection of VAE differs with the patients' condition of being awake or anesthetized. In awake patients who undergo surgery for DBS, TEE cannot be used. Since the invasive monitoring techniques may be of limited use in those patients, etCO$_2$ monitoring is recommended to be used via a nasal cannula, although coughing and shortness of breath may become the only symptoms to occur without any change in etCO$_2$. Hence, the symptoms and signs should be observed attentively to detect VAE and prevent further air entrainment into the circulation.[1] The timing of coughing in relation to the placement of the burr hole and opening of the dura should immediately prompt suspicion of VAE. The coughing combined with derangement in vital signs or chest pain or nausea should raise suspicion for VAE and measures to treat and prevent further air entrance should be taken immediately. The differentiation of a cough due to VAE from a regular spontaneous one mainly depends on clinical experience. The mechanism of cough has not been clearly established yet; however, it may be due to bronchial irritation caused by pulmonary venous congestion. In the study conducted by Chang et al.,[1] the presence of cough associated with a significant decrease in etCO$_2$, hypotension, or an additional coughing episode was accepted to indicate a higher probability of VAE whereas a single episode was accepted to indicate a lower probability. In both situations, all measures were recommended to be taken to prevent worsening of the event.[1] In the case of a PAE event, it is vital to detect the left-sided cardiac air by using TEE or pcDoppler to prevent poor neurological outcome.[2]

Besides its catastrophic hemodynamic and neurologic consequences, VAE was also shown to be associated with coagulopathy and thrombocytopenia; the platelet count was shown to be associated with the grade of VAE.[12,15] In a study on swine, 47% decrease in platelet count was reported following an average of 4.6 mL/kg of air infused.[16] This decrease in platelet count may have several pathophysiological mechanisms including the following: (1) air bubbles are covered with platelets via direct binding and are stabilized in conglomerates, and (2) air in the pulmonary vasculature causes gaps between endothelial cells, which results in mediator release activating both complement and platelets. The conglomerates formed by platelets and air interfere with air reabsorption. Moreover, the prolonged obstruction to pulmonary blood flow increases the RV afterload, leading to cardiovascular compromise. Coagulation variables were shown to be poor indicators for VAE-induced coagulation anomalies. However, rotational thromboelastometry and impedance aggregometry were shown to indicate VAE-induced platelet dysfunction with high sensitivity in swine.[16]

How to treat VAE

As the quantity and frequency of air embolisms are directly related to the clinical consequence and outcome, treatment of VAE mostly focuses on prevention of the episodes and further air entrainment.

Acute management in VAE includes several measures to be taken simultaneously: aspiration of air from RA, waxing the open venous channels of the bone, flooding the operation site with saline, lowering the patient's head, discontinuing N$_2$O, raising FiO$_2$ to 1, and increasing cerebral venous pressure.[4] Controlled fluid load and direct compression of jugular veins raises cerebral venous pressure to prevent further air entrance.[5,17] This maneuver also helps surgeon to identify open vessels. However, the efficacy of manual compression may not be sufficient to increase the pressure and may cause adverse events such as decrease in cerebral blood flow due to direct compression of carotid arteries. In a study on swine, intrajugular balloon catheters have recently been proposed to be used as a safe and effective alternative.[17] PEEP and the Valsalva maneuver are not used anymore because they increase the risk of PAE and the superiority of direct compression on jugular veins to raise the cerebral venous pressure has been confirmed. PEEP >5 cmH$_2$O has been shown to raise the hazard of VAE.[2,18] Similarly, in a large prospective study, PEEP of 10 cmH$_2$O has been shown to cause adverse cardiopulmonary effects without any change in the incidence of VAE.[19] In the presence of cardiovascular dysfunction caused by VAE, a sudden application of PEEP may further cause deterioration by impairing the systemic venous return.[5] Besides the avoidance of PEEP and the Valsalva maneuver, it should be kept in mind that bilateral jugular vein compression may not help identify the source of air entrance in cervical spinal procedures even as high as C$_2$; moreover, this watershed region may have different routes for drainage. In cervical spinal surgeries, waxing venous lacunae of spongiosa, packing paravertebral venous plexuses with hemostatic material, coagulation of nonbleeding veins, and dural tenting gain importance.[4]

When VAE causes sustained hemodynamic derangement, the patient should be placed in a lateral position with the right side up. This position allows the air in the RA to remain attainable by right atrial catheter and prevents the development of an air lock in the right ventricle. However, this position is impossible with a patient in a pin head holder. Additionally, enough data are not available to prove the efficacy of this maneuver in terms of hemodynamic benefit. A right-heart catheter provides immediate evacuation of air, which makes it indispensable in patients operated on in a sitting position.

The management of VAE in awake patients undergoing surgery for DBS is similar to the patients under general anesthesia with a few other measures to be considered. A major concern is that the risk of a VAE event occuring in these patients is often underestimated, leading to a delay in recognition. In a study undertaken by Chang et al.,[1] an algorithm for VAE management in awake patients was presented. This algorithm defines the probability of the development of a VAE according to the severity of symptoms and signs, which begin with coughing. If a VAE event reveals transient symptoms or signs and there is no suspicion for further air entrance, the procedure can be continued safely.

If inotropic support and aspiration of air from RA become imperative, then the incision should be closed as soon as possible an the procedure should not proceed.

References

1. Chang EF, Cheng JS, Richardson RM, Lee C, Starr PA, Larson PS. Incidence and management of venous air embolisms during awake deep brain stimulation surgery in a large clinical series. *Stereotact Funct Neurosurg* 2011;89:76–82.
2. Fathi AR, Eshtehardi P, Meier B. Patent foramen ovale and neurosurgery in sitting position: A systematic review. *Br J Anaesth* 2009;102(5):588–596.
3. Spektor S, Fraifeld S, Margolin E, Saseedharan S, Eimerl D, Umansky F. Comparison of outcomes following complex posterior fossa surgery performed in the sitting versus lateral position. *J Clin Neurosci* 2015;22:705–712.
4. Basaldella L, Ortolani V, Corbanese U, Sorbara C, Longatti P. Massive venous air embolism in the semi-sitting position during surgery for a cervical spinal cord tumor: Anatomic and surgical pitfalls. *J Clin Neurosci* 2009;16:972–975.
5. Drummond JC, Patel PM, Lemkuil BP. Anesthesia for neurologic surgery. In: Miller RD, editor. *Miller's Anesthesia*, 8th ed. Philadelphia, PA: Elsevier; 2015, pp. 2158–2199.
6. Swank K. A 54-year-old trauma patient with cardiovascular collapse. In: Duke J, editor. *Anesthesia Pearls*. Philadelphia, PA: Hanley & Belfus; 2003, pp. 143–146.
7. Kumar R, Goyal V, Chauhan RS. Venous air embolism during microelectrode recording in deep brain stimulation surgery in an awake supine patient. *Br J Neurosurg* 2009;23(4):446–448.
8. Girard F, Ruel M, McKenty S et al. Incidences of venous air embolism and patent foramen ovale among patients undergoing selective peripheral denervation in the sitting position. *Neurosurgery* 2003;53:316–320.
9. Feigl GC, Decker K, Wurms M et al. Neurosurgical procedures in the semi-sitting position: Evaluation of the risk

Acute Management of a VAE Event

- Pack the surgical field with saline-soaked gauze.
- Apply wax to the bone edges.
- Cauterize the possible sources of bleeding.
- Discontinue N_2O, apply 100% O_2 (with facial mask in awake patients).
- Manually compress the jugular veins to increase JVP, to prevent further entrance of air and to localize the source of air entry.
- If possible, change the patient's position to lower the head to the level of the heart, in order to lower the gradient between the operating site and the RA in the presence of a major VAE event.
- Attempt aspiration of air from the RA via CVC.
- Start vasopressors and volume infusion in case of hemodynamic instability.
- Avoid PEEP and the Valsalva maneuver.

of paradoxical venous air embolism in patients with a patent foramen ovale. *World Neurosurg* 2014;81:159–164.

10. Jadik S, Wissing H, Friedrich K, Beck J, Seifert V, Raabe A. A standardized protocol for the prevention of clinically relevant venous air embolism during neurosurgical interventions in the semi-sitting position. *Neurosurgery* 2009;64:533–539.

11. Gracia I, Fabregas N. Craniotomy in sitting position: Anesthesiology management. *Curr Opin Anesthesiol* 2014;27:474–483.

12. Schafer ST, Sandalcioglu IE, Stegen B, Neumann A, Asgari S, Peters J. Venous air embolism during semi-sitting craniotomy evokes thrombocytopenia. *Anaesthesia* 2011;66:25–30.

13. Ganslandt O, Merkel A, Schmitt H et al. The sitting position in neurosurgery: Indications, complications and results. A single institution experience of 600 cases. *Acta Neurochir* 2013;155:1887–1893.

14. Wei S, Chen D. Catastrophic venous air embolism during craniotomy in the supine position: The bleeding pattern as a warning sign? *J Craniofac Surg* 2013;24 (3):e228–e229.

15. Moningi S, Kulkarni D, Bhattacharjee S. Coagulopathy following venous air embolism: A disastrous consequence. *Korean J Anesthesiol* 2013;65(4):349–352.

16. Schafer ST, Neumann A, Lİndemann J, Gorlinger K, Peters J. Venous air embolism induces both platelet dysfunction and thrombocytopenia. *Acta Anaesth Scand* 2009;53:736–741.

17. Eckle VS, Neumann B, Greiner TO, Wendel HP, Grasshoff C. Intrajugular balloon catheter reduces air embolism in vitro and in vivo. *Br J Anaesth* 2015;114(6):973–978.

18. Bithal PK, Pandia MP, Dash HH, Chouhan RS, Mohanty B, Padhy N. Comparative incidence of venous air embolism and associated hypotension in adults and children operated for neurosurgery in the sitting position. *Eur J Anaesthesiol* 2004;21:517–522.

19. Giebler R, Kollenberg B, Pohlen G, Peters J. Effect of positive end-expiratory pressure on the incidence of venous air embolism and on the cardiovascular response to the sitting position during neurosurgery. *Br J Anaesth* 1998;80:30–35

29

Postoperative pain

ZULFIQAR ALI, MAJID JEHANGIR, and HEMANSHU PRABHAKAR

Introduction

Acute postoperative pain is defined as the pain that occurs within the first 24–48 h after a craniotomy. This pain, if severe and untreated, may lead to sympathetic stimulation and may precipitate secondary intracranial hemorrhage.[1] Patients having postoperative pain are usually presumed to have a lower intensity of pain due to lesser number of pain receptors in the dura, pain insensitivity of the brain, and reduced pain fiber density along the incision lines.[2] De Benedittis et al.[3] conducted a pilot study and found that around 60% of postcraniotomy patients had moderate-to-severe postoperative pain. Subtemporal and suboccipital craniotomies were associated with the highest incidence of postoperative pain, which was observed mainly 48 h after surgery.[4–7] Despite several studies in the treatment of acute pain, a gold standard for analgesic therapy in this subgroup of patients is still lacking.[8,9]

Anatomical and physiological basis of pain following craniotomy

The brain is enclosed and protected by calvarium. The lower part of the skull is formed by the facial skeleton, which articulates with the mandible. The scalp is composed of five layers: skin, subcutaneous tissue, epicranium, subaponeurotic areolar tissue, and the pericranium. The interior of the cranium is lined with a fibrous membrane known as the endocranium. The endocranium forms the outer zone of the dura mater. It becomes continuous with the periosteum on the outer surface of the skull, which is called the pericranium. Three layers of meninges—the dura mater, the arachnoid, and the pia mater—enclose the brain. The scalp and the dura are innervated (Figure 29.1a and b) mainly by the following:

1. The trigeminal nerve, and its three principal divisions (mandibular, maxillary, and ophthalmic) along with their branches.

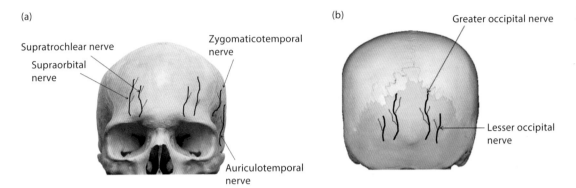

Figure 29.1 Nerves of the scalp distributed (a) frontal and temporal regions and (b) occipital region.

2. The upper three cervical nerves and the cervical sympathetic trunk.
3. Minor branches from the vagus, hypoglossus, facial, and glossopharyngeal nerves.

The anterior scalp is innervated by the branches of the frontal nerve, which are mainly the supraorbital and the supratrochlear nerves. The temporal region is supplied by the zygomaticotemporal, temporomandibular, and auriculotemporal nerves (branches of the trigeminal nerve; Figure 29.1a). The occipital region receives the sensory innervations from the greater auricular and the greater and lesser occipital nerves (originating from the cervical plexus). The dura mater is innervated by nerves that accompany the meningeal arteries.

The surgical approaches to the skull are mainly supratentorial and infratentorial. Supratentorial craniotomies are mainly frontal, frontotemporal, temporal, and pterional. In addition to supratentorial and infratentorial craniotomies, various minimally invasive endoscopic procedures have been in use for the last two decades.

Pathogenesis of postcraniotomy pain

Postcraniotomy pain is superficial in character,[3] suggesting a somatic rather than a visceral origin. The pain mainly originates from the pericranial muscles and soft tissues. The highest incidence of pain is seen in suboccipital and subtemporal craniotomies. This could be mainly due to the nociceptive pain from surgical incision of the major muscles such as temporal, splenius capitis, and cervicis. Since the skull does not have any sensory innervations, it can be drilled and opened without any discomfort to the patient. The surgical dissection of the

brain tissue does not lead to any pain by itself.[3,10] Clinical and experimental evidence shows that noxious stimuli may sensitize the central neural structures involved in pain perception. This is contrary to the traditional theory of pain perception in which it was believed that pain is directly transmitted from somatic receptors to the brain. Experimental evidence shows the development of sensitization, windup, or expansion of receptive fields of neurons in the central nervous system.

Characteristics of acute pain following craniotomy

Postcraniotomy pain is usually pulsating or pounding in nature, similar to tension headaches. Sometimes it can be steady and continuous. A higher incidence is observed in women and young patients compared to other groups.[11,12] The pain is a consequence of surgical incision and is somatic in origin as it depends on the number of pericranial muscles and soft tissues of the scalp. Suboccipital and subtemporal approaches involving considerable dissection of major muscles such as temporal, splenius capitis, and cervicis are associated with the highest incidence of pain.[13] Skull base surgeries using these approaches produce a higher degree of postoperative pain.[14] Dunbar et al.[2] however observed that patients who had undergone frontal craniotomy reported higher pain scores. Meningeal irritation is also a contributive factor to postsurgical pain. Overall, the intensity of postcraniotomy pain depends on the amount of tissue damage rather than the location of surgery.[15] Another causative factor for headache is that postsurgical cerebrospinal fluid (CSF) leakage can occur following skull base surgeries. Such headaches are orthostatic in nature, which aggravate while in an upright position and decrease with recumbency.[16]

Classification and assessment of postcraniotomy pain

The International Classification of Headache Disorders (ICHD-3) has classified postcraniotomy headache into acute and persistent types. The description of the types is as follows:

Acute headache attributed to craniotomy

Description: When the headache follows a surgical craniotomy and has a duration of less than 3 months.
Diagnostic criteria: They are as follows:

A. Any headache fulfilling criteria C and D.
B. Surgical craniotomy has been performed.
C. Headache is reported to have developed within 7 days after one of the following:
   1. The craniotomy
   2. Regaining of consciousness following the craniotomy
   3. Discontinuation of medications that impair ability to sense or report headache following the craniotomy
D. Either of the following:
   1. Headache has resolved within 3 months after the craniotomy.
   2. Headache has not yet resolved but 3 months have not yet passed since the craniotomy.
E. Not better accounted for by another ICHD-3 diagnosis.

Persistent headache attributed to craniotomy

Description: Headache of less than 3 months' duration caused by surgical craniotomy.[17]
Diagnostic criteria: They are as follows:

A. Any headache fulfilling criteria C and D.
B. Surgical craniotomy has been performed.
C. Headache is reported to have developed within 7 days after one of the following:
   1. The craniotomy
   2. Regaining of consciousness following the craniotomy
   3. Discontinuation of medication that impairs ability to sense or report headache following the craniotomy

D. Either of the following:
   1. Headache has resolved within 3 months after the craniotomy.
   2. Headache has not yet resolved but 3 months have not yet passed since the craniotomy.
E. Not better accounted for by another ICHD-3 diagnosis.[17]

There is a limitation in quantification of pain in postcraniotomy patients, as the patients may not be capable of perceiving and expressing pain following the neurosurgical procedures. Subjective assessments by observing acute pain behavior may be required. However, alert and oriented patients can be asked to rate their pain numerically such as using the visual analog scale (VAS).[18]

Preemption of pain

Wall suggested the concept of preemptive analgesia[19] while as Wilder et al found that the effects of preemptive analgesia may even outlast the presence of drugs.[20] Severe or prolonged acute pain in the postoperative period may lead to increased nociception. This may lead to development of the chronic pain.

Treatment of acute pain

Infiltration with local anesthetic

Local anesthetic scalp infiltration prior to incision blunts the hemodynamic responses to craniotomy. It minimizes bleeding from the skin incision due to the vasoconstrictive properties of the adrenaline added to the local anesthetic. Bloomfield et al.[21] showed that the infiltration of the scalp for skeletal fixation, skin incision, and wound closure has been found to reduce postoperative pain scores, without exerting any effect on hemodynamics. There has been reduction in postcraniotomy pain even up to 48 h with a scalp block using ropivacaine[22] (Table 29.1). The advantages of the scalp block include the ability to perform an accurate neurological assessment postoperatively as it does not affect motor or sensory modalities. The scalp block has shown to decrease the frequency of rescue analgesics, in the initial postoperative phase.[23] Local anesthetics decrease the postcraniotomy pain[24] by a selective action on A δ and C fibers, which innervate the

Table 29.1 Commonly Used Drugs and the Doses Used for Postcraniotomy Pain

Local anesthetics and the doses that can be used for scalp blocks			
Agent	Concentration available	Maximum dose (mg/kg)	Typical duration of the nerve block
Bupivacaine	0.25%, 0.5%, 0.75%	3	Long
Lidocaine (Lignocaine)	0.2%, 1%, 1.5%, 2%, 4%	4.5 7 (with epinephrine)	Medium
Mepivacaine	1%, 1.5%, 2%, 3%	4.5 7 (with epinephrine)	Medium
Ropivacaine	0.2%, 0.5%, 0.75%	3	Long
Opioids			
Agent	Dose and duration	Route of administration	Lockout interval (min)
Codeine phosphate	30–60 mg 4 hourly	Oral/rectal Intramuscular[17,18]	
Morphine	Intravenously through PCA pump	1–1.5 mg	8–10 min with a 4 h limit of 40 mg[20]
Fentanyl	Intravenously through PCA pump	(0.2 µg/kg/h)	6–8 mi with a 4 h limit of 300 µg[30]
Tramadol PCA set to deliver 10-mg boluses with a 5-min lockout and an 4-h limit of 200 mg.		10 mg	5-min lockout and a 4-h limit of 200 mg[31]

PCA, patient-controlled anesthesia

scalp. Various studies have shown a reduced stress response with lower plasma cortisol and adrenocorticotropic hormone levels seen with the scalp block when compared with local infiltration at pin sites using 0.5% bupivacaine.[25–27]

Use of opioids

Parenteral opioids are mainly used for intraoperative pain during craniotomy surgeries. Their postoperative use in spontaneously breathing patients is limited due to fears of excessive sedation and respiratory depression, which may lead to carbon dioxide retention, increased blood flow, and increased intracranial pressure.[28] Patient-controlled analgesia (PCA) with morphine or oxycodone may be effective for postcraniotomy pain.[29] However, the occurrence of postoperative sedation may be troublesome because of the need of frequent postoperative neurological examinations. Morphine, when used for postcraniotomy pain, may produce miosis, sedation, nausea, and respiratory

depression. However, in various published studies, none of these effects have been seen to be of clinical significance. Also, there are no clinical studies to date that have evaluated the safety of intravenous morphine in clinical doses that provide adequate postcraniotomy pain control.

Codeine phosphate, 30–60 mg 4 hourly, is used in the immediate postoperative period by oral, rectal, or intramuscular routes because of its ceiling to its respiratory depressant effects.[30,31] It has an added advantage that it does not mask pupillary signs. Following absorption, codeine undergoes demethylation with a cytochrome P450 enzyme to form morphine. Patients with a cytochrome *P450* gene with inactivating mutations are poor metabolizers. They have a severely compromised ability to metabolize codeine. The traditional use of codeine has shown to have inadequate analgesia.[32] Williams et al.[32] and Stoneham et al.[33] recommend the use of PCA with morphine as a better alternative to codeine. Jellish et al.[34] published their experience of morphine use over 2 years by PCA. The authors found that a dosing regimen of 1.5 mg morphine with a lockout period of 8 min was associated with no incidence of respiratory depression or reintubation. The authors recommended that the total dose of morphine in 4 h should not exceed 40 mg.[34] Goldsack et al.[35] compared the use of intramuscular morphine with that of intramuscular codeine in a double-blind trial. The authors found that 10 mg of intramuscular morphine was more efficacious than 60 mg of intramuscular codeine in terms of pain relief. None of their patients showed any form of respiratory depression, sedation, pupillary constriction, or unwanted cardiovascular effects.

Fentanyl is a more lipophilic and faster-acting drug than morphine. Because of its short duration of action, it is administered via PCA in the postoperative period. Morad et al.[36] and Na[37] demonstrated that pain control is superior when fentanyl was used through PCA either alone or in conjunction with nonsteroidal anti-inflammatory drugs (NSAIDs).[37] Increased lucidity and patient comfort are the additional advantages with fentanyl usage in the postoperative period. Though transdermal fentanyl application has been introduced into clinical practice, it has disadvantages in the treatment of acute pain relief due to its delay in onset, unpredictable drug delivery, and prolonged elimination half-life.[38] The safety of transdermal fentanyl is questionable in neurosurgical patients as subcutaneous absorption of fentanyl continues to occur for a substantial period of time following patch removal.[38]

Tramadol is a synthetic analgesic that provides analgesia via a μ receptor agonist as well as a nonopioid agonist, increasing central neuronal synaptic levels of serotonin and noradrenaline. The analgesic efficacy of tramadol is lesser than that of morphine. However, the advantages of tramadol are that repeated administration does not lead to dependence, the ceiling effect is absent, and respiratory depression is rare. Addition of tramadol to other narcotics in the postoperative period reduces postoperative pain, decreases side effects of other opioids, decreases length of stay, and reduces overall hospitalization costs.[39] However, due to the probability of distressing nausea and vomiting[40] and rare incidence of seizures[41] following bolus administration, its use merits caution.

Nonsteroidal anti-inflammatory drugs

The use of NSAIDs for postoperative pain relief mainly after a craniotomy may lead to: (1) platelet dysfunction and risk of bleeding, (2) altered myocardial function, and (3) renal toxicity. These concerns are mainly from data collected from studies conducted in patients receiving NSAIDs from a few days to several weeks or months preoperatively.[42] Palmer et al.[43] found that the incidence of postoperative hematoma was 1.1% in a retrospective series of 6668 neurosurgical procedures. NSAID use in the 2 weeks preceding surgery was reported as a possible cause of postoperative hematoma. All but one patient with postoperative wound hematoma received either aspirin or NSAIDs within 2 weeks before surgery.[43] There is a significant difference between nonselective NSAIDs and COX-2 inhibitors with regard to their potential to cause hemostatic complications. The likelihood of developing various complications was higher by 5.8 times for patients using NSAIDs 24 h before surgery.[44] In contrast to nonselective NSAIDs, celecoxib in doses of 1200 mg per day administered for 10 consecutive days in healthy adults demonstrated no effect on platelet aggregation or bleeding time.[45] More clarity is required with regard to the safety and efficacy of NSAIDs for postcraniotomy pain relief. It seems to be clear that preoperative NSAIDs should be stopped prior to intracranial surgery. Also, COX-2 inhibitors in the postoperative period should be avoided in patients with cardiac disease. Repeated use of paracetamol may not be sufficient for adequate pain relief in adult postcraniotomy patients unlike that in the pediatric population.[8]

NMDA receptor antagonist

This is involved in pain modulation at the level of the spinal cord and sensitization of nociceptors. A previous review has shown a reduction in postoperative pain and analgesic requirement using dextromethorphan and ketamine.[46] Using ketamine in postcraniotomy patients seems injudicious considering the undesirable ICP raise, but dextromethorphan may prove to be an important constituent in the multimodal analgesia regimens following craniotomy.[47]

Gabapentin

This is a new-generation antiepileptic that possesses antinociceptive or antihyperalgesic properties. Investigation carried out by Türe et al.[48] has shown that preoperative administration of gabapentin leads to reduced pain scores, lower opioid consumption, and lower incidence of nausea and vomiting in the postoperative period. However, the disadvantages seen were higher levels of sedation and delayed tracheal extubation.

α2 Adrenoceptor agonist

Dexmedetomidine is a potent presynaptic α2 adrenoceptor antagonist that provides sedation without affecting respiration. Investigations involving dexmedetomidine claim a reduction of postoperative opioid consumption by as much as 60% in intra-abdominal and orthopedic procedures.[49] Preemptive analgesic activity of this drug has also been postulated.[50] However, delayed recovery and longer discharge times from the post-anesthesia care unit (PACU) have been observed in patients receiving perioperative dexmedetomidine infusions.[51]

Chronic pain following craniotomy

Persistent pain after suboccipital craniotomy is a debilitating condition that impairs the professional and social life of the subject. Various causes attributed to development of chronicity include dural traction,[52,53] cervical muscle destruction,[53] nerve entrapment,[54] or CSF leakage.[55] Chronic pain may also result from uneventful supratentorial craniotomies affecting a sizeable number of patients.[56] In the retrosigmoid approach, replacement of bone flap or direct dural closure leads to higher incidence of pain.[57] Application of fibrin glue or drilling possibly leading to aseptic meningitis can be the genesis chronic pain.[58,59] Postcraniotomy headache can also occur following scar tissue formation, which involves the occipital nerves or development of fibrous adhesions that bind neck muscles to the dura. Neck movement causes traction on the dura and leads to generation of pain.[60] Chronic headache is a common aftermath following head injury afflicting a sizeable proportion of patients.[61]

Chronic postcraniotomy pain can be treated using nonpharmacological (transelectrical nerve stimulation, acupuncture, radiofrequency or cryoablation, physiotherapy, etc.) or pharmacological therapies. Combination of the two therapies can also be tried to obtain favorable outcomes. The common medications prescribed are NSAIDs, paracetamol, or narcotics (codeine, hydrocodone, and oxycodone).[62] Local anesthetics in the form of trigger point injections or topical gels and patches are viable alternatives in selected cases. Along with the routine analgesics, combination therapy with newer antiepileptics such as gabapentin, lamotrigine,[63] topiramate, and tiagabine has been tried. In neuropathic pain associated with allodynia and hyperalgesia, gabapentin has shown promising results. Other anticonvulsants like sodium valproate are effective in migraine-like headaches associated with craniotomy of posthead trauma.[64,65] Newer drugs like sumatriptan (5HT1 agonist) have been found useful in patients with persistent headache following acoustic neuroma excision.[66]

Newer prospects for treating postcraniotomy pain

Electromyography provides a noninvasive means to detect muscular imbalance in patients following craniotomy.[67] Application of this technique can help in titrating the pharmacological management according to the individual patients. Cryotherapy has emerged as an attractive option whereby application of ice packs on wounds and periorbital areas significantly alters pain intensity in subjects with postcraniotomy pain.[68] Voltage-gated sodium channels, especially the tetrodotoxin (TTX)-resistant channels (NaV1.8), are implicated in the development of various chronic pain syndromes. Development of drugs specifically targeting the functions of these channels will aid immensely in providing relief from chronic postcraniotomy pain.

Postcraniotomy pain management in the pediatric population

There are little data about analgesia use or pain experienced in children after neurosurgical procedures. Because of presumed lack of need, and a concern that opioids will adversely affect postoperative outcome and interfere with the neurologic examination, children undergoing neurosurgical procedures may be inadequately treated. A study by Maxwell et al.[69] in 284 pediatric patients found that the commonly used analgesics in the postoperative period were oral oxycodone and/or acetaminophen. Pain scores in the studied children were low, side effects were minimal, and parental satisfaction was high.[69] Another study conducted by Teo et al.[70] in 52 children to assess the degree of pain experienced by children after neurosurgery over a period of 72 h found that there was no significant pain in these children with median pain scores of 0.7 and 1.3, and 42% of these children had at least one episode of a pain score >3.[70] Postoperatively, 71% of children received parenteral morphine, 92% of children received paracetamol, 35% oxycodone, 19% oral codeine, 4% tramadol, and 2% ibuprofen. Using multivariate regression, it was found that duration of procedure was the only factor associated with parenteral morphine use for >24 h, and older age was the only factor associated with having an episode of pain scoring >3. Commonly used drugs and their doses in the pediatric neurosurgical population are summarized in Table 29.2. Paracetamol is used in neurosurgical patients but may cause increased bleeding time due to dysfunction of the platelet. Therefore, paracetamol should be used carefully in the early postcraniotomy period to avoid devastating bleeding after neurosurgery.

Table 29.2 Drugs and Their Doses in the Pediatric Neurosurgical Population

Drug	Route	Dose
Paracetamol	Suspension Tablets Suppositories	20 mg/kg 6 hourly PO/PR for 48 h, then reduce to 15 mg/kg 6 hourly Maximum daily dose 75 mg/kg, not exceeding 4 g/day
Intravenous paracetamol	Only to be prescribed if oral route not available 50 mL–500 mg 100 mL–1 g	≤10 kg–7.5 mg/kg 6 hourly >10 kg–15 mg/kg 6 hourly >50 kg–1 g max 6 hourly
Morphine	Oramorph: 10 mg/5 mL Tablets: 10, 20 mg Injection: 15 mg/mL	Orally ≤12 months: 50 µg/kg 4 hourly >12 months: 100–300 µg/kg 4 hourly Intravenous ≤6 months: 100 µg/kg 6 hourly >6 months: 100 µg/kg 6 hourly Oramorph >12 months: 100 µg/kg 6 hourly If OSA/altered respiratory drive: 50 µg/kg 6 hourly
Intravenous morphine infusion		
Any patient requiring a morphine infusion with complex medical or surgical problems requires admission in a high-dependency unit	Ensure adequate loading dose of 100 µg/kg	0–1 month: maximum of 5 µg/kg//h 1–3 months: maximum of 10 µg/kg/h Over 3 months: maximum of 40 µg/kg/h Maximum infusion rate should be 2 mL/h, which is equal to 40 µg/kg/h
Morphine patient-controlled analgesia (PCA)		
For use in 4 years and above; usually have the ability to understand and push the button	Loading dose: 100 µg/kg Bolus: 20 µg /kg Lockout: 5 min.	

OSA, obstructive sleep apnea

Conclusion

Perioperative pain management in neurosurgical patients has not been satisfactorily recognized and treated. However, better understanding of pain modulation and increased awareness have led to improved practices and a better perioperative outcome following craniotomy. Assessment of neurological function is the biggest challenge in managing postcraniotomy pain while providing adequate analgesia with minimal respiratory depression, for which a multimodal approach to analgesia using various drugs and techniques may be practiced. Randomized controlled trials are needed so as to determine the best combination of drugs or techniques for treating perioperative pain in this patient population.

References

1. Basali A, Mascha EJ, Kalfas L, Schubert A. Relation between perioperative hypertension and intracranial hemorrhage after craniotomy. *Anesthesiology* 2000;93(1):48–54.
2. Dunbar PJ, Visco E, Lam AM. Craniotomy procedures are associated with less analgesic requirements than other surgical procedures. *Anesth Analg* 1999;88(2):335–340.
3. De Benedittis G, Lorenzetti A, Migliore M et al. Postoperative pain in neurosurgery: A pilot study in brain surgery. *Neurosurgery* 1996;38:466–469.
4. Klimek M, Ubben JF, Ammann J et al. Pain in neurosurgically treated patients: A prospective observational study. *J Neurosurg* 2006;104:350–359.
5. Gottschalk A, Berkow LC, Stevens RD et al. Prospective evaluation of pain and analgesic use following major elective intracranial surgery. *J Neurosurg* 2007;106:210–216.
6. Quiney N, Cooper R, Stoneham M et al. Pain after craniotomy. A time for reappraisal? *Br J Neurosurg* 1996;10:295–299.
7. Mordhorst C, Latz B, Kerz T et al. Prospective assessment of postoperative pain after craniotomy. *J Neurosurg Anesthesiol* 2010;22:202–206.
8. Nemergut EC, Durieux ME, Missaghi NB et al. Pain management after craniotomy. *Best Pract Res Clin Anaesthesiol* 2007;21:557–573.
9. Hansen MS, Brennum J, Moltke FB et al. Pain treatment after craniotomy: Where is the (procedure-specific) evidence? A qualitative systematic review. *Eur J Anaesthesiol* 2011;28:821–829.
10. Fishman SM, Ballantyne JC, Rathmell JP editors. Supraspinal mechanisms of pain and nociception. In: *Bonicas Management of Pain*, 4th ed. Philadelphia, PA: Lippincott Williams and Wilkins; 2010, pp. 61–73.
11. Notermans SL, Tophoff MM. Sex differences in pain tolerance and pain perception. *Psychiatr Neurol Neurochir* 1967;70(1):23–39.
12. Woodrow KM, Friedman GD, Siegelaub AB, Collen MF. Pain tolerance: Differences according to age, sex and race. *Psychosom Med* 1972;34(6):548–556.
13. de Gray LC, Matta BF. Acute and chronic pain following craniotomy: A review. *Anaesthesia* 2005;60(7):693–704.
14. Vijayan N. Postoperative headache in acoustic neuroma. *Headache* 1995;35(2):98–100.
15. Talke PO, Gelb AW. Postcraniotomy pain remains a real headache! *Eur J Anaesthesiol* 2005;22(5):325–327.
16. Mokri B. Posture-related headaches and pachymeningeal enhancement in CSF leaks from craniotomy site. *Cephalalgia* 2001;21(10):976–979.
17. Headache Classification Committee of the International Headache Society (IHS). The International Classification of Headache Disorders, 3rd edition (beta version). *Cephalalgia* 2013;33(9):629–808.
18. Kim YD, Park JH, Yang S-H et al. Pain assessment in brain tumor patients after elective craniotomy. *Brain Tumor Res Treat* 2013;1(1):24–27.
19. Wall PD. The prevention of postoperative pain. *Pain* 1988;33:289–290.
20. Wilder-Smith OHG, Tassonyi EC, Ben JP, Arendt-Nielsen L. Quantitative sensory testing and human surgery: Effects of analgesic management on postoperative neuroplasticity. *Anesthesiology* 2003;98:1214–1222.
21. Bloomfield EL, Schubert A, Secic M, Barnett G, Shutway F, Ebrahim ZY. The influence of scalp infiltration with bupivacaine on haemodynamics and postoperative pain in adult patients undergoing craniotomy. *Anesth Analg* 1998;87:579–582.

22. Nguyen A, Girard F, Boudreault D et al. Scalp nerve blocks decrease the severity of pain after craniotomy. *Anesth Analg* 2001;93:1272–1276.

23. Migliore M, Spagnoli D, Lorenzetti A. Perioperative pain management following neurosurgery. *J Neurosurg* 2005;101:356–370.

24. Nguyen A, Girard F, Boudreault D et al. Scalp nerve blocks decrease the severity of pain after craniotomy. *Anesth Analg* 2001;93(5):1272–1276.

25. Ayoub C, Girard F, Boudreault D, Chouinard P, Ruel M, Moumdjian R. A comparison between scalp nerve block and morphine for transitional analgesia after remifentanil-based anesthesia in neurosurgery. *Anesth Analg* 2006;103(5):1237–1240.

26. Geze S, Yilmaz AA, Tuzuner F. The effect of scalp block and local infiltration on the haemodynamic and stress response to skull-pin placement for craniotomy. *Eur J Anaesthesiol* 2009;26:298–303.

27. Nemergut EC, Missaghi NB, Durieux ME, Himmelseher S. Pain management after craniotomy. *Best Pract Res Clin Anaesthesiol* 2007;21(4):557–573.

28. Cold GE, Felding M. Even small doses of morphine might provoke "luxury perfusion" in the postoperative period after craniotomy (letter). *Neurosurgery* 1993;32:327.

29. Jellish WS, Leonetti JP, Sawicki K, Anderson D, Origitano TC. Morphine/ondansetron PCA for postoperative pain. Nausea and vomiting after skull base surgery. *Otolaryngol Head Neck Surg* 2006;135:175–181.

30. MacEwan A, Sigston PE, Andrews KA. A comparison of rectal and intramuscular codeine phosphate in children following neurosurgery. *Paediatr Anaesth* 2000;10:189–193.

31. Cunliffe M. Codeine phosphate in children: Time for re-evaluation? *Br J Anaesth* 2001;86:329–331.

32. Williams DG, Hatch DJ, Howard RF. Codeine phosphate in paediatric medicine. *Br J Anaesth* 2001;86:413–421.

33. Stoneham MD, Cooper R, Quiney NF, Walters FJ. Pain following craniotomy: A preliminary study comparing PCA morphine with intramuscular codeine phosphate. *Anaesthesia* 1996;51:1176–1178.

34. Jellish WS, Murdoch J, Leonetti JP. Perioperative management of complex skull base surgery. *Neurosurg Focus* 2002;12(5).

35. Goldsack C, Scuplak SM, Smith M. A double blind comparison of codeine and morphine for postoperative analgesia following intracranial surgery. *Anaesthesia* 1996;51:1029–1032.

36. Morad AH, Winters BD, Yaster M et al. Efficacy of intravenous patient-controlled analgesia after supratentorial intracranial surgery: A prospective randomized controlled trial—clinical article. *J Neurosurg* 2009;111(2):343–350.

37. Na H-S, An S-B, Park H-P et al. Intravenous patient-controlled analgesia to manage the postoperative pain in patients undergoing craniotomy. *Korean J Anesthesiol* 2011;60(1):30–35.

38. Gottschalk A, Yaster M. Pain management after craniotomy. *Neurosurg Q* 2007;17(1):64–73.

39. Rahimi SY, Alleyne CH Jr, Vernier E, Witcher MR, Vender JR. Postoperative pain management with tramadol after craniotomy: Evaluation and cost analysis: Clinical article. *J Neurosurg* 2010;112(2):268–272.

40. Sudheer PS, Logan SW, Terblanche C, Ateleanu B, Hall JE. Comparison of the analgesic efficacy and respiratory effects of morphine, tramadol and codeine after craniotomy. *Anaesthesia* 2007;62(6):555–560.

41. Kahn LH, Alderfer RJ, Graham DJ. Seizures reported with tramadol. *JAMA* 1997;278(20):1661.

42. Umamaheswara Rao GS, Gelb AW. To use or not to use: The dilemma of NSAIDs and craniotomy. *Eur J Anaesthesiol* 2009;26(8):625–626.

43. Palmer JD, Sparrow OC, Iannotti F. Postoperative hematoma: A 5-year survey and identification of avoidable risk factors. *Neurosurgery* 1994;35:1061–1064.

44. Robinson CM, Christie J, Malcom-Smith N. Nonsteroidal antiinflamatory drugs, perioperative blood loss, and transfusion requirements in elective hip arthroplasty. *J Arthroplasty* 1993;8:607–610.

45. Leese PT, Hubbard RC, Karim A et al. Effects of celecoxib, a novel cyclooxygenase-2 inhibitor, on platelet function in healthy adults: A randomized, controlled trial. *J Clin Pharmacol* 2000;40:124–132.

46. McCartney CJL, Sinha A, Katz J. A qualitative systematic review of the role of *N*-methyl-D-aspartate receptor antagonists in preventive analgesia. *Anesth Analg* 2004;98(5):1385–1400.

47. Helmy SAK, Bali A. The effect of the preemptive use of the NMDA receptor antagonist dextromethorphan on postoperative analgesic requirements. *Anesth Analg* 2001;92(3):739–744.

48. Türe H, Sayin M, Karlikaya G, Bingol CA, Aykac B, Türe U. The analgesic effect of gabapentin as a prophylactic anticonvulsant drug on postcraniotomy pain: A prospective randomized study. *Anesth Analg* 2009;109(5):1625–1631.

49. Arain SR, Ruehlow RM, Uhrich TD, Ebert TJ. The efficacy of dexmedetomidine versus morphine for postoperative analgesia after major inpatient surgery. *Anesth Analg* 2004;98(1):153–158.

50. Unlugenc H, Gunduz M, Guler T, Yagmur O, Isik G. The effect of pre-anaesthetic administration of intravenous dexmedetomidine on postoperative pain in patients receiving patient-controlled morphine. *Eur J Anaesthesiol* 2005;22(5):386–391.

51. Turgut N, Turkmen A, Ali A, Altan A. Remifentanil-propofol vs dexmedetomidine-propofol—anesthesia for supratentorial craniotomy. *Middle East J Anesthesiol* 2009;20(1):63–70.

52. Schessel DA, Nedzelski JM, Rowed DW, Feghali JG. Pain after surgery for acoustic neuroma. *Otolaryngol Head Neck Surg* 1992;107(3):424–429.

53. Schessel DA, Rowed DW, Nedzelski JM, Feghali JG. Postoperative pain following excision of acoustic neuroma by the suboccipital approach: Observations on possible cause and potential amelioration. *Am J Otol* 1993;14(5):491–494.

54. Cohen NL. Retrosigmoid approach for acoustic tumor removal. *Otolaryngol Clin North Am* 1992;25(2):295–310.

55. Finegold H, Stacey BR. Epidural blood patch to treat persistent headache after retromastoid craniectomy. *Reg Anesth* 1996;21(6):602–603.

56. Kaur A, Selwa L, Fromes G, Ross DA. Persistent headache after supratentorial craniotomy. *Neurosurgery* 2000;47(3):633–636.

57. Schaller B, Baumann A. Headache after removal of vestibular schwannoma via the retrosigmoid approach: A long-term follow-up-study. *Otolaryngol Head Neck Surg* 2003;128(3):387–395.

58. Schessel DA, Rowed DW, Nedzelski JM, Feghali JG. Postoperative pain following excision of acoustic neuroma by the suboccipital approach: Observations on possible cause and potential amelioration. *Am J Otolaryngol* 1993;14(5):491–494.

59. Harner SG, Beatty CW, Ebersold MJ, Rhoton AL Jr, Samii M. Impact of cranioplasty on headache after acoustic neuroma removal. *Neurosurgery* 1995;36(6):1097–1100. doi:10.1227/00006123-199506000-00005.

60. Hack GD, Hallgren RC. Chronic headache relief after section of suboccipital muscle dural connections: A case report. *Headache* 2004;44(1):84–89.

61. Spierings ELH, Ranke AH, Schroevers M, Honkoop PC. Chronic daily headache: A time perspective. *Headache* 2000;40(4):306–310.

62. Gee JR, Ishaq Y, Vijayan N. Postcraniotomy headache. *Headache* 2003;43(3):276–278.

63. Backonja M-M. Use of anticonvulsants for treatment of neuropathic pain. *Neurology* 2002;59(5):S14–S17.

64. Packard RC. Treatment of chronic daily posttraumatic headache with divalproex sodium. *Headache* 2000;40(9):736–739.

65. Perucca E. Pharmacological and therapeutic properties of valproate: A summary after 35 years of clinical experience. *CNS Drugs* 2002;16(10):695–714.

66. Levo H, Pyykko I, Blomstedt G. Postoperative headache after surgery for vestibular schwannoma. *Ann Otol Rhinol Laryngol* 2000;109(9):853–858.

67. Oncins MC, Douglas CR, Paiva G. A eletromiografia como auxílio na conduta terapêutica após cirurgia de craniotomia fronto-temporal: Relato de caso. *Revista CEFAC* 2009;11:457–465.

68. Shin YS, Lim NY, Yun S-C, Park KO. A randomised controlled trial of the effects of cryotherapy on pain, eyelid oedema and facial ecchymosis after craniotomy. *J Clin Nurs* 2009;18(21):3029–3036.

69. Maxwell LG, Buckley GM, Kudchadkar SR et al. Pain management following major intracranial surgery in pediatric patients: A prospective cohort study in three academic children's hospitals. *Paediatr Anaesth* 2014;24:1132–1140.

70. Teo JH, Palmer GM, Davidson AJ. Post-craniotomy pain in a paediatric population. *Anaesth Intensive Care* 2011;39:89–94.

30

Postoperative nausea and vomiting

KIRAN JANGRA and VINOD K GROVER

Introduction

Nausea is defined as an unpleasant sensation with an urge to vomit, while vomiting is the forceful expulsion of the stomach contents. Postoperative nausea and vomiting (PONV) is classified as early (0–2 h after surgery) and late (2–24 h after surgery). Various studies have reported an incidence of post-craniotomy nausea and vomiting ranging from 55% to 70%.[1–3]

The complications associated with PONV include fluid and electrolyte imbalance, airway compromise, venous hypertension, wound dehiscence, and surgical site hematoma. Increase in intra-abdominal and intrathoracic pressures during the ejection phase (up to >100 mmHg) is directly transmitted to the intracranial cavity.[4] Besides this, neurosurgical patients might be at risk of aspiration due to depressed neurological status or weakened airway reflexes.[5] PONV also adversely affects the outcome after intracranial procedures and delays hospital discharge. Therefore, it is important to identify the patients at risk for PONV and the goal should be to reduce the incidence and to implement intervention in time.

Pathophysiology of vomiting

The vomiting center (VC) and chemoreceptor trigger zone (CTZ) are the centers in brain that are involved in PONV (Figure 30.1). The VC is located in the lateral reticular formation of brain stem and coordinates with the smooth and striated muscles in the genesis of vomiting. The CTZ is situated in the area postrema on the floor of fourth ventricle. It is not covered by blood–brain barrier, so it is sensitive to the chemical stimulation such as drugs and toxins. Various neurotransmitters are known to be involved in the vomiting pathway, such as histamine, serotonin, dopamine, acetylcholine, and, recently discovered, substance P. These neurotransmitters act via the H_1 receptor, dopamine receptor D_2, 5-hydroxytryptamine (5-HT_3) receptors, muscarinic receptors, and neurokinin-1 (NK-1) receptors, respectively.[6] The VC receives afferents from higher cortical centers, cerebellum, vestibular apparatus, vagal and glossopharyngeal nerves and the efferents travel through the glossopharyngeal, vagus, hypoglossal, trigeminal, and facial nerves to the gut, diaphragm, and abdominal muscles to complete the vomiting reflex.

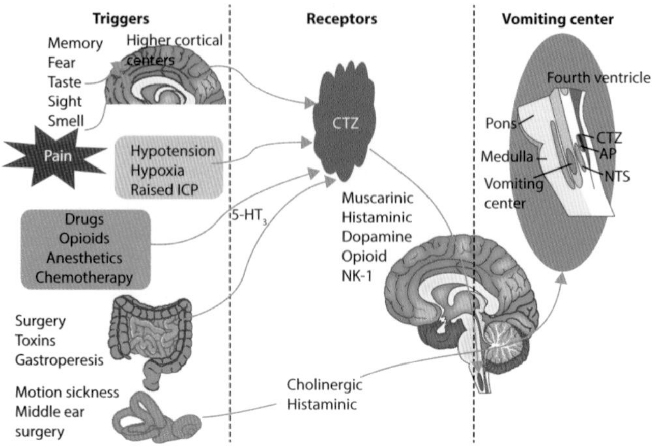

Figure 30.1 Pathophysiology of nausea and vomiting: triggers, receptors, and vomiting center. (ICP, intracranial pressure; 5-HT$_3$, 5-hydroxytryptamine; NK-1, neurokinin-1; CTZ, chemoreceptor trigger zone; AP, area postrema; NTS, nucleus tractus solitarius.)

Risk factors for PONV

In general surgical populations, the risk factors for PONV have been described as patient factors, surgical factors, and anesthetic factors (Table 30.1).[7,8] Apfel et al[9] have suggested a simplified score to identify the patients at risk of PONV. This score includes four predictors: female gender, history of motion sickness or PONV, nonsmoking status, and use of postoperative opioids. Here, each factor was given a score of 1 and the total score of 0, 1, 2, 3, or 4 predicts the incidence of PONV as 10%, 20%, 40%, 60%, and 80%, respectively. The validity of this score is not proven for neurosurgery, which is considered an independent risk factor for PONV by itself. If a neurosurgical patients also have other established risk factors, then the risk of PONV increases by manifolds. There are no well-established risk factors for neurosurgical patients, but a few probable risk factors described in various studies are enumerated in Table 30.2.

Table 30.1 Risk Factors for PONV in General Anesthesia

Risk factors	Established risk factors for general surgeries	Level of evidence[8]
Patient factors	Female after puberty	B1
	Childhood >3 years	B1
	Adulthood	B1
	Nonsmoker	B1
	History of PONV	B1
	History of motion sickness	B1
Surgical factors	Gynecological surgery	B1
	Ear, nose, and throat surgeries	B1
	Strabismus surgery	B1
	Intra-abdominal procedures	B1
	Neurosurgery	B1
	Longer duration of surgery	B1
Anesthetic factors	Volatile anesthetic agents	A1
	Nitrous oxide	A1
	Long-acting opioids	A1
	Muscle relaxant antagonists	A1 (conflicting)
	General anesthesia > regional anesthesia	A1

Table 30.2 Risk Factors for PONV in Neurosurgical Patients

Gender	Female
Anatomical location	Infratentorial surgery
	Cranial nerve V decompression > cranial nerve VII, IX, X decompression
	Acoustic neuroma
	Spine surgery
Duration of surgery	Procedure >6 h
Type of anesthesia	General anesthesia > awake craniotomies at 4 h
	Inhalational > TIVA
Transnasal surgeries	Fat graft for cerebral spinal fluid leak
	Intraoperative use of a lumbar drain
	Craniopharyngioma > nonfunctioning pituitary tumor

TIVA, total intravenous anesthesia.

There are various studies in the literature describing that infratentorial surgeries are more at risk than supratentorial surgeries.[5,10,11] The risk is even more during cranial nerve V decompression than for the cranial nerve VII, IX, or X.[12] The hypothesis described for these results states that the manipulation VC during the resection of infratentorial lesions aggravate PONV. The resection of acoustic neuromas may manipulate the vestibular apparatus and increase the risk of PONV.[13] Some studies[14] have reported that PONV is more common after spinal surgeries as compared to the intracranial surgeries, while other studies[15,16] did not find such difference.

The incidence of PONV was also affected by anesthetic techniques such as awake versus general anesthesia. Manninen and Tan[11] observed that PONV was significantly less after awake anesthesia than after general anesthesia. This difference remained only for the first 4 h after surgery; thereafter no difference was observed. The patient undergoing awake craniotomy received more propofol, which is known to have inherent antiemetic effects. The patients in whom craniotomy was performed under general anesthesia received more intraoperative opioids, nitrous oxide, and neostigmine contributing to the higher incidence of PONV in this group.

Among the patients undergoing endonasal transsphenoidal procedures, those who required intraoperative fat graft or intraoperative lumbar drain were found to have a greater risk of PONV.[17] This suggests the role of low cerebral spinal fluid (CSF) pressure or changes in CSF dynamics in triggering the PONV.

Apfel et al[18] reported that TIVA leads to 18.9% absolute risk reduction of PONV in high-risk general surgical patients. In that trial, neurosurgical patients were not included; hence, these findings cannot be extrapolated to this population. TIVA was found to decrease the incidence of PONV only in patients undergoing supratentorial craniotomy but not in those undergoing infratentorial surgeries.[13]

Management of PONV

Use of antiemetic prophylaxis is a matter of debate. One should weigh the risk of side effects and unnecessary cost against the harm caused by vomiting in neurosurgical patients. In general surgical patients, a risk-dependent antiemetic approach is used. Use of risk scores such as the simplified Apfel score,[9] as described wide supra, stratifies the risk of PONV. The patients with 0–1, 2, and 3 or more risk factors are classified as low, medium, and high risk, respectively.[8] In the low-risk category, prophylaxis is usually not required while medium- and high-risk categories require one or more antiemetics. Moreover, for the patients in whom consequences of vomiting are undesirable, such as mandibular wiring, esophageal surgery, and raised intracranial pressure (ICP) or ocular pressure, prophylaxis should be instituted. The multidisciplinary international panel of the Society for Ambulatory Anesthesia has updated guidelines to successfully manage PONV:

1. Identify the patients at risk for PONV.
2. Establish factors that reduce the baseline risks for PONV.
3. Determine the most effective antiemetic single-drug and combination therapy regimens for

PONV prophylaxis, including pharmacological and nonpharmacological approaches.
4. Ascertain the optimal approach to the treatment of PONV.
5. Manage the patients with prophylaxis failure who are undergoing treatment for PONV.

Management of PONV as per guidelines in neurosurgical patients

1. *Identify the patients at risk:* This goal is achieved by using general risk scores as well as neurosurgical risk factors as described in the section "Risk factors for PONV."
2. *Establish factors that reduce the baseline risks for PONV:* Strategies to reduce the baseline risk decrease the incidence of PONV significantly. Expert penal recommendations to decrease baseline risk are enumerated in Table 30.3.[8]

PONV is less common if propofol is used for both induction and maintenance, and nitrous oxide is avoided. Hypotension decreases the cerebral blood flow and causes brain stem (VC and CTZ) ischemia that induces nausea and vomiting. Good hydration has been shown to reduce the incidence of PONV. Pain itself increases the incidence of PONV and opioid analgesics multiply it further. Hence, we should control pain with multimodal analgesics and techniques, such as regional blocks that reduces the dose of perioperative opioid. Sudden postural changes such as sudden head-up or head rotations may trigger vomiting by stimulation of the vestibular apparatus. Controlled movement, reduction in noise, and brightness can reduce the risk of PONV.

3. *Determine the most effective antiemetic single drug and combination therapy regimens for PONV prophylaxis, including pharmacological and nonpharmacological approaches:* The prevalence of PONV is reported to be more than 70% in the absence of prophylaxis in neurosurgical patients.[2] Vomiting is triggered through the multiple pathways and a multimodal approach should be used to prevent it.[19] The recommended antiemetics for PONV prophylaxis in adults include 5-HT$_3$ receptor antagonists, NK-1 receptor antagonists, corticosteroids, butyrophenones, antihistamines, and anticholinergics, but none of the drugs is efficacious as a single agent in high-risk patients for PONV.[8] The drug dosage, mechanism of action (MOA), and common side effects of these drugs are enumerated in Table 30.4.

5-HT$_3$ receptor antagonists are the most commonly used antiemetic in neurosurgical patients. These drugs are effective for vomiting and also lack the side effects of sedation and extrapyramidal signs. None of the 5-HT$_3$ antagonists are superior to or have lesser side effects than any other drug of this class. Dexamethasone is an effective antiemetic drug and its onset is delayed but prolonged. It can cause hyperglycemia that can be deleterious for neurosurgical patients. Hence, blood sugar should be closely monitored while using this drug.

For those patients who are at moderate to high risk, combination therapy has shown to be more efficacious for PONV prophylaxis. Combination therapy should include drugs having different mechanisms and sites of action. As neurosurgeries are considered moderate to high risk, triple therapy regimens have been tried in various studies.[20–22] Some antiemetics (anticholinergics, antihistamines, benzamides, and butyrophenones) can cause sedation and interfere with neurocognitive monitoring, which precludes the use of such drugs in neurosurgical patients.

Table 30.3 Strategies to Reduce Risk for PONV

Strategies	Level of evidence
Avoidance of general anesthesia by using regional anesthesia (awake versus general anesthesia in neurosurgery)	A1
Use of propofol for induction and maintenance of anesthesia (found to be effective only in supratentorial surgeries)	A1
Avoidance of nitrous oxide	A1
Avoidance of volatile anesthetics	A2
Minimization of intraoperative and postoperative opioids	A2 and A1
Adequate hydration	A1

Table 30.4 PONV Drugs List

Drugs	Dosage	Timing	MOA	Common side effects
5-HT₃ receptor antagonists				
Ondansetron	4 mg/8 mg IV	At the end of surgery	Blocks both peripheral (in GUT) and central 5-HT₃ receptors (in CTZ) leading to decrease in visceral afferents and CTZ stimulation of VC; most effective and considered first-line drug for antiemesis	Headache, elevated liver enzymes, constipation, prolonged QTc interval
Ramosetron	0.3 mg IV			
Dolasetron	12.5 mg IV			
Granisetron	0.35–3 mg IV			
Tropisetron	2 mg IV			
Palonosetron	0.075 mg IV			
NK-1 receptor antagonists				
Aprepitant	40 mg per os	1–3 h before induction	Antagonize substance P in VC; effective against cytotoxic chemotherapy	Headache, obstipation, elevated transaminases, dry mouth, drowsiness
Casopitant	150 mg per os			
Rolapitant	70–200 per os			
Corticosteroid				
Dexamethasone	4–5 mg IV	After anesthesia induction	Exact MOA is unclear but could be due to inhibition of central prostaglandin inhibition, blockade of the corticoreceptors in the nucleus tractus solitarius, release of endorphins, and reduction in the serotonin concentration in the brain and the gut; strong anti-inflammatory action, which reduces the ascending impulses to the VC	Increased risk of postoperative infection; increases in blood glucose, hypertension; adrenal insufficiency; immunosuppression not associated with a single dose
Methylprednisolone	40 mg IV			
Antihistamine				
Dimenhydrinate	1 mg/kg IV	Not known	Block H₁ and muscarinic receptors in the VC	Drowsiness, dry mouth, tachycardia, QT prolongation, visual disturbances, dysuria
Meclizine	50 mg per os	1 h before induction	Effective in managing PONV associated with activation of vestibular pathway	
Promethazine	6.25–12.5 mg IV			

(Continued)

Table 30.4 PONV Drugs List (Continued)

Drugs	Dosage	Timing	MOA	Common side effects
Anticholinergics				
Scopolamine	Transdermal patch	4 h before surgery or 6 h before the end of anesthesia	Inhibit stimulation of VC by mainly blocking the action of acetylcholine at muscarinic receptors in the vestibular system; effective against nausea vomiting arising from vestibular pathway	Visual disturbances, dry mouth, confusion, hallucinations, urinary retention
Others				
Propofol	20 mg in PACU	Induction/ maintenance/ PACU		Associated with sedation, shorter duration of action; weak and short-lived effect on nausea
Alpha 2-agonists				
Clonidine			Direct antiemetic properties of alpha 2-agonists or their opioid-sparing effect	
Dexmedetomidine				
Mirtazapine	30 mg per os	Before surgery	Noradrenergic and specific serotonergic antidepressant	
Gabapentin	600 mg per os	2 h before surgery		
Midazolam	2 mg IV	30 min before end of surgery		
Nonpharmacological therapy				
P-6 point stimulation	5 cm proximal to the ventral wrist crease between flexor carpi radialis and palmaris longus	Before anesthesia induction	Release of endogenous β-endorphin in the CSF or a change in serotonin transmission, via the activation of serotonergic and noradrenergic fibers	Not effective as mainstay of treatment; works as adjuvant

One of the triple therapy regimens studied in neurosurgery includes droperidol, promethazine, and dexamethasone, which allows smaller doses of each agent when used together.[20] This practice was affected by the increased warnings and contraindications for droperidol issued by the Food and Drug Administration (FDA). Even though droperidol has been issued a black box warning, studies have shown that QTc prolongation is equal to ondansetron in clinically relevant dosage.[21] Droperidol was replaced by transdermal scopolamine (TDS) in the triple therapy regimen along with dexamethasone and ondansetron.[22] Scopolamine was found to be equally or more effective but was associated with certain undesirable side effects, such as dry mouth, dizziness, blurred vision, and disorientation.

Recently, a new drug category, NK-1 receptor inhibitors, is being tried in neurosurgical patients. Tsutsumi et al.[23] found that NK-1 receptor antagonists are more efficacious in preventing PONV in neurosurgical patients. Bergese et al[24] included aprepitant in triple-drug therapy along with promethazine and dexamethasone, and compared it with the ondansetron, promethazine, and dexamethasone combination. The results of this trial are awaited.

Certain nonpharmacological treatments, such as acupuncture, acupressure, and electrical stimulation at the P-6 point, were also found to be a good adjuvant with standard antiemetic treatment.[25] Various mechanisms have been described through which P-6 stimulation prevents PONV. These are endogenous β-endorphin release in the CSF or a change in serotonin transmission via activation of serotonergic and noradrenergic fibers. The timing of stimulation has no effect on efficacy in preventing PONV.

4. *Ascertain the optimal approach to treatment of PONV*: If the patient presents with PONV, look for the contributing factors first, including opioid patient-controlled analgesia (PCA) pumps, blood trickling down the throat, or an abdominal obstruction. After excluding the offending agents, rescue antiemetic therapy should be instituted. The anesthesia chart must be reviewed to assess whether the patient had received antiemetic prophylaxis or not. If the patient did not receive any antiemetic prophylaxis, low-dose 5-HT$_3$ antagonists (ondansetron 4 mg) can be used for the treatment of PONV.[26,27] Other treatment options

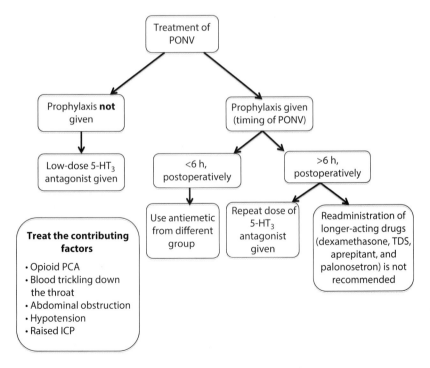

Figure 30.2 Treatment protocol for postoperative nausea and vomiting (PONV). (h, hours; TDS, transdermal patch; PCA, patient-controlled analgesia; ICP, intracranial pressure.)

for PONV include dexamethasone 2–4 mg IV, droperidol 0.625 mg IV, or promethazine 6.25–12.5 mg IV.[28–30] A bolus dose of propofol 20 mg can be considered for rescue therapy in the postanesthesia care unit (PACU) and is as effective as ondansetron.[31,32] There are a few limitations associated with the use of propofol, including sedation that hampers the neurological assessment and its brief duration of action.

5. *Manage the patients with prophylaxis failure and undergoing treatment of PONV:* Previous studies observed that patients who received ondansetron prophylaxis and developed PONV within the first 4 postoperative hours(h) did not respond to a second dose of ondansetron or to crossover with granisetron.[33,34] If PONV develops 6 h postoperatively, a second dose of a 5-HT$_3$ antagonists or butyrophenones (droperidol or haloperidol) can be effective. Readministration of longer-acting drugs, for example, dexamethasone, TDS, aprepitant, and palonosetron, is not recommended. (Figure 30.2). It is appropriate.

Summary

PONV in neurosurgical patients can lead to dreaded consequences, such as increase in ICP, intracranial hemorrhage, increased mortality and morbidity, and prolonged hospital stay. We should identify high-risk patients and try to minimize the risk of PONV. As the mechanism of PONV involves multiple receptors, multimodal management and combination of drugs should be used for its prophylaxis. The combination should include the drugs that act on different receptors. Drugs with sedative side effects should be avoided in neurosurgical patients as these might interfere with neurocognitive assessment. If the patients present with PONV within 6 h postoperative, then 5-HT$_3$ receptor antagonists are used in those patients who did not receive prophylaxis. For patients who received prophylaxis and complain of vomiting in less than 6 h, drugs of different group should be considered. Vomiting occurring 6 h later can be treated with a repeat dose of 5-HT$_3$ receptor antagonists but the drugs with longer duration of action should not be repeated.

References

1. Meng L, Sullivan EA, Meno KM. Postoperative nausea and vomiting: A retrospective analysis in patients undergoing retromastoid craniectomy with microvascular decompression of cranial nerves. *Anesthesiology* 2003;99:A314.

2. Fabling JM, Gan TJ, El-Moalem HE, Warner DS, Borel CO. A randomized, double-blinded comparison of ondansetron, droperidol, and placebo for prevention of postoperative nausea and vomiting after supratentorial craniotomy. *Anesth Analg* 2000;91:358–361.

3. Kathirvel S, Dash HH, Bhatia A, Subramaniam B, Prakash A, Shenoy S. Effect of prophylactic ondansetron on postoperative nausea and vomiting after elective craniotomy. *J Neurosurg Anesthesiol* 2001;13:207–212.

4. Andrews PLR. Physiology of nausea and vomiting. *Br J Anaesth* 1992;69(7 Suppl 1): 2S–19S.

5. Fabling JM, Gan TJ, Guy J, Borel CO, el-Moalem HE, Warner DS. Postoperative nausea and vomiting. A retrospective analysis in patients undergoing elective craniotomy. *J Neurosurg Anesthesiol* 1997;9(4):308–312.

6. Iqbal IM, Spencer R. Postoperative nausea and vomiting. *Anaesth Intensive Care Med* 2012;13(12):613–616.

7. Chatterjee S, Rudra A, Sengupta S. Current concepts in the management of postoperative nausea and vomiting. *Anesthesiol Res Pract* 2011;2011:748031. doi:10.1155/2011/748031.

8. Gan TJ, Diemunsch P, Habib AS et al. Consensus guidelines for the management of postoperative nausea and vomiting. *Anesth Analg* 2014;118:85–113.

9. Apfel CC, Laara E, Koivuranta M, Greim CA, Roewer N. A simplified risk score for predicting postoperative nausea and vomiting: Conclusions from cross-validations between two centers. *Anesthesiology* 1999;91(3):693–700.

10. Kurita N, Kawaguchi M, Nakahashi K et al. Retrospective analysis of postoperative nausea and vomiting after craniotomy. *Masui* 2004;53(2):150–155.

11. Manninen PH, Tan TK. Postoperative nausea and vomiting after craniotomy for tumor surgery: A comparison between awake craniotomy and general anesthesia. *J Clin Anesth* 2002;14(4):279–283.

12. Meng L, Quinlan JJ. Assessing risk factors for postoperative nausea and vomiting: A retrospective study in patients undergoing retromastoid craniectomy with microvascular decompression of cranial nerves. *J Neurosurg Anesthesiol* 2006;18(4):235–239.

13. Tan C, Ries CR, Mayson K, Gharapetian A, Griesdale DE. Indication for surgery and risk of postoperative nausea and vomiting after craniotomy: A case-control study. *J Neurosurg Anesthesiol* 2012;24(4):325–330.

14. Manninen PH, Raman SK, Boyle K, el-Beheiry H. Early postoperative complications following neurosurgical procedures. *Can J Anaesth* 1999;46(1):7–14.

15. Irefin SA, Schubert A, Bloomfield EL, DeBoer GE, Mascha EJ, Ebrahim ZY. The effect of craniotomy location on postoperative pain and nausea. *J Anesth* 2003;17(4):227–231.

16. Leslie K, Troedel S, Irwin K, et al. Quality of recovery from anesthesia in neurosurgical patients. *Anesthesiology* 2003;99(5):1158–1165.

17. Flynn BC, Nemergut EC. Postoperative nausea and vomiting and pain after transsphenoidal surgery: A review of 877 patients. *Anesth Analg* 2006;103(1):162–167.

18. Apfel C, Korttila K, Abdalla M et al. A factorial trial of six interventions for the prevention of postoperative nausea and vomiting. *N Engl J Med* 2004;350:2441–2451.

19. Habib AS, Gan TJ. Combination therapy for postoperative nausea and vomiting—a more effective prophylaxis? *Ambul Surg* 2001;9:59–71.

20. Gan TJ, Meyer T, Apfel CC et al. Consensus guidelines for managing postoperative nausea and vomiting. *Anesth Analg* 2003;97:62–71.

21. Charbit B, Albaladejo P, Funck-Brentano C, Legrand M, Samain E, Marty J. Prolongation of QTc interval after postoperative nausea and vomiting treatment by droperidol or ondansetron. *Anesthesiology* 2005;102:1094–1100.

22. Bergese SD, Antor MA, Uribe AA, Yildiz V, Werner J. Triple therapy with scopolamine, ondansetron, and dexamethasone for prevention of postoperative nausea and vomiting in moderate to high-risk patients undergoing craniotomy under general anesthesia: A pilot study. *Front Med (Lausanne)* 2015;2:40.

23. Tsutsumi YM, Kakuta N, Soga T et al. The effect of intravenous fosaprepitant and ondansetron for the prevention of postoperative Nausea and vomiting in neurosurgery patients: A prospective, randomized, double-blinded study. *Biomed Res Int* 2014;2014:307025. doi:10.1155/2014/307025.

24. Bergese S, Viloria A, Uribe A, Antor A, Fernandez S. Aprepitant versus ondansetron in preoperative triple-therapy treatment of nausea and vomiting in neurosurgery patients: Study protocol for a randomized controlled trial. *Trials* 2012;3(13):130.

25. Lipp A, Kaliappan A. Focus on quality: Managing pain and PONV in day surgery. *Curr Anaesth Crit Care* 2007;18:200–207.

26. Kazemi-Kjellberg F, Henzi I, Tramèr MR. Treatment of established postoperative nausea and vomiting: A quantitative systemic review. *BMC Anesthesiol* 2001;1(1):2.

27. Meyer TA, Roberson CR, Rajab MH, Davis J, McLeskey CH. Dolasetron versus ondansetron for the treatment of postoperative nausea and vomiting. *Anesth Analg* 2005;101:373–377.

28. Habib AS, Gan TJ. The effectiveness of rescue antiemetics after failure of prophylaxis with ondansetron or droperidol: A preliminary report. *J Clin Anesth* 2005;17:62–65.

29. Chia YY, Lo Y, Liu K, Tan PH, Chung NC, Ko NH. The effect of promethazine on

postoperative pain: A comparison of preoperative, postoperative, and placebo administration in patients following total abdominal hysterectomy. *Acta Anaesthesiol Scand* 2004;48:625–630.

30. Habib AS, Reuveni J, Taguchi A, White WD, Gan TJ. A comparison of ondansetron with promethazine for treating postoperative nausea and vomiting in patients who received prophylaxis with ondansetron: A retrospective database analysis. *Anesth Analg* 2007;104:548–551.

31. Gan TJ, Glass PS, Howell ST, Canada AT, Grant AP, Ginsberg B. Determination of plasma concentrations of propofol associated with 50% reduction in postoperative nausea. *Anesthesiology* 1997;87:779–784.

32. Gan TJ, El-Molem H, Ray J, Glass PS. Patient-controlled antiemesis: A randomized, double-blind comparison of two doses of propofol versus placebo. *Anesthesiology* 1999;90:1564–1570.

33. Kovac AL, O'Connor TA, Pearman MH et al. Efficacy of repeat intravenous dosing of ondansetron in controlling postoperative nausea and vomiting: A randomized, double-blind, placebo-controlled multicenter trial. *J Clin Anesth* 1999;11:453–459.

34. Candiotti KA, Nhuch F, Kamat A et al. Granisetron versus ondansetron treatment for breakthrough postoperative nausea and vomiting after prophylactic ondansetron failure: A pilot study. *Anesth Analg* 2007;104:1370–1373.

31

Postoperative respiratory complications

ZULFIQAR ALI, YASIR N. SHAH, and HEMANSHU PRABHAKAR

Introduction

Postoperative pulmonary complications (PPCs) are a major cause of morbidity, mortality, and prolonged hospital stay in the neurosurgical population with an incidence of about 23% in elective intracranial procedures.[1] They manifest mainly as pneumonia, bronchitis, atelectasis, and respiratory failure.

Pneumonia

Pneumonia is a common PPC in the neurosurgical population. It is defined as an inflammatory condition of the lungs due to bacterial, viral, or fungal infection. Prolonged endotracheal intubation and duration of ventilation significantly increase the incidence of pneumonia. Noninvasive ventilation (NIV) reduces the incidence of pneumonia. The routine use of NIV is not feasible because of the altered sensorium in the neurosurgical population.

The criteria laid down by the American Thoracic Society[2] suggest that the diagnosis of pneumonia should be considered in any patient with new or progressive radiological infiltrates and the following clinical features that suggest infection:

- Fever (core temperature >38°C)
- Leukocytosis (>10,000 mm^{-3}) or leukopenia (<4,000 mm^{-3})
- Purulent tracheal secretions
- Increased oxygen requirements, reflecting new or worsening hypoxemia

The American Thoracic Society and the Infectious Diseases Society of America laid down the definitions[2] for hospital-acquired pneumonia (HAP), health care-associated pneumonia, and ventilator-associated pneumonia (VAP), which were published in 2005. These definitions are summarized in Table 31.1.

Early onset HAP is mainly caused by community-acquired pathogens (*Streptococcus pneumonia* and *Haemophilus influenza*). It usually responds to antibiotic therapy. In contrast, late onset HAP occurs mainly after 5 days of admission. It is caused by drug-resistant organisms such as

Table 31.1 Definitions of HAP, HCAP, and VAP

HAP	Pneumonia that occurs 48 h or more after admission, which was not incubating at the time of admission
HCAP	Pneumonia developing in any patient who was hospitalized in an acute care hospital for 2 or more days within 90 days of the infection, received recent intravenous antibiotic therapy, chemotherapy, or wound care within the past 30 days of the current infection or attended a hemodialysis clinic
VAP	Pneumonia that arises more than 48–72 h after endotracheal intubation Early VAP/HAP is defined as pneumonia occurring within first 4 days of hospitalization Late VAP/HAP is defined as pneumonia occurring after 5 days of hospitalization

Source: American Thoracic Society. Am J Respir Crit Care Med 2005;171:388–416.
HAP, hospital-acquired pneumonia; HCAP, health care-associated pneumonia; VAP, ventilator-associated pneumonia

Table 31.2 Causative Organisms in HAP/VAP

Pathogen	Examples
Staphylococcus aureus	Methicillin-sensitive (MSSA) or methicillin-resistant (MRSA)
Enterobacteriaceae	Klebsiella, Escherichia coli, Proteus, Enterobacter, Serratia
Streptococcus spp.	Streptococcus pneumonia
Haemophilus spp.	Haemophilus influenzae
Pseudomonas aeruginosa	
Acinetobacter spp.	
Neisseria spp.	

Table 31.3 Risk Factors Associated with the Development of Pneumonia

Patient factors	Advanced age, immunosuppression, severe acute illness, coexisting chronic illness as chronic lung disease, malnutrition
Factors that enhance colonization of the oropharynx and stomach	Recent antibiotic therapy, bolus enteral feeding, gastric acid suppression, prolonged or recent hospital admission, poor oral hygiene
Conditions predisposing to aspiration or reflux	Tracheal intubation (especially frequent reintubations), insertion of nasogastric tube, supine positioning, coma, paralysis
Prolonged periods of mechanical ventilation	Development of ARDS

ARDS, acute respiratory distress syndrome

Pseudomonas aeruginosa and methicillin-resistant *Staphylococcus aureus* (MRSA). Fungal infections are seen usually in immunocompromised patients. The most common causative organisms are summarized in Table 31.2.

Pathogenesis and risk factors

Pneumonia occurs due to colonization of the lower respiratory tract by the microbial organisms from microaspiration from the oropharynx or the gastrointestinal (GI) tract. Hematogenous spread occurs from a distant site of infection.

The risk factors for the development of pneumonia are summarized in Table 31.3.

Preventive measures

The American Thoracic Society and the National Institute of Clinical Excellence (the United Kingdom) recommend a care bundle,[2,3] which is summarized in Table 31.4.

Selective decontamination of the digestive tract (SDD) involves the use of local and systemic antibiotics to prevent colonization of the GI tract. A recent Cochrane review[4] found that SDD was associated

Table 31.4 Care Bundle Proposed by the American Thoracic Society (US) and the National Institute of Clinical Excellence (UK) for Prevention of Pneumonia

Prevention of transmission of microorganisms
1. Good hand hygiene measures
2. Wear gloves for contact with patient or contaminated secretions
3. No routine changing of ventilator circuits/heat and moisture exchangers unless specifically indicated (malfunction or visible contamination)

Prevention of aspiration related to endotracheal intubation
1. Early weaning and daily sedation breaks to reduce the duration of endotracheal intubation and mechanical ventilation as much as possible
2. Avoidance of repeated reintubations
3. Control of endotracheal cuff pressures between 20 and 30 cmH$_2$O
4. Use of endotracheal tubes with subglottic drainage ports
5. Use of noninvasive ventilation if clinically appropriate

Prevention of aspiration associated with enteral feeding
1. Semirecumbent positioning (30–45° head up) if possible
2. Confirm correct placement of nasogastric tube prior to use

Prevention of oropharyngeal colonization
Oral hygiene strategy for patients at risk of hospital-acquired pneumonia, including the use of an oral antiseptic agent, e.g., chlorhexidine gel

with a reduction in both the incidence of HAP and overall mortality. However, SDD is not practiced at many medical centers as it may lead to the emergence of drug-resistant bacteria as *Clostridium difficile*, causing pseudomembranous colitis.[5]

Management

Choice and duration of antibiotic therapy

In the initial phase of the disease, broad-spectrum empirical antibiotics are administered. After 48–72 h, de-escalation to a narrower spectrum is performed, which is determined by the culture results.[6]

Initially, the antibiotics are administered intravenously. After a good clinical response, oral antibiotics are started if there is a functioning GI tract. Table 31.5 summarizes the specific regimens used for HAP.[6]

Duration of antibiotic therapy

A large, multicenter randomized control trial showed that there was no difference in outcomes in patients with non-multidrug-resistant (NMDR) organisms whether they were treated for 8 or 15 days.[7] Patients with multidrug-resistant (MDR) pathogens in the 8-day group were more likely to develop a recurrent infection than those in the 15-day group.[6]

Antibiotics are mainly administered for approximately 7–10 days in patients with sensitive organisms whereas resistant organisms need 14–21

days of antibiotic therapy. Clinical parameters of resolution of infection are more important than the radiographic or microbiological parameters.

A clinical pulmonary infection score (CPIS; Table 31.6) is helpful in diagnosis of suspected VAP. It takes into consideration the clinical, radiographic, physiological (PaO$_2$/FiO$_2$), and microbiologic data, and translates it into a single numerical result. A CPIS >6 has a good correlation with the presence of pneumonia when correlated with quantitative cultures of bronchoscopic, nonbronchoscopic, and bronchoalveolar lavage specimens.[8] Clinical improvement takes at least 48–72 h. A falling score on day 3 indicates a response to treatment and can help identify patients who may be suitable to receive shorter courses of antibiotics. Of all the components of CPIS, an improvement in arterial oxygenation indicated by the PaO$_2$/FiO$_2$ ratio is the most valuable factor in predicting response to treatment.[9]

Neurogenic pulmonary edema

Neurogenic pulmonary edema (NPE) is an acute onset of pulmonary edema resulting from central nervous system (CNS) injury due to subarachnoid hemorrhage, severe head injury,[10] and status epilepticus. It results in higher intracranial pressures (ICPs) and low cerebral perfusion pressures.[11] The "blast injury" phenomenon causes a

Table 31.5 Suggested Empirical Antibiotic Regimens

Onset	Empirical antibiotic therapy	Examples
Early onset	Second-/third-generation cephalosporin or β-Lactam/β-lactamase inhibitor or Fluoroquinolone	Cefuroxime/ceftriaxone Amoxicillin + clavulanic acid Ciprofloxacin/levofloxacin
Late onset or Risk factors for MDR pathogen	Antipseudomonal cephalosporin or Antipseudomonal carbapenem or Broad-spectrum β-lactam/β-lactamase inhibitor and either Aminoglycoside or Fluoroquinolone If MRSA suspected Glycopeptide or Oxazolidinone	Ceftazidime Meropenem Piperacillin + tazobactam Gentamicin Ciprofloxacin/levofloxacin Vancomycin Linezolid

MDR, multidrug resistant; MRSA, methicillin-resistant *Staphylococcus aureus*
Linezolid may have better tissue penetration than vancomycin in VAP

Table 31.6 Clinical Pulmonary Infection Score

Points	0	1	2
Tracheal secretions	Minimal	Abundant	Purulent
Chest X-ray	No infiltrates	Diffuse infiltrates	Localized infiltrates
Temperature (°C)	36.5–38.4	38.5–38.9	≥ 39 or ≤ 36
Leukocytes (mm^{-3})	4,000–11,000	<4,000 or >11,000	<4,000 or >11,000 plus band forms >500
PaO_2/FiO_2 ratio (mmHg)	>240 or ARDS		<240 and no ARDS
Microbiology	Negative		Positive

surge in adrenergic response, leading to an increase in capillary pressures in the lung bed and endothelial damage. This leads to a capillary leak into the alveoli and pulmonary interstitium[12] associated with production of inflammatory mediators such as interleukin-6 (IL-6).[13,14] A "double hit" model has been proposed in patients with a brain injury. The "first hit" may be the result of a combination of an adrenergic surge and systemic production of inflammatory mediators, making the lung more susceptible to injury, and a "second hit" may be from extracorporeal variables such as infections, transfusions, and mechanical ventilation.[15]

The diagnostic investigations include the chest X-ray, electrocardiogram (ECG), transthoracic echocardiography (TTE), and cardiac output monitoring. The chest X-ray shows bilateral pulmonary infiltrates with increased vascular shadowing. ECG may be normal or may have T-wave inversion, ST segment changes, and arrhythmias. Elevated plasma troponin levels are frequently observed.

TTE may show myocardial stunning, reduced ejection fraction (as low as 20%–30%), impaired contraction, and wall motion abnormalities. Cardiac output monitoring with pulmonary artery catheter studies shows a reduced cardiac index (<2.5 L/min/m^2), with increased mean pulmonary arterial pressure and systemic vascular resistance (SVR). Pulmonary capillary wedge pressure (PCWP) may be elevated (>20 mmHg) or normal.

Management

The initial step in management is the identification and definitive treatment of the precipitating cause. The main aim is to reverse the pathophysiological disturbance with supportive management. The edema usually resolves within 24–48 h with appropriate treatment; however, some cases need intensive care for many days. Some cases may progress to acute lung injury or acute respiratory distress syndrome (ARDS).

Management strategies may include taking care of the airway, breathing, and circulation. Dobutamine has been suggested as a first-line inotrope in the treatment of severe neurogeneic pumonary edema (NPO).[16]

Lung atelectasis

This occurs in the neurosurgical population due to respiratory depression and impaired consciousness leading to aspiration.[17] Weakness of thoracoabdominal muscles due to cervical and thoracic spine injuries may lead to hypoventilation and bronchial obstruction from mucous plugs. Associated injuries such as traumatic pneumothorax and hemothorax may be contributing factors.

The investigations used for the diagnosis of atelectasis are summarized in Table 31.7.

Management

Prevention of atelectasis is better than attempts to reopen the collapsed lung. Evidence-based studies on the management of atelectasis are lacking.

Perioperative management

The initiation of physiotherapy, bronchodilators, cessation of smoking, and antibiotics a week before the elective surgery helps in optimizing respiratory function.

During anesthesia, application of continuous positive airway pressure (CPAP) can prevent the formation of atelectasis. Positive pressure ventilation with positive end-expiratory pressure (PEEP) may be helpful.

Suggested recruitment manoeuvres[18] include the following: (a) vital capacity maneuver using an inflation pressure of 40 cmH_2O sustained for 10–15 s, and (b) increasing PEEP to 15 cm H_2O and then increasing tidal volumes to achieve peak inspiratory pressure of 40 cmH_2O for 10 breaths.

Postoperative pain interferes with spontaneous deep breathing and coughing, resulting in decreases

Table 31.7 Summary of the Investigations Used for Diagnosis of Collapse

Chest X-ray	Direct signs (related to loss of lung volume and collapsed lobes):
	1. Increased opacification in the area of atelectasis
	2. Displacement of fissures occurs with large degree of collapse
	3. Loss of aeration. If the collapsed lung is adjacent to the mediastinum or diaphragm, then loss of definition of these structures indicates loss of aeration (the silhouette sign)
	4. Vascular signs. In partial collapse, crowding of vessels may be seen
	Indirect signs (occurring as a result of compensatory changes due to volume loss):
	1. Elevation of a hemidiaphragm
	2. Mediastinal displacement to the side of collapse. Some contents of the mediastinum that are easily seen on plain chest X-rays include the trachea, tracheal tube, central venous catheters in the superior vena cava, and nasogastric tubes in the esophagus
	3. Hilar displacement. The hilum may be elevated in the upper lobe collapse, and depressed in the lower lobe collapse.
Computerized tomography (CT) scan	Atelectasis on CT has been defined as pixels with attenuation values of −100 to +100 Hounsfield units
Ultrasound	Obstructive atelectasis on ultrasound shows as an area of homogenous low echogenicity. An important role for ultrasound is to distinguish basal lung collapse from a loculated pleural effusion

in functional residual capacity (FRC), leading to atelectasis. Good postoperative pain control minimizes PPCs by enabling earlier ambulation and improving the patient's ability to take deep breaths.

Management in critical care

Ventilation strategies

Typical recruitment measures used in intensive care[19] include the following: (a) three consecutive volume-limited breaths per minute with a plateau pressure of 45 cmH_2O (also called sigh). (b) PEEP increased by 5 cmH_2O every 30 s with a 2 mL/kg decrease in tidal volume. When PEEP reaches 25 cmH_2O, CPAP at 30 cmH_2O is used for 30 s. (c) Application of CPAP: 35–40 cmH_2O for 30 s.

Pulmonary thromboembolism

This is common in the neurosurgical population due to chronic immobility or paraplegia. It manifests as acute onset dyspnea, hypoxemia, or hypotension. Initial screening by D-dimer, lower limb compression ultrasound, or multidetector computed tomography (MDCT) angiography is helpful. Neurosurgical patients should receive thromboprophylaxis by mechanical or pharmacological means. It has been seen that the majority of deep venous thrombi (DVTs) occurred within the first week after a neurosurgical

procedure.[20] Use of early subcutaneous heparin (at either 24 or 48 h) causes a significant (43%) reduction of a lower-extremity DVT, with no increase in surgical site hemorrhage.[20,21] After craniotomy, low-dose subcutaneous heparin (5000 U BID or TID) starting after the second day significantly reduces the frequency of venous thromboembolism, without any incidence in intracranial bleeding.[22] Treatment with low molecular weight heparin (i.e., enoxaparin 40 mg daily) is equally efficacious as unfractionated heparin.[23] In the presence of contraindications to heparin, the use of inferior vena cava filters may be necessary in the short term.[21] Pulmonary embolectomy is helpful to relieve acute obstruction in massive pulmonary embolism (PE) or when the thrombolytic treatment is contraindicated because of bleeding risks.

Acute respiratory distress syndrome and acute lung injury

Acute respiratory distress syndrome and acute lung injury are frequently observed in the neurosurgical population. The European Society of Intensive Care Medicine with endorsement from the American Thoracic Society and the Society of Critical Care Medicine gathered evidence through a panel of experts[24] in Berlin and proposed a revised set of criteria for the diagnosis of ARDS. These guidelines[24] (Table 31.8) were later published in June 2012.

Table 31.8 Acute Respiratory Distress Syndrome (Berlin Definition)

Timing		Within 1 week of a known clinical insult or new or worsening respiratory symptoms	
Chest imaging[a]		Bilateral opacities—not fully explained by effusions, lobar/lung collage, or nodules	
Origin of edema		Respiratory failure not fully explained by cardiac failure of fluid overload. Need objective assessment (e.g.., echocardiography) to exclude hydrostatic edema if no risk factor present	
	Mild	Moderate	Severe
Oxygenation[b]	$200 < PaO_2/FiO_2 \leq 300$ with PEEP or CPAP ≥ 5 cmH_2O[c]	$100 $ y$ PaO_2/FiO_2 \leq 200$ with PEEP or CPAP ≥ 5 cmH_2O	$PaO_2/FiO_2 \leq 100$ with PEEP or CPAP ≥ 5 cmH_2O

CPAP, continuous positive airway pressure; FiO_2, fraction of inspired oxygen; PaO_2, partial pressure of arterial oxygen; PEEP, positive end-expiratory pressure

a Chest radiograph or computed tomography scan

b If attitude is higher than 1000 m, the correction factor should be calculated as follows: [PaO_2/FiO_2 × (barometric pressure/760)]

c This may be delivered noninvasively in the mild acute respiratory distress syndrome group.

Management

Ventilation strategy

With the exception of low tidal volumes, there is little evidence of survival benefit for any particular ventilation strategy; however volume-controlled ventilation is often used. The targets for ventilation strategy are summarized in Table 31.9.

Pressure-controlled inverse ratio ventilation (PC-IRV) and ventilation in prone position may be used in refractory cases. In PC-IRV, the inspiratory time (I) is prolonged until it is equal to or greater than expiratory time (E), for example, using an I/E ratio of 1:1, 2:1, or 3:1. The physiological rationale of prone ventilation is that it optimizes lung recruitment and ventilation perfusion matching while preventing alveolar overinflation and allowing better postural drainage. Dramatic improvements in oxygenation are often observed in patients who are turned into the prone position for several hours, and this improvement may be sustained when they are returned to the supine position. The technique should be used for 12–24 h. However, there are practical difficulties in turning the critically ill patient and in nursing the patient in the prone position.

A number of advanced techniques are available, but there is little evidence of increased survival with any of them.

Nebulized prostacyclin

Nebulized prostacyclin produces pulmonary vasodilation, dilating those vessels in well-ventilated parts of the lung, thus improving ventilation/perfusion matching. Because it is removed from the circulation rapidly, it does not cause systemic hypotension.

Inhaled nitric oxide

Like prostacyclin, this is a selective pulmonary vasodilator.

Corticosteroids

A regimen of methylprednisolone 2 mg/k daily may suppress ongoing inflammation during the fibroproliferative phase. The response may be apparent usually after 3–5 days.[25] A more recent meta-analysis by Peter et al.[26] found a possible reduced mortality when steroids were started after the onset of ARDS, but preventative steroids increased the risk of ARDS.

Surfactant therapy

This aims to replace surfactant lost from the lung and thus improve compliance and alveolar stability, and decrease lung water. However, early results have been disappointing.

High-frequency oscillation ventilation

This can be used to raise mean airway pressure without dangerous increases in peak airway

Table 31.9 Targets for Ventilation Strategy in Acute Respiratory Distress Syndrome

FiO_2 0.5–0.6 to minimize oxygen toxicity.

PaO_2 ≥8 kPa (SaO_2 ≥90%). Do not attempt to achieve higher values.

$PaCO_2$ < 10 kPa as long as pH > 7.2. Do not achieve lower values if this requires excessively high tidal volumes ("permissive hypercapnia").

Tidal volumes 6–8 mL/kg to minimize alveolar distension and volutrauma.

Plateau pressures of 30 cmH_2O to minimize alveolar distension and volutrauma.

Positive end-expiratory pressure (PEEP) titrated to achieve best oxygen delivery—commonly 10–15 cmH_2O.

This increases functional residual capacity, recruits alveoli, and puts the lung on the steeper part of the compliance curve.

Higher levels of PEEP should be avoided, as they decrease venous return and thus cardiac output—PEEP should be set to maximize oxygen delivery rather than oxygenation alone

Recruitment maneuvers. This is the use of a high level of CPAP (30–40 cmH_2O) for 30 s in an apneic patient via a ventilator. The aim is to recruit collapsed alveoli, and its occasional use may lead to marked improvements in oxygenation.

pressure. It is expensive and only available in specialist centers.

Extracorporeal membrane oxygenation

Extracorporeal membrane oxygenation (ECMO) consists of a pump oxygenator that performs gas exchange, allowing the lungs to be "rested." This is only available in specialist centers.

Strategies for prevention of postoperative pulmonary complications following craniotomy

The strategies that may be helpful for preventing postoperative respiratory complications include thromboprophylaxis by mechanical and pharmacological means. Prophylactic strategies for venous thromboembolism should be started within the first postoperative week.[20] American College of Physicians guidelines[27] have graded evidence for strategies to reduce risk for PPCs. Postoperative lung expansion modalities (incentive spirometry, deep breathing exercises, intermittent positive-pressure breathing, and CPAP) are the only strategies that are supported by good evidence for reduction in PPCs. Selective rather than routine use of nasogastric tubes and short-acting neuromuscular blockade decrease the risk of PPCs.[28]

Early tracheostomy should be considered in patients with a high cervical spinal cord injury and in those with a need for prolonged duration of mechanical ventilation. Bedside percutaneous dilatational tracheostomy is becoming the popular technique for tracheostomy in neurosurgical patients[29] with a low incidence of complications in neurosurgical patients.

Areas for future research

Most neurological patients have lower Glasgow Coma Scale (GCS) scores on admission. During their hospital stay, they have more intensive care unit (ICU) and ventilator days, with more early tracheostomies and more VAP rates when compared with those of non-neurological patients.[30] However, studies have shown that the rate of reintubation is similar to that of non-neurological patients. Hence, mental status and GCS may not be the only predictors for successful extubation.[31] It is not clear as to why neurological patients are more

likely to get "stuck" on the ventilator or may need early reintubation. The other factors that need to be addressed in this scenario are age, neurological diagnosis, characteristics of tracheobronchial secretions, cranial nerve involvement, pupillary abnormalities, and absence of gag reflex.[32] These questions can be answered by formulating well-designed multicentric prospective clinical trials. Meanwhile the clinical expertise of a neurointensivist may guide the best approach to a particular patient.

References

1. Sogame LC, Vidotto MC, Jardim JR, Faresin SM. Incidence and risk factors for postoperative pulmonary complication in elective intracranial surgery. *J Neurosurg* 2008;109:222–227.
2. American Thoracic Society. Guidelines for the management of adults with hospital-acquired, ventilator-associated, and healthcare associated pneumonia. *Am J Respir Crit Care Med* 2005;171:388–416.
3. Masterton RG, Galloway A, French G et al. Guidelines for the management of hospital-acquired pneumonia in the UK. *J Antimicrob Chemot* 2008;62:5–34.
4. Liberati A, D'Amico R, Pifferi S, Torri V, Brazzi L, Parmelli E. Antibiotic prophylaxis to reduce respiratory tract infections and mortality in adults receiving intensive care. *Cochrane Database Syst Rev* 2009;4:CD000022.
5. National Institute for Health and Clinical Excellence (NICE), National Patient Safety Agency (NPSA). Technical patient safety solutions for ventilator-associated pneumonia in adults. August 2008, Ref: NICE/NPSA/2008/PSG002. Available at: http://guidance.nice.org.uk/PSG002/Guidance/pdf/English
6. McCormick B. Hospital-acquired pneumonia. Update in Anesthesia. *J World Fed Soc Anaesthesiol* 2012;28:188–191.
7. Chastre J, Wolff M, Fagon JY et al. Comparison of 8 vs 15 days of antibiotic therapy for ventilator-associated pneumoniain adults: A randomized trial. *JAMA* 2003;290:2588–2598.

8. Pugin J, Auckenthaler R, Mili N, Janssens JP, Lew PD, Suter PM. Diagnosis of ventilator-associated pneumonia by bacteriologic analysis of bronchoscopic and nonbroncho-scopic "blind" bronchoalveolar lavage fluid. *Am Rev Respir Dis* 1991;143:1121–1129.

9. Zilberberg MD, Shorr AF. Ventilator-associated pneumonia: The clinical pulmonary infection score as a surrogate for diagnostics and outcome. *Clin Infect Dis* 2010;51(Suppl. 1):S131–S135.

10. Rogers FB, Shackford SR, Trevisani GT, Davis JW, Mackersie RC, Hoyt DB. Neurogenic pulmonary edema in fatal and nonfatal head injuries. *J Trauma* 1995;5:860–868.

11. Touho H, Karasawa J, Shishido H, Yamada K, Yamazaki Y. Neurogenic pulmonary edema in the acute stage of hemorrhagic cerebrovascular disease. *Neurosurgery* 1989;5:762–768.

12. Theodore J, Robin ED. Speculations on neurogenic pulmonary edema (NPE). *Am Rev Resp Dis* 1976;4:405–411.

13. Ott L, McClain CJ, Gillespie M, Young B. Cytokines and metabolic dysfunction after severe head injury. *J Neurotrauma* 1994;5:447–472.

14. Mckeating EG, Andrews PJ, Signorini DF, Mascia L. Transcranial cytokine gradients in patients requiring intensive care after acute brain injury. *Br J Anaesth* 1997;5:520–523.

15. Mascia L. Acute lung injury in patients with severe brain injury: A double hit model. *Neurocrit Care* 2009;3:417–426.

16. Deehan SC, Grant IS. Haemodynamic changes in neurogenic pulmonary oedema: Effect of dobutamine. *Intensive Care Med* 1996;22:672–676.

17. Guleria R, Madan K. Pulmonary complications in neurosurgical patients. *Indian J Neurosurg* 2012;1:175–178.

18. Ray K, Bodenham A, Paramasivam E. Pulmonary atelectasis in anaesthesia and critical care. *Contin Educ Anaesth, Crit Care Pain* 2014;5:236–245.

19. Rival G, Patry C, Floret N, Navellou JC, Belle E, Capellier G. Proneposition and recruitment manoeuvre: The combined effect improves oxygenation. *Crit Care* 2011;15:R125.

20. Khaldi A, Helo N, Schneck MJ, Origitano TC. Venous thromboembolism: Deep venous thrombosis and pulmonary embolism in a neurosurgical population. *J Neurosurg* 2011;114:40–46.

21. Guyatt GH, Akl EA, Crowther M, Gutterman DD, Schuunemann HJ. Executive summary: Antithrombotic therapy and prevention of thrombosis, 9th ed: American College of Chest Physicians Evidence-Based Clinical Practice Guidelines. *Chest* 2012;141:7S-47S.

22. Boeer A, Voth E, Henze T, Prange HW. Early heparin therapy in patients with spontaneous intracerebral haemorrhage. *J Neurol Neurosurg Psychiatry* 1991;54:466–467.

23. Cook D, Meade M, Guyatt G et al. Dalteparin versus unfractionated heparin in critically ill patients. *N Engl J Med* 2011;364:1305–1314.

24. ARDS Definition Task Force, Ranieri VM, Rubenfeld GD et al. Acute respiratory distress syndrome: The Berlin definition. *JAMA* 2012;307:2526–2533.

25. Meduri GU, Headley AS, Golden E et al. Effect of prolonged methylprednisolone therapy in unresolving acute respiratory distress syndrome. A randomized controlled trial. *JAMA* 1998;280:159–165.

26. Peter JV, John P, Graham PL et al. Corticosteroids in the prevention and treatment of acute respiratory distress syndrome (ARDS) in adults: Meta-analysis. *BMJ* 2008;336:1006–1009.

27. Qaseem A, Snow V, Fitterman N et al. Clinical Efficacy Assessment Subcommittee of the American College of Physicians. Risk assessment for and strategies to reduce perioperative pulmonary complications for patients undergoing non cardiothoracic surgery: A guideline from the American College of Physicians. *Ann Intern Med* 2006;144:575–580.

28. Smetana GW. Postoperative pulmonary complications: An update on risk assessment and reduction. *Cleve Clin J Med* 2009;76:S60–S65.

29. Browd SR, MacDonald JD. Percutaneous dilational tracheostomy in neurosurgical patients. *Neurocrit Care* 2005;2:268–273.

30. Pelosi P, Ferguson ND, Frutos-Vivar F et al. Management and outcome of mechanically ventilated neurologic patients. *Crit Care Med* 2011;39:1482–1492.

31. Coplin WM, Pierson DJ, Cooley KD, Newell DW, Rubenfeld GD. Implications of extubation delay in brain injured patients meeting standard weaning criteria. *Am J Respir Crit Care Med* 2000;161:1530–1536.

32. Karanjia N, Nordquist D, Stevens R, Nyquist P. A clinical description of extubation failure in patients with primary brain injury. *Neurocrit Care* 2011;15:4–12

32

Postoperative blindness

KIRAN JANGRA and VINOD K. GROVER

Introduction

Postoperative vision loss (POVL) is a rare but devastating complication with an incidence ranging from 0.002% to 0.2%.[1-3] It is defined as partial or complete vision loss after nonophthalmic surgeries. POVL is known to occur after various surgeries such as cardiac, spine, orthopedic, endonasal, and urological procedures.[2-5] There are a few case reports of blindness after transsphenoidal surgeries[6] and embolization of head and neck arteriovenous malformation.[7] Owing to the increased number of complex spinal procedures, the incidence of POVL is one rise following these surgeries.

Clinical anatomy of the visual pathway

Visual sensations are transmitted from the retina to the brain via the visual pathway. The visual pathway starts from the cornea and lens, which focus images on the retina. From the retina, optic nerve fibers carry the visual sensations through optic chiasm to the lateral geniculate body of thalamus, and finally these optic radiations terminate in the occipital lobe. The optic nerve carries fibers from ipsilateral retina only until the optic chiasm where medial fibers decussate. Any pathology causing interruptions in this visual pathway leads to blindness (Figure 32.1).

Arterial supply of the optic nerve

The eye is predominantly supplied by the ophthalmic artery (OA), the first intracranial branch of the internal carotid artery. Posterior ciliary arteries, the central artery of the retina, and pial arteries along the course of optic nerve, emerge from the OA. In addition to these arteries, the anterior portion of the optic nerve also receives blood supply from the posterior ciliary arteries and circle of Zinn-Haller formed by the choroidal and posterior ciliary arteries. Neighboring carotid and hypophyseal arteries strengthen the blood supply of the posterior segment of the optic nerve. The middle segment of the optic nerve receives only small pial arteries, keeping this portion of the optic nerve at risk of ischemia (Figure 32.2).

Causes and pathophysiology of POVL

The causes of POVL after spinal surgery can be categorized into six groups:

1. *External ocular injury*: Direct trauma to the glob or prolonged exposure of the cornea can lead to exposure keratitis, corneal abrasions or lacerations, and glob perorations. These injuries vary in severity from self-limiting injuries to severe trauma necessitating the surgical

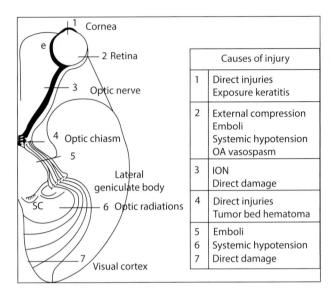

Figure 32.1 Clinical anatomy of the visual pathway and causes of vision loss at different levels of the pathway. Solid lines indicate sites of injuries leading to vision loss. (OA, ophthalmic artery; ION, ischemic optic neuropathy.)

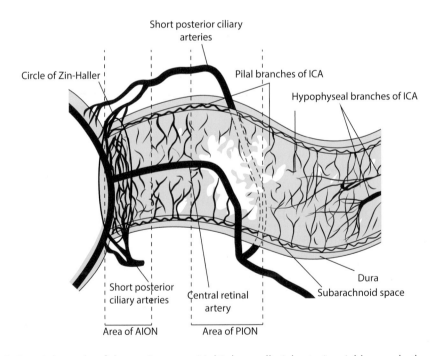

Figure 32.2 Arterial supply of the optic nerve. Multiple small pial arteries richly supply the anterior optic nerve along with branches from the circle of Zinn Haller. The posterior part of the optic nerve also receives supply from the adjacent hypophyseal artery while the midorbital optic nerve is supplied by only the small pial branches making it vulnerable for PION. (ICA, internal carotid artery; AION, anterior ischemic optic neuropathy; PION, ischemic optic neuropathy.)

interventions. External ocular injuries are extremely painful and usually preventable.

2. *Retinal ischemia*: The causes of retinal ischemia include central retinal artery occlusion (CRAO), severe systemic hypotension, or orbital venous outflow obstruction (Figure 32.3).[8] CRAO occurs due to direct compression on the glob and emboli that are either injected near the facial vessels[9] or enter through surgical field during spine surgeries. CRAO cuts off the blood supply of the entire retina while a branch retinal artery occlusion (BRAO) causes a localized injury to the small portion of retina. This complication is mostly observed after major cardiac[3] and vascular surgeries, but after spinal surgeries it occurs due to improper patient positioning causing external compression of the glob.[10] Certain facial anomalies, such as altered facial anatomy, osteogenesis imperfecta, exophthalmos, and lower nasal bridges in the patients belonging to Asian descent, increase the vulnerability to external compression.[11] Patients present with the painless vision loss and abnormal pupil reactivity. At the cellular level, retinal ischemia incites excitotoxicity,[12] hyperemia, and hypoperfusion, which aggravate blindness. Lignocaine and adrenaline "infiltration" of nasal mucosa during endonasal surgeries might cause intense vasospasm of the retinal artery leading to retinal ischemia.[13]

3. *Ischemic optic neuropathy*: Ischemic optic neuropathy (ION) is the most common cause of sudden visual loss in patients undergoing posterior spinal fusion. Anatomical and developmental variations make children more vulnerable for ION.[3] Two types of IONs are described in the literature: anterior ischemic optic neuropathy (AION) and posterior ischemic optic neuropathy (PION). ION is termed as "arteritic" when it occurs secondary to inflammations of blood vessels, as seen in autoimmune disorders, and "nonarteritic" if it occurs due to noninflammatory causes. Perioperatively, nonarteritic PION is more common. AION is usually observed after autoimmune disorders. PION is reported commonly after instrumental spinal fusion operations and head and neck surgeries.[14,15]

The exact etiology of ION is unknown, but a few risk factors are described by the POVL study group (Table 32.1).[16] The vascular risk factors include hypertension, coronary artery disease, diabetes,

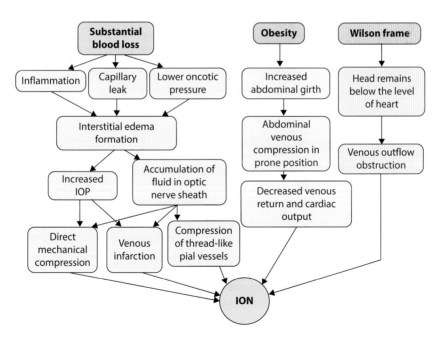

Figure 32.3 Pathophysiology of retinal ischemia. (IOP, intraocular pressure; CRAO, central retinal artery occlusion.)

Table 32.1 Summary of Practice Advisory for Postoperative Visual Loss

	Parameter evaluated	Expert's statements
I	**Preoperative**	
	Evaluation and preparation	Identify the patient characteristics to predict perioperative ION
		There is no neuroophthalmic evaluation to identify the patients at risk
		Small but unpredictable risk factors include prolonged procedures and/or substantial blood loss
II	**Intraoperative management**	
	Blood pressure management	Invasive blood pressure monitoring should be performed in high-risk patients
		Deliberate hypotensive techniques during spine surgery are not associated with the risk of POVL and can be planned on a case-specific basis
	Management of intraoperative fluids	Central venous pressure monitoring should be considered in high-risk patients
		During substantial blood loss, colloids should be used along with crystalloids to maintain intravascular volume
	Management of anemia	Hemoglobin or hematocrit values should be monitored in high-risk patients who had substantial blood loss
		Transfusion threshold and lower limit of hemoglobin concentration associated with the development of POVL are not yet established
	Use of vasopressors	Current evidence is insufficient to guide the use of α-adrenergic agonists in high-risk patients during spine surgery
		Decision should be made on a case-specific basis
III	**Patient positioning**	Facial edema is not associated with perioperative ION
		Direct ocular compression is not associated with isolated perioperative anterior ION or posterior ION but should be avoided to prevent CRAO
		Patient's head should be either at the level of or higher than the heart whenever possible
		Head position should be maintained in a neutral position (i.e., without significant neck flexion, extension, lateral tilt, or rotation)
IV	**Staging of surgical procedures**	In high-risk patients complex spinal procedures should be performed
V	**Postoperative management**	Vision should be assessed as soon as the patient becomes alert
		Once detected, urgent ophthalmologic consultation should be obtained to determine the cause
		Supportive management includes optimizing hemoglobin or hematocrit values, hemodynamic status, and arterial oxygenation
		Magnetic resonance imaging is considered to rule out intracranial pathology
		There is no role of antiplatelet agents, steroids, or intraocular pressure-lowering agents in the treatment of perioperative ION

Source: American Society of Anesthesiologists Task Force on Perioperative Visual Loss. *Anesthesiology* 116:274–285, 2012.

obesity, peripheral vascular disease, and tobacco use while perioperative factors include preoperative anemia, prolonged surgical duration, significant blood loss, excessive crystalloid use for blood loss replacement, and use of the Wilson frame (Figure 32.4).[17] According to the American Society Anesthesiologists (ASA) Registry, the procedures were considered prolonged when they exceed an average duration of 6.5 h, and substantial blood loss was defined as an average loss of 44.7% of estimated blood volume.[16] A few case reports mentioned that the use of vasopressors such as epinephrine and phenylephrine intraoperatively might increase the risk of POVL.[18,19] However, the experimental studies suggested that α-adrenergic receptors are not located in the optic nerve and blood–brain barrier prevents the entry of systemically administered agents in optic nerve, except the prelaminar zone. Therefore, association between the risk of ION and vasopressors use remains unknown.

4. *Cortical blindness*: The causes of cortical blindness include global or focal ischemia, cardiac arrest, hypoxemia, vascular occlusion, intracranial hypertension, exsanguinating hemorrhage, and emboli.[3] Patients may present with the signs of stroke in the parieto-occipital region and agnosia, that is, inability to interpret sensory stimuli. The vision might recover within days, but impairment in spatial perception and in the relationship between sizes and distances may remain for a longer period.[20]

5. *Acute congestive glaucoma*: Acute congestive glaucoma might flare after general anesthesia usually in the prone position for a prolonged period.[21] Patients present with painful red eye, cloudy vision, and headache accompanied by nausea and vomiting. Acute glaucoma might mimic corneal abrasion (painful vision loss but without the pupillary signs) and increased intraocular pressure (IOP) in the presentation.

6. *Posterior reversible encephalopathy syndrome*: Posterior reversible encephalopathy syndrome is also known as reversible posterior leukoencephalopathy syndrome. Presentation of PRES is quite variable ranging from mild neurological symptoms including headaches to altered mental status/function, seizures, and loss of vision. There is symmetric edema in the subcortical white matter and cortices of the occipital and parietal lobes. Though PRES is better known in the obstetric literature and was initially described in

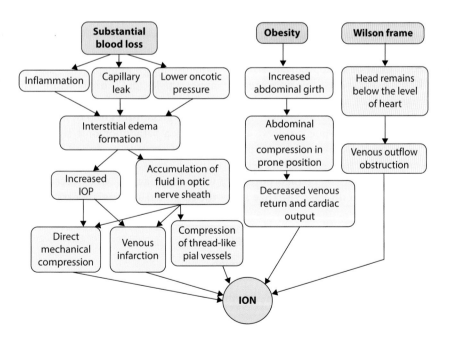

Figure 32.4 Pathophysiology of ischemic optic neuropathy (ION). (IOP, intraocular pressure; CAD, coronary artery disease.)

1996,[22] later it was also described in nonobstetric surgery such as a video-assisted thoracoscopic wedge resection,[23] hysterectomy, lumbar fusion,[24] and Chiari malformation.[25] The exact pathophysiology of PRES is still unknown but two theories are described in the literature. These are hypertensive episodes exceeding the autoregulatory capacity of the cerebral vasculature causing breakthrough brain edema, and cytotoxic drugs or diseases causing endothelial injury leading to edema formation.

Prevention

Once established, POVL has a very dreaded prognosis as the recovery is either partial or absent. So, every effort should be made to prevent this complication. Prevention strategies are summarized in Table 32.2. Corneal injuries can be prevented by a common practice of taping the patient's eyes prior to positioning.[26] To prevent CRAO, the anesthesiologist must avoid compression of the globe. Pressure on the eyes can result from large face masks, use of head rests during the prone position for surgery, and use of goggles as eye shields. A foam or gel headrest should be preferred and eyes should be properly placed such that they are free from pressure. If a horseshoe headrest is used, it must be of appropriate size as a smaller headrest can exert excessive pressure on the eyes. During cervical spine surgeries, head movement by the surgeon might change head position relative to the horseshoe headrest and can cause compression of the eyes. Hence, a pin-type head holder should be preferred during cervical spine surgeries. A mirror can be incorporated underneath the headrest to directly visualize the

eyes. The position of the eyes should be checked intermittently every 20 min by palpation or visualization.[27] During supratentorial surgeries optic nerve handing can cause direct optic nerve damage, and during skull base surgeries, the surgeon can compress the eyeball. So, the anesthesiologist should remain vigilant for oculocardiac reflex during such surgeries as it indirectly reflects glob and optic nerve handling. The maneuvers that decrease the chances of embolization should be used to prevent cortical blindness.[28]

Diagnosis

Vision should be assessed postoperatively in all patients undergoing surgeries that are at risk for POVL as soon as patient regains consciousness. Those patients who present with partial or complete vision loss should be assessed by the ophthalmologist immediately after the detection. The diagnosis is made by a combination of signs and symptoms, examination, and investigations (Table 32.3).

Fundoscopic examination shows either normal disc (Figure 32.5a) in PION and cortical blindness or edematous disc in AION (Figure 32.5b). In the later phase of ION, there can be disc atrophy. In BRAO appearance of the disc varies as per the content of emboli. Cholesterol emboli appear bright yellowish, glistening; calcific emboli are white, nonglistening; and platelet and fibrin emboli appear pale (dull, dirty white) (Figure 32.5c). A "cherry-red spot" on the retina with a pale ground-glass background and attenuated arterioles is a pathognomonic sign of CRAO (Figure 32.5d). Complete occlusion of the retinal artery gives the pale appearance to retina on fundoscopy while the macula, which receives blood through the choroidal arteries, appears red.

Table 32.2 Strategies to Prevent Postoperative Blindness

1. Eyes should be kept closed by simple eye taping
2. External pressure on the eyes should be avoided
3. Optic nerve handling should be minimized intraoperatively and surgeon should be notified immediately of oculocardiac reflex
4. Avoid systemic insults such as severe hypotension, hypoxia, anemia, excessive crystalloids (as a replacement to blood loss), and prolong head-down position
5. Avoid extreme neck positions
6. Complex spinal pathologies should be operated on in stages

Table 32.3 Diagnosis for Postoperative Vision Loss

Cause of blindness	Signs and symptoms	Examination			
		Local	Light reflex	Fundoscopy	Radiology brain and orbit
External corneal injuries	Pain Watering Photophobia Foreign body sensation Burring/clouding of vision	Visible trauma to glob	N	N	N
CRAO	Complete blindness Loss of light perception Signs of trauma near the eye Periorbital and eyelid edema Chemosis, proptosis, and ptosis Paresthesias of supraorbital region Corneal abrasion Loss of eye movements	Chemosis Abrasions	A or RAPD	Cherry-red spot	Proptosis Extraocular muscle swelling
BRAO	Partial painless loss of vision Scotomas	N	N or RAPD	Pale emboli of platelet fibrin Attenuated vessels	Normal
ION	Painless scotomas Partial/complete blindness (in PION, neither patient nor doctor can see anything)	N	A or RAPD	*AION* Optic disc edema Hemorrhages *PION* Initially, normal Later, atrophy	Normal
Cortical blindness	Painless Hemianopia Scotomas	N	N	Normal	Infarct Edema Hemorrhages in occipital lobe
Acute glaucoma	Painful red eye Cloudy or blurred vision Headache Nausea Vomiting Often bilateral	Red watering eye	A	N	Normal
PRES	Seizures Cortical blindness Homonymous hemianopia Blurred vision Decreased level of consciousness Headaches Nausea and vomiting Brainstem symptoms Hemiplegia	N	N	Papilledema	Symmetrical edema in occipital and parieto-occipital cortices and subcortical white matter and posterior frontal lobes

N, normal; RAPD, relative afferent pupillary defect; A, absent; CRAO, central retinal artery occlusion; BRAO, bramch retinal artery occlusion; ION, ischemic optic neuropathy; PRES, posterior reversible encephalopathy syndrome.

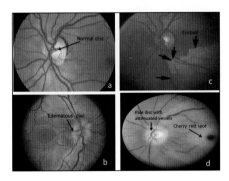

Figure 32.5 Fundoscopic appearance of normal disc (a), Edematous disc seen in anterior ischemic optic neuropathy (b), emboli in attenuated vessels (c), cherry red spot with pale retina in central retinal artery occlusion (d).

Computed tomography (CT) or magnetic resonance imaging (MRI) of the brain is usually not required but if intracranial pathology is suspected, then the radiology helps in localizing the lesion.

Treatment

There is no definitive treatment for POVL and only supportive therapy is used in all of cases (Table 32.4). Mild corneal injuries can be treated with topical lubricants and antibiotics while severe injuries need surgical interventions such as repair or corneal transplant. Treatment of CRAO[29] includes ocular massage, use of arterial dilators, and embolectomy. POVL secondary to ION is treated with supportive treatments to decrease IOP such as diuretics,[30] head-up position, correction of hemodynamics and anemia, and orbital decompression in the presence of intraocular compartment syndrome. There is no role of steroids in the treatment of POVL. There are a few case reports showing benefits of hyperbaric oxygen, use of neuroprotective agents,[31] and drugs that lower IOP, but without any proven efficacy in improving the vision.

Acute congestive glaucoma is an ophthalmological emergency and treatment includes β-adrenergic antagonists, α-adrenergic agonists, carbonic anhydrase inhibitors, cholinergic agonists, corticosteroids, and peripheral iridectomy.[32]

To conclude, perioperative vision loss is a serious complication with medicolegal implications but it is preventable to a great extent. Early diagnosis and timely treatment can preserve vision but recovery is not always complete. Anesthetists, especially those involved in complex spinal procedures in the prone position, must take adequate precautions during positioning and maintain adequate hematocrit and intravascular volumes.

Table 32.4   Treatment of Postoperative Vision Loss

Cause of blindness	Treatment
External corneal injuries	*Mild injury*: lubrication ointments/plugs/artificial tears/contact lenses, antibiotic ointments
	Severe injuries: corneal repair/transplants
Retinal ischemia CRAO/BRAO	(a) *Ocular massage*: to dislodge emboli and decrease IOP
	(b) *Arteriolar dilators*:
	Carbogen inhalation (5% CO_2, 95% O_2; for 10 min, every 2 h for 48 h)
	Pentoxyphylline
	Increases erythrocyte flexibility
	Reduces blood viscosity
	Increases microcirculatory flow and tissue perfusion
	(c) Hyperbaric oxygen (begin within 2–12 h of symptom onset for 10 min every 2 h for 48 h)
	(d) *Embolectomy*:
	Mechanical
	Nd:YAG laser

Cause of blindness	Treatment
ION	No definitive treatment
	Supportive therapy:
	Head-up position
	Correct hypotension and anemia
	Lateral canthotomy—for ocular compartment syndrome
	IOP lower agents (efficacy not proven):
	Diuretics
	Mannitol
	Acetazolamide
	Furosemide
	*No role of steroids
Cortical blindness	Supportive treatment
Acute glaucoma	β-Adrenergic antagonists
	α-Adrenergic agonists
	Carbonic anhydrase inhibitor
	Cholinergic agonists
	corticosteroids
	Peripheral iridectomy
PRES	Treat causative factor
	Cerebral decongestants
	Mechanical ventilation

IOP, intraocular pressure; CRAO, central retinal artery occlusion; BRAO, bramch retinal artery occlusion; h, hours; ION, iscemic optic neuropathy; Nd:YAG, neodymium-doped yttrium aluminum garnet

References

1. Chang SH, Miller NR. The incidence of vision loss due to perioperative ischemic optic neuropathy associated with spine surgery: The Johns Hopkins Hospital Experience. *Spine* 2005;30:1299–1302.
2. Patil CG, Lad EM, Lad SP, Ho C, Boakye M. Visual loss after spine surgery: A population-based study. *Spine* 2008;33:1491–1496.
3. Shen Y, Drum M, Roth S. The prevalence of perioperative visual loss in the United States: A 10-year study from 1996 to 2005 spinal, orthopedic, cardiac, and general surgery. *Anesth Analg* 2009;109:1534–1545.
4. Halvorsen H, Ramm-Pettersen J, Josefsen R et al. Surgical complications after trans-sphenoidal microscopic and endoscopic surgery for pituitary adenoma: A consecutive series of 506 procedures. *Acta Neurochir* 2014;156:441–449.
5. Moslemi MK, Soleimani M, Faiz HR, Rahimzadeh P. Cortical blindness after complicated general anesthesia in urological surgery. *Am J Case Rep* 2013;20:376–379.
6. Tong H, Wei S, Zhou D, Zhu R, Pan L, Jiang J. Vision deterioration after trans-sphenoidal surgery for removal of pituitary adenoma. *Zhonghua Wai Ke Za Zhi* 2002;40:7468.
7. Kim DJ, Kim DI, Lee SK, Kim SY. Homonymous hemianopia after embolization of an aneurysm-associated AVM supplied by the anterior choroidal artery. *Yonsei Med J* 2003;44:1101–1105.
8. Crockett AJ, Trinidade A, Kothari P, Barnes J. Visual loss following head and neck surgery. *J Laryngol Otol* 2012;126:418–420.
9. Park SW, Woo SJ, Park KH, Huh JW, Jung C, Kwon OK. Iatrogenic retinal artery occlusion caused by cosmetic facial filler injections. *Am J Ophthalmol* 2012;154(4):653–662.
10. Delattre O, Thoreux P, Liverneaux P et al. Spinal surgery and ophthalmic complications: A French survey with review of 17 cases. *Spinal Disord Tech* 2007;20:302–307.
11. Bradish CF, Flowers M. Central retinal artery occlusion in association with osteogenesis imperfecta. *Spine* 1987;12:193–194.

12. Roth S, Pietrzyk Z. Blood flow after retinal ischemia in cats. *Invest Ophthalmol Vis Sci* 1994;35:3209–3217.

13. Awad J, Awad A, Wong Y, Thomas S. Unilateral visual loss after a nasal airway surgery. *Case Rep* 2013;6:119–23.

14. Ho VTG, Newman NJ, Song S, Suzan S, Ksiazek S, Steven Roth. Ischemic optic neuropathy following spine surgery. *J Neurosurg Anesthesiol* 2005;17:38–44.

15. Özkiriş M, Akin I, Özkiriş A, Adam M, Saydam L. Ischemic optic neuropathy after carotid body tumor resection. *J Craniofac Surg* 2014;25(1):58–61.

16. American Society of Anesthesiologists Task Force on Perioperative Visual Loss. Practice advisory for perioperative visual loss associated with spine surgery: An updated report by the American Society of Anesthesiologists Task Force on Perioperative Visual Loss. *Anesthesiology* 2012;116:274–285.

17. Lorri AL. Perioperative visual loss and anesthetic management. *Curr Opin Anesthesiol* 2013;26:375–381.

18. Lee LA, Deem S, Glenny RW et al. Effects of anaemia and hypotension on porcine optic nerve blood flow and oxygen delivery. *Anesthesiology* 2008;108:864–72.

19. Lee LA, Lam AM. Unilateral blindness after prone lumbar surgery. *Anesthesiology* 2001;95:793–795.

20. Grover VK, Jangra K. Perioperative vision loss: A complication to watch out. *J Anaesth Clin Pharmacol* 2012;28:11–16.

21. Singer MS, Salim S. Bilateral acute angle closure glaucoma as a complication of facedown spine surgery. *Spine J* 2010;10(9):7–9.

22. Hinchey J, Chaves C, Appignani B et al. A reversible posterior leukoencephalopathy syndrome. *N Engl J Med* 1996;334:494–500.

23. Eran A, Barak M. Posterior reversible encephalopathy syndrome after combined general and spinal anesthesia with intrathecal morphine. *Anesth Analg* 2009;108:609–612.

24. Yi JH, Ha SH, Kim YK, Choi EM. Posterior reversible encephalopathy syndrome in an untreated hypertensive patient after spinal surgery under general anesthesia. *Korean J Anesthesiol* 2011;60:369–372.

25. Hansberry DR, Agarwal N, Tomei KL, Goldstein IM. Reversible encephalopathy syndrome in a patient with a Chiari malformation. *Surg Neurol Int* 2013;4:130.

26. Grover VK, Kumar KV, Sharma S, Sethi N, Grewal SPS. Comparison of methods of eye protection under general anaesthesia. *Can J Anaesth* 1998;45:575–577.

27. Roth S. Postoperative vision loss. In: Miller RD, editor. *Textbook of Anesthesia*, 7th ed. New York: Elsevier; 2010, p. 2826.

28. Pugsley W, Klinger L, Paschalis C, Treasure T, Harrison M, Newman S. The impact of microemboli during cardiopulmonary bypass on neuropsychological functioning. *Stroke* 1994;25:1393–1399.

29. Cugati S, Varma DD, Chen CS, Lee AW. Treatment options for central retinal artery occlusion. *Curr Treat Options Neurol* 2013;15:63–77.

30. Hayreh SS. Anterior ischaemic optic neuropathy: III, Treatment, prophylaxis, and differential diagnosis. *Br J Ophthalmol* 1974;58:981–989.

31. Arnold AC, Levin LA. Treatment of ischemic optic neuropathy. *Semin Ophthalmol* 2002;17:39–46.

32. Emanuel ME, Parrish RK, Gedde SJ. Evidence-based management of primary angle closure glaucoma. *Curr Opin Ophthalmol* 2014;25(2):89–92.

PART IX

Basics of neuroradiology

33

Understanding neuroradiology

S. LEVE JOSEPH DEVARAJAN

Introduction

The neuroradiology of today is multifaceted. On the clinical front it serves two important roles, namely diagnostic and therapeutic (or interventional). On the basic science aspect, it is indispensable in the fields of neurobiology, pharmacology, neurolinguistics, and behavioral science, among others. This chapter reviews the clinical aspects of neuroradiology in two parts: diagnostic neuroradiology and interventional neuroradiology.

Diagnostic neuroradiology

The modalities

We present here a modality-wise overview of diagnostic neuroradiology.

Plain radiography

1. Skull radiography is almost obsolete, yet its basic principles such as positioning, projections, various anatomical landmarks, and lines are fundamental to the understanding and practice of other higher imaging modalities, especially angiography.

2. Some peripheral centers still use skull radiographs to evaluate bony sella and skull injuries.
3. Plain radiographs of the spine, especially the dynamic ones are, however, the mainstay of the various abnormalities of the spine and postsurgical assessment.
4. Flexion and extension views of the craniovertebral junction (CVJ) are a must in the presurgical evaluation of the CVJ anomalies. Similarly, radiographs with axial loading are very useful in the evaluation of degenerative spine, scoliosis, listheses, and so on.

Myelograms are occasionally useful in the postoperative settings.

Ultrasonography and color Doppler

1. Antenatal ultrasonography is helpful in the diagnosis of congenital anomalies, for example, myelomeningocele, holoprosencephaly, and vein of Galen aneurysmal malformation.
2. Neurosonography is a very useful investigation in neonatal conditions such as hypoxic ischemic encephalopathy, germinal matrix hemorrhage, and vein of Galen aneurysmal malformation.

3. Carotid ultrasound and Doppler are screening tools for atherosclerotic carotid disease. Carotid stenosis and dissection can be evaluated.[1] Other major vessels in the neck and their abnormalities can also be noninvasively evaluated.

4. Transcranial Doppler is an indispensable tool for monitoring for vasospasm in patients with subarachnoid hemorrhage (SAH). It can also help diagnose patent foramen ovale and forms a part of stroke workup.

Computerized tomography

Physical principles

A thin beam of X-rays from an X-ray tube is passed across an object (patient). A row of detectors placed on the other side of the object receives the rays and calculates their attenuation, which is proportional to the density of the object. Rotation of this tube-detector assembly allows the user to obtain multiple such projections. Complex mathematical algorithms are used by the computer to reconstruct a cross-sectional image of the object from multiple projections.

Indications

Computed tomography (CT) scan has become such a basic tool in the practice of clinical neurosciences that a comprehensive description of its indications here is not practical. However, we present a classified description of indications based on the relative importance or utility of CT in various clinical situations.

1. When CT scan is essential:
   a. In acute head trauma: To assess for bony and brain parenchymal injuries.
   b. In acute stroke: To rule out intracranial bleed. In the case of an ischemic stroke, to locate and assess the extent of parenchymal involvement. To identify arterial occlusion if possible.
   c. In SAH: Location of the sentinel hematoma, grading, complications such as hydrocephalus and infarcts secondary to vasospasm
   d. In Figure 33.1(i) central nervous system (CNS) infection: Meningitis and complications such as hydrocephalus, brain abscess, subdural empyema, CNS tuberculosis, and neurocysticercosis (NCC). Contrast CT may be needed in these conditions.
   e. Brain tumors: To assess the number, location, mass effect, and tumor matrix for calcification, hemorrhage and necrosis. Density may indicate cellularity and hence sometimes the histological type (Figure 33.1(iii)).
   f. Evaluation of bony skull in congenital anomalies, infections, and tumors.
   g. Evaluation of an unconscious patient when a structural cause is suspected.
   h. Patient follow-up: Postoperative follow-up, monitoring ventricle size in shunted patients, for example, monitoring treatment response in chronic infections such as tuberculosis (TB) and NCC.
   i. Spine CT: Evaluation of congenital anomalies including CVJ anomalies, diastematomyelia, and segmentation anomalies; primary or secondary vertebral neoplasms; degenerative spinal diseases.

2. When CT scan can be a useful initial investigation:
   a. In the evaluation of chronic headache.
   b. Epilepsy: CT can identify granulomas, benign cortical tumors, calcifications, and gross anomalies.
   c. In cases of metabolic encephalopathy.
   d. Cranial neuralgias.
   e. Degenerative diseases.

Advanced CT applications

Recent technological advances in CT hardware have ushered in multislice CT and dual-energy CT. In a single gantry rotation, multislice CT allows acquisition of multiple slices, which may be 16, 64, 128, 256, or even 512 in some of the advanced scanners, which effectively means that in a very short span of time (in seconds), longer length, hence larger volume, of a patient can be scanned along the z-axis, that is, head–foot axis. This, combined with ever advancing computational power and software techniques, has resulted in effective and exquisite clinical CT applications. Some of them have been described here.

1. *CT angiography (CTA):* The entire arterial tree starting from the arch of aorta until the distal intracranial arteries can be imaged with high spatial resolution and without much venous contamination by injecting only 50–60 mL of contrast intravenously. This is made possible by rapidity of the scanning (as described in the previous paragraph),

Illustrative CT images

IMAGING IN SAH

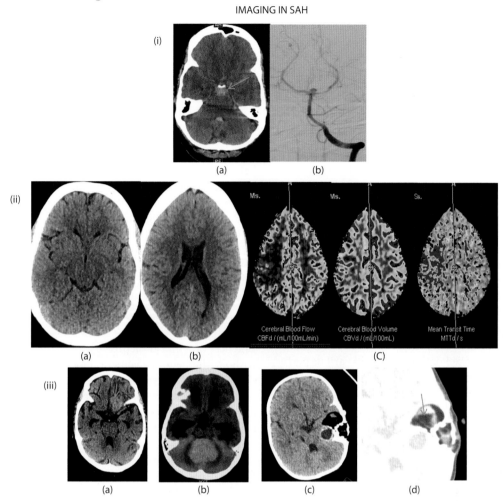

Figure 33.1 Imaging in SAH (i) CT reveals SAH with extension in fourth ventricle. Larger hematoma in the prepontine cistern (arrow), called sentinel hematoma, can indicate the location of the aneurysm. DSA revealed basilar top aneurysm. (ii) A 56-year-old man presented with acute left hemiparesis within 3 hours of onset. NCCT did not reveal any obvious infarct. CT perfusion revealed decreased CBF, normal CBV, increased MTT, indicating the presence of penumbra, which means potentially salvageable brain parenchyma. (iii) CT attenuation better correlates with histology. In a proven case of CNS lymphoma, plain CT reveals a hyperdense mass lesion (arrow in a). Hyperdensity of the mass lesion on plain CT suggests high cellularity. Subpart (b) shows a hyperdense cerebellar lesion in a child proved later to be a medulloblastoma. Fat containing lesion with calcification (c and d) s/o teratoma. Arrow in (d) indicates fat component.

contrast bolus tracking technique, and state-of-the-art injectors that permit contrast injection in a tight bolus followed by saline chase. The following are the clinical applications of CTA:

a. *In acute stroke:* The presence and site of large vessel occlusion can be known in a matter of seconds. Further, multiphasic CTA permits collateral scoring, which can be useful for selecting patients for mechanical thrombectomy.[2]

b. In patients with *recent or old stroke* and those with *transient ischemic attacks*, CTA is the choice for vascular imaging if contrast administration is otherwise not contraindicated.

c. *In SAH:* Aneurysms can be detected and evaluated for planning intervention though digital subtraction angiography (DSA) is the gold standard investigation for the purpose.

d. *Intracranial arteriovenous malformations (AVMs):* DSA is better; however CTA can be conducted in a case of intracranial bleed of uncertain etiology.

e. *Other applications:* Moyamoya disease, follow-up of bypass shunts such as external carotid artery (ECA)/internal carotid artery (ICA) and ECA/middle cerebral artery (MCA), spinal vascular diseases, in skull base tumors to assess vascular encasement, and in cervical spinal anomalies—for presurgical evaluation of vertebral artery anatomy.

2. *CT perfusion:* The first pass of an iodinated contrast agent through the cerebral vasculature after an IV bolus is monitored by multiple dynamic scans. Complex deconvolution analysis of the time–density curves obtained for the arterial and venous regions of interest (ROIs) and each pixel of the brain yield various perfusion parameters such as cerebral blood volume, cerebral blood flow, and mean transit time. CT perfusion applications in neuroradiology are given next.

   a. *In acute stroke:* Perfusion parameters help to assess the presence and volume of the penumbra, that is, potentially salvageable hypoperfused tissue (Figure 33.1(ii)).[3]

   b. *Tumor:* To assess tumor neovascularity, differentiate between radiation necrosis and glioma recurrence.

   c. *In vasospasm:* In SAH setting, vasospasm and its response to treatment can be monitored.

3. *Dual-energy CT:* This uses X-ray beams of two energies, for example, 80 and 140 keV, which are differentially attenuated by tissue depending on their material content. This in turn can be used to probe tissues for their content or nature. Examples of clinical applications include differentiation between hemorrhage and contrast enhancement (iodine) and between iodine and calcium in a contrast-enhanced CT (CECT) of the brain.

CT-guided interventions

CT-guided biopsy of vertebral and paravertebral lesions is part of a routine of any busy neuroradiology department. With the advent of CT fluoroscopy, procedures such as vertebroplasty, kyphoplasty, and even some external spinal fixations are performed under CT guidance. CT myelograms are sometimes used in the evaluation of postoperative spine and in locating a cerebrospinal fluid (CSF) leak in cases of CSF rhinorrhea or otorrhea.

Radiation dose

CT scan involves substantial radiation exposure. The relative radiation doses to the patient from various CT examinations are given in the table below. Hence, CT scans should be used judiciously in clinical practice.

a. Background radiation is 3 mSv/year
b. CXR = 0.1 mSv
c. CT head = 2 mSv
d. CT chest = 8 mSv
e. CT abdomen and pelvis = 20 mSv

Magnetic resonance imaging

Practice of clinical neurology or neurosurgery without the help of magnetic resonance imaging (MRI) is virtually unimaginable today. Apart from providing excellent soft tissue contrast and anatomic detail, MRI is capable of giving functional information also. Understanding the working of MRI requires a grasp of higher physics including quantum mechanics and higher mathematics among other things quite alien to a medical practitioner.[4] Detailing of physical principles of MRI is hence beyond the scope of this chapter. However, a basic description of various MR sequences and the appearance of normal brain structures and common pathology are given in the next section.

Basic MRI sequences

T1-weighted image

Gray matter appears gray and white matter appears relatively white; ventricles and CSF spaces are dark on T1. T1 images are better suited for studying anatomy. The majority of pathologies appear hypointense or dark on T1 images. A few things that appear bright on T1 are fat, hemorrhage, soft calcification, melanin, and protein.

T2-weighted image

Gray matter appears gray and white matter appears relatively dark; ventricles and CSF spaces are bright on T2. T2 images are better suited for studying pathology in a given case. The majority of pathologies appear hyperintense or bright on T1 images. A few things that appear dark on T2 are hemorrhage, soft calcification, melanin, and protein.

Fluid-attenuated inversion recovery

A fluid-attenuated inversion recovery (FLAIR) sequence is basically a T2-weighted image in which CSF (water) signal has been selectively suppressed. Therefore, ventricles and CSF spaces are dark on FLAIR images whereas pathological fluid appears bright.

Susceptibility-weighted imaging

Susceptibility-weighted imaging (SWI) is used in clinical practice for detection of calcification and bleed. Both show blooming (increased dark signal) on SWI images.

Diffusion-weighted image

Diffusion-weighted image (DWI) forms a powerful tool in the assessment of hydrogen motion. Entrapped water molecules (hydrogen atoms) show restricted diffusion and appear bright on DWI images.

Short tau inversion recovery

A short tau inversion recovery (STIR) sequence suppresses bright T1 signal. It is used to suppress fat signal and is useful in spine imaging.

Post-contrast enhanced MRI

T1-weighted post gadolinium images are used to characterize lesions based on their enhancement pattern.

Advanced MRI techniques

Magnetic resonance spectroscopy

Magnetic resonance spectroscopy (MRS) enables us to determine the biochemical nature of either lesions or brain parenchyma. It is a very useful technique in assessment of conditions such as brain abscess, tumor, and metabolic diseases.

MR perfusion

MRI perfusion with or without contrast is used to characterize cerebral perfusion, as is done by CT perfusion.

Functional MRI

Functional MRI (FMRI) helps us in localizing various functional areas such as the motor or speech area in relation to a given pathology. This provided invaluable information for presurgical planning, thereby minimizing postoperative neurological deficit.

Diffusion tensor imaging

Diffusion tensor imaging (DTI) is used for identifying various white matter tracts and understanding their relation to the cerebral or spinal lesion.

Indications for MRI

MRI can be useful virtually in any of the neurological or neurosurgical conditions. The role may vary such as making a diagnosis or differential diagnoses, evaluating the disease process, planning treatment, and assessing treatment response. The following is a list of common indications for MRI.

1. *Congenital*: MRI is useful is diagnosing various cranial and spinal congenital malformations with the help of volumetric sequences. MRI has also enabled us in to make these diagnoses antenatally.
2. *Brain tumors*: Basic MR sequences in conjunction with MRS and MR perfusion are required for diagnosis, grading, treatment planning, follow-up, and prognostication in patients with brain tumors.
3. *Stroke:* DWI imaging helps in an early and accurate detection of infarct. Diffusion–perfusion mismatch allows estimating penumbra in acute stoke cases.[5] MR angiography and vessel wall imaging are part of the vascular workup of a stroke case.
4. *Infections*: MRI helps in detection and characterization of granulomas, abscess, and pachymeningeal and leptomeningeal diseases.
5. *Degenerative*: Degenerative disease of the spine is adequately evaluated with MRI. It allows for assessment of disc bulge, ligament or facet joint hypertrophy, spinal or nerve root compression, and postoperative changes. In degenerative diseases of the brain and spinal cord, MRI can assess disease extent, severity, and progression.
6. *Metabolic conditions*: MRI is indispensable in the evaluation of neurometabolic conditions

which can be congenital, for example, enzyme deficiencies or acquired in nature.

7. *Demyelinating diseases*: Evaluation and follow-up of primary or secondary demyelinating diseases.

8. *Psychiatric diseases*: MRI, especially its advanced applications such as FMRI and DTI, can prove useful in the imaging of the brain as well. Some of the well-known psychiatric conditions like schizophrenia have been recently found to have structural correlates.

Illustrative MRI cases

See Figures 33.2–33.5.

Interventional neuroradiology

The practice of interventional neuroradiology comprises diagnostic neuroangiography and neurointerventional procedures. Since it is based on plain radiography, it evolved early in the history of neuroradiology, well before the advent of cross-sectional imaging. The technique of cerebral angiography was first developed in 1927 by the Portuguese physician Egas Moniz at the University of Lisbon. The practice of therapeutic neurointervention started in the 1960s and has made rapid strides in recent decades.

Neuro cath lab

A biplane angiosuite, that is, one with two C-arms, is recommended for neurovascular work. The A plane, usually floor mounted, is provided with the capability of 3D rotational angiography. The B plane is ceiling mounted and moves on rails. The following, though not exhaustive, is the list of essentials to be present in a neuro cath lab.

1. An array of monitors or a large single monitor with multiformat viewing
2. A programmable power injector synced with the main machine
3. Mobile translucent radiation barriers
4. Multiple cupboards housing the various hardware (catheters, guide wires, coils, etc.) and drugs used in angiography or neurointervention
5. A state-of-the-art anesthesia machine
6. One set of anesthesia monitors mounted in the console (outside the main radiation area)

Neuroangiography

DSA of the brain and spine, named neuroangiography, is the gold standard investigation for the diagnosis and evaluation of the most neurovascular disorders. It generally includes evaluation of aortic arch and extracranial head and neck vasculature also. Successful performance of neuroangiography in any patient requires careful planning and meticulous techniques, and hence should always be performed by a skilled angiographer.[6] Attention should be paid to each of the steps discussed in the following:

Clinical assessment
Patient preparation
Vascular access
Procedure: technique
Interpretation
Post-procedure care

Clinical assessment

The following simple questions should be raised before embarking on neuro-DSA in a given patient: Why has this examination been ordered? How will it affect management? What is the current neurological status of the patient? Answering these questions requires a quick evaluation of the history and clinical status. In particular understanding the indication for the DSA is essential to plan and tailor the examination. The common indications and their usual clinical presentations are given in Table 33.1. Uncooperative patients, particularly those with altered consciousness, may require general anesthesia (GA). There would be a common inertia to administer GA for the sake of a diagnostic procedure. However, taking an early decision in favor of GA will ultimately save time and prove safe too.

Neuroangiography: How to perform?

As indicated earlier in the "Neuroangiography" section, neuroangiography requires careful execution of precise techniques. In fact, each institution has its own methods of practice and tries to inculcate certain "good habits" in its fellows and residents performing neuroangiography. In general, a cerebral or spinal DSA examination comprises sequential execution of the following steps:

1. *Patient preparation*: Time should be spent to explain to the patient and/or the family about the procedure and possible complications such

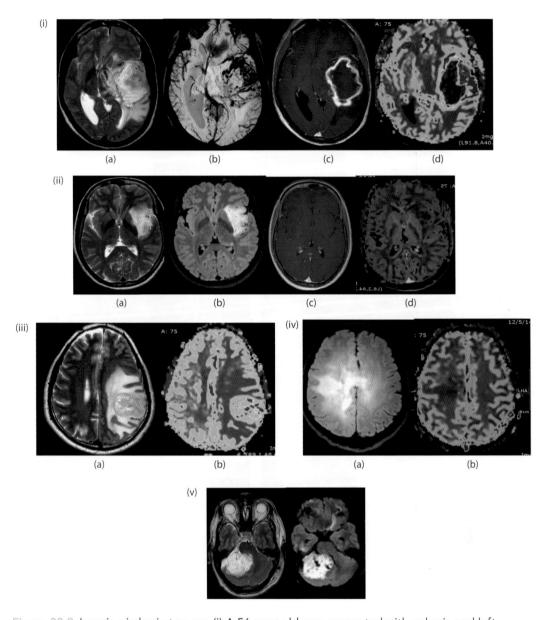

Figure 33.2 Imaging in brain tumors. (i) A 56-year-old man presented with aphasia and left hemiparesis. MRIs reveal mass with heterogeneous signal on T2 (a), irregular peripheral enhancement on post gad (c), blooming on SWI (b), and high perfusion on CBV maps (d). Histology: glioblastoma multiforme. (ii) A 30-year-old woman presented with seizures. MRIs reveal mass with homogenous hyperintense mass on T2 and FLAIR (a, b), no enhancement on post gad images (c), and low perfusion on CBV maps (d). Histology: low-grade astrocytoma. (iii) A 67-year-old woman presented with seizures. MRIs reveal heterogeneous mass with perilesional edema on T2 (a) and increased perfusion on CBV maps (b). Histology: metastasis. (iv) A 47-year-old man presented with headache. MRIs reveal mass heterogeneous infiltrative mass on T2 (a) and no increase in perfusion on CBV maps (b). Histology: gliomatosis cerebri. (v) A 35-year-old woman presented with ataxia. MRIs reveal a hyperintense mass (a) with diffusion restriction on DWI (b) Histology: epidermoid.

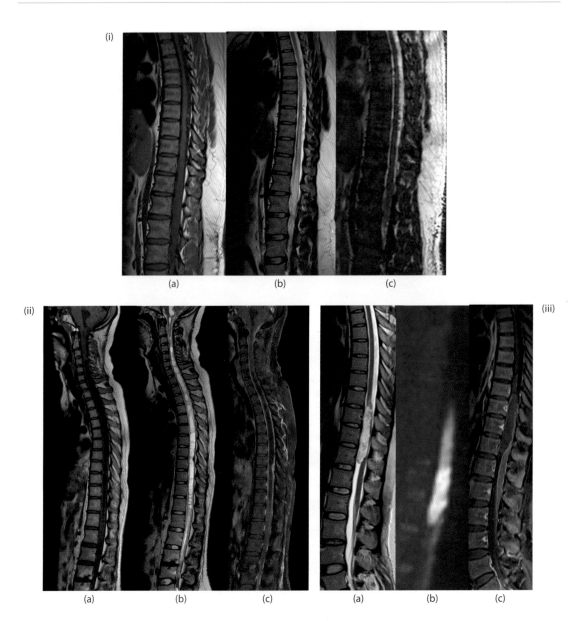

Figure 33.3 Imaging in spinal pathologies. (i) A 45-year-old man with H/O gradually progressive paraparesis, involuntary jerks, and bladder bowel incontinence for 1 year. MRIs reveal long segment intramedullary T2 hyperintensity (b) with multiple vascular flow voids along surface of cord on T2 and heavily volumetric T2 image (b and c), suggesting spinal vascular malformation. DSA (not shown here) proved it to be a spinal dural AVF. (ii) MRI in a 34-year-old woman with progressive myelopathy over 6 months. T1 (a) and T2 (b) images showing extensive cord cavitation and signal changes with loss of CSF–cord interface. Post-contrast image (c) shows extensive irregular surface enhancement. These features are consistent with *arachnoiditis*, often tubercular in etiology in endemic countries. (iii) Diffusion restriction (b) in a focal nonenhancing lower dorsal lesion (a, c) in a young man. It was proved to be *epidermoid*, in which diffusion restriction is a consistent finding.

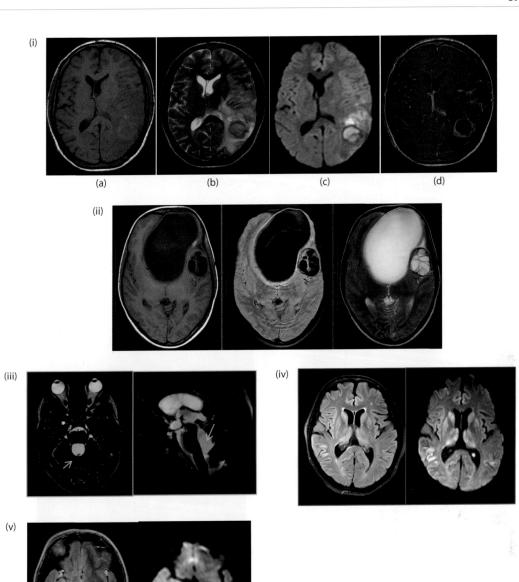

Figure 33.4 Imaging in brain infections. (i) Focal left parietal lesion with surrounding edema in a young lady presenting with seizure. The walls of the ring enhancing (d) lesion were subtly bright on T1 (a) and dark on T2 (b) images with the core of the lesion showing diffusion restriction (c). Adjacent meninges also show enhancement (d). A diagnosis of CNS tuberculosis was made, which was later proved by surgery. (ii) Multilocular cystic lesions in left frontal lobe in a middle-aged man. Proved to be hydatid cyst on surgery. (iii) Intraventricular neurocysticercosis. Heavily T2-weighted volumetric images nicely depict the cyst with eccentric scolex in the IV ventricle. (iv) A case of Creutzfeldt–Jakob disease (CJD), which typically affects basal ganglia and cortices. FLAIR shows hyperintensity in these areas (a) where diffusion restriction is also noted (arrow in b). (v) A case of herpes simplex encephalitis in which temporal lobe, insula, and cingulate gyrus (limbic system) are typically affected.

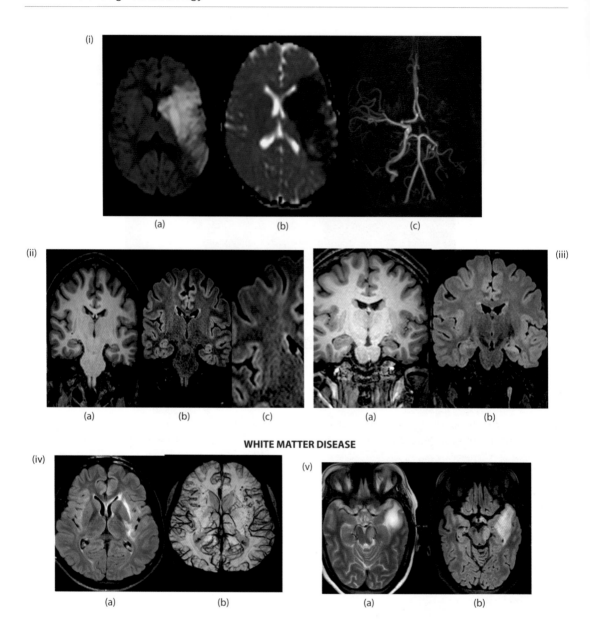

Figure 33.5 Imaging in acute infarct. (i) MRIs in a 42-year-old man with acute-onset right hemiparesis reveal a large area of diffusion restriction in left MCA territory (a and b) with nonvisualization of left MCA on MR angiography images. (ii) Coronal MRIs of a 22-year-old man with intractable epilepsy reveal cortical thickening with subcortical hyperintensity in left superior frontal sulcus consistent with focal cortical dysplasia. (iii) Coronal MRIs of an 18-year-old man with intractable epilepsy reveal atrophy with FLAIR hyperintensity in left hippocampus, consistent with left MTS. Coronal images better depict hippocampal anatomy. (iv) MRIs reveal FLAIR hyperintensities (a) with multiple foci of blooming on SWI (b) both in lesion and normal appearing brain parenchyma, consistent with CNS vasculitis. (v) Large areas of T2 and FLAIR hyperintensity (a and b) with minimal mass effect as compared to extent of the lesion; findings favor diagnosis of tumefactive demyelination.

Table 33.1 Indications for Neuroangiography

1. Cerebral
   a. Evaluation of intracranial aneurysms presenting with SAH or mass effect or incidentally detected on imaging
   b. Dissecting aneurysms, vascular dysplasias
   c. Extracranial aneurysms like posttraumatic dissecting aneurysms of carotid artery
   d. Intracranial AVMs—presenting with bleed or chronic symptoms
   e. Dural sinus pathologies—sinus thrombosis, dural AVMs
   f. Posttraumatic high-flow fistulas in head and neck, for example, carotid-cavernous fistula (CCF), vertebral-venous fistula, carotid-jugular fistula
   g. Acute stroke
   h. Recurrent stroke, TIAs—evaluation of neck vessels and intracranial vessels
   i. Tumors—to asses vascularity, vascular encasement, patency of circle of Willis
   j. Other neurovascular pathologies—vasculitis, Moyamoya disease, scalp AVMS, orbital AVMs, and so on.

2. Spinal
   To evaluate for spinal vascular malformations that can present such as:
   a. Progressive myelopathy in the middle-aged or older population
   b. Acute myelopathy, frequently with hematomyelia in adolescents and young adults
   c. Intradural macrofistulas or rarely AVMS in young kids
   d. Syndromic conditions with metameric malformations, for example, Klippel–Trenaunay syndrome

as contrast reaction and embolism though they are very rare. The following is the checklist one should pay attention to before taking a patient for DSA.

   a. Blood investigations such as serum creatinine, B urea, electrolytes, prothrombin time (PT), and international normalized ratio (INR).
   b. Patient counselling and informed consent.
   c. Part preparation (shaving of lower abdomen, groins, and upper thigh).
   d. At least 6 hours of fasting.
   e. Bowel preparation in the case of spinal DSA when the suspected malformation is in the lower thoracic or lumbar region.
   f. Possibility of interventional treatment in the same sitting, if it exists, should be discussed beforehand.

2. *Vascular access*: Femoral artery at the groin, usually on the right side, is the preferred site for vascular access. Radial or brachial artery puncture or direct carotid puncture may be performed when femoral access is impossible or contraindicated. A local anesthetic agent (6–8 mL) is injected under the skin at the puncture site and also deeply on either side of the common femoral artery. The modified Seldinger (single puncture) technique is used for femoral artery puncture. A long 18 G (or thinner one in children) beveled needle is used for this purpose. Subsequently, a short 6 F femoral sheath is deployed in the iliac–femoral artery over a guide wire. A 4 F sheath is used in pediatric patients. Bilateral femoral access may be needed for some interventional procures or when balloon test occlusion is planned during diagnostic angiography. Bolus heparin is given at a dose of 50 IU/ kg once the sheath is placed.

3. *Selective catheterization*: For a complete cerebral DSA, all six major arteries in the neck, namely the internal carotid artery, external carotid artery, and vertebral arteries on each side should be selectively catheterized sequentially. Usually a 5 F diagnostic catheter is used in adults. Six-to-eight milliliters of 50% nonionic iodinated contrast is injected by hand in each vessel while the corresponding intracranial vasculature is imaged by DSA. Care should be taken to include venous phase in each run. Conscious patients should be clearly instructed beforehand not to shake or move their head during an angiographic run when they may feel a warm sensation in the head. Movement blur in the images can rob vital information. Quick evaluation should be made after each angiographic run. Any suspicion of abnormality should

trigger further focused evaluation. Any indication of presence of an aneurysm in a particular angiographic run warrants a 3D rotational angiography of that vessel. A complete spinal angiography requires injection of bilateral subclavian and vertebral arteries, all the intercostals and lumbar arteries, and bilateral internal iliac arteries, especially when searching for a spinal dural A-V fistula. However, a targeted examination may be sufficient when a preprocedural diagnosis is made with reasonable confidence by other noninvasive means.

4. *Post-procedure care*: The femoral sheath should be carefully removed and the puncture site should be compressed until complete hemostasis is obtained. The usual compression time is 10–15 min but may be prolonged in some patients, especially those receiving antiplatelets. Nowadays puncture site closure devices are also available. The (punctured) lower limb should be kept straight for at least 6 h. Adequate hydration should be maintained. Mobile patients can resume normal activity in 24 h.

Neurointerventional procedures

Rapid technological advances in the past one and half decades, especially in the materials used in the neurointervention, have revolutionized the practice of interventional neuroradiology. The expanse and effectiveness of neurointervention have increased phenomenally. It is beyond the scope of this chapter to dwell in detail on the multitude of neurointerventional procedures. Following are some of the general points pertinent to neurointervention followed by illustrated examples of a few major procedures:

- Most of the neurointerventional procedures are performed under GA because absolute immobility of the patient is needed during the entire procedure, such as aneurysm coiling and glue injection in AVMs, which may sometimes last for several hours.
- Since the patient is under GA, the anesthetist assumes the prime role in the monitoring of vitals and neurophysiological parameters. Invasive blood pressure monitoring is advisable. Usually the anesthetist is the first one to alarm about any intraprocedural mishaps like aneurysm rupture.

- The anesthetist may be called on to alter the blood pressure favorably. Intentional hypotension may be required in AVM embolization during the injection of glue.
- Bradyarrhythmias, requiring prompt reaction, can occur during angioplasty of carotid stenosis or secondary to trigeminocardiac reflex in certain intracranial interventions.
- Intracranial aneurysm treatment:
  - The International Subarachnoid Aneurysm Trial (ISAT) trial proved the superiority of endovascular coiling over surgical clipping.[7]
  - Aneurysms with narrow neck (<3 mm) or with favorable dome/neck ratio (>1.6) are treated by simple coiling.
  - Wide-necked aneurysms can be treated by balloon- or stent-assisted coiling. Recent introduction of "flow diverters" has made even aneurysms with unfavorable anatomy like very wide necked, fusiform aneurysms and dysplastic aneurysms amenable to endovascular treatment.
    - Such technological advances have made it possible to treat more than 90% of aneurysms with endovascular means. The concerns of aneurysm recurrence raised in the ISAT have also been addressed.
- *Intracranial AVM treatment*:
  - Liquid embolic agents used are N-butyl cyanoacrylate (glue) and ethylene vinyl alcohol (EVOH).
    - A microcatheter is advanced as close as possible to the nidus, which is then permeated with liquid embolics.
- Acute stroke treatment: Recent trials have proved the superiority of mechanical thrombectomy over IV thrombolysis or conservative treatment.[8]
- Dural AVF treatment: Complete understanding of angioarchitecture venous drainage and altered hemodynamics is essential to treat these rather difficult conditions. Endovascular embolization is the mainstay of treatment for these lesions.
- Some therapeutic interventions such as carotid artery stenting and balloon embolization of carotid-cavernous fistulas are performed under local anesthesia with anesthetic monitoring.

Illustrative neurointervention cases

See Figures 33.6 through 33.9.

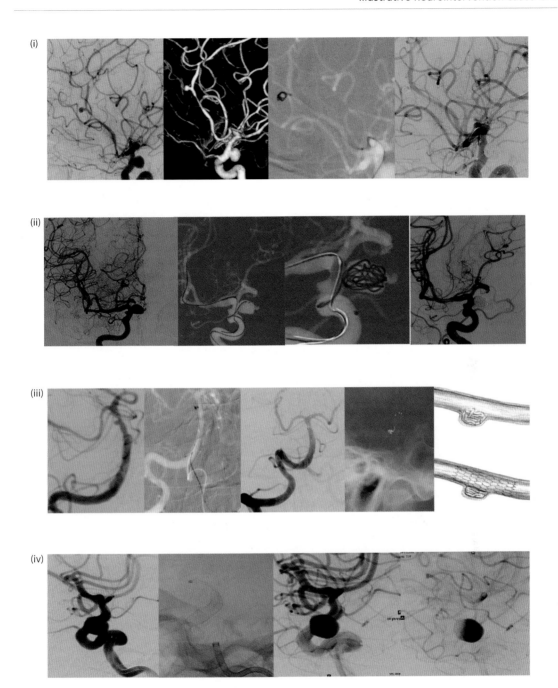

Figure 33.6 Various ways to treat aneurysms. (i) Direct coiling of distal ACA aneurysm. (ii) Balloon-assisted coiling of superior hypophyseal aneurysm. (iii) Stent-assisted coiling of mid basilar aneurysm. (iv) Flow diverter placement in large superior hypophyseal aneurysm.

Intracranial AVMs

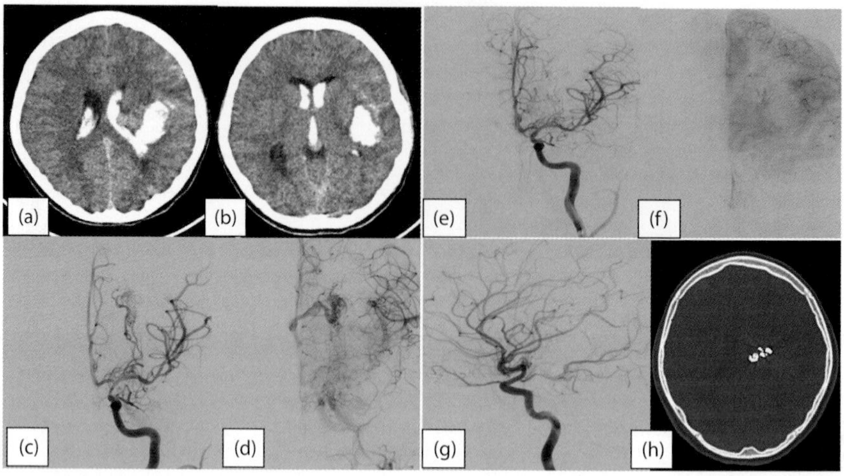

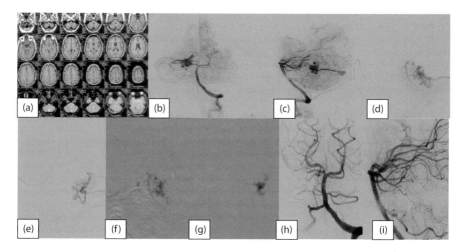

Figure 33.7 A 15-year-old boy presented with sudden-onset severe headache followed by loss of consciousness. Plain CT (a, b) showed left basal ganglia bleed with intraventricular extension. Initial DSA (c and d) showed left striatal AVM with major feeder from left lateral lenticulostriate artery. Glue embolization of AVM was performed through a single pedicle. Post embolization check runs (e, f, and g) showed complete obliteration of AVM. Post-embolization CT (h) showed the glue cast.

Figure 33.8 A 50-year-old man with history of severe headache and vomiting. (a) MRI shows bleed in the right superior cerebellar hemisphere. (b and c) Right superior cerebellar AVM with feeding artery pseudoaneurysm. (d and e) Microcatheter injections show two different compartments of AVM nidus. (f and g) Glue cast in feeding a. pseudoaneurysm and nidal component. (h and i) Check angiogram shows complete obliteration of AVM and pseudoaneurysm.

Dural AVF

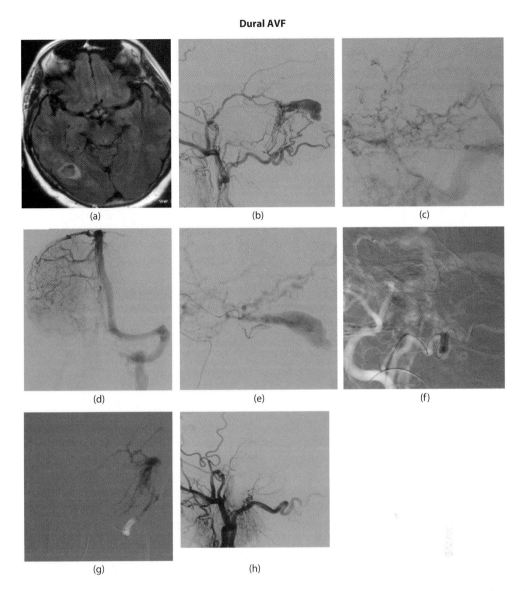

(a) (b) (c)

(d) (e) (f)

(g) (h)

Figure 33.9 (a–h) A 63-year-old woman presented with sudden-onset headache. The MRI (a) showed intraparenchymal hemorrhage with adjacent abnormal vascular flow voids in the right parietotemporal region. DSA (b, c, and d) performed 1 month later showed right transverse DAVF with isolated sinus and secondary cortical venous reflux (Cognard type 2b) with congestive cortical venous strain. Right transverse sinus was thrombosed. (e and f) Embolization was performed through transarterial route with a microcatheter in the middle meningeal artery and flow arrest with balloon occlusion of the right occipital artery. (g) Subsequent glue embolization was performed from the middle meningeal artery. (h) Check angiogram showed complete occlusion of fistula. The patient was stable with no neurological symptoms on follow-up after 18 months.

References

1. Qureshi AI, Suri MF, Ali Z et al. Role of conventional angiography in evaluation of patients with carotid artery stenosis demonstrated by Doppler ultrasound in general practice. *Stroke* 2001;32:2287–2291.

2. V. Nambiar, Sohn SI, Almekhlafi MA et al. CTA collateral status and response to recanalization in patients with acute ischemic stroke. *Am J Neuroradiol* 2014;35:884-890.

3. Vo KD, Yoo AJ, Gupta A et al. Multimodal diagnostic imaging for hyperacute stroke. *Am J Neuroradiol* 2015;36:2206–2213.

4. Westbrook C. *Handbook of MRI Technique,* 4th ed. Hoboken, NJ: Wiley-Blackwell; 2014.

5. Wintermark M, Ko NU, Smith WS, Liu S, Higashida RT, Dillon WP. Vasospasm after subarachnoid hemorrhage: Utility of perfusion CT and CT angiography on diagnosis and management. *AJNR Am J Neuroradiol* 2006;27:26–34.

6. Morris P. *Practical Neuroangiography,* 3rd ed. Philadelphia, PA: Lippincott Williams & Wilkins; 2013.

7. Molyneux A, International Subarachnoid Aneurysm Trial (ISAT) Collaborative Group. International Subarachnoid Aneurysm Trial (ISAT) of neurosurgical clipping versus endovascular coiling in 2143 patients with ruptured intracranial aneurysms: A randomised trial. *Lancet* 2002;360:1267–1274.

8. Yarbrough CK, Ong CJ, Beyer AB, Lipsey K, Derdeyn CP. Endovascular thrombectomy for anterior circulation stroke: Systematic review and meta-analysis. *Stroke* 2015;46:3177–3183.

Basics of neurointensive care

34

Basic principles of neurointensive care

SWAGATA TRIPATHY

Introduction

The critically ill patient with a primary neurologic disorder is best managed in a neurocritical care unit. The specialized care provides an interface between the brain and the various other organ systems of the body while catering to the unique requirements of a deranged physiology.

The basic tenets of neuroprotection such as optimizing cerebral perfusion pressure (CPP) with improved oxygen delivery and minimizing cerebral metabolic oxygen requirement, which have presumably begun in the emergency room or operating theater, have to be maintained in the critical care unit. Time has to be given after this for the "damaged, but protected brain" to heal itself. This difference in the duration of stay of the patient in a compromised status is where lies the role of neurocritical care—in preventing further neurologic (and other systemic) injury, and recognizing and treating ongoing and new onset threats. All this has to be done while maintaining normal homeostasis in the hitherto *normal* organs surrounded by abnormal milieu.

Critical care for specific neurologic conditions

1. *Cerebrovascular accident*: A common cause of admission in the critical care unit, acute stroke usually presents with sudden onset weakness. Rapid classification and thrombolization may improve outcome as time is brain.[1-5]
   a. *Resuscitation*: Airway protection if Glasgow Coma Scale (GCS) score is less than or equal to 8, ensuring normoxia and normocarbia. Care to be taken against intubation-related raised intracranial pressure (ICP) by giving adequate induction agents.

Rules of airway management

- Gentle intubation with good preoxygenation
- Adequate suppression of airway reflexes with drugs as needed
- No tube ties, allow good jugular venous drainage
- Regular blood gases and ventilation adjusted to keep $PaO_2 > 100$ mmHg and $PaCO_2$ 30–40 mmHg
- Gentle suctioning (on demand)

---

b. Urgent noncontrast computed-tomography (CT) scan to rule out intracerebral hemorrhage (ICH)—go to step "h" in case of hemorrhagic stroke.

c. *Management of hemodynamics*: If planned for thrombolysis, target a blood pressure (BP) less than 185/110 mmHg. If not, target for less than 220/110 mm Hg. Any reduction must be gradual, using monitored infusion of agents such as labetalol and sodium nitroprusside.

d. If received within 3 h (4.5 in nondiabetic patients without history of previous stroke, less than 80 years of age) of stroke onset, consider thrombolysis with tissue plasminogen activator (tPA): 90 mg/kg body weight, 10% given as bolus over 1 min followed by infusion over 1 h. Proper patient selection for thrombolytic therapy is vital as is close neurologic monitoring in the intensive care unit (ICU) after thrombolysis; any decrease in the GCS score must be assumed to be due to hemorrhage and thrombolysis should be stopped. Invasive procedures such as nasogastric tube/urinary catheter insertion may be delayed until 24 h after thrombolysis. Antiplatelets and anticoagulants are also started after 24 h after a normal follow-up noncontrast head CT scan.

e. After 24 h of thrombolytic therapy (or at presentation in patients who are not thrombolysed), antiplatelet therapy with 325 mg aspirin followed by 150–325 mg daily is started. If the patient is allergic, then 75 mg clopidogrel is recommended.

f. Monitor in ICU with basic neurologic bundles; anticipate neurologic deterioration due to any of three complications: infarct expansion, infarct-related edema, or hemorrhagic transformation of the ischemic stroke. Infarct expansion would warrant less aggressive correction of hypertension, edema medical ICP management, and hemorrhagic transformation withholding antiplatelets and anticoagulants.

g. Investigate and treat for risk factors of stroke such as lipid, vasculitis, and thrombophilia profile in young patients with stroke, echocardiogram (for embolic source), carotid Doppler study (for critical carotid stenosis), HbA1c, and Holter monitoring for paroxysmal atrial fibrillation.

h. In hemorrhagic stroke confirmed by a noncontrast CT scan of the brain, resuscitation and general ICU care follows the neurocritical care bundle and step a. BP will need to be reduced judiciously: aggressive reduction if >200 systolic blood pressure (SBP) or >150 mean arterial pressure (MAP) = (SBP + 2DBP)/3, where DBP is diastolic blood pressure.

i. Raised ICP if suspected (or measures as per the unit protocol) needs to be managed medically or surgically if indicated.

j. In patients with coagulopathy, fresh frozen plasma, platelets, or activated factor VII may be considered.

k. Electroencephalogram (EEG)-proven or new onset seizures need to be treated with antiepileptic drugs. Prophylaxis is not warranted.

l. In young, nonhypertensive patients, cerebral angiography may be considered.

m. Surgical management may be considered in cerebellar hemorrhage, brain stem compression, and hydrocephalus or for ICP management in the form of external ventricular drain (EVD) placement of decompressive craniotomy.

n. General care as per neurocritical care bundle (NCC) bundle.

Neurocritical care bundle

1. PaO_2 > 100 mmHg
2. $PaCO_2$ < 40 >30 mmHg
3. Blood sugar < 150 mg%
4. Normothermia
5. Euvolemia
6. Adequate nutrition approx. 20–30 kcal/kg/day with 1-2 g/kg protein with aspiration prophylaxis
7. Bowel and bladder care
8. Bedsore prevention and care
9. Skin and eye care
10. Deep vein thrombosis (DVT) prophylaxis (chemical or mechanical)
11. Stress ulcer prophylaxis
12. Normal serum electrolytes
13. ICP < 20 mm Hg, CPP > 60 mm Hg (CPP= MAP – ICP), where ICP is

intracranial pressure, MAP is mean arterial pressure, and CPP is cerebral perfusion pressure

14. Medical management of raised ICP with bolus therapy of mannitol 10–20% (1 g/kg IV) over 10–20 min repeated as needed, hypertonic saline bolus, and elevation of head end of the bed by 30°

15. Safe intrahospital transport

2. *Subarachnoid hemorrhage (SAH):* Most commonly due to a ruptured aneurysm, SAH may also be seen in trauma, arteriovenous malformation (AVM), hemorrhagic infarction, and hypertensive hemorrhage. The patient usually presents with severe headache, nausea, and photophobia with altered mental status. A high degree of suspicion and rapid diagnosis is related to better outcome.[6–8]

   a. Resuscitation and airway protection to ensure normocarbia and avoid hypoxia in obtunded patients.

   b. Focused history about sentinel headaches, trauma, hypertension, anticoagulant/antiplatelet intake, and cocaine abuse.

   c. Urgent noncontrast CT of head may be followed by a lumbar puncture (xanthochromia and crenated red blood cells [RBCs]) if in doubt. Sensitivity of CT in detecting SAH decreases with time.

   d. If confirmed as SAH, severity assessment with the Hunt and Hess scale or the World Federation of Neurosurgical Societies (WFNS) classification may predict prognosis.

The Hunt and Hess scale

1. Asymptomatic or mild headache, and slight neck rigidity
2. Moderate-to-severe headache, neck rigidity, no neurological deficit other than cranial nerve palsy
3. Drowsiness/confusion, mild focal neurological deficit
4. Stupor, moderate-to-severe hemiparesis
5. Coma, decerebrate positioning

The WFNS classification

1. GCS 15, no motor deficit
2. GCS 13 or 14, no motor deficit
3. GCS 13 or 14, motor deficit present
4. GCS 7–12, motor deficit absent or present
5. GCS 3–6, motor deficit absent or present

   e. Initial treatment will consist of bed rest to prevent rebleed of aneurysm with adequate analgesia. Titration of BP to avoid rebleed while maintaining a good perfusion pressure will need to be closely monitored along with the neurologic status in the ICU. Mannitol administration has been known to precipitate rebleed by affecting aneurysm transmural gradient.

   f. These patients need to be closely monitored for neurologic deterioration, which may be difficult to detect when the patients are sedated and ventilated. Monitoring of cerebrospinal fluid (CBF), cerebral oxygenation, and CPP should go along with routine ICU monitoring. ICP monitoring is desirable along with a jugular bulb catheter, cerebral function analysis, near-infrared spectroscopy, and cerebral microdialysis where available.

   g. A four-vessel cerebral digital subtraction angiography (DSA) is the gold standard among imaging modalities: if not feasible, an initial CT or magnetic resonance (MR) angiogram may be considered.

   h. A decision on endovascular coiling versus microsurgical clipping may be made in a multidisciplinary setup with an interventional radiologist and a neurosurgeon depending upon the patient and aneurysm characteristics and available services at the center—evidence suggests better outcomes with endovascular coiling in patients equally suited for both types of treatment.[6]

   i. After definitive treatment, ICU care is for preventing, detecting, or treating vasospasm—the notoriously dreaded complication after SAH. Onset typically starts at days 3–5, peaking over days 5–14, and resolving over 2–4 weeks thereafter. Risk factors include age, higher grade of SAH, and amount of blood. Oral nimodipine

60 mg 4 hourly for 21 days is administered at this stage and is known to decrease poor outcomes from SAH. It is important at this stage of care to avoid dehydration, aiming for euvolemia, inducing hypertension (keeping MAP > 110 mmHg with titrated vasopressor infusion), and keeping the hematocrit around 30%. The typical triple-H therapy is controversial with increased cardiopulmonary complications.[7] Bedside transcranial Doppler (TCD) studies allow early detection of vasospasm in the ICU.

j. Acute hydrocephalus or delayed ventriculomegaly may be another complication in patients with SAH. This manifests as change in the GCS score and is detected by a noncontrast CT scan. Careful drainage (to prevent rebleed due to sudden decompression) or CSF diversion may be required.

k. Hyponatremia may occur in patients with SAH due to syndrome of inappropriate antidiuretic hormone (SIADH) or cerebral salt-wasting syndrome. The two may be differentiated clinically: the patient with SIADH appears euvolemic and needs carefully titrated fluid restriction (to avoid ischemic deficits), whereas the patient with cerebral salt-wasting syndrome is treated with volume repletion using isotonic fluids.

l. Deranged autonomic control and raised ICP seen in SAH may cause cardiac (arrhythmias, nonspecific ECG changes, etc.) and pulmonary (neurogenic pulmonary edema) dysfunction. Management involves treating the underlying cause and symptomatic support such as mechanical ventilation.

m. Seizure prophylaxis may be warranted before aneurysm is secure. Long-term prophylaxis is not recommended.

n. General care as per the NCC bundle.

3. *Acute head injury*: Head injury is an important cause of mortality and morbidity in patients 15–45 years of age. Good outcomes, defined as Glasgow Outcome Scale (GOS) 1 or 2 < vary widely. The magnitude of primary injury depends on the severity of impact and mechanism of injury. Intracranial hematoma, contusion, or axonal injury leads to activation of an injury cascade consisting of inflammation, ischemia, and release of excitatory amino acids, calcium ions, and oxidants. This causes secondary neurologic damage—cell swelling, synaptic dysfunction, and breakdown of the blood–brain barrier (BBB). The goal of critical care of traumatic brain injury (TBI) is to minimize secondary injury and allow recovery of the damaged tissue.[9]

Glasgow Outcome Scale

1 = Good recovery
2 = Moderate disability
3 = Severe disability
4 = Vegetative state
5 = Dead

Good outcome = 1 and 2
Poor outcome = 3–5

---

a. Resuscitation and airway control with cervical spine control as required. Primary and secondary survey as per trauma care guidelines.

b. Imaging with noncontrast CT head and cervical spine to evaluate the injury.

c. Proceed to surgery if amenable for surgical evacuation (extradural or subdural hematoma or contusion with midline shift).

d. Institute ICP monitoring along with invasive arterial line monitoring and central venous catheter.

e. Establish TCD or other multimodality monitor as per institute protocol.

f. Seizure prophylaxis (with phenytoin or carbamazepine) to reduce early posttraumatic epilepsy.

g. Keep ICP < 20 mm Hg with CPP > 70 mmHg with the following:
   i. Medical management with 20% mannitol (2 mL/kg three times or till plasma 320 mOsm/L), hypertonic saline 3%/7.5% until serum sodium 155 mEq/dL; increase MAP with fluids or vasopressors.

ii. Ensure normothermia with surface or endovascular cooling modalities. Diagnose and treat subclinical seizures.

iii. Sedation and paralysis as per unit protocol (with monitoring of bispectral index).

iv. Hypothermia may be instituted[10] up to 33°C.

v. Consider surgical decompression (results controversial) in the case of intracranial hypertension refractory to all medical management.

vi. Hyperventilation to reduce $PaCO_2$ to <30 mmHg may be attempted for short durations (in impending herniation); prolonged hyperventilation is contraindicated as it results in deleterious vasoconstriction.

h. There is no role of steroids in the management of TBI.

i. General care as per the NCC bundle.

Causes of secondary brain injury

- Hypotension (SBP < 90 mmHg)
- Hypoxemia (PaO_2 < 60 mmHg; O_2 saturation < 90%)
- Hypocapnia ($PaCO_2$ < 35 mmHg)
- Hypercapnia ($PaCO_2$ > 45 mmHg)
- Hypertension (SBP > 160 mmHg or MAP > 110 mmHg)
- Anemia (hemoglobin [Hb] < 100 g/L or hematocrit [Ht] < 0.30)
- Hyponatremia (serum sodium < 142 mEq/L)
- Hyperglycemia (blood sugar > 10 mmol/L)
- Hypoglycemia (blood sugar < 4.6 mmol/L)
- Hypoosmolality (plasma osmolality [POsm] < 290 mOsm/kg H2O)
- Acid-base disorders (acidemia, pH < 7.35; alkalemia, pH > 7.45)
- Fever (temperature > 36.5°C)
- Hypothermia (temperature < 35.5°C)

---

4. *Postoperative care*: Postoperative care after neurosurgery in the ICU may have many indications—preoperative cardiopulmonary disease; prolonged surgery with severe blood loss; need for ICP monitoring; need for ventilation; need for induced hypertension for CPP maintenance or hypotension after AVM surgery; recovery from hypothermia, coagulopathy, or unstable hemodynamics.

a. Close neurologic monitoring in the postoperative period—continuous monitoring of ICP, MAP, arterial blood gases, and half hourly monitoring of GCS. TCD, EEG, and evoked potentials may be monitored if indicated.

Advances in multimodality monitoring including near-infrared spectroscopy, jugular bulb saturation, cerebral microdialysis, and so on, may be used as available. Although strong evidence is lacking, multimodal monitoring may improve outcomes in critically ill patients by individualized targeting of the pathophysiology.[11]

b. Ventilation and sedation—Compromised central ventilatory drive due to drug or disease is to be anticipated. Ventilation must maintain normoxia and avoid hyper- or hypocapnia: both are deleterious. Well-titrated sedation and analgesia will improve management of blood gases in the desired range. Continuous sedoanalgesia with fentanyl, sufentanil, and propofol in various combinations may be used as per the unit protocol. Prolonged propofol infusion beyond 48–72 h has to be monitored for lipid load. Midazolam infusion may be used but is associated with delayed awakening as compared to propofol. Dexmedetomidine infusion has been tried in recent times and is showing promising results in the ICU, especially in reducing ventilator days and delirium. The Richmond Agitation Sedation Scale (RASS) along with the Confusion Assessment Method for ICU (CAM-ICU) are popular (among others) tools for assessment of sedation and delirium in ICU patients.[12,13]

c. Postoperative pain and appropriate analgesia is an important consideration for first 48–72 h. Subtemporal and suboccipital routes are associated with maximum postoperative pain. Assessment can be as per ICU protocol, with the Numeric Pain Scale or the Wong–Baker FACES Pain Rating Scale. Intravenous paracetamol up to 4 g in 24 h and diclofenac 75 mg 8 hourly (in the absence of bleeding or renal problems) may be given in brain surgeries: morphine sulfate works well in spinal surgeries.

d. Hemodynamic monitoring—Invasive arterial pressure is routine in the neuro-ICU. Central venous pressures and pulmonary artery catheterization (PAC) have limited indications. PAC may be replaced by the less-invasive continuous cardiac output monitoring where available.

e. Common complications in the postoperative patient include specific ones such as intracranial bleed, seizures, and fluid–electrolyte imbalance. Nonspecific complications include cardiac arrhythmias, myocardial infarction, and cardiac failure; infections such as ventilator-associated pneumonia (VAP), central line infections, urinary tract infections, and meningitis from external ventricular drains; deep vein thrombosis (DVT); and pulmonary embolism. All neurosurgical patients must be on mechanical DVT prophylaxis in the intra- and postoperative periods: systemic heparinization in case of DVT or pulmonary embolism is contraindicated and a caval filter may be required to prevent recurrence.

5. *Status epilepticus*: A continuous generalized convulsive seizure of more than 5-min duration or two or more seizures during which the patient does not return to baseline consciousness is defined as convulsive status epilepticus (CSE).

   a. Begin resuscitation and airway control.
   b. 50% Dextrose, 50 mL and thiamine 100 mg IV.
   c. Lorazepam 4 mg IV, repeated 2 mg after 10 min.
   d. Phenytoin 20 mg/kg (50 mg/min) or fosphenytoin 15–20 mg.
   e. Repeat phenytoin (or fosphenytoin at equivalent dose) 5–10 mg/kg if seizures persist.
   f. Midazolam 0.2 mg/kg loading dose followed by infusion 0.1–2.0 mg/kg/h: propofol 1–2 mg/kg loading may also be used followed by infusion 2–10 mg/kg/h.

Observe and manage for hypotension and loss of airway control. End point of sedation is an EEG burst suppression. May taper and stop if patient remains seizure free for 24 h.

   g. General ICU support and care.
   h. Investigate for underlying cause and treat.

6. *Acute flaccid paralysis*: Patients with neuromuscular weakness due to any cause are usually admitted to the ICU for respiratory failure, which is usually progressive in nature and requires ventilator support. A detailed neurologic examination and investigations such as electromyogram, nerve conduction studies, CSF examination, and nerve or muscle biopsies are required for a diagnosis.[14] Complete details are outside the scope of this text.

   a. Guillain–Barré syndrome (GBS) is more commonly associated with an acute gastrointestinal or respiratory tract infection; history of recent immunization, surgery, or organ transplant may be sought.
   Symmetric ascending motor paralysis with loss of deep tendon reflexes and minimum sensory involvement is a hallmark. Autonomic dysfunction, bulbar palsy, and respiratory failure may be fatal.
   By the second week of the disease, a CSF study may reveal albumin cytologic dissociation with normal glucose. Features of demyelination may appear in electrodiagnostic studies.
   Treatment—Plasmapheresis three to five cycles (40–50 mL/kg per exchange) or intravenous immunoglobulin (IVIG) 400 mg/kg/day for 5 days. The choice may be one of availability, although IVIG is preferred in hemodynamically unstable patients, and may be reserved for after plasmapheresis. There is no role of the use of corticosteroids in GBS.[15]

   b. Myasthenia gravis—An autoimmune disease in which antibodies are directed against the acetylcholine receptors of the neuromuscular junction. The disease usually progresses from affecting the extraocular muscles to generalized weakness involving limb, facial, and oropharyngeal muscles.
   Treatment—Acetylcholinesterase inhibitors and immunomodulators such as

steroids or azathioprine are used for treatment. Myasthenia gravis presenting as respiratory failure for the first time to the neuro-ICU is uncommon. Usually, a patient who is a known case of myasthenia and on medications has an acute crisis and respiratory compromise following a stress like an infection, surgery, or anesthesia. Cholinergic crisis (due to excessive usage of therapeutic drugs) may confound the diagnosis and can be differentiated by the Tensilon test—if a cholinergic crisis, 1 mg IV edrophonium worsens the patient's condition. Management in the ICU includes care of the respiratory failure by invasive or noninvasive mechanical ventilation, treatment of the precipitating disease, and administering plasmapheresis to help tide over the crisis by washout of the offending antibodies. The role of IVIG is less clear in this disease. General care as per the NCC bundle.

c. Critical illness neuropathy and myopathy—Weakness, muscle wasting, and loss of deep tendon reflexes with relative facial sparing is the common finding of critical illness neuropathy (CIN). This usually follows sepsis and multiorgan dysfunction and has also been described in trauma, burns, and so on. Diagnosis may be confirmed by nerve conduction studies (reduced compound muscle action potentials) and electromyography (fibrillation and sharp waves in proximal and distal muscles). Critical illness myopathy (CIM) includes a wide range of diseases from disuse atrophy to necrotizing muscle disease. Prolonged neuromuscular paralysis with muscle relaxants along with use of steroids has been implicated in this disease. Treatment for both CIN and CIM are supportive and nonspecific.

References

1. Warburton LA. Management of acute ischemic stroke. In: Matta BF, Menon DK, Turner JM, editors. *Textbook of Neuroanesthesia and Critical Care*. Oxford: Greenwich medical media; 2002, pp. 353–369.
2. The National Institute of Neurological Disorders and Stroke rt-PA Stroke Study Group. Tissue plasminogen activator for acute ischemic stroke. *N Engl J Med* 1995;333:1581–1587.
3. Chan S, Hemphill JC 3rd. Critical care management of intracerebral hemorrhage. *Crit Care Clin* 2014;30:699–717.
4. Morgenstern LB, Hemphill JC 3rd, Anderson C et al. Guidelines for the management of spontaneous intracerebral hemorrhage: A guideline for healthcare professionals from the American Heart Association/American Stroke Association. *Stroke* 2010;41(9):2108–2129.
5. Connolly ES Jr, Rabinstein AA, Carhuapoma JR et al. Guidelines for the management of aneurysmal subarachnoid hemorrhage: A guideline for healthcare professionals from the American Heart Association/American Stroke Association. *Stroke* 2012;43(6):1711–1737.
6. Diringer MN, Bleck TP, Hemphill JC 3rd, et al. Critical care management of patients following aneurysmal subarachnoid hemorrhage: Recommendations from the Neurocritical Care Society's Multidisciplinary Consensus Conference. *Neurocrit Care* 2011;15(2):211–240.
7. Dankbaar JW, Slooter AJ, Rinkel GJ, Schaaf IC. Effect of different components of triple-H therapy on cerebral perfusion in patients with aneurysmal subarachnoid haemorrhage: A systematic review. *Crit Care* 2010;14: R23.

Anterior horn cells and nerves	Neuromuscular junction	Myopathies
Guillain–Barré syndrome (GBS)	Myasthenia gravis	Periodic paralysis
Toxic neuropathies	Lambert–Eaton syndrome	Mitochondrial diseases
Amyotrophic lateral sclerosis	Botulism	Metabolic myopathies
Critical illness polyneuropathy	Drugs	Polymyositis
		Critical illness myopathy

8. Tripathy S, Mahapatra AK. Targeted temperature management in brain protection: An evidence-based review. *Indian J Anaesth* 2015;59(1):9–14.

9. Le Roux P, Menon DK, Citerio G et al. Consensus summary statement of the International Multidisciplinary Consensus Conference on Multimodality Monitoring in Neurocritical Care: A statement for healthcare professionals from the Neurocritical Care Society and the European Society of Intensive Care Medicine. *Neurocrit Care* 2014;21(Suppl. 2):S1–S26.

10. Joseph B, Haider A, Rhee P. Traumatic brain injury advancements. *Curr Opin Crit Care* 2015;21(6):506–511.

11. Erdman MJ, Doepker BA, Gerlach AT, Phillips GS, Elijovich L, Jones GM. A comparison of severe hemodynamic disturbances between dexmedetomidine and propofol for sedation in neurocritical care patients. *Crit Care Med* 2014 Jul;42(7):169–702.

12. Teitelbaum JS, Ayoub O, Skrobik Y. A critical appraisal of sedation, analgesia and delirium in neurocritical care. *Can J Neurol Sci* 2011 Nov;38(6):815–825.

13. Teitelbaum JS, Ayoub O, Skrobik Y. A critical appraisal of sedation, analgesia and delirium in neurocritical care. *Can J Neurol Sci* 2011 Nov;38(6):815–825.

14. Chawla R, Todi S (editor). *ICU Protocols: A Stepwise Approach*. India: Springer; 2012.

15. Review. Tripathy S. Nutrition in the neurocritical care unit. *J Neuroanaesthesiol Crit Care* 2015;2:88–96

Special considerations

35

Pregnancy

VASUDHA SINGHAL

Introduction

Pregnancy poses a unique challenge to a neuroanesthesiologist in that the principles of management for neurosurgery and pregnancy are contradictory. While one warrants a slow controlled induction, the other demands a rapid-sequence induction to tackle the full-stomach situation. Moreover, both the maternal and the fetal well-being should be taken into consideration.

Requirement of neurosurgery during pregnancy

1. *Intracranial hemorrhage (ICH):*
   a. Overall incidence: 6.1 per 100,000 deliveries—7.1% of all pregnancy-related mortality[1]
   b. Risk of ICH greatest in postpartum period
   c. Most common are the following:
      i. Subarachnoid hemorrhage (SAH) due to ruptured arterial aneurysms
      ii. Arteriovenous malformations (AVM)—risk of rebleeding 25% during the same pregnancy (3%–6% risk during the first year in the general population)
   d. *Risk factors:*
      i. Advanced maternal age
      i. African American race
      ii. Hypertensive diseases
      iii. Coagulopathy
      iv. Tobacco abuse[2]
   e. Parity may confer a moderate long-term protective effect on the risk of SAH.[3]
2. *Brain tumors:*
   a. Incidence not increased in the pregnant population.
   b. Meningiomas may become symptomatic during pregnancy due to water retention, engorgement of vessels, and the presence of sex hormone receptors on tumor cells.[4]
   c. Choriocarcinoma—an aggressive gestational tumor—metastasizes to the brain.

d. Clinical diagnosis challenging—symptoms may mimic hyperemesis gravidarum in early pregnancy and eclampsia in late pregnancy.

e. Urgent surgery may be required in:
    i. Malignancies
    ii. Active hydrocephalus
    iii. Benign brain tumors associated with signs of impending herniation or progressive neurological deficit

f. Increased incidence of VP (ventriculo-peritoneal) shunt complications—shunt displacement and occlusion—due to increased intraabdominal pressure and anatomical changes.[5]

3. *Spinal tumors*:
    a. Symptomatic disc herniation—1:10,000 pregnancies[6]
    b. Severe backache common—due to ligamentous laxity caused by high serum levels of relaxin and by extra mechanical stress
    c. 85% patients with symptomatic disc herniation due to nerve root compression improve with conservative management within 6 weeks[5]
    d. Urgent surgery may be indicated in:
        i. Disc herniation with worsening neurological deficit, or cauda equina symptoms
        ii. Newly symptomatic spinal tumors
        iii. Spontaneous spinal epidural hematoma (SSEH), vertebral canal abscess, or spinal AVMs—uncommon indications[7–9]

4. *Traumatic brain injury*:
    a. Leading non-obstetric cause of maternal death[10]
    b. Primary goals of management:
        i. Aggressive resuscitation of the mother
        ii. Maintenance of uteroplacental perfusion and fetal oxygenation, by avoidance of
            A. Hypoxia
            B. Hypotension
            C. Hypocapnia
            D. Acidosis
            E. Hypothermia

Timing and method of delivery

Urgent neurosurgical intervention in a pregnant patient has to proceed, and the timing of delivery of the fetus would be determined by the gestational age:

- <24 weeks: proceed with surgery—all care to optimize maternal hemodynamics so as to preserve fetal well-being
- >24 weeks: one of the following three—
    - Cesarean delivery followed by neurosurgery in the same sitting
    - Cesarean followed by neurosurgery at a later date
    - Neurosurgery with an aim to maintain pregnancy
- >32 weeks: delivery proceeded by surgery

> Whatever the timing of delivery, the basic fundamentals of avoiding maternal hypoxemia, hypotension, and acidosis should always be remembered.

Maternal and fetal physiology

Physiological alterations during pregnancy

The major physiological alterations produced during pregnancy to meet the increasing metabolic demands of the fetus and to prepare the mother for delivery present a considerable challenge to the anesthesiologist. The attending anesthesiologist needs to take into account the implications of these changes while taking care of the pregnant patient. Some of the important considerations while administering anesthesia to a pregnant patient are the following:

- *Risk of hypoxemia* during induction and emergence due to increased oxygen consumption and reduced functional residual capacity—adequate preoxygenation (at least 2 min) mandatory prior to induction.[10]
- *Difficult airway* due to soft tissue edema and capillary engorgement of respiratory mucosa—gentle laryngoscopy and small-sized endotracheal tubes (6–7 mm ID) may be needed.[11]
- *Aortocaval compression* by the gravid uterus, when combined with the hypotensive effects of anesthesia, may produce fetal asphyxia—left uterine displacement by tilting the operating table 30° to the left or placing a roll under the patient's right hip should be done.

- *High risk for regurgitation and pulmonary aspiration* due to reduced gastroesophageal sphincter tone by the elevated progesterone levels, and upward displacement of the stomach by gravid uterus—all pregnant patients treated as full stomach and adequate aspiration prophylaxis given as a rule.
- *Elevated risk of deep vein thrombosis (DVT)* due to hypercoagulability caused by increased clotting factors, and chronic partial caval obstruction by the pregnant uterus.
- *Decrease in the requirement of inhalational anesthetics* due to surge in endorphin levels, decreasing the minimum alveolar concentration (MAC) of inhalationals by ~40%.[12,13]
- *Reduction in the dose of local anesthetics by ~30%* due to reduced volume of cerebrospinal fluid (CSF) secondary to epidural venous engorgement and resultant cephalad spread of the local anesthetic in the subarachnoid space.

Teratogenic potential of anesthetic drugs

Teratogenicity of a drug[14,15] is determined by the following:

- Dose of the drug administered
- Route of administration of the drug
- Timing of exposure of the drug to the fetus:
  - First 15 days: all or none phenomena—fetus lost or preserved fully intact
  - Time of organogenesis (15–56 days): structural abnormalities in the fetus
  - 57 days to delivery: functional changes observed—structural abnormalities rare

Moreover, anesthetic drugs are usually administered for such brief periods that their potential for harm would as such be minimal.

Local anesthetics, volatile anesthetics, induction agents, muscle relaxants, and opioids are not teratogenic when normal maternal physiology is maintained.

> Derangements in maternal physiology, such as maternal hypotension and hypoxemia, are teratogenic themselves. All care should therefore be taken to maintain oxygenation and hemodynamic stability in the mother.

Nitrous oxide

- Known to affect DNA synthesis and have teratogenic potential in animals.[16]
- Human studies have failed to show an association between nitrous oxide use in settings with modern scavenging techniques and adverse pregnancy outcome.[17,18]
- Best to avoid nitrous oxide during pregnancy because its use is not necessary to provide safe and effective anesthesia.

Recent controlled studies have invalidated the association between benzodiazepine use, cleft palate, and cardiac anomalies.[19,20]

Factors associated with neonatal depression

The following three major factors decrease uterine flow during pregnancy:

1. Systemic hypotension
2. Uterine vasoconstriction
3. Uterine contractions

Measures to optimize uterine blood flow and minimize fetal depressions are the following:

- *Minimize:*
  - Aortocaval compression
  - Hypovolemia
  - Anesthetic overdose
  - Vasodilators
  - Excessive positive pressure ventilation, which leads to hypotension and subsequent fetal distress during anesthesia
- Appropriate IV fluids—proportionate to the surgical blood loss.
- Ephedrine, which was considered the drug of choice for maternal hypotension, is now known to be associated with neonatal acidosis, as compared to phenylephrine or other α-agonists.[21]

> Recent clinical trials have proven that phenylephrine or other α-agonists (e.g., metaraminol) are safe and generally more effective than ephedrine alone to prevent maternal hypotension and its sequelae (e.g., nausea and vomiting).[22,23]

Uteroplacental drug transfer

Uteroplacental drug transfer depends largely on molecular size, lipid solubility, and degree of ionization of the drug:

- *Drugs that freely cross placenta:*
  - Inhalational agents (low molecular weight/high lipid solubility)
  - Induction agents—thiopentone, propofol, etomidate, and ketamine (highly lipophilic and low degree of ionization)—rapid distribution and metabolism limit effect on the fetus
  - Local anesthetics and opioids (lipid soluble/low degree of ionization)
  - Atropine
  - Warfarin—teratogenic potential—contraindicated in pregnancy
    - β-Blockers—esmolol infusions implicated in causing persistent fetal bradycardia[24]

> Labetalol is the drug of choice for treating maternal hypertension as it is relatively safe for the fetus.

- *Drugs that do not cross the placental barrier:*
  - Muscle relaxants—both depolarizing and nondepolarizing
  - Reversal agents—neostigmine and edrophonium
  - Glycopyrrolate (due to its quaternary ammonium structure)
    - Heparin—anticoagulant of choice during pregnancy

Radiation exposure and fetus

The International Commission on Radiological Protection (ICRP) suggests that at doses under 100 mGy (1 Gy = 1 Sv):

Lethal effects in preimplantation period of embryonic development: infrequent

Risks of malformations after in utero exposure: not expected

Any effects on IQ following in utero exposure to less than 100 mGy: of no practical significance

Lifetime cancer risk similar to that following irradiation in early childhood[25]

A typical computed tomography (CT) of the head exposes a fetus to 0.01–0.1 mSv radiation.

Therapeutic procedures such as coiling or embolization result in a greater radiation dose: 2–10 mSv exposure to the mother.

> ICRP concludes that prenatal doses from most correctly performed diagnostic procedures do not increase the risk of prenatal or postnatal death, developmental damage including malformation, or impairment of mental development over the background incidence of these abnormalities.

Anesthetic management during pregnancy

Optimal planning with a multidisciplinary approach, involving the neurosurgeon, neuroanesthesiologist, neuroradiologist, neurologist, obstetrician, neonatologist, and neurointensivist, is the key to successful management in pregnant patients.

Premedication

Sedation: only in highly anxious patients—in the preoperative area with adequate monitoring—hypoventilation, hypercarbia, and rise in intracranial pressure (ICP) may be a risk, as in any other neurosurgical patient

- *Aspiration prophylaxis*: to reduce the acidity and volume of gastric secretions—sodium citrate/metoclopramide/ranitidine
- *Anticonvulsant therapy*: may need to be started or continued in the preoperative phase—therapeutic levels need to be monitored

Induction

Goals of induction contradictory: rapid-sequence induction to reduce the risk of aspiration compared to slow neuroinduction to reduce ICP.

Modified rapid-sequence induction in pregnant patients:

- Patient is placed supine with a wedge under the right hip or a 15° leftward tilt of the operating table.

- Adequate preoxygenation for 3–5 min.
- Difficult airway equipment kept handy to tackle at risk situations.
- Head up "ramped" position for obese, pregnant females—by elevation of the shoulders with a pillow underneath.
- Induction: thiopentone 4–6 mg/kg, or propofol 2 mg/kg.
- Short-acting opioids to blunt pressor responses to laryngoscopy: fentanyl (2–5 µg/kg) or remifentanil (1 µg/kg given over 60 s).
- Lignocaine 1 mg/kg may be used concomitantly.
- Nondepolarizing muscle relaxant like rocuronium 0.9–1.2 mg/kg: modification of rapid-sequence induction (as succinylcholine is avoided in neurosurgery due to concerns about a transient increase in ICP).
- Cricoid pressure applied: maintained until intubation confirmed by capnography and cuff inflated.
- Gentle ventilation by a mask may be done in a modified rapid-sequence induction.

> Magnesium sulfate (30–60 mg/kg) is the drug of choice for blunting the response to laryngoscopy in patients with eclampsia and preeclampsia.

Maintenance

Inhalational anesthetics: end-tidal concentration of 1% isoflurane and 1.5% sevoflurane.[26]

- Opioids such as fentanyl 1–2 µg/h.
- Nondepolarizing muscle relaxant.
- Thiopental or propofol infusions (5–6 mg/kg/h) may be administered to reduce ICP in cases of tight brain.

Hemodynamic considerations

- Invasive blood pressure (BP) monitoring indicated prior to induction: to avoid and treat excessive swings in BP
- Large bore intravenous access
- Central venous pressure monitoring, if indicated

Ventilation

- Hyperventilation to maintain maternal $PaCO_2$ between 25 and 30 mmHg

> Lower $PaCO_2$ levels may be associated with cerebral ischemia and impaired oxygen dissociation from hemoglobin, along with uterine artery vasoconstriction leading to fetal distress.

Mannitol: concern about increased maternal osmolality and resultant fetal dehydration—doses of 0.25– 0.5 mg/kg have however been used in individual case reports and appear safe..[27,28]

Intravenous fluid replacement: glucose-free isotonic crystalloid or colloid solutions, to prevent brain edema and increased ICP.

Steroids

- Short-term use of dexamethasone (4 mg IV, 6 hourly) indicated to reduce peritumor edema—also acts to accelerate fetal lung maturity by increasing surfactant production.
- Continued use of steroids during pregnancy, especially during third trimester, results in fetal adrenal suppression and neonatal hypoadrenalism.[29]

Temperature regulation

- Body temperature to be monitored with a temperature probe (nasopharyngeal/esophageal/axillary)
- Normothermia to be maintained with the use of forced warm air blankets

Perioperative fetal heart rate (FHR) monitoring

Useful after 26 weeks of gestation to indicate fetal well-being.[30]

Clinical utility only if there are expert personnel to interpret acute changes in the FHR and intervention is feasible (in terms of staff and facility) if need arises.

May serve as a guide to search for potential reversible causes of fetal distress, such as maternal hypotension and hypoxemia.

Emergence

- Early extubation favored to facilitate early neurological evaluation
- Extubation only after the patient is fully awake and airway reflexes intact—to prevent aspiration

- Airway stimulation and bucking on the endotracheal tube prevented by lidocaine, fentanyl, or sedative doses of propofol
- Indications of postoperative ventilation:
  - Poor preoperative neurologic status
  - Eventful intraoperative course: bleeding, cerebral edema, or ischemia

Surgery in prone position during pregnancy

- Prone position provides good uteroplacental perfusion.
- Challenging—with respect to fetal monitoring, emergent cesarean delivery, and increased epidural venous bleeding.

Combined caesarean delivery and neurosurgery

Possibility of uterine atony causing postpartum hemorrhage during the subsequent neurosurgery:

Synthetic oxytocin can be used in patients with intracranial tumors—may cause transient hypotension and tachycardia.[31]

Ergometrine: may lead to hypertension and increased ICP, given only when other treatments are insufficient and in the lowest possible dose.

Inhalational-based anesthesia: concerns over uterine atony, used without incidence in most neurosurgical cases.[32]

Regional anesthesia

- May be appropriate to use when cesarean delivery is performed subsequent to recent successful and uncomplicated neurosurgery—in awake, alert, and cooperative patients.[26]
- Contraindicated in patients with evidence of raised ICP—dural puncture causes acute CSF leakage, which decreases CSF pressure and may produce cerebellar herniation[33] or hemorrhage in uncorrected vascular malformations.
- Epidural and caudal anesthesia also contraindicated in patients with increased ICP because of the risk of accidental dural puncture.
  - ICP may be further increased by injection of local anesthetic solution into the epidural space.[34]

Postoperative care

Pain management

Good postoperative analgesia for maternal comfort and mobility, and to reduce undesirable hemodynamic disturbances.

Multimodal analgesia using local infiltration of the incision site/scalp blocks, IV paracetamol, and opioids such as fentanyl and morphine in controlled doses.

Tramadol discouraged as it lowers seizure threshold.

Nonsteroidal anti-inflammatory drugs (NSAIDs) avoided because of:

Antiplatelet effect—tendency to cause potential bleeding after intracranial surgery[35]

Potential fetal complications (renal failure, necrotizing enterocolitis, and persistent fetal circulation after birth) when used in the last trimester[36]

Deep vein thrombosis prophylaxis

Intermittent pneumatic leg compression devices or elastic stockings to be used peri- and postoperatively in all patients.

Pharmacological prophylaxis with low molecular weight heparin to be started as early as feasible in the postoperative period after discussing with the neurosurgeon.

Anesthesia for interventional neurosurgical procedures

Endovascular treatment may be needed during pregnancy for the coiling of ruptured intracerebral aneurysms, embolization of AVMs, or thrombolysis of acute thromboembolic strokes.

- General anesthesia preferred for coiling—principles of management same as those of craniotomy.
- Invasive BP monitoring indicated for BP control—hypotension may compromise uteroplacental perfusion/hypertension may risk aneurysm rupture.[37]
- FHR monitoring may be useful to guide the range of BP to be maintained for an adequate uterine perfusion and oxygen delivery.

Cerebral vasospasm:

Pregnant patients somewhat protected from vasospasm because of their hemodiluted and hypervolemic state.

Nimodipine has been shown to increase the risk of intrauterine growth retardation and congenital abnormalities in animal studies—no human studies so far.

Benefits of nimodipine in preventing spasm outweigh any potential risk to the fetus and should be administered as clinically indicated.[38]

> Magnesium sulfate, the drug of choice for preventing and treating eclampsia, has been shown to reduce the severity of vasospasm after SAH.[39]

References

1. Bateman BT, Schumacher HC, Bushnell CD et al. Intracerebral hemorrhage in pregnancy: Frequency, risk factors, and outcome. *Neurology* 2006;67(3):424–429.
2. Kittner SJ, Stern BJ, Feeser BR et al. Pregnancy and the risk of stroke. *N Engl J Med* 1996;335:768–774.
3. Gaist D, Pedersen L, Cnattingius S, Sorensen HT. Parity and risk of sub-arachnoid hemorrhage in women. *Stroke* 2004;35:28–33.
4. Kanaan I, Jallu A, Kanaan H. Management strategy for meningioma in pregnancy: A clinical study. *Skull Base* 2003;13(4): 197–203.
5. Ng J, Kitchen N. Neurosurgery and Pregnancy. *J Neurol Neurosurg Psychiatry* 2008;79:745–752.
6. Fast A, Shapiro D, Ducommun EJ, Friedmann LW, Bouklas T, Floman Y. Low back pain in pregnancy. *Spine* 1987;12:368–371.
7. Bose S, Ali Z, Rath GP, Prabhakar H. Spontaneous spinal epidural haematoma: A rare cause of quadriplegia in the post-partum period. *Br J Anaesth* 2007;99(6):855–857.
8. Szkup P, Stoneham G. Case report: Spontaneous spinal epidural hematoma during pregnancy: Case report and review of the literature. *Br J Radiol* 2004;77:881–884.
9. Cywinski JB, Parker BM, Lozada LJ. Spontaneous spinal epidural hematoma in a pregnant patient. *J Clin Anesth* 2003;16:371–375.
10. Weinberg L, Steele RG, Pugh R, Higgins S, Herbert M, Story D. The pregnant trauma patient. *Anaesth Intensive Care* 2005;33:167–180.
11. Reitman E, Flood P. Anaesthetic considerations for non-obstetric surgery during pregnancy. *Br J Anaes* 2011;107:72–78.
12. McClelland SH, Bogod DG, Hardman JG. Pre-oxygenation in pregnancy: An investigation using physiological modeling. *Anaesthesia* 2008;63:259–263.
13. Boutonnet M, Faitot V, Keïta H. Airway management in obstetrics. *Ann Fr Anesth Reanim* 2011;30(9):651–664.
14. Van De Velde M, De Buck F. Anesthesia for non-obstetric surgery in the pregnant patient. *Minerva Anestesiol* 2007;73:235–240.
15. Kress HG. Effects of general anaesthetics on second messenger systems. *Eur J Anaesth* 1995;12:83–97.
16. Sturrock JE, Nunn JF. Mitosis in mammalian cells during exposure to anesthetics. *Anesthesiology* 1975;43:21–33.
17. Fujinaga M, Baden JM. Methionine prevents nitrous oxide-induced teratogenicity in rat embryos grown in culture. *Anesthesiology* 1994;81:184–189.
18. Hemminki K, Kyyronen P, Lindbohm ML. Spontaneous abortions and malformations in the offspring of nurses exposed to anaesthetic gases, cytostatic drugs, and other potential hazards in hospitals, based on registered information of outcome. *J Epidemiol Community Health* 1985;39:141–147.
19. Rosenberg L, Mitchell AA, Parsells JL et al. Lack of relation of oral clefts to diazepam use during pregnancy. *N Engl J Med* 1983;309:1282–1285.
20. Ornoy A, Arnon J, Shectman S et al. Is benzodiazepine use during pregnancy really teratogenic? *Reprod Toxicol* 1998;12:511–515.

21. Ngan Kee WD, Khaw KS, Tan PE, Ng FF, Karmakar MK. Placental transfer and fetal metabolic effects of phenylephrine and ephedrine during spinal anesthesia for cesarean delivery. *Anesthesiology* 2009;111:506–512.

22. Ngan Kee WD, Lee A, Khaw KS, Ng FF, Karmakar MK, Gin T. A randomized double-blinded comparison of phenyleph-rine and ephedrine infusion combinations to maintain blood pressure during spinal anes-thesia for cesarean delivery: The effects on fetal acid base status and hemodynamic control. *Anesth Analg* 2008;107:1295–1302.

23. LaPorta RF, Arthur GR, Datta S. Phenylephrine in treating maternal hypotension due to spinal anaesthesia for caesarean delivery: Effects on neonatal catecholamine concentrations, acid base status and Apgar scores. *Acta Anaesthesiol Scand* 1995;39:901–905.

24. Eisenach JC, Castro MI. Maternally administered esmolol produces fetal beta-adrenergic blockade and hypoxemia in sheep. *Anesthesiology* 1989;71:718–722.

25. Wrixon AD. New recommendations from the International Commission on Radiological Protection—A review. *Phys Med Biol* 2008;53(8):R41–R60.

26. Wang LP, Paech MJ. Neuroanesthesia for the pregnant woman. *Anesth Analg* 2008;107:193–200.

27. Bruns PD, Linder RO, Drose VE, Battaglia F. The placental transfer of water from fetus to mother following the intravenous infusion of hypertonic mannitol to the maternal rabbit. *Am J Obstet Gynecol* 1963;86:160–167.

28. Biggs JSG, Allan JA. Medication and pregnancy. *Drugs* 1981;21:69–75.

29. Lee BH, Stoll BJ, McDonald SA, Higgins RD, National Institute of Child Health and Human Development Neonatal Research Network. Adverse neonatal outcomes associated with antenatal dexamethasone versus antenatal betamethasone. *Pediatrics* 2006;117:1503–1510.

30. Tuncali B, Aksun M, Katircioglu K, Akkol I, Savaci S. Intraoperative fetal heart rate monitoring during emergency neurosurgery in a parturient. *J Anesth* 2006;20:40–43.

31. Thomas JS, Koh SH, Cooper GM. Haemodynamic effects of oxytocin given as i.v. bolus or infusion on women undergoing caesarean section. *Br J Anaesth* 2007;98:116–119.

32. Al-areibi A, Coveny L, Sing S, Katsiris S. Case report: Anesthetic management for sequential Caesarean delivery and laminectomy. *Can J Anaesth* 2007;54:471–474.

33. Neal JM, Bernards CM, Hadzic A, Hebl JR, Hogan QH, Horlocker TT, Lee LA, Rathmell JP, Sorenson EJ, Suresh S, et al. ASRA Practice Advisory on Neurologic Complications in Regional Anesthesia and Pain Medicine. *Reg Anesth Pain Med* 2008;33(5):404–415.

34. Hilt H, Gramm J, Link J. Changes in intracranial pressure associated with extradural anaesthesia. *Br J Anaesth* 1986;58:676–680.

35. Palmer J, Sparrow O, Iannotti F. Postoperative hematoma: A 5-year survey and identification of possible risk factors. *Neurosurgery* 1994;35:1061–1064.

36. Ostensen ME, Skomsvoll JF. Anti-inflammatory pharmacotherapy during pregnancy. *Expert Opin Pharmacother* 2004;5:571–580.

37. Marshman LAG, Aspoas AR, Rai MS, Chawda SJ. The implications of ISAT and ISUIA for the management of cerebral aneurysms during pregnancy. *Neurosurg Rev* 2007;30:177–180.

38. Marsh C, Shinde S. Neurosurgery and the parturient anaesthesia—Tutorial of the week 253. *ATOTW* 2012.

39. Veyna RS, Seyfried D, Burke DG et al. Magnesium sulphate after aneurysmal subarachnoid hemorrhage. *J Neurosurg* 2002;96:510–514.

36

Pediatrics

FARZANA AFROZE, HELENA OECHSNER, and MELISSA EHLERS

Introduction

Caring for infants and children undergoing neurosurgical procedures presents unique challenges to both neurosurgeons and anesthesiologists. To provide anesthesia safely and effectively, anesthesiologists need to have a thorough understanding of pediatric neurophysiology and age-dependent variables that are distinctive to the pediatric population. This chapter highlights the key points of the common pediatric neurological disorders and reviews the age-dependent physiologic differences and their effects on anesthetic management for neurosurgical procedures.

Neurophysiology and pathophysiology

Developmental considerations

1. The development of the central nervous system (CNS) starts very early intra-utero, but is incomplete at birth and does not mature until the end of the first year of life.[1]
2. Two concepts distinguish infants and children from adults: (1) age-dependent differences in cerebrovascular physiology, and (2) cranial bone maturation. The CNS undergoes major structural changes during the first 2 years of life, which contributes to physiologic changes

and thus affects anesthetic management for intracranial pathology.[2]

3. The cranial vault of an infant is in a state of flux. The skull of an infant is not fully ossified and is more compliant due to the open fontanelles and cranial sutures (Figure 36.1). The posterior fontanelle generally closes between 2 and 3 months of age, and the anterior fontanelle closes between 12 and 24 months of age.

Intracranial pressure

1. Normal intracranial pressure (ICP) in a full-term infant is 2–6 mmHg and is likely lower in premature infants. In children and adults ICP is 10–15 mmHg.[2,3]

2. High ICP >15–20 mmHg is considered pathological and warrants treatment; severe uncontrolled intracranial hypertension with ICP >40 mmHg may lead to catastrophic brain herniation and eventually death.[4]

3. Clinical signs of elevated ICP can be variable in children and can be undiagnosed until late in the disease process.

4. The cranium of the infants has the ability to expand at the open fontanelles and nonfused sutures; therefore, ICP in infants and children may remain normal and may not show any signs of elevated ICP even in the presence of significant intracranial pathology. Gradual increase in volume can lead to increase in heard circumference, which can be the first sign of intracranial pathology. See Table 36.1 for chronic and late signs of elevated ICP.

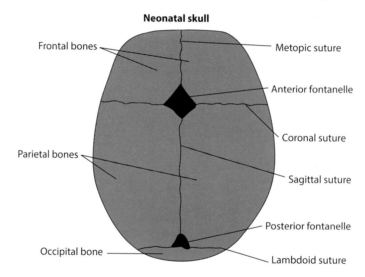

Neonatal skull

Frontal bones — Metopic suture — Anterior fontanelle — Coronal suture — Parietal bones — Sagittal suture — Posterior fontanelle — Occipital bone — Lambdoid suture

Figure 36.1 Normal cranial sutures and fontanelles during infancy.

Table 36.1 Chronic and Late Signs of Elevated ICP

Signs of chronic ICP elevation	Late signs of elevated ICP
• Increased head circumferences and widened cranial sutures (may be an early sign in infants) • Bulging fontanelles (may be an early sign in infants) • Nausea and vomiting (especially in the morning) • Irritability • Headaches • New onset of seizures • Decreased oral intake/failure to thrive	• Lethargy • Altered level of consciousness or mental status • HTN/bradycardia (Cushing's) • Mydriasis • Papilledema • Abnormal response to painful stimuli

5. Imaging with computed tomography (CT) or magnetic resonance imaging (MRI) is warranted for patients with any of these symptoms and often reveals a decrease in the size or complete obliteration of the ventricles or basilar cisterns, hydrocephalus, intracranial masses, midline shift, and diffuse cerebral edema when increased ICP is associated with closed head injury, encephalopathy, or encephalitis.[3,5]

6. Placing a ventricular catheter is the most common and accurate way to measure ICP, with the additional benefit of draining cerebrospinal fluid (CSF) for diagnostic or therapeutic purposes. Other methods used in adults such as a subdural bold, epidural catheter, and subdural catheter to monitor ICP can be used and have been used effectively in children as well.[5]

Cerebrospinal fluid

1. The volume of CSF is smaller in children due to the smaller subarachnoid space, but larger on mL/kg basis.

2. The rate of CSF production is similar to the rates observed in adults, which is 0.35 mL/min or 500 mL/day.[6,7]

Cerebral blood flow and cerebral blood volume

1. As in adults, cerebral blood flow (CBF) is tightly coupled with cerebral metabolic demand. Other regulators of CBF are the partial pressure of oxygen (PaO_2), partial pressure of carbon dioxide ($PaCO_2$), blood viscosity, and cerebral autoregulation.

2. In the pediatric population, CBF and the percentage of cardiac output (CO) to the brain varies with age. In contrast to adults, infants and children have a higher percentage of CO to the developing brain.

3. According to Wintermark et al.,[8] in the first 6 months of life CBF is between 10% and 20% of the CO, peaks at 55% between 2 and 4 years, then settles to adult levels of 15% by 7 and 8 years of age.[8] This likely indicates preferential high blood flow to the growing brain during the critical stage of the development.

4. The CBF in healthy awake children (3–12 years) is approximately 100 mL/100 g/min.[9]

5. From 6 months to 3 years, CBF believed to be 90 mL/ 100 g/min.[10]

6. Neonates and premature infants have less CBF 40 mL/100 g/min compared to adults and children.[11]

Cerebral metabolic rate

1. Children have a higher global cerebral metabolic rate (CMR) than adults. The CMR for oxygen consumption ($CMRO_2$) is 5.8 in children compared to 3.5 mL/100 g/min in adults and glucose consumption is 6.8 in children compared to 5.5 mL/100 g/min in adults.[9]

2. Conversely, neonates tend to have a lower $CMRO_2$, 2.3 mL/100 g/min and a lower CBF with a relative tolerance to hypoxemia.[10]

Cerebral autoregulation

1. Owing to a lack of controlled manipulation of blood pressure in the human neonate, the lower limit of autoregulation (LLA) in the neonate and premature infant is not known with certainty.[12] The cerebral autoregulation in a healthy newborn is believed to be in a narrow range between 20 and 60 mmHg.[13] A general rule of thumb when caring for newborn or premature infants is that the lower limit of acceptable mean arterial pressure (MAP) is approximately the gestational age.[3]

2. Current evidence suggests cerebral autoregulation is preserved in healthy full-term neonates but absent in term and preterm infants who are neurologically impaired. These sick premature neonates have pressure passivity, resulting in a linear correlation between systemic pressure and CBF.[14,15]

3. The autoregulatory slope of the neonatal CBF/BP has a shorter plateau curve and is shifted more toward the left (Figure 36.2). This indicates that sudden hypotension or hypertension at either end of the autoregulatory curve places the neonate at increased risk for cerebral ischemia and intraventricular hemorrhage (IVH).

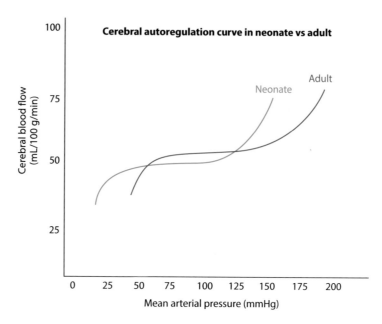

Figure 36.2 Autoregulation curve of cerebral blood flow in children and adults. The slope of the autoregulatory curve drops and rises significantly at the lower and upper limits of the curve and is shifted to further left in neonates and infants (left curve) when compared with adults (right curve).

Preoperative evaluation and surgical preparation

Though organ-based evaluation and consideration of underlying neurological disorders for risk stratification to minimize perioperative morbidity and mortality is crucial, the most essential preoperative evaluation is to have a thorough understanding of the underlying neurological pathology and coexisting disease and their potential physiologic derangements during the perioperative period.

History

1. Review presenting neurological symptoms, for example, seizure, headache, weakness, vision changes, mental status changes, and vomiting. On the basis of these symptoms, a clinician should estimate the degree of increase in ICP.
2. Current medications, coexisting chronic illness and severity of the diseases, and poor nutritional status may further complicate the perioperative course (Table 36.2).

Physical examination

1. Brief age-appropriate neurologic evaluation, which includes level of consciousness, motor and sensory functions, normal and pathologic reflexes, integrity of the cranial nerves, and signs and symptoms of intracranial hypertension.
2. Assessment of intravascular access and intravascular volume status.
3. A thorough evaluation of the airway is essential, because certain craniofacial anomalies are associated with a difficult airway and may need special airway management.

Laboratory and radiologic evaluation

1. For minor surgeries no laboratory work is usually warranted. For major surgeries with expected blood loss, determination of baseline hemoglobin hematocrit and blood typing and cross matching is valuable.
2. Additional studies such as coagulation parameters, serum electrolytes, osmolality, kidney and liver function tests, blood gas analysis, chest radiograph, and electrocardiography should be performed if indicated from the patient's past medical history.
3. Most neurosurgical patients will have some type of radiologic imaging, either an MRI or a CT scan of the head or spine as part of their preoperative evaluation.
4. Review of the imaging studies preoperatively can provide important information to the

Table 36.2 System-Based Evaluation for Coexisting Conditions

• Cardiovascular system	• Congenital heart disease, hypoxia, arrhythmias, paradoxical emboli, congestive heart failure associated with large A-V malformation, electrolyte abnormalities
• Respiratory system	• BPD, chronic lung disease (CLD), aspiration pneumonia, postoperative apnea, vocal cord paralysis
• Gastrointestinal system	• GERD, nausea, vomiting
• Urinary system	• Latex sensitivity, infection
• Nervous system	• Seizures, mental status changes, neurologic deficits
• Endocrine system	• Diabetes insipidus, SIADH, adrenal insufficiency in pituitary or hypothalamic lesions, electrolyte abnormalities
• Airway evaluation	• Craniofacial anomaly or syndromes associated with difficult airway anatomy

BPD, bronchopulmonary dysplasia; SIADH, syndrome of inappropriate antidiuretic hormone

anesthesiologists in planning for the induction and maintenance of anesthesia for the procedure.

Preoperative discussion

1. Preoperative communication is essential to the neurosurgical team, regarding their concern for the specific patient and surgical plan, for example, intraoperative somatosensory evoked potential (SSEP) and motor evoked potential (MEP) monitoring, positioning patient, anticipated blood loss, need for invasive monitoring, and postoperative care and discharge.

Premedication

1. Preoperative anxiety is due to different reasons in different stages of development:
   a. Separation anxiety from parents in small children around 9 months to 5 years of age
   b. Anxiety of needle and pain in patients 6–12 years of age
   c. Anxiety about surgery and self-image in adolescence
2. Anxiety leading to intense crying and fighting can cause significant elevation in ICP; conversely, oversedation can cause raise in $EtCO_2$ and then ICP.
3. When it is indicated, midazolam 0.25–0.5 mg/kg (maximum 20 mg) orally, administered 10–20 min before surgery, is effective to relieve preoperative anxiety. If an indwelling IV catheter is in place, a small dosage of IV midazolam can be titrated to effect.
4. Children with developmental delay or neurologic impairment may not need any premedication.

5. Premedication with narcotics is best avoided as they may cause nausea or respiratory depression, especially in children with elevated ICP, and may further increase the ICP.
6. Ketamine increases CBF and CMR, which further increase the ICP and thus should be avoided as premedication.

Fasting guidelines in children

According to an updated report by the American Society of Anesthesiologists,[16] fasting guidelines prior to surgery in infants and children to minimize the risk of pulmonary aspiration are the following:

Clear liquids	2 h
Breast milk	4 h
Formula/nonhuman milk	6 h

Intraoperative management

Induction of anesthesia

There is no standard way to induce anesthesia in children for neurosurgical procedures. The choice of anesthetic induction should be dictated by the patient's neurological status and coexisting medical issues.

1. In the presence of intracranial hypertension, the primary goal of a smooth anesthetic induction is to avoid further increase in ICP and ischemia due to hypoxia, hypercapnia, volatile anesthetic-induced increase in CBF, and hypotension.[10]

2. As a general rule, all volatile anesthetics increase CBF and decrease CMR, and all intravenous agents, except ketamine, decrease CBF and CMR.

3. As most patients coming from home for scheduled neurosurgical procedures are less likely to have severely elevated ICP, mask induction with sevoflurane followed by obtaining IV access and airway management is well tolerated by them.

4. Sodium thiopental (4–8 mg/kg) is the drug of choice for IV induction in countries where it is available. Propofol (2–4 mg/kg) is most commonly used for IV induction in children in the United States. Etomidate and ketamine can be used in patients, who are hemodynamically unstable, but etomidate can cause central nervous excitation and ketamine is known to increase CBF, CMR, and ICP; therefore, these drugs are typically not recommended.

5. Nondepolarizing muscle relaxants, short- and fast-acting narcotics, for example, fentanyl (1–2 μg/kg) or remifentanil (0.5–1 μg/kg), and lidocaine (1–1.5 mg/kg) are commonly used to blunt the sympathetic response from direct laryngoscopy and to facilitate securing the airway safely.

6. Patients with altered mental status and somnolence with elevated ICP are at risk for aspiration and will require intravenous rapid sequence induction (RSI) with cricoid pressure. For RSI, the use of succinylcholine may be necessary and the small increase in ICP from succinylcholine may be attenuated by the use of nondepolarizing neuromuscular agents and opiates. In patients in which succinylcholine is contraindicated, rocuronium can also be used.

Airway management

1. Anatomically, the pediatric airway is different than adults, which can make airway management challenging. The following is a quick review of the main pediatric airway anatomical differences:
   a. Large occiput compared to the rest of the body, large tongue and short mandible.
   b. Larynx funnel shaped and elongated.
   c. Cricoid cartilage is the narrowest portion of the airway—leading to subglottic

stenosis after prolonged intubation due to mucosal swelling from a tight cuffed tube.
   d. Short trachea—changes in head position with extension/flexion risk migration of the tube causing inadvertent extubation or endobronchial intubation.

2. Either an oral or a nasal tube is appropriate for small children. A nasal tube offers more stability, especially in prone patients and may be more comfortable for children when prolonged postoperative intubation is necessary. In either case, the endotracheal tube (ETT) should be meticulously secured and bilateral breath sounds should be auscultated after final patient positioning.

3. A cuffed ETT is not contraindicated in small children, but the cuff should be inflated with caution with minimum pressure requiring sealing and the air leak needs to be checked prior to extubation or checked frequently if the patient remains intubated for a long period. A half-size ETT is recommended when a cuffed tube is used.

4. Another consideration is that an orotracheal tube can kink at the base of the tongue when the head is flexed, resulting in airway obstruction and pressure injury to the tongue.[17]

5. Small children are especially at risk for significant facial and airway edema leading to postoperative airway obstruction after prolonged prone or craniofacial surgeries and procedures involving heavy blood loss requiring large volume replacement.[2]

Positioning

1. Positioning patients for lengthy neurosurgical procedures is an important concept for both neurosurgeons and anesthesiologists and is even more important for pediatric patients.

2. Planning and communication with the operating room staff is crucial. Operating room table extensions can be removed from both the head and leg ends to make the table short and to have better access to small pediatric patients.

3. The physiological effects of the prone and lateral positions are similar to those of adults.

4. Be meticulous about padding and stabilization of the extremities to prevent stretch and pressure injuries.

Vascular access and monitoring

1. Since the patient may not be accessible after draping, especially small children, mandatory good venous accesses are essential prior to the start of the procedure.
2. For short procedures with minimal blood loss, one functioning IV is adequate. Major surgeries, for example, craniotomies, craniofacial reconstructive surgeries, and spine surgeries, when significant blood loss and/or sudden hemodynamic changes are expected due to hemorrhage, venous air embolism (VAE), and herniation syndrome need at least two large-bore IVs and an arterial line (A-line) for frequent blood gas sampling.
3. If adequate peripheral IV access is difficult to obtain, consider a central venous catheter (CVC). Placement of a CVC is not routine and before placing one in a small child consider the risks versus benefits of it. A femoral catheter is probably a better option for small children undergoing craniotomies as it is easy to access and there are less chances of the catheter kinking during head positioning.
4. A radial A-line is suitable for most children. If possible, avoid the femoral A-line as it can be associated with lower extremity ischemia in infants and small children. Another option for A-line placement is the dorsalis pedis artery.
5. An appropriate-sized Foley catheter for the bladder is necessary for fluid management and urine output monitoring.
6. Neonates and small children are especially at risk for hypothermia under general anesthesia in the operating room. An oral or rectal tem-perature robe should be placed as it is crucial to avoid hypothermia to avoid hypothermia-related complications, such as bleeding, infection, and arrhythmias.

Venous air embolism

The standard neurosurgical mild head-up position to optimize CSF drainage for better surgical exposure is a potential risk for intraoperative VAE. Infants and small children undergoing craniotomies are at a greater risk for VAE because their head is larger in relation to the body and rests above the heart in both the supine and prone positons.[17]

Other risk factors for VAE in small children are highly vascular nature of the infant scalp, rapid blood loss leading to a pressure gradient between the right atrium and surgical site favoring air entrainment, and the presence of a persistent foramen ovale in 50% of children under 5 years of age.[18]

There are several methods to detect VAE but a precordial Doppler probe is a sensitive, inexpensive, and practical way of detecting VAE. In addition to its characteristic sound in the presence of VAE, the clinical picture will typically show sudden hypotension, a decrease in $EtCO_2$, ischemic changes on the electrocardiogram (EKG), and in severe cases, arrhythmias and cardiac arrest.[17]

Treatment of a suspected VAE involves flooding the surgical field; head drop; left lateral position, if possible; and inotropic support, if needed.

Neurophysiologic monitoring

Many neurosurgical procedures around the posterior fossa, cerebellum, and spinal cord will require neurophysiological monitoring with the aim to immediately detect and treat any potential intraoperative neural damage or ischemia.

Anesthesia management to facilitate SSEP and MEP monitoring is the same as that in adults.

Maintenance of anesthesia

1. Maintenance of anesthesia in children is similar to that in adults; a balanced technique with the combination of opiates, volatile anesthetics, and neuromuscular blockade is typically used.
2. Anesthetic goals are to decrease ICP, preserve cerebral autoregulation, and maintain organ perfusion with stable hemodynamics, adequate intraoperative analgesia and amnesia, and rapid emergence for quick postoperative neurological assessment without agitation.
3. These goals can be achieved with volatile anesthetic gas concentration for <0.5 MAC for the age, short-acting narcotic infusion, for example, fentanyl, sufentanil, or remifentanil, and propofol infusion for adequate amnesia. Dexmedetomidine infusion is an alternative option and can be continued postoperatively

if sedation is required.[19] Neuromuscular blockade can be used if intraoperative motor function is not being assessed.

4. Nitrous oxide (N_2O) is best avoided since neurosurgical procedures have a relative high risk of postoperative nausea and vomiting and VAE. In addition, N_2O increases CBF and $CMRO_2$, which have unfavorable effects on ICP.

Fluid and blood administration

1. Careful fluid management is essential for infants and children for neurosurgical procedures. Immature renal function leading to inability to readily handle excessive fluid and solute load and immature cardiorespiratory physiology in infants and small children makes fluid management challenging.

2. Because of preoperative conservative fluid management and diuretic therapy to decrease ICP, intraoperative hemodynamic instability and cardiovascular collapse from low intravascular volume can occur; a fluid bolus is indicated in these cases.

3. There is no standard formula for fluid management in children for neurosurgical procedures. Intraoperative fluid management is basically a balance of maintaining normovolemia to avoid hypoperfusion of the brain and other vital organs while not contributing to further cerebral edema and serum glucose concentration. Things to consider are the following: the proposed procedure, an assessment of preoperative volume status, consideration of coexisting conditions, and finally, the age and estimated circulating blood volume and the estimation of the allowable blood loss (ABL).

Estimated circulating blood volume (ECBV)

Preterm neonate	100 mL/kg
Term neonate	90 mL/kg
Infant	80 mL/kg
Children and adolescents	70–75 mL/kg
Adults	70 mL/kg

To calculate maximal allowable blood loss:
$$ECBV \times [Hb_{start} - Hb_{lowest}]/Hb_{start}$$

4. Isotonic crystalloids such as Lactated Ringer's (LR) or 0.9% normal saline (NS) can be used like any other surgical procedures. However, 0.9% NS is most commonly used because of its slightly hyperosmolar nature, which may minimize cerebral edema. Large quantities of NS administration are associated with hyperchloremic metabolic acidosis. A colloid like 5% albumin can be used when the blood–brain barrier is intact. But there is no evidence that resuscitation with colloids improves outcome.

	Osmolarity (mOsm/L)	Chloride (mEq/L)	pH
Serum	285–290	–	7
NS	308	154	5.7
LR	273	130	6.6

5. Nonchemical strategies to decrease cerebral edema are careful hyperventilation and head elevation. In severe cases, and also to optimize the surgical field, the administration of osmotic diuretics such as mannitol (0.25–0.5 g/kg) or hypertonic saline (2% or 3%) and loop diuretics, such as furosemide, are useful. All these drug therapies may cause hypovolemia and electrolyte derangements in the perioperative period and interfere with the ability to use urine output as a guide to intravascular volume status.

6. Estimation of blood loss is difficult during neurosurgical procedures, and frequently blood is hidden under the drape or behind the head and it is difficult to visualize the surgical field. Infants and small children are more vulnerable to sudden acute blood loss and resultant hypotension.

7. There is no clear blood transfusion guideline in the pediatric patient. The decision for transfusion should be based on the type of surgery, estimation of current/ongoing blood loss, calculation of ABL for the age, evaluation of hemodynamic status, and drawing intraoperative blood gases if possible.

8. An infusion of packed red blood cells (PRBC) 10 mL/kg will raise the hematocrit levels by 10% or by three points. Acute blood loss can also be replaced either with 3 mL NS for 1 mL blood loss or a colloid solution,

such as 5% albumin, equal to the volume of blood loss.

9. Maintenance fluid should be administered based on the weight using the 4-2-1 rule:

First 10 kg	4 mL/kg/h up to 10 kg
Second 10 kg (10–20 kg)	40 mL + 2 mL/kg/h over 10 kg
≥20 kg	60 mL + 1 mL/kg/h over 20 kg

Blood loss, urine output, and insensible loss of body fluid should be replaced with isotonic crystalloid administration at 3–10 mL/kg/h, depending on the length of the surgery and exposure of the surgical field.

10. Perioperative glucose homeostasis is critical for neurosurgical patients. Infants and neonates with limited glycogen storage are at risk for intraoperative hypoglycemia, thus they require infusion of a glucose-containing solution at 5–6 mg/kg/min to maintain normal serum glucose levels.[17]

11. Many neurosurgical patients, especially patients with intracranial tumor, are on an exogenous steroid to decrease vasogenic edema. The stress from the acute illness and the surgery, along with exogenous steroid administration, may make these patients insulin resistant and thus hyperglycemic. Although there is evidence that hyperglycemia in children is associated with poor outcome, it is still unclear if a tight glycemic control with insulin therapy offers any significant benefit.[20–22] On the basis of the current evidence, it is advised that hyperglycemia should be avoided, and until further prospective clinical trials with better glycemic guidance in children are available, a conservative approach with frequent perioperative serum glucose measurement to keep glucose <180 mg/dL is probably the best approach.[23]

12. Other causes of perioperative fluid electrolyte derangements to consider are syndrome of inappropriate antidiuretic hormone (SIADH), diabetes insipidus (DI), and cerebral salt-wasting syndrome. Diagnosis can be made with correlation of the clinical picture along with serum and urine electrolytes and osmolarity.

Postoperative care

1. Appropriate postoperative care varies on the setting, patient comorbidities, and the type of surgery.

2. After major intracranial and craniofacial surgeries patients will require the intensive care unit for further observation and frequent neurological assessment.

3. After any neurosurgical procedures quick emergence from anesthesia is desirable for immediate neurological assessment, thus longer-acting analgesics are avoided. Postoperative pain control is dictated by the type of surgery, but typically oral acetaminophen around the clock and a small dose of narcotics as needed is adequate.

Anesthetic approach to common pediatric neurosurgical procedures

Brain tumors

1. After leukemias, brain tumors are the most common solid tumors in children, and the second most common childhood cancer.

2. Location of these tumors varies with age. Younger patients tend to have cerebellar and brainstem involvements whereas older patients tend to have cerebral/supratentorial involvement.

3. Two-thirds of all childhood brain tumors are located infratentorially, in the posterior fossa region, which allows them to substantially grow in size before clinical symptoms are manifested.

4. The posterior fossa tumors include medulloblastoma, cerebellar astrocytoma, brainstem gliomas, and ependymomas of the fourth ventricles.

5. Craniopharyngiomas are the most common perisellar tumor in children and adolescents. Although benign in nature, they may be associated with hypothalamic and pituitary dysfunctions. Patients are generally on steroid replacement therapy with dexamethasone or hydrocortisone because the integrity of the hypothalamic–pituitary–adrenal axis is uncertain. These patients may present with visual impairment due to optic nerve impingement, growth failure, and endocrine abnormalities. Preoperative thyroid and

adrenal functions should be investigated. DI is also common in the perioperative period. DI is a common preoperative and postoperative finding, but rarely occurs intraoperatively.[24]

6. Anesthetic concerns for the perioperative periods include elevated ICP, cerebral edema, intraoperative blood loss and VAE, fluid and electrolyte imbalances, patient positioning, and loss of protective airway reflexes due to compression of the brainstem region.

7. The anesthetic goal should be directed toward minimizing ICP and maintaining adequate cerebral perfusion pressure and CBF, and toward a rapid emergence at the end of the procedure for a thorough neurological assessment.

Hydrocephalus

1. Hydrocephalus is probably the most common pediatric neurosurgical condition that results from either increased CSF production or obstruction of normal CSF flow.

2. The etiology can be either congenital as in aqueductal stenosis, Dandy–Walker syndrome, and Arnold–Chiari malformation or acquired as in IVH of prematurity, brain tumor, infection, and myelomeningocele.[24]

3. Most children with hydrocephalus will have some degree of elevated ICP and intracranial hypertension, and the urgency of the surgery will depend on the degree of ICP.

4. Children typically present with headaches and irritability, but can also present with seizure, lethargy, vomiting, and opthalmoplegia.[25]

5. Surgical treatment includes insertion of a shunt to divert CSF from the ventricle to another part of the body cavity (peritoneal, pleural, or right atrium), and a ventriculoperitoneal (VP) shunt is most commonly used. Shunts may require revision due to malfunction, blockage, infection, or natural growth of the child.[10,24]

6. Anesthesia planning, depending on the degree of the ICP and intracranial hypertension, RSI, and tracheal intubation, may be necessary. Anesthesia can be maintained with muscle relaxants, a small dose of short-acting narcotics, for example, fentanyl, and volatile anesthetics. The most stimulating portion of the procedure is the tunneling portion of the procedure, which can be managed with a small dose of narcotics along with increasing the depth of anesthesia.[26] This procedure requires exposure of the significant portion of the body, thus heat conservation strategies are needed. Blood loss is pretty minimal, thus one functioning IV is sufficient. Like any other neurosurgical procedures, rapid emergence for a neurological assessment is desirable. Postoperatively, the pain is typically well controlled with oral acetaminophen and a small dose of narcotics as needed.

Seizure

1. Children with intractable seizure disorder, who have failed medical treatment, may need surgical treatments such as vagal nerve stimulator placement, craniotomy for resection of the brain area with the seizure foci, hemispherectomy, and corpus callosotomy.

2. A vagal nerve stimulator is a small device implanted subcutaneously around the collar bone and uses a wire to electrically stimulate the vagus nerve round the neck. With recent advances in nerurophysiological monitoring, now craniotomy and focal resection of an area of the brain generating seizures is possible. Corpus callosotomy and hemispherectomy are rarely performed. With corpus callosotomy the two hemispheres of the brain are surgically separated to diminish the severity of the seizure activity, and in hemispherectomy, one side of the brain is disconnected from the other to decrease signal.[24,26] Surgical treatments are invasive and used to treat and minimize the severity of certain types of seizures, which are unresponsive to medical treatment with anticonvulsants and are debilitating to the patients.[26]

3. Anesthetic considerations for these patients include underlying coexisting diseases, developmental delay, perioperative seizures, effects of anticonvulsants therapy on certain anesthetic drug metabolism from liver enzyme induction, and drug interaction between the anesthetic agents and anticonvulsants medications.

4. Awake craniotomy is an option for older/mature children with the benefit of intraoperative electrocorticographic mapping and resection of the specific brain area only.

Spinal cord surgery

1. Commonly performed pediatric spinal cord neurosurgical procedures are dorsal rhizotomy and intrathecal baclofen pump placement to treat spasticity and tethered cord release.[26] Although spinal cord tumors are rare in the pediatric population, accounting for 1%–10% of all pediatric CNS tumors, they may need surgical resection.[27]
2. A tethered cord can result from either congenital developmental abnormality around the spinal cord such as spinal cord lipoma or surgeries around the spinal cord as in after myelomeningocele repair, which basically means entrapment of the nerves of the cauda equine.
3. Anesthetic consideration includes underlying neurologic condition, developmental status, and coexisting diseases. Positioning can be challenging due to spasticity and contractures. Many spinal cord surgeries use intraoperative nerve conduction monitoring, so muscle relaxants should be avoided and maintenance of anesthesia may need to be modified to facilitate intraoperative sensory and motor monitoring.

Neuroradiology

1. The most common neuroradiological studies include CT scans and MRIs and can be performed with light sedation, but children who failed light sedation or uncooperative and with coexisting comorbidities will require general anesthesia.
2. ETT is appropriate for small children and older children can be done with laryngeal mask airways (LMAs).
3. Anesthetic concerns include remote location, MRI-compatible monitors and equipment, and comorbidities.

Traumatic brain injury

1. Traumatic brain injuries (TBIs) are the leading cause of death in pediatric populations.[25] Acute head trauma can cause intracranial hematoma, diffuse cerebral edema and axonal injury, impaired autoregulation and intracranial compliance, and unstable hemodynamics.[10,24]

2. Perioperative concerns include the following: (1) cervical spine stability, (2) management of a traumatized airway, (3) aspiration of gastric content, (4) evolving intracranial hypertension due to bleeding and cerebral edema, (5) cerebral ischemia from secondary hypoxia or hypotension, (6) anemia secondary to acute blood loss, (7) coagulopathy, (8) stress-induced hyperglycemia or hypoglycemia, and (9) hemodynamic collapse.
3. Emergent decompressive craniotomy may be required for decompression and evacuation of the hematoma. Communication among teams is crucial and all the measures to decrease ICP should be taken.

Chiari malformation

Chiari malformation is a congenital condition defined by anatomic anomalies of the craniocervical junction with downward displacement of the cerebellar structures through the foramen magnum, frequently associated with syringomyelia (spinal cord cavitation). With any of the Chiari malformations, additional abnormalities may be observed. These include atlas assimilation, atlanto-occipital dislocation, or Klippel–Feil anomaly.[28] Depending on severity, the malformation is classified into four types with the recent addition of type 0 and type 1.5. These are the following:

CM type 0: Syringomyelia with the absence of cerebellar tonsillar herniation.[28]

CM type I: This is the most common form, characterized by abnormally shaped cerebellar tonsils, which are displaced below the level of the foramen magna. It is frequently diagnosed in adolescence or even in adulthood; the presenting symptoms may vary depending on age.

CM type 1.5: This is a CM II-like malformation without spina bifida.[29]

CM type II: The classic Chiari malformation (also known as Arnold–Chiari) is commonly associated with myelomeningocele. It is characterized by downward displacement of the cerebellar vermis and tonsils and brainstem malformation.

CM type III: This is a rare, most severe form with cerebellum displacement into a high cervical or occipital encephalocele, where the brain stem and fourth ventricle are herniating into the spinal canal.

CM type IV: This is a rare congenital cerebellar hypoplasia.

Indications for surgical treatment of CM type I are the presence of syringomyelia, scoliosis, ataxia, sensory loss, motor loss, lower cranial nerve palsies, myelopathy, cerebellar symptoms, severe neck pain, or occipital headache.[30] Accidental findings with no clinical symptoms may be managed conservatively with an MRI surveillance.[31]

The goals of surgical treatment are to decompress the craniocervical junction and to restore the normal flow of CSF through the foramen magnum.[30] Posterior decompression with or without duraplasty via suboccipital craniectomy is the most common procedure.[32] Other procedures include anterior decompression of the foramen magnum by odontoidectomy and shunting procedure.[33,34]

For CM type II and CM type III, surgical interventions include closure of open neural tube defects shortly after birth, treatment of hydrocephalus, and decompression of posterior fossa structures.

Arteriovenous malformation

Pediatric vascular CNS malformations include specific lesions found in children as well as anomalies seen in adults. These include arteriovenous malformations (AVMs), cavernous malformations, and dural arteriovenous fistulas (AVF). They may, however, have some distinct characteristics in children.[35] Vascular malformation can present as a space-occupying lesion, a source of intracranial hemorrhage, or a cause of high-output cardiac failure.

Pediatric-specific lesions are commonly associated with other conditions and certain genetic mutations only recently described.

Infantile hemangiomas present as strawberry red lesions and show rapid growth right after birth with spontaneous regression in preschool years. They are benign vascular tumors of infancy affecting mostly females.[36] Evidence supports use of propranolol as a first-line therapy, being more effective and having fewer side effects compared to systemic steroids or laser ablation therapy.[37,38] Hemangiomas can present as a part of a broader condition, PHACES (posterior fossa, hemangioma, arterial lesions, cardiac abnormalities, eye abnormalities), which includes posterior fossa, arterial, cardiac, eye, and sternal anomalies.

Vein of Galen malformation is unique to pediatric populations. This malformation, prior to development of endovascular technique, had a very high morbidity and mortality with or without surgical therapy. Clinical manifestation may include parenchymal brain loss and calcification, high-output heart failure, refractory pulmonary hypertension, hydrocephalus, facial and scalp venous prominence, intracranial venous hypertension, and neurocognitive decline.

Dural sinus malformation presents prenatally or early in neonatal period with enormous enlargement of one of the dural venous sinuses. The enlarged vascular structure can cause brain volume loss, intracranial hemorrhage, and thrombosis.

Several of the arteriovenous syndromes including Parkes–Weber syndrome, vein of Galen malformation, spinal arteriovenous lesions, and pial AVF show an association with *mutation in the RASA1 gene* and thus are genetically linked.[39–41]

The endovascular approach has significantly improved outcomes with a demonstrated survival rate of 76.9% for embolization of vein of Galen lesions.[42] Most centers use the transarterial approach for embolization with a nest of coils and subsequent liquid embolic agent injection using the femoral artery or umbilical artery for vascular access.[36,43] Increased use of the endovascular technique helped to speed development of catheters suitable for very small sheets while still allowing the use of balloons and other devices.[44]

Anesthesia for endovascular coiling and the embolization procedure present unique challenges. Vascular radiology suites are usually very cold and the space is limited due to vital but bulky X-ray equipment with added anesthesia paraphernalia. This requires that our equipment setup has to be well thought out. General anesthesia with endotracheal intubation is usually needed to prevent unwanted movement and control of respiration. Extensions for the breathing circuit and intravenous tubing may be added and an underbody warming blanket should be used to prevent hypothermia. Blood products should be ordered and readily available. Maintenance of anesthesia may need to accommodate the use of intraoperative neuromonitoring. Additional monitoring such as an A-line is occasionally warranted. Rigid blood pressure control both during the procedure and upon emergence is typically indicated as well and may prompt postoperative admission to the pediatric intensive care unit (PICU).

Myelomeningocele

Myelomeningocele is the most common form of the open neural tube defect, presenting as a posterior midline bone defect with exposed meninges and flat plate of dysplastic neural tissue (neural placode). This defect is a result of failure of caudal neurulation during fourth week of gestation.[45,46]

Over the past 50 years, the incidence has decreased with improved prenatal care and early folate supplementation.

It is a multisystem disease resulting from severe CSN injury early in gestation. The multisystemic morbidity presents a significant economical and psychological burden over the patient's lifetime. Patients are frequently evaluated for ventriculoperitoneal shunt, symptomatic tethered cord, urinary deficits, foot and spinal deformities, lower limb weakness, and difficulty in ambulation (Table 36.3).[47]

Primary myelomeningocele repair aims to eliminate CSF leak, prevent infection, preserve neural function, and prevent secondary tethering of the spinal cord. The surgery is performed within the first 48 h after initial stabilization and evaluation of the newborn.[48]

Surgery is performed in the prone position, so ETT should be very carefully secured. Temperature monitoring and use of active warming with an underbody forced-air warming

Table 36.3 Conditions Frequently Encountered with Myelomeningocele Defect

Arnold–Chiari type II malformation
Hydrocephalus
Tethered cord
Motor and sensory deficits below the
   level of lesion
Cognitive delay and learning disabilities
Depression
Sexual dysfunction
Urinary tract infection
Gastrointestinal dysfunction
Latex allergy

Source: Ferschl M. et al., *Anesthesiology* 118, 1211–1223, 2013.

blanket, warm ambient air, and warming lights are recommended to prevent hypothermia. Blood loss can be significant with large defects where complete skin closure requires freeing of a larger area of skin. Latex-free equipment should be used to prevent allergic reactions due to subsequent frequent exposures.

During induction of general anesthesia and intubation of the trachea, special care has to be taken to avoid direct pressure on the meningomyelocele by supporting the uninvolved part of the back or using a "donut" ring. Airway management can be difficult in patients with significant hydrocephalus.

Open fetal repair is a developing option showing improved motor outcome at 30 months of age and decreased need for ventriculoperitoneal shunt during the Management of Myelomeningocele Study (MOMS).[49] It aims to reduce the "second hit" caused by exposure of neural tissue to the uterine environment. However, open fetal repair was noted to carry risk for both mother and the fetus. Preterm birth and partial or complete uterine dehiscence were the most common risk factors. A multidisciplinary approach in the perioperative care is key to optimal outcome.[50]

Craniosynostosis

Premature closure of the scull sutures causes failure of normal bone growth perpendicular to the suture, resulting in an abnormal head shape. This is mostly an isolated condition but about 15%–40% of cases present as a part of a syndrome.[50] There are more than 180 syndromes associated with craniosynostosis (Table 36.4).[51]

Almost 50% of patients with Apert, Crouzon, or Pfeiffer syndromes develop obstructive sleep apnea.[52,53] Scaphocephaly (caused by sagittal synostosis) is the most common form of nonsyndromic craniosynostosis accounting for about 50% cases.

Any untreated craniosynostosis can lead to elevated ICP, abnormal intellectual and neurological development, and significant psychosocial implications.

Surgical approaches include open strip craniectomy, endoscopic strip craniectomy with postoperative helmet therapy, spring-mediated cranioplasty, and complex cranial vault reconstruction.

Open cranioplasty is a complex procedure with significant (and difficult to judge) blood loss.

Table 36.4 Most Common Syndromes Associated with Craniosynostosis

Apert syndrome	Brachycephaly, midface hypoplasia, maxillary retrusion, hypertelorism, syndactyly, cleft palate
Crouzon syndrome	Midface hypoplasia, mandibular prognathism, strabismus, beaked nose, conductive hearing loss, often normal intelligence
Pfeiffer syndrome	Hypertelorism, midface hypoplasia, nasopharyngeal stenosis, strabismus, hearing loss, often normal intelligence
Saethre–Chotzen syndrome	Short statue, facial asymmetry, low frontal hairline, ptosis, partial syndactyly, cardiac defects, deafness, often normal intelligence
Carpenter syndrome	Brachycephaly with synostosis of coronal, lambdoid, sagittal suture, cardiac and renal defects, optic atrophy, hearing loss
Cutis gyrata syndrome	Midface hypoplasia, cloverleaf skull, hydrocephalus, developmental delay, associated with increased paternal age
Muenke syndrome	Macrocephaly, unicoronal or bicoronal synostosis, ptosis, high-arched palate, hearing loss, developmental delay

Source: Stricker PA, Fiajoe J. *Anesthesiol Clin* 32, 215–235, 2014; Panigrahi I. *Indian J Hum Genet* 17, 48–53, 2011.

The airway is inaccessible during the surgery and the infant's proportionally large body surface is exposed to the cold operating-room environment, predisposing the patient to hypothermia.

Open procedures have significant blood loss and many techniques are used to decrease the likelihood or the amount of transfusion as well as promote homeostasis:

- Preoperative erythropoietin administration and iron supplementation
- Local anesthetic with epinephrine solutions infiltration
- Application of scalp clips
- Temporary locking scalp sutures placed anteriorly and posteriorly to the incision
- Continuous infusion of tranexamic acid (antifibrinolytic therapy)
- Cell salvage
- Acute normovolemic hemodilution
- Prophylactic administration of fresh-frozen plasma (FFP)

Endoscopic strip procedures usually have minimal blood loss but there is still a potential for inadvertent dural venous sinus entry or emissary vein disruption and large hemorrhage, so good intravenous access and immediate blood availability is a necessity. After surgery, the infant is fitted with cranial orthotics. Patients wear their helmet 22 h daily for about 6 months to assure normal skull shape with subsequent growth.

Spring-mediated cranioplasty

During this procedure, simple strip craniectomy is performed with insertion of specific springs between the edges of bone. This promotes cranial expansion and normalization of growth. Just like endoscopic strip craniectomy, it is usually performed on infants less than 6 months of age, with isolated sagittal synostosis. It is a shorter procedure with minimal blood loss and a short hospital stay. Patients are not required to wear a helmet after this procedure, but do need to return for a second operation to remove the springs.

Following are the intraoperative complications to watch out for during these procedures:[54]

- Hyponatremia
- Hypocalcemia
- VAE
- Intracranial hypertension
- Hypothermia
- Positioning and eye protection

Conclusion

Providing anesthesia for neurosurgical procedures for infants and children presents with unique challenges for the anesthesiologist because of the anatomic, physiologic, and developmental growth differences. Also as discussed briefly in this chapter, certain conditions are more common in pediatric populations. The anesthesiologist must consider all the developmental stage differences to be able to care for these patients safely.

References

1. Bissonnett B. Anesthesia for neurosurgical procedures. In: Gregory GA, editor. *Pediatric Anesthesia*. New York: Churchill Livingstone; 1994, pp. 375–419.

2. Vavilala MS, Soriano SG. Anesthesia for neurosurgery. In: Davis PJ, Cladis FP, Motoyama EK, editors. *Smith's Aesthesia for Infants and Children*. Philadelphia, PA: Elsevier; 2011, pp. 713–744.

3. McClain GD, Soriano SG. The central nervous system: Pediatric neuroanesthesia. In: Holzman RS, Mancuso TJ, Polaner DM, editors. *A Practical Approach to Pediatric Anesthesia*. Philadelphia, PA: Lippincott Williams & Wilkins; 2008, pp. 177–214.

4. Abraham M, Singhal V. Intracranial pressure monitoring. *J Neuro Anesthiol Crit Care* 2015;2:193–203.

5. Mcclain GD, Soriano SG, Rockoff MA. Pediatric neurosurgical anesthesia. In: Cote CJ, Lerman J, Anerson BJ, editors. *A Practice of Anesthesia for Infants and Children*. Philadelphia, PA: Elsevier; 2013, pp. 510–532.

6. Minns RA, Brown JK, Engleman HM. CSF production rate: "real time" estimation. *Z Kinderchir* 1987;42:36–40.

7. Blomquist HK, Sundin S, Ekstedt J. Cerebrospinal fluid hydrodynamic studies in children. *J Neurol Neurosurg Psychiatry* 1986;49:536–548.

8. Wintermark M, Lepori D, Cotting J et al. Brain perfusion in children: Evolution with age assessed by quantitative perfusion computed tomography. *Pediatrics* 2004;113:1642–1652.

9. Kennedy C, Sokoloff L. An adaptation of the nitrous oxide method to the study of cerebral circulation in children: Normal values for cerebral blood flow and cerebral metabolic rate in childhood. *J Clin Invest* 1957;36:1130–1137.

10. Fury C, Howell T. Paediatric neuroanesthesia. *Cont Educ Anesth Crit Care Pain* 2010;10:172–176.

11. Cross KW, Dear PR, Hathorn MK et al. An estimation of intracranial blood flow in the new-born infant. *J Physiol* 1979;289:329–345.

12. Greisen G. Autoregulation of cerebral blood flow in newborn babies. *Earl Human Dev* 2005;81:423–428.

13. Pryds O. Control of cerebral circulation in the high-risk neonate. *Ann Neurol* 1991;30:321–329.

14. Boylan GB, Young K, Panerai RB et al. Dynamic cerebral autoregulation in sick newborn infants. *Pedi Res* 2000;48:12–17.

15. Tsuji M, Saul JP, du PA et al. Cerebral intravascular oxygenation correlates with mean arterial pressure in critically ill premature infants. *Pediatrics* 2000;106:625–632.

16. American Society of Anesthesiologists Committee. Practice guidelines for preoperative fasting and the use of pharmacologic agents to reduce the risks of pulmonary aspiration: Application to healthy patients undergoing elective procedures. *Anesthesiology* 2011;3:495–511.

17. Soriano SG, McManus ML. Pediatric neuroanesthesia and critical care. In: Cottrell JE, Young WL, editors. *Cottrell and Young's Neuroanesthesia*. Philadelphia, PA: Mosby Elsevier; 2010, pp. 327–342.

18. Faberowski LW, Black S, Mickle JP. Incidence of venous air embolism during craniotomy for craniosynostosis repair. *Anesthesiology* 2000;92:20–23.

19. Mason KP, Lerman J. Dexmedetomidine in children: Current knowledge and future applications. *Anesth Analg* 2011;113:1129–1142.

20. Branco RG, Tasker RC. Glycemic level in mechanically ventilated children with bronchiolitis. *Pediat Crit Care Med* 2007;8:546–550.

21. Sharma D, Jelacic J, Chennuri R et al. Incidence and risk factors for perioperative hyperglycemia in children with traumatic brain injury. *Anesth Analg* 2009;108:81–89.

22. Klein GW, Hojsak JM, Rapaport R. Hyperglycemia in the pediatric intensive care unit. *Curr Opin Clin Nutr Metab Care* 2007;10:187–192.

23. Branco RG, Garcia PC, Piva JP et al. Glucose level and risk of mortality in pediatric septic shock. *Pediat Crit Care Med* 2005;5:470–472.
24. Rath GP, Dash HH. Anesthesia for neurosurgical procedures in paediatric patients. *Indian J Anaesth* 2012;56:502–510.
25. Deshpande JK. Anesthesia for neurosurgery in infants and children. Available at: www.sld.cu/galerias/pdf/sitios/anestesiologia/neuro_anest_ped.pdf
26. Vuksanaj D, Deshpande JK. Anesthesia for neurosurgery in infants and children. *ASA Refresh Courses Anesthesiol* 2008;36:215–216.
27. Wilson PE, Oleszek JL, Clayton GH. Pediatric spinal cord tumors and masses. *J Spinal Cord Med* 2007;30:s15–s20.
28. Sarnat HB. Disorders of segmentation of the neural tube: Chiari malformations. *Handb Clin Neurol* 2008;87:89.
29. Tubbs RS, Iskendar BJ, Bartolucci AA, Oakes WJ. Critical analysis of the Chiari 1.5 malformation. *J Neurosurg* 2004;101:179.
30. Hankinson TC, Klimo P, Feldstein NA et al. Chiari malformations, syringohydromyelia and scoliosis. *Neurosurg Clin N Am* 2007;18:549–568.
31. Novegno F, Caldarelli M, Massa A et al. The natural history of the Chiari Type I anomaly. *J Neurosurg Pediatr* 2008;2:179.
32. Tubbs RS, McGirt MJ, Oakes WJ. Surgical experience in 130 pediatric patients with Chiari I malformations. *J Neurosurg* 2003;99:291.
33. Hwang SW, Heilman CB, Riesenburger RI, Kryzanski J. C1–C2 arthrodesis after transoral odontoidectomy and suboccipital craniectomy for ventral brain stem compression in Chiari I patients. *Eur Spine J* 2008;17:1211.
34. Hankinson TC, Grunstein E, Gardner P et al. Transnasal odontoid resection followed by posterior decompression and occipitocervical fusion in children with Chiari malformation Type I and ventral brainstem compression. *J Neurosurg Pediatr* 2010;5:549.
35. Lizuka Y, Rodesch G, Garcia-Monaco R et al. Multiple cerebral arteriovenous shunts in children: Report of 13 cases. *Childs Nerv Syst* 1992;8:437–444.
36. Burch EA, Orbach DB. Pediatric central nervous system vascular malformations. *Pediatr Radiol* 2015;45:S463–S472.
37. Ghosh PS, Ghosh D. Infantile intraspinal and extensive cutaneous hemangioma: Excellent response to propranolol. *Neurology* 2011;76:1771.
38. Liu X, Qu X, Zheng J, Zhang L. Effectiveness and safety of oral propranolol versus other treatments for infantile hemangiomas: A meta-analysis. *PLoS One* 2015;10(9):e0138100.
39. Johnston IH, Whittle IR, Besser M, Morgan MK. Vein of Galen malformation: Diagnosis and management. *Neurosurgery* 1987;20:747–758.
40. Earola I, Boon LM, Mulliken JB et al. Capillary malformation–arteriovenous malformation, a new clinical and genetic disorder caused by *RASA1* mutations. *Am J Hum Genet* 2003;73:1240–1249.
41. Revencu N, Boon LM, Mulliken JB et al. Parkes Weber syndrome, vein of Galen aneurysmal malformation, and other fast-flow vascular anomalies are caused by RASA1 mutations. *Hum Mutat* 2008;29:959–965.
42. Thiex R, Mulliken JB, Revencu N et al. A novel association between RASA1 mutations and spinal arteriovenous anomalies. *Am J Neuroradiol* 2010;31:775–779.
43. Berenstein A, masters LT, Nelson PK et al. Transumbilical catheterization of cerebral arteries. *Neurosurgery* 1997;41:846–850.
44. Gross BA, Orbach DB. Addressing challenges in 4F and 5F arterial access for neurointerventional procedures in infants and young children. *J Neurointerv Surg* 2014;6:308–313.
45. Wagner W, Schwarz M, Perneczky A. Primary myelomeningocele closure and consequences. *Curr Opin Urol* 2002;12:465–468.
46. Tulipan N, Bruner JP. Intrauterine myelomeningocele repair. In: McLone DG, editor. *Pediatric Neurosurgery. Surgery of the Developing Nervous System.* Philadelphia, PA: WB Saunders; 2001, pp. 1281–1293.
47. Ferschl M, Ball R, Lee H, Rollins MD. Anesthesia for in utero repair of

myelomeningocele. *Anesthesiology* 2013;118:1211–1223.

48. Park TS. Meylomeningocel. In: Albright AL, Pollack IF, Adelson PD, editors. *Principles and Practice of Pediatric Neurosurgery.* Stuttgart: Thieme; 1999, pp. 291–320.

49. Adzick NS, Thom EA. MOMS investigators: A randomized trial of prenatal versus postnatal repair of myelomeningocele. *N Engl J Med* 2011;364:993–1004.

50. Stricker PA, Fiajoe J. Anesthesia for craniofacial surgery in infancy. *Anesthesiol Clin* 2014;32:215–235.

51. Panigrahi I. Craniosynostosis genetics: The mystery unfolds. *Indian J Hum Genet* 2011;17:48–53.

52. Thomas K, Hughes C, Johnson D, Das S. Anesthesia for surgery related to craniosynostosis: A review. Part 1. *Pediatr Anesth* 2012;22:1033–1041.

53. Moore M. Upper airway obstruction in the syndromal craniosynostoses. *Br J Plast Surg* 1993;46:355–362.

54. Hughes C, Thomas K, Johnson D, Das S. Anesthesia for surgery related to craniosynostosis: A review. Part 2. *Pediatr Anesth* 2012;23:22–27.

Geriatrics

M. V. S. SATYA PRAKASH

Introduction

Patients who are aged more than 65 years are called elderly, old-age, or geriatric patients. Because of the improved medical facilities and public health facilities throughout the world, the geriatric population is increasing each year. As the geriatric population is increasing, a subgroup is emerging called the oldest old, who are more than 80 years old.[1]

Physiological changes in old age

The process of aging causes many changes in the physiological function of all the organ systems. Whether it is programmed theory or error theory which explains the process of aging, all say that aging causes a progressive decline in the normal function, the reserve capacity of the organs, and the ability to respond to intrinsic and extrinsic stimuli.[2]

Central nervous system

As age increases, there is decrease in brain volume (4% every year), dopamine levels (10% every decade), and cerebral metabolic rate in the brain.

At the same time, there is an increase in blood–brain barrier permeability, increase in arterial wall thickness, and increase in monoamine oxidase activity. All these changes occur after 40 years of age. As there is reduction in brain volume, it is more loss in the white matter than the gray matter. There is decrease in memory of the episodic type.[3] As dopamine and serotonin levels decline during old age, cognitive and motor performances also decrease. As monoamine oxidase increases during old age, it causes more release of free radicals from reactions that exceed the antioxidant reserves of the brain leading to cell damage. As the blood–brain barrier permeability increases with age, it allows inappropriate passage of mediators from the plasma into the brain, leading to increased inflammatory response and structural damage to the brain. The denseness of the capillaries decreases and intimal thickness increases with age (from the fifth decade of life) in the brain, leading to increase in vascular resistance, and decrease in perfusion pressure, thereby decreasing neurocognitive function. There is progressive decline in central nervous system (CNS) activity and loss of neurons in cerebral cortex, leading to decrease in slow-wave sleep (stage 4), susceptibility to delirium

(<1 month), nocturnal respiratory dysfunction (sleep apnea syndrome), Alzheimer's syndrome, dementia, and global cognitive impairment. All these changes lead to increase in the prevalence of postoperative cognitive dysfunction and delirium after anesthesia.

Cardiovascular system

As age increases, the connective tissue within the arteries, veins, and the myocardium stiffens due to cessation of elastin production leading to replacement with less flexible collagen causing them to become less compliant. Arterial stiffening leads to systolic hypertension, impaired impedance matching, and myocardial hypertrophy. The combination of myocyte hypertrophy and increased left ventricular afterload prolongs myocardial contraction. This extended contraction leads to a delay in ventricular relaxation and results in early diastolic filling rates declining by approximately 50% between the second and the eighth decades. But the end-diastolic volume is preserved secondary to late diastolic filling and becomes more dependent on atrial contribution for effective filling. Ventricular myocardial stiffening and hypertrophy, therefore, render the heart dependent on atrial filling pressures. All these increase susceptibility to diastolic heart failure due to diastolic dysfunction in old age with preserved ejection fraction. As age increases, there is increase in sympathetic system activity, leading to increase in the release of norepinephrine levels at the nerve endings. Beta-receptor response to the stimulation decreases with age due to decrease in the intracellular coupling with adenylate cyclase. This leads to decrease in chronotropic and ionotropic responses to the beta-receptor stimulation to the intrinsic and extrinsic drugs. There is decrease in nitric oxide production leading to increase in the damage due to the free radicals in the vessels and myocardium. This causes impairment of the flow in the microvasculature thus increasing the risk for organ dysfunction. All the earlier mentioned changes lead to more hypotension and more hemodynamic instability during anesthesia in old age.

Respiratory system

The maximal functional status of the lung is achieved by the third decade. Lung function starts decreasing after the third decade due to old age. Like that of the CVS, the elastin production decreases with age leading to reduction in the elastic recoil of the alveoli. This leads to decrease in the lung volume at a rate of 0.1–0.2 cmH_2O per year. The alveolar surface area decreases from 75 to 30–60 m^2 by 70 years of age. The structural changes in the intercostal muscles, joints, ribs, and their articulations with the vertebrae lead to decrease in the compliance of the chest wall. As age increases, there is increase in the ventilation perfusion mismatch, chest wall rigidity, work of breathing, residual volume, and closing volume, and decrease in respiratory muscle strength, functional alveolar surface area, vital capacity, and gas exchange. All these lead to increased chances for postoperative respiratory complications such as prolonged mechanical ventilation. At the same time, there is decrease in response to hypoxia and hypercapnia.

Gastrointestinal system

There is decrease in esophageal motility, decrease in gastric acid secretions, and increase in gastric emptying time, leading to increased chances for aspiration during general anesthesia. As age increases, secondary atrophic gastritis develops, which leads to decreased bioavailability of calcium and decreased absorption of vitamin B_{12}. As age increases, the hepatic blood flow, hepatic blood volume, microsomal demethylation pathway, and drug metabolism decrease, leading to decrease in the metabolism of all the anesthetic drugs.

Renal system

In old age, the number of functional nephrons decreases, leading to decrease in glomerular filtration rate and renal blood flow. All these lead to decrease in the ability to concentrate urine and maintain electrolyte homeostasis in the body (especially sodium and potassium). The renin–angiotensin system activity decreases with age, leading to decrease in plasma renin and angiotensin when compared to angiotensin II.[4] All these decrease systemic clearance of drugs in old age and increase the chances of perioperative acute kidney injury.

Endocrine system

There is no change in the serum thyroxine levels and female luteinizing hormone in old age. There is impaired glucose tolerance with age due to increased insulin resistance, leading to more lability in the glucose levels in the perioperative period. As there is decrease in the endocrine function in old age, tissue responsiveness to drugs decreases.[5] Endocrine responses to elective surgical procedures is not altered in geriatric patients.

There is depression in the immune function in old age. So they have an initial hyperactive response followed by delayed termination of the inflammatory response to surgery and anesthesia. The magnitude of surgical stress response depends on duration of surgery, type of anesthesia, surgical technique, age and comorbidity of the patient, frailty, and malnutrition of the patient.

Pharmacokinetics

As age increases, there is decrease in total body water by 10%–15%, leading to increase in the plasma concentrations of water-soluble drugs in the initial period of administration. There is increase in total body fat, leading to increase in the volume of distribution of the lipophilic drugs and prolonged action of these drugs. There is increase in circulating $\alpha 1$ glycoprotein and decrease in plasma albumin in old age, leading to changes in the free and active part of the administered anesthetic drugs. As age increases, there is decrease in renal clearance, decrease in hepatic clearance, and increase in volume of distribution, leading to increase in elimination half-life. Patients are vulnerable to cumulative effects of a drug with repeated doses.

Pharmacodynamics

As age increases, sensitivity of drugs increases due to loss of neuronal tissue and other systems in the body. Thus, the amount of a drug that is required for the same effect when compared to a younger patient is decreased. At the same time, as the metabolism and excretion also decrease, there is increase in duration of action of drugs. So it is advised to use those drugs that are not dependent on body metabolism, such as cisatracurium, or decrease the dosages or use those drugs that are short acting.[6] As age increases, the MAC requirement to achieve adequate depth of anesthesia for inhalation drugs decreases. Thus, an 80-year-old patient who is on 66% N_2O requires only 0.3% sevoflurane to achieve a minimum alveolar concentration (MAC) of 1. Meperidine and benzodiazepines cause more postoperative delirium when compared to their younger counterparts. Thus, according to the Beers criteria, it is advised not to use them in geriatric patients. Alternative medications should be used.

Preoperative evaluation of the patient

Guidelines for preoperative assessment of a geriatric patient were released by the American College of Surgeons (ACS) in 2012, the National Surgical Quality Improvement Program (NSQIP), and the American Geriatrics Society (AGS).[7] Their guidelines are given in Table 37.1. These assessments are in addition to the routine examination of the patient.

As per the ACS, the NSQIP, and the AGS guidelines, a complete neurological evaluation has to be done before surgery in terms of a patient's ability to understand the surgery and its consequences, his/her capacity for decision-making, and risk factors for postoperative delirium. The Mini-Cog test (Table 37.2) and clock drawing are recommended as tools to assess a patient's cognitive impairment and dementia. Neurological assessment also includes assessing a patient's ability to make a decision practically and legally and assessing whether the patient can give consent for surgery legally. Risk factors for postoperative delirium are given in Table 37.3. The CAGE test is conducted to determine the patient's depression and substance abuse. If the results are positive, then consider preoperative withdrawal prophylaxis or refer to a detoxification or abstinence program. Preoperative cognitive assessment can be done by the Mini–Mental State Examination. If preoperative cognitive function decreases, then the chances for postoperative delirium and pulmonary complications increase. If the patient has preoperative depression, then there are increased chances for major complications and discharge of the patient to other than home and increased mortality.

Cardiac evaluation should be performed according to the American College of Cardiology (ACC)/ American Heart Association (AHA) guidelines.

A preoperative risk calculator is developed based on type of surgery, functional status, creatinine level, American Society of Anaesthesiologists (ASA) class, and age of the patient. It provides probable chances for development of intraoperative myocardial infarction or cardiac event. Likewise, a risk calculator is developed for determining the postoperative respiratory failure or pulmonary complications. It includes type of surgery, emergency nature of the surgery, functional status, infection, and ASA class of the patient. The additional risk factors for postoperative pulmonary complications are chronic obstructive pulmonary disease (COPD), congestive heart failure (CHF), obstructive sleep apnea (OSA), preoperative abnormal creatinine and urea levels, general anesthesia, and preoperative transfusion.

Frailty of the patient can be assessed by many scores. It is recommended that the patient is at least assessed by one frailty score. The more frailty, the more the chances for developing intra- and

Table 37.1 Guidelines for Preoperative Assessment in the Elderly by the ACS, the NSQIP, and the AGS

- Assessing patients' cognitive ability and capacity to understand the anticipated surgery.
- Screening for depression, alcohol, and other substance abuse or dependence.
- Identifying the risk factors in the patient for the development of postoperative delirium.
- Performing cardiac and pulmonary evaluation as per the ACC/AHA guidelines, identifying the risk factors for postoperative pulmonary complications, and developing strategies for their prevention.
- Documenting the functional status and history of falls.
- Determining the baseline frailty score.
- Assessing patients' nutritional status.
- Enquiring about the detailed medical and pharmacological history.

Table 37.2 Mini-Cog Test

1. Get the patient's attention, then say:
   - "I am going to say three words that I want you to remember now and later. The words are banana, sunrise, chair. Please say them for me now."
   - Give the patient three attempts to repeat the words. If unable after three attempts, go to the next item.
2. Say all the following phrases in the order indicated:
   - "Please draw a clock in the space below. Start by drawing a large circle. Put all the numbers in the circle and set the hands to show 11:10 (10 past 11)."
   - If the patient has not finished the clock drawing in 3 min, discontinue and ask for recall of items.
3. Say: "What were the three words I asked you to remember?"
   - If the patient cannot recall all three items or if the patient is able recall one to two items and the clock drawing test is abnormal, then the patient is said to be demented.
   - If the patient is able to recall all three items or if the patient is able to recall one to two items and the clock drawing test is normal, then the patient is said to be normal.

Table 37.3 Risk Factors for Postoperative Delirium

- Cognitive and behavioral disorders such as cognitive impairment, depression, alcohol abuse or use, and sleep deprivation or disturbance.
- Diseases such as aortic procedures, hip fracture, infection, renal insufficiency, improper control of pain, anemia, hypoxia, and hypercarbia.
- Metabolic problems such as poor nutrition, dehydration, and electrolyte abnormalities such as hypo- or hypernatremia.
- Functional impairments such as hearing or visual impairment, poor functional status, or immobilized or partially immobile patient.
- Others such as age more than 65 years, polypharmacy especially psychotropic medications, urinary retention, constipation, and presence of urinary catheter.

postoperative complications. A few frailty scores are given in Table 37.4.

Functional status of the patient has to be assessed to know the baseline physical capacity. This determines the probability for developing postoperative complications. A few assessment tools are given in Table 37.5.

Nutritional status of the patient should be assessed by measuring height, weight, body mass index (BMI), serum albumin and prealbumin levels, and history of unintentional weight loss in the last 12 month. If the patient is malnourished, this has to be corrected to the possible level before an elective surgery. Nutritional status can

Table 37.4 Frailty Scores

Canadian study of health and aging frailty index (modified frailty index)	Hopkins frailty index
History of diabetes mellitus History of congestive heart failure History of hypertension requiring medication History of either transient ischemic attack or cerebrovascular accident Functional status 2 (not independent) History of myocardial infarction History of either peripheral vascular disease or rest pain History of cerebrovascular accident with neurological deficit History of either COPD or pneumonia History of prior PCI, PCS, or angina History of impaired sensorium Functional status measured in the 30 days prior to surgery. The presence of each variable was scored as 1. The score ranges from 0–11. Score 0 represents absence of frailty, while a score of 11 represents highest degree of frailty	Weight loss ≥10 pounds in the last year, decreased grip strength, exhaustion, low physical activity ascertained by inquiring about leisure time activities, slowed walking speed measured by the speed at which patient could walk 15 feet Additional criteria include age, race, gender, comorbidities, cancer surgery, preoperative residence, type of procedure (moderate or major surgery), type of surgery (laparoscopic or open surgery), site of surgery (intra- or extra-abdominal) Each parameter has a score of 0–1. A patient is said to be not frail if the score is 0–1, intermediately frail if the score is 2–3, and frail if the score is 4–5

COPD, chronic obstructive pulmonary disease; PCI, percutaneous coronary intervention; PCS, previous cardiac surgery.

Table 37.5 Tools for Assessing Functional Status of the Patient

Tool	Descriptions	Strengths	Limitations
Timed Up and Go Test (TUGT)	The time that a person takes to rise from a chair, walk 3 m, turn around, walk back to the chair, and sit down. During the test, the person is expected to wear his/her regular footwear and use any mobility aids that he/she would normally require. If the patient completes this test in less than 15 s, then the patient is said to be of good functional status	Easy to assess, reliable, and validated	Need a chair at the right height, difficult for patients with dementia, Parkinson, and visual impairments

(Continued)

Table 37.5 Tools for Assessing Functional Status of the Patient (*Continued*)

Tool	Descriptions	Strengths	Limitations
Modified Elderly Mobility Scale (MEMS)	Seven items are tested. Each is given a score and a combined score is used to determine the functional status of the patient. The items are a sitting patient is asked to lie down, a lying patient is asked to sit, a sitting patient is asked to stand, and a standing patient is asked to sit, along with gait of the patient, time to walk 5 m, and functional reach of the patient	Quick, easy to administer, reliable, and validated	No self-care component is present, needs to be assessed immediately after admission, needs controlled environment, functional reach component is difficult to assess
Tinetti Assessment Tool	This consists of a balance section and gait section. The balance section consists of nine factors. Each is given a score and a total of 16 score is given. The gait section consists of eight components. Each is given a score and a total of 12 score is given. The total of the two components is used to determine the functional status of the patient. A score of ≤18 is high, 19–23 moderate, and ≥24 low chances for fall	Simple and easy to administer and had good inter-rater reliability	Validity is not reported, no self-care component, and not enough to pick up some functional changes

be assessed by the Mini Nutritional Assessment score (Table 37.6). Total medication history has to be reviewed. Consider discontinuing nonessential medications. Identify the medications that need to be discontinued just on the morning of the day of surgery or 24 h before surgery. Avoid starting benzodiazepines as they increase the risk of developing postoperative delirium. Limit prescribing new medications. Adjust the dose of drugs that are excreted by kidney based on glomerular filtration rate rather than serum creatinine alone. Even though serum creatinine remains the same because of decreased muscle mass in old age, the glomerular filtration rate decreases.

Geriatric patients require baseline investigations such as hemoglobin level, renal function, albumin level, electrocardiogram (ECG), and chest X-ray. Cardiac evaluation should be done as per the ACC/AHA guidelines. Testing has to be done depending on the presence of a disease or symptoms or signs. Unnecessary investigation leads

to confusion and problems. The patient has to be counseled and prepared properly for the surgery so that the patient undergoes the surgery with less anxiety and less postoperative complications.

A complete review of the comorbid conditions has to be done. The Charlson Comorbidity Index determines the 10-year mortality rate for a patient who has many comorbid conditions. More comorbidities preoperatively indicate that there are more chances for developing more postoperative complications and more chances for morbidity and mortality. Try to optimize the comorbid conditions to the optimum levels before taking up for surgery.

Intraoperative management

A majority of neurosurgery cases are given general anesthesia as a majority of surgeries are performed on the brain. But some surgeries are performed by neurosurgeons that do not require general anesthesia, such as awake craniotomy. It is found that

MAC with light sedation is preferable to regional anesthesia and regional anesthesia is preferable to general anesthesia as there are less chances of developing postoperative complications.[8,9] Cai et al.[10] performed a randomized controlled study in which they compared inhalational maintenance (TIMA) and total intravenous anesthesia (TIVA). They concluded that TIVA is associated with lesser activation of stressor response than TIMA as there was less serum cortisol, norepinephrine, epinephrine, and growth hormone levels and less heart rate variability in TIVA. But there were many limitations in this study and the inhalational levels that were maintained were at higher levels than usually followed. At the same time, there are no such studies comparing TIVA with TIMA for postoperative complications in elderly patients. Thus at present, we cannot comment on which of the two techniques has fewer postoperative complications. Geriatric patients are generally on polypharmacy.[11] So an anesthesiologist should be careful in choosing drugs so that there are no interactions between the drugs. The anesthesiologist should administer drugs keeping in mind that in older patients there is delayed onset of action and prolongation of duration of action, so that there should not be stacking of doses, which may lead to overshooting of the doses leading to prolonged postoperative complications. To avoid dose stacking, try to induce slowly titrating to the effect and reduce the amount of drug that is given to get the desired response as per the age of the patient. Geriatric patients are more prone to comorbid conditions than their young counterparts. This should be kept in mind while devising the plan for anesthesia.

Postoperative management

There is decreased physiological reserve in geriatric patients. This leads to increased chances of postoperative complications. A proper preoperative assessment and preparation of the patient reduces postoperative complications. Postoperative complications that can occur are increased length of stay, increased chances of ICU stay, increased hours of elective ventilation, unanticipated postoperative ventilation, development of postoperative cognitive dysfunction, postoperative delirium, increased duration of cardiovascular instability, and so on. A majority of these complications can be reduced by properly treating pain.

Pain should be treated in geriatric patients using a multimodal approach consisting of opioids, nonopioid analgesics (e.g., paracetamol, nonsteroidal anti-inflammatory drugs [NSAIDs], tramadol, and gabapentinoids), regional anesthesia techniques, and peripheral nerve blocks. It should be kept in mind that geriatric patients have increased sensitivity to drugs leading to prolongation of their duration of action. Intravenous patient-controlled analgesia

Table 37.6 Mini Nutritional Assessment

Parameter to be assessed	Points to be allotted
Has food intake decreased over the past 3 months?	0, severe decrease; 1, moderate decrease; 2, no decrease
Weight loss during the last 3 months?	0, greater than 3 kg; 1, does not know; 2, weight loss between 1 and 3 kg; 3, no weight loss
Mobility	0, bedridden or chair bound; 1, able to get out of bed or chair but cannot go out; 2, goes out
Any psychological stress or acute disease in the past 3 months?	0, yes; 2, no
Neuropsychological problems	0, severe dementia or depression; 1, mild dementia; 2, no psychological problem
BMI (kg/m^2)	0, BMI < 19; 1, 19–21; 2, 21–23; 3, 23 or greater
If BMI cannot be measured then calf circumference (cm) should be measured	0, less than 31; 3, more than 31
A maximum score of 14 is available. If a patient scores 12–14 points, this is considered normal nutritional status, 8–11 points is at risk for malnutrition, and 0–7 points is said to be malnourished	

BMI, body mass index.

and patient-controlled epidural analgesia are more preferred than intermittent or continuous administration of drugs as they produce less complications. Drugs that are supposed to cause harmful effects in geriatric patients when compared to their younger counterparts were stratified into risk groups by the AGS using the Beers criteria.[12] These criteria help the clinician in making a full risk–benefit assessment in choosing an analgesic.

References

1. Aurini L, White PF. Anesthesia for the elderly outpatient. *Curr Opin Anaesthesiol* 2014;27:563–575.
2. Schmucker DL. Age-related changes in liver structure and function: Implications for disease? *Exp Gerontol* 2005;40:650–659.
3. Peters R. Ageing and the brain. *Postgrad Med J* 2006;82:84–88.
4. Epstein M. Aging and the kidney. *J Am Soc Nephrol* 1996;7:1106–1122.
5. Alvis BD, Hughes CG. Physiology considerations in geriatric patients. *Anesthesiol Clin* 2015;33:447–456.
6. Akhtar S, Ramani R. Geriatric pharmacology. *Anesthesiol Clin* 2015;33:457–469.
7. Chow WB, Rosenthal RA, Merkow RP et al. Optimal preoperative assessment of the geriatric surgical patient: A best practices guideline from the American College of Surgeons National Surgical Quality Improvement Program and the American Geriatrics Society. *J Am Coll Surg* 2012;215(4):453–466.
8. Kim S, Brooks AK, Groban L. Preoperative assessment of the older surgical patient: Honing in on geriatric syndromes. *Clin Interv Aging* 2014;10:13–27.
9. Lester L. Anesthetic considerations for common procedures in geriatric patients: Hip fracture, emergency general surgery, and transcatheter aortic valve replacement. *Anesthesiol Clin* 2015;33:491–503.
10. Cai Y, Hu H, Liu P et al. Association between the apolipoprotein E4 and post-operative cognitive dysfunction in elderly patients undergoing intravenous anesthesia and inhalation anesthesia. *Anesthesiology* 2012;116(1):84–93.
11. Wehling M. Guideline-driven polypharmacy in elderly, multimorbid patients is basically flawed: There are almost no guidelines for these patients. *J Am Geriatr Soc* 2011;59:376–377.
12. American Geriatrics Society 2012 Beers Criteria Update Expert Panel. American Geriatrics Society updated Beers Criteria for potentially inappropriate medication use in older adults. *J Am Geriatr Soc* 2012;60(4):616–631.

38

Traumatic brain injury

SHOBHA PUROHIT and RADHIKA DUA

Introduction

Traumatic brain injury (TBI) is a silent global epidemic and is a major cause of morbidity and mortality.[1] The incidence is steadily increasing and affecting the younger generation because of high-speed motorcycles, and is becoming a serious public health problem.

Nowadays in this era of modern science and technology, TBI should be managed by a multidisciplinary team of neurointensivists, neuroanesthesiologists, and neurosurgeons, so as to prevent the development of secondary injury and for better outcomes.

Other causes of TBI include falls and assault. TBI is of two types: primary injury and secondary injury. Primary injury occurs within the first few milliseconds and consists of the biomechanical effects of the forces applied to the brain. These can range from mild scalp lacerations to hematoma (extradural and subdural) or contusions. The secondary injury takes a few minutes, hours, or days to develop after the trauma. The contributory factors of secondary injury are hypoxia, hypotension, hyper- or hypoglycemia, and raised intracranial pressure (ICP).

Pathophysiology

TBI can be divided into two categories:

1. Primary injury, which occurs within milliseconds and is due to the biomechanical effects of trauma. The outcome depends on the degree of primary injury.
2. Secondary injury, which takes a few minutes to days to set in and is due to cerebral hypoxia and hypotension.

Primary injury

Static and dynamic mechanical forces in road traffic accidents lead to primary injury of the brain. Dynamic force injuries are seen more frequently than injuries due to static force. Car accidents and injuries are an example of dynamic loading and may result in depressed, linear, or basilar skull fractures, extradural hematomas, and coop contusions. Static loading occurs when slow-moving vehicles collide or during earthquakes. These cause multiple comminuted fractures of the vault or base of skull.

Types of primary injury

1. *Skull fractures*: These may be vault or basilar in location. Vault fractures may extend into the sinuses while basal skull fractures may be associated with injuries to the cranial nerves and discharge from ear, nose, or throat. The fractures are also classified as stellate, closed or open, depressed or nondepressed, and simple or compound fractures.

2. *Intracranial hemorrhages*: These are classified as epi- or extradural hematoma, subdural hematoma, Intra cerebral, intraventricular or subarachnoid hemorrhage.

   a. *Epi- or extradural hematomas (EDHs)*: These usually occur as a result of linear squamous temporal skull fractures with laceration of a branch of the middle meningeal artery. They can also be caused by laceration of dural arteries or veins, or by diploic veins in the skull's marrow. The potential space between the dura and the bone is expanded by the hematoma which creates a convex lens configuration. This gives the classical biconvex appearance on the CT scan (Figure 38.1). This is typically associated with a lucid interval following trauma. EDHs occur commonly in younger age groups, accounting for 66% patients under 20 years of age and only 5% patients aged over 50 years. An EDH is a surgical emergency and can be fatal if not evacuated urgently.

   b. *Subdural hematomas (SDHs)*: These are a collection of blood accumulating in the potential space between the dura and the arachnoid mater. These are due to stretching and tearing of bridging cortical veins as they cross the subdural space to drain into an adjacent dural sinus. These are the most common mass lesions resulting from head trauma. These can be acute (less than 3 days), subacute (4–21 days), or chronic (more than 21 days). They are typically crescent-shaped, and are usually more extensive than EDHs. In contrast to EDHs, SDHs are not limited by sutures but are limited by dural reflections, such as the falx cerebri, tentorium, and falx cerebelli. These lesions evolve rapidly and require urgent evacuation. Chronic SDHs are usually seen in infants and adults more than 60 years of age, and very often history of trauma is not elicited.

   c. *Intracerebral hemorrhages*: These occur within the cerebral parenchyma secondary to laceration or contusion of the brain with injury to larger deeper cerebral vessels associated with cortical contusion.

   d. *Intraventricular hemorrhages*: These have been found to occur in 35% moderate-to-severe TBI cases. These usually occur with extensive associated damage and so are associated with an unfavorable prognosis.[2,3]

   e. *Subarachnoid hemorrhage (SAH)*: Trauma is the most common cause of SAH. It may be caused by laceration of superficial microvessels in the subarachnoid space.

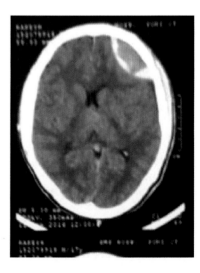

Figure 38.1 Computed tomographic scan showing classical biconvex appearance of large extradural hematoma.

Communicating or noncommunicating hydrocephalus may develop if blood products obstruct the arachnoid villi or blood clots obstruct the third or fourth ventricle, respectively.

3. *Coup and contrecoup contusions*: Coup contusions occur at the area of direct impact to the skull. These occur because of the creation of negative pressure when the skull, distorted at the site of impact, returns to its normal shape. Contrecoup contusions are located opposite the site of direct impact.

The amount of energy dissipated at the site of impact determines whether the ensuing contusion will be coup or contrecoup. Impact with a small, hard object results in a coup contusion, whereas a larger object will cause less injury at the impact site leading to a contrecoup contusion.

4. *Concussion*: This is the most common type of TBI and is caused by deformity of deep structures of the brain. It can lead to neurological dysfunction ranging from impaired consciousness to coma.

5. *Diffuse axonal injury*: High-speed acceleration/deceleration causes strain in tentorium and falx leading to extensive damage to white matter of the brain.

6. *Penetrating head injuries*: Gunshot wounds and missile/nonmissile projectiles cause many penetrating head injuries. High-velocity missiles tend to cause the most profound damage.

Secondary injury

This sets within minutes to days, but is preventable, and is mainly due to hypoxia or hypotension. A single episode of hypotension may increase the morbidity and mortality of patients (impact study). So, secondary injury can be minimized by avoiding cerebral ischemia and maintenance of adequate cerebral blood flow (CBF) and mean arterial pressure (MAP). The other factors that should be taken care of include blood glucose, PCO_2, temperature, anemia, and seizures.

The normal CBF is 50 mL/min/100 g and cerebral perfusion pressure (CPP) is 50–70 mmHg. The autoregulation ensures the maintenance of constant CBF with a varied range of CPP. This autoregulation is disrupted following severe TBI so that CBF becomes proportional to CPP. Immediately after head injury, the CBF decreases significantly and may decrease to 18 mL/min/100 g, further increasing the cerebral ischemic damage. Since CBF is difficult to measure, CPP is used as a marker for cerebral perfusion. CPP is determined by subtracting ICP or CVP (whichever is higher) from MAP (CPP = MAP − ICP). So, any increase in ICP will result in a decrease in CPP. Normal ICP is 5–15 mmHg. A rise in ICP of >20 mmHg is alarming and measures should be taken to reduce it.

Secondary injury is attributable to further cellular damage from the effects of primary injury. It is mediated through various neurochemical mediators such as excitatory amino acids (EAAs), including glutamate and aspartate causing cell swelling, vacuolization, and cell death. Endogenous opioids may also contribute to neurological damage by modulating the presynaptic release of EAA neurotransmitters. Heightened metabolism in the injured brain is stimulated by an increase in the circulating levels of catecholamines from TBI-induced stimulation of the sympathoadrenomedullary axis and serotonergic system with associated depression in glucose utilization, contributing to further brain injury.

Other biochemical processes leading to a greater severity of injury include an increase in extracellular potassium, leading to edema; an increase in cytokines, contributing to inflammation; and a decrease in intracellular magnesium, contributing to calcium influx.[3,4] These factors combined, along with the primary injury, lead to a vicious cycle of cerebral hypoxia with ischemia leading to depletion of ATP, inflammation, and blood–brain barrier (BBB) leak causing cerebral edema and raised ICP, which in turn decreases CBF and hypoxia. Tissue death occurs if CBF decreases below 8–10 mL/100 g/min.

Outcome

Analyzing the outcome of patients with head injury is quite difficult and depends on the type of injury, associated injuries, age, and the treatment received by the patients.

Lennett and Bond categorized the patient outcome under five groups:

Group I: Good recovery
Group II: Moderate disability
Group III: Severe disability

Group IV: Persistent vegetative state
Group V: Death

Classification

The classification of severity of TBI is based on Glasgow Coma Scale (GCS) score, which is used to assess consciousness and neurologic functioning of the patient duration of loss of consciousness (LOC), and posttraumatic amnesia (PTA) (Table 38.1).

The scoring is based on best motor response, best verbal response and eye opening.

Eye opening (Spontaneous = 4, To speech = 3, To painful stimulus = 2, No response = 1)

Best verbal response (Oriented to person, place and date = 5, Converses but is disoriented = 4, Inappropriate words = 3, Incomprehensible sound = 2, No response = 1)

Best motor response (Follows commands = 6, Localises pain = 5, Withdraws from pain = 4, Flexor (decorticate) posturing to pain = 3, Extensor (decerebrate) posturing to pain = 2, No response = 1)

It is the time from the moment of injury till the time the patient is able to demonstrate a continuous memory of things around them.

Initial assessment and management

Initial assessment of all trauma victims is carried out according to the tenets of Advanced Trauma Life Support (ATLS), followed by a specific neurological exam that includes GCS score, pupillary response, other cranial nerves examination, motor and sensory system examination, and attention to secondary injury mechanisms.

The main aim of management is maintenance of CBF to prevent hypoxia and ischemia. The Brain Trauma Foundation guidelines are given in Table 38.2.

Table 38.1 Classification of Severity of Traumatic Brain Injury

Severity	GCS	LOC	PTA
Mild	13–15	<20 min to 1 h	<24 h
Moderate	9–12	1–24 h	>24 h to < 7 days
Severe	3–8	>24 h	>7 days

Table 38.2 Brain Trauma Foundation Guidelines

Resuscitation of blood pressure and oxygenation	Avoid SBP < 100 mmHg and PaO_2 < 60 mmHg
ICP monitoring	Severe head injury with abnormal CT scan or normal CT with two or more factors: Age > 40 years SBP < 90 mmHg Unilateral/bilateral posturing
ICP monitoring technique	Ventricular catheter connected to external strain gauge
ICP treatment threshold	Treatment initiated at an upper limit of 22 mmHg
CPP	60–70 mmHg
Hyperventilation	Prophylactic hyperventilation (<25 mmHg) to be avoided in first 24 h
Hyperosmolar therapy	Mannitol (0.25–1 g/kg) effective for control of raised ICP
High-dose barbiturates	In hemodynamically stable patients with refractory intracranial hypertension not responsive to all medical and surgical therapies
Steroids	Not recommended
Antiseizure prophylaxis	Not recommended for prevention of late posttraumatic seizures

Nutrition	Replacement of 140% of REE in nonparalytic patients and 100% REE in paralytic patients with at least 15% calories as proteins by day 7

SBP, systolic blood pressure; CT, computed tomography; ICP, intracranial pressure; CPP, cerebral perfusion pressure; REE, resting energy expenditure.

Perioperative management

The initial assessment and resuscitation is started in the emergency room before the patient is transferred for CT scan and other interventions.

A CT scan is indicated in all patients with severe head injury. In the case of minor head injury, the New Orleans Criteria can be followed that state that CT scan is required if the patient meets two or more of the following conditions:[5]

- Headache
- Vomiting
- Age > 60 years
- Drug or alcohol intoxication
- Persistent anterograde amnesia (short-term memory deficits)
- Visible trauma above the clavicle
- Seizures

The resuscitative measures should continue while the patient is being transported to the operation theater. Any new onset of hypotension, anemia, hemodynamic instability, or hypoxia should prompt one to look for associated thoracic, abdominal, spinal, or long-bone injuries that are evolving after initial assessment.

Airway management

It has been reported that there is a higher incidence of cervical spine injury in patients with TBI, especially in those with severe TBI as determined by low GCS score and unconsciousness.[6,7]

Airway management is complicated by additional factors such as urgency of the situation due to hypoxia, presence of vomitus, blood or debris in the oral cavity, or skull base fracture. Criteria for intubation include the following:

- GCS score ≤ 8
- Risk of raised ICP due to agitation (sedation requirement)
- Loss of protective laryngeal reflexes

- A decrease of ≥2 points on motor component of GCS
- Optimization of oxygenation and ventilation
- Seizures
- Bleeding into mouth/airway
- Bilateral fractured mandible

Rapid sequence intubation is required while maintaining cervical spine immobilization using manual in-line stabilization. Various aids anticipating difficult airway situation should be available, such as video laryngoscope, fiberoptic laryngoscope, and laryngeal mask airways (LMAs).

Anesthetic management

The main goals of anesthetic management are as follows:

1. Provision of adequate analgesia and amnesia.
2. Maintenance of CPP.
3. Prevention and treatment of increased ICP.
4. Avoidance of secondary injury, such as hypoxemia, hypotension, hypo- or hypercapnia, and hypo- or hyperglycemia.

Anesthetic agents

Craniotomies are most commonly performed for evacuation of epidural, subdural, or intracerebral hematomas and contusion. Intravenous anesthetics decrease CBF, decrease cerebral metabolic rate ($CMRO_2$), and do not have an adverse effect on ICP, and as such are preferred over volatile anesthetics, which are cerebral vasodilators. The order of cerebral vasodilating property potency is halothane >> enflurane > desflurane > isoflurane > sevoflurane.

Thiopentone decreases CBF, $CMRO_2$, and ICP. It causes greater decrease in $CMRO_2$ than CBF. However, it may cause bronchospasm, and may decrease arterial pressure, stroke volume, and cardiac output which may be deleterious. It has been the induction agent of choice for years and is considered the gold standard.[8]

Etomidate also has neuroprotective effects in addition to being cardiac stable, showing minimal cardiodepressant effect. Therefore, it may be beneficial in patients with coexisting conditions such as hypertension, congestive heart failure, or previous myocardial infarction.

Propofol has similar properties of neuroprotection with the added advantage of rapid onset and short duration of action. It decreases systemic blood pressure and has a greater negative inotropic effect than both thiopentone and etomidate.

Autoregulation and carbon dioxide (CO_2) responsiveness is also generally maintained with intravenous agents.

Nitrous oxide (N_2O) is a cerebral vasodilator as well and is most potent when used as the sole agent. Its vasodilatory effect is least when it is combined in a balanced anesthesia technique with narcotics, benzodiazepines, or propofol.

Muscle relaxants with a propensity to release histamine (atracurium, mivacurium) should be used in divided doses. Succinylcholine also causes increase in ICP transiently, but rapid control of airway and ventilation should be given precedence over prevention of rise in ICP. Rapid intubation can also be achieved with high dose of rocuronium in patients in whom succinylcholine is contraindicated.

Monitoring

All the monitors that are part of the American Society of Anesthesiologists (ASA) standards should be used. In addition, an arterial catheter for invasive blood pressure and blood gas analysis may be inserted. Central venous catheterization may be performed for fluid resuscitation and vasopressor administration. However, these procedures should not delay the evacuation of expanding hematomas.

ICP monitoring may be done in accordance with the Brain Trauma Foundation guidelines.[9]

Depressed skull fractures over the sagittal sinus may warrant the placement of precordial Doppler and a right heart catheter for risk of venous air embolism.

Jugular venous oxygen saturation monitoring ($SjvO_2$) is not a widespread intraoperative application. Inadequate CBF results in an increased oxygen extraction, increased arteriovenous content difference, and reduced $SjvO_2$ value.

A normal $SjvO_2$ value is between 55% and 75%. Values <50% for 5 min are indicative of jugular desaturation. Various interventions such as increasing MAP, reducing hyperventilation, or inducing hypervolemia result in improvement in $SjvO_2$ value. It indicates global oxygen extraction and might have limited use in focal events.

Brain tissue oxygen monitoring ($PBtO_2$) is not generally used intraoperatively. It is more useful in the intensive care unit (ICU) during the postoperative period. It can be measured by inserting a flexible microcatheter usually in the frontal white matter, fixed to a special bolt. The normal value of $PBtO_2$ is around 40 mmHg and it is reflective of CBF. Values less than 22 mmHg are indicative of ischemia. Its limitation is that it might give information about the regional blood flow, where the catheter is inserted, which might not reflect global blood flow or ischemia.[10–14]

Ventilation

The patient should be ventilated to maintain PaO_2 of >60 mmHg. Hypercarbia must be avoided; however, hypocarbia should not be used indiscriminately. The target range of PaO_2 should be >100 mmHg and $PaCO_2$ should be kept in the low normal range between 35 and 39 mmHg. There is no role of prophylactic hyperventilation. The Brain Trauma Foundation guidelines state that hyperventilation should be avoided in the first 24 h after injury when CBF is critically reduced. It should be used to treat raised ICP, preventing or reversing herniation, to facilitate surgical access, and to minimize retractor pressure all of which are important in the management of patients with TBI. Excessive hyperventilation may cause vasoconstriction and lead to ischemia. End-tidal CO_2 is not a reliable indicator and arterial PCO_2 values should be monitored.[15]

Intravenous fluid management

The general principles for fluid management are maintenance of normovolemia to maintain MAP and to prevent reduction in serum osmolarity to prevent cerebral edema. The fluids most commonly used intraoperatively are normal saline or lactated Ringer's solution. Normal saline has osmolarity of 308 mOsm/L, which is slightly hypertonic with respect to plasma (295 mOsm/L) and in large volumes may cause hyperchloremic metabolic acidosis.[16] Lactated Ringer's solution, being slightly hypotonic (273 mOsm/L), is not ideal for replacement of both blood and third space loss, but serves as a compromise for meeting both needs simultaneously and is suitable at most times. However, large volume replacement with lactated Ringer's solution may lead to cerebral edema.[17] Thus, in the settings of large-volume fluid administration, it may be advisable to alternate both fluids.

The role of colloids versus crystalloids is a controversial one. Although the transcapillary pressure gradients due to reduction of colloid oncotic pressure are very small as compared to those produced by reduction in serum osmolarity, they might have the potential to augment edema.[18] So, it would be prudent to select a combination of isotonic crystalloid and colloid in the face of administration of a large volume of fluids such as in patients of multiple trauma.

The type of colloid solution to be used has been a subject for debate. A recent analysis of patients in the Saline versus Albumin Fluid Evaluation (SAFE) trial with severe head injury revealed increased mortality and unfavorable neurological outcome at 24 months in patients receiving albumin.[19] The dextran-containing solutions should generally be avoided because of their effects on platelet function. The starch-containing solutions may be used, but their cautious use is advised because they interfere with platelets and factor VIII complex and also cause dilutional reduction of coagulation factors. The recommended dose should not be exceeded while using these (20 mL/kg/24 h).[20]

There is current interest in the use of hypertonic saline as a resuscitation fluid in patients with TBI because it increases intravascular volume and decreases ICP. A double-blind randomized controlled trial comparing prehospital resuscitation of hypotensive TBI patients with hypertonic saline using standard fluid resuscitation protocols found no difference in neurological outcome at 6 months.[21]

For the time being, the choice of fluid for administration should be made on the basis of effect on the systemic circulation, because restoring systemic hemodynamics is likely to be advantageous to the injured brain.

Blood pressure management and vasopressor use

Vasopressors are used to treat hypotension or to increase CPP. There are very few studies comparing the effects of various vasopressors in patients of TBI. Although the studies showed there were no differences in mean cerebral flow velocity and cerebral oxygenation or metabolism between the two vasopressors, norepinephrine had a more predictable and consistent effect while dopamine use led to higher ICP.[22] Current evidence does not support the use of one vasopressor over another.

Blood transfusion

Both anemia and red blood cell (RBC) transfusion are associated with a poor neurological outcome. Anemia is associated with increased hospital mortality and lower hospital discharge GCS score.[23,24]

RBC transfusion can lead to acute lung injury and is also associated with longer hospital and ICU stay and mortality. Although it increases the oxygen-carrying capacity of blood, it also increases circulating volume and may increase CBF in patients with impaired cerebral autoregulation secondary to TBI. It is thus advocated that a liberal transfusion strategy (transfusion when Hb < 10 g/dL) should not be used in these patients.

Coagulopathy and factor VII

Coagulation disorder occurs commonly after TBI. A recent review has found that the prevalence of coagulopathy was more than 60% in severe TBI and was also associated with an increased mortality and poor outcome.[25]

Due to the release of tissue factor (TF) subsequent to brain injury, procoagulant factors are activated resulting in thrombin formation and conversion of fibrinogen to fibrin. Antithrombotic mechanisms are also activated to counter fibrin formation. Disseminated intravascular coagulation (DIC) inhibits the antithrombotic mechanism, causing imbalance of coagulation and fibrinolysis. Currently, there are no guidelines for management of coagulopathy in TBI. Hemostatic drugs including antifibrinolytic agents such as tranexamic acid and procoagulant drugs such as recombinant activated factor VII (rFVIIa) are sometimes used in treatment of coagulopathy after TBI.

The Clinical Randomization of an Antifibrinolytic in Significant Hemorrhage (CRASH-2) trial, evaluating the effect of tranexamic acid on death, vascular occlusion events, and blood transfusion in adult trauma patients, demonstrated that tranexamic acid was associated with a reduction of mortality.[26]

Hyperosmolar therapy

Diuretics have been widely used to reduce the volume of intracellular and extracellular fluid compartments of the brain. Mannitol is the preferred osmotic diuretic and is used in doses from 0.25 to 1.0 g/kg. It lowers ICP via two mechanisms. Early plasma expansion decreases blood viscosity and improves cerebral microvascular circulation and oxygenation. The delayed effect is due to osmotic gradient, drawing water from cerebral extracellular space into the vasculature, thereby reducing cerebral edema. An intact BBB is mandatory for osmotic action of mannitol otherwise edema may be worsened. It is administered over 10–15 min because sudden exposure to extreme hyperosmolarity may cause vasodilation worsening brain edema. Mannitol may cause hypotension, electrolyte imbalance, and rebound cerebral edema.

A combined administration of loop diuretic and osmotic diuretic may be used. It is based on the rationale that mannitol would draw out fluid from brain parenchyma and furosemide by excretion of water from intravascular compartment facilitating the maintenance of the gradient.

In patients with severe TBI and elevated ICP refractory to mannitol treatment, 7.5% hypertonic saline can increase cerebral oxygenation and improve cerebral and systemic hemodynamics.

Glycemic control

Hyperglycemia after TBI is associated with increased morbidity and mortality.[27–29] Secondary brain injury from hyperglycemia can occur, leading to an increase in glycolytic rates as shown by increased lactate/pyruvate ratio, causing metabolic acidosis, overproduction of reactive oxygen species, and neuronal cell death. However, more recent studies have failed to demonstrate the mortality benefit of intensive insulin therapy and also found an increased risk of hypoglycemia. Given the current evidence for glucose control for TBI in perioperative period, a target glucose range of 80–180 mg/dL is deemed reasonable.

Anticonvulsant therapy

Posttraumatic seizures can be immediate (within 24 h), early (within 7 days), and late (>7 days). Prophylaxis of early seizures reduces brain metabolism thereby reducing ICP.[30] The current literature supports the use of antiepileptics for prophylaxis of early posttraumatic seizures. Phenytoin has been extensively used and recommended in the first week after TBI. Levetiracetam is alternative therapy. The Brain Trauma Foundation guidelines do not recommend prophylaxis for late seizures.

Therapeutic hypothermia and steroids

Hypothermia reduces cerebral metabolism during stress, reduces excitatory neurotransmitters release, attenuates BBB permeability, and has been used for brain protection in patients with TBI for decades. However, clinical evidence in terms of mortality and functional outcomes is still inconclusive. A recent meta-analysis reported statistically insignificant reduction in mortality and increased favorable neurological outcome with hypothermia in TBI.[31] The benefits of hypothermia were greater when cooling was maintained for more than 48 h, but the potential benefits of hypothermia may be offset by various complications such as pneumonia, coagulopathy, and dysrhythmias.

Steroids have not been shown to improve outcomes or lower ICP in TBI. In fact, findings from a randomized multicenter study on the effect of corticosteroids (MRC CRASH trial) showed that administration of methylprednisolone within 8 h of TBI was associated with higher risk of death, and the risk of death or severe disability was more compared to placebo.[31,32] Therefore, the use of high-dose methylprednisolone is contraindicated in patients with moderate or severe TBI.

Postoperative management in the ICU

The decision to extubate a patient at the end of craniotomy is based on the severity of TBI and the anesthetic agents used. Patients with severe TBI as based on the GCS score are ventilated postoperatively and shifted to the ICU for further management. Those with mild-to-moderate head injury may be extubated at the end of the procedure, after confirming the reversal of neuromuscular blockade and recovery of the patient's airway protective reflexes. Further management in the ICU of the ventilated patients is based on the Brain Trauma Foundation guidelines, in addition to the general daily care received by all the patients, such as the following:

1. Head end of the bed should be elevated by 30°–45°. This, in addition to lowering ICP and improving CPP, also lowers the risk of ventilator-associated pneumonia (VAP).[33]
2. Head and neck of the patient should be kept in a neutral position to facilitate cerebral venous drainage and prevent rise of ICP.
3. Patients' position should be changed frequently to prevent development of pressure sores.
4. Provision should be made to ensure skin and mouth hygiene and eye care.
5. Central line bundle and VAP bundle should be implemented.[34]

Summary

TBI is a major cause of morbidity and mortality worldwide. The management of TBI focuses on prevention and treatment of secondary injury. Evidence-based guidelines and protocol-driven management have improved outcome in patients with TBI. A multidisciplinary team of the emergency department, neurosurgeons, and neuroanesthesiologists should be involved in the patient care.

References

1. Gururaj G. Epidemiology of traumatic brain injuries: Indian scenario. *Neurol Res* 2002;24(1):24–28.
2. Barkley JM, Morales D, Hayman LA, Diaz-Marchan PJ. Static neuroimaging in the evaluation of TBI. In: Zasler ND, Katz DI, Zafonte RD, editors. *Brain Injury Medicine: Principles and Practice.* New York, NY: Demos Medical Publishing; 2006, pp. 140–143.
3. Choi DW. Ionic dependence of glutamate neurotoxicity. *J Neurosci* 1987;7(2):369–379.
4. Meier R, Bechir M, Ludwig S et al. Differential temporal profile of lowered blood glucose levels (3.5 to 6.5 mmol/l versus 5 to 8 mmol/l) in patients with severe traumatic brain injury. *Crit Care* 20084;12(4):R98.
5. Haydel MJ, Preston CA, Mills TJ, Luber S, Blaudeau E, DeBlieux PM. Indications for computed tomography in patients with minor head injury. *N Engl J Med* 2000;343:100–105.
6. Holly LT, Kelly DF, Counelis GJ, , McArthur DL, Cryer HG. Cervical spine trauma associated with moderate and severe head injury: Incidence, risk factors, and injury characteristics. *J Neurosurg* 2002;96:285–291.
7. Demetriades D, Charalambides K, Chahwan S et al. Nonskeletal cervical spine injuries: Epidemiology and diagnostic pitfalls. *J Trauma* 2000;48:724–727.
8. Katzung BG. *Basic and Clinical Pharmacology.* New York, NY: Lange Medical Books/McGraw-Hill; 2001.
9. Bratton SL, Chestnut RM, Ghajar J et al. Guidelines for the management of severe traumatic brain injury. VI. Indications for intracranial pressure monitoring. *J Neurotrauma* 2007;24:S37–S44.
10. Meixensberger J, Dings J, Kihniqk H, Roosen K. Studies of tissue PO2 in normal and pathological human brain cortex. *Acta Neurochir Suppl (Wien)* 1993;59:58–63.

11. van den Brink WA, Haitsma IK, Avezaat CJ, Houtsmuller AB, Kros JM, Maas AI. Brain parenchyma/pO2 catheter interface: A histopathological study in the rat. *J Neurotrauma* 1998;15:813–824.
12. Leniger-Follert E. Oxygen supply and microcirculation of the brain cortex. *Adv Exp Med Biol* 1985;191:3–19.
13. Hoffman WE, Charbel FT, Edelman G, Hannigan K, Ausman JI. Brain tissue oxygen pressure, carbon dioxide pressure and pH during ischemia. *Neurol Res* 1996;18:54–56.
14. Doppenberg EM, Zauner A, Watson JC, Bullock R. Determination of the ischemic threshold for brain oxygen tension. *Acta Neurochir Suppl* 1998;71:166–169.
15. Bratton SL, Chestnut RM, Ghajar J et al. Guidelines for the management of severe traumatic brain injury. XIV. Hyperventilation. *J Neurotrauma* 2007;24:S87–S90.
16. Kellum JA. Saline-induced hyperchloremic metabolic acidosis. *Crit Care Med* 2002;30:259–61.
17. Tommasino C, Moore S, Todd MM. Cerebral effects of isovolemic hemodilution with crystalloid or colloid solutions. *Crit Care Med* 1988;16:862–868.
18. Drummond JC, Patel PM, Cole DJ, Kelly PJ. The effect of reduction of colloid oncotic pressure, with and without reduction of osmolality, on post traumatic cerebral edema. *Anesthesiology* 1998;88:993–1002.
19. Myburgh J, Cooper DJ, Finfer S et al. Saline or albumin for fluid resuscitation in patients with traumatic brain injury. *N Engl J Med* 2007;357:874–884.
20. Kozeck-Langenecker SA. Effects of hydroxyethyl starch solutions on hemostasis. *Anesthesiology* 2005;103:654–660.
21. Cooper DJ, Myles PS, McDermott FT, et al. Prehospital hypertonic saline resuscitation of patients with hypotension and severe traumatic brain injury: A randomized controlled trial. *JAMA* 2004;291:1350–1357.
22. Ract C, Vigué B. Comparison of the cerebral effects of dopamine and norepinephrine in severely head-injured patients. *Intensive Care Med* 2001 Jan;27(1):101–106.
23. Alvarez M, Nava JM, Rué M, Quintana S. Mortality prediction in head trauma patients: Performance of Glasgow Coma Score and general severity systems. *Crit Care Med* 1998 Jan;26(1):142–148.
24. Carlson AP, Schermer CR, Lu SW. Retrospective evaluation of anemia and transfusion in traumatic brain injury. *J Trauma* 2006;61(3):567–571.
25. Harhangi BS, Kompanje EJ, Leebeek FW, Maas AI. Coagulation disorders after traumatic brain injury. *Acta Neurochir (Wien)* 2008;150:165–175.
26. Shakur H, Roberts I, Bautista R et al.. Effects of tranexamic acid on death, vascular occlusive events, and blood transfusion in trauma patients with significant haemorrhage (CRASH-2): A randomised, placebo-controlled trial. *Lancet* 2010;376:23–32.
27. Liu-DeRyke X, Collingridge DS, Orme J et al. Clinical impact of early hyperglycemia during acute phase of traumatic brain injury. *Neurocrti Care* 2009;11:151–157.
28. Jeremitsky E, Omert LA, Dunham CM, Wilberger J, Rodriguez A. The impact of hyperglycemia on patients with severe brain injury. *J Trauma* 2005;58:47–50.
29. Sharma D, Jelacic J, Chennuri R, Chaiwat O, Chandler W, Vavilala MS. Incidence and risk factors for perioperative hyperglycemia in children with traumatic brain injury. *Anesth Analg* 2009;108:81–89.
30. Practice parameter: Antiepileptic drug treatment of posttraumatic seizures. Brain Injury Special Interest Group of the American Academy of Physical Medicine and Rehabilitation. *Arch Phys Med Rehabil* 1998 May;79(5):594–597.
31. Peterson K, Carson S, Carney N. Hypothermia treatment for traumatic brain injury: A systematic review and meta-analysis. *J Neurotrauma* 2008;25:62–71.
32. Edwards P, Arango M, Balica L et al. Final results of MRC CRASH, a randomised placebo-controlled trial of intravenous corticosteroid in adults with head injury-outcomes at 6 months. *Lancet* 2005;365:1957–1959.

33. Ng I, Lim J, Wong HB. Effects of head posture on cerebral hemodynamics: Its influences on intracranial pressure, cerebral perfusion pressure, and cerebral oxygenation. *Neurosurgery* 2004;54(3):593–597.

34. Tablan OC, Anderson LJ, Besser R et al. Guidelines for preventing health-care–associated pneumonia, 2003: Recommendations of CDC and the Healthcare Infection Control Practices Advisory Committee. *MMWR Recomm Rep* 2004;53(RR-3):1–36.

39

Myasthenia gravis

PRASANNA U. BIDKAR and NARMADHA LAKSHMI K.

Introduction

Myasthenia gravis (MG), also called "Erb–Goldflam syndrome," is a chronic autoimmune neurological disorder. It is caused by formation of autoantibodies against postsynaptic cholinergic receptors at the motor end plate. Incidence of the disease is found to be 50–142 cases per million.[1] Its prevalence in the United States is reported to be around 20 cases per 100,000 population.[2] Exact data on its prevalence in India is not known. It is characterized by increasing weakness and fatigability as work increases and improvement in muscle strength with rest. The disease proposes a significant challenge to anesthesiologist not only because of the disease process but also from the medications used to treat it (acetylcholinesterase inhibitors, steroids, etc.).

Pathophysiology of myasthenia gravis

The disease is caused by destruction of postsynaptic acetylcholine receptors (AChRs) by autoantibodies at the neuromuscular junction (NMJ).

Conventionally, acetylcholine is released presynaptically that binds with postsynaptic receptors and generates muscle action potential. In MG, the number of postsynaptic receptors available to generate muscle action potential becomes insufficient. With continuous work, as the muscle gets stimulated repeatedly, the acetylcholine release decreases with stimulation and correlates with the characteristic fatigability. Immunoregulatory defect and association of the disease with other autoimmune diseases have been reported. The role of the thymus in the pathogenesis of MG is not entirely clear, but 85% patients with MG have thymic hyperplasia and 15% have thymoma.

Forty percent of patients with MG possess anti-MuSK (muscle-specific tyrosine kinase) antibodies instead of anti-AChR antibodies. MuSK is essential for maintenance of agrin/rapsyn-dependent AChR clusters in postsynaptic membrane. The interaction of anti-MuSK antibodies and the receptor may lead to complement activation, subsequently damage and reduction of the number of AChRs.

Classification of myasthenia gravis

Osserman classified patients with MG into five grades:

Grade I: Only eyes affected
Grade IIa: Mild generalized MG responding well to therapy
Grade IIb: Moderate generalized MG responding less well
Grade III: Severe generalized disease
Grade IV: Myasthenic crisis requiring mechanical ventilation[3]

The most widely accepted classification of MG is the one given by the Myasthenia Gravis Foundation of America Clinical Classification,[4] which is the modification of original Osserman classification[5]:

- Class I: Any eye muscle weakness; possible ptosis; no other evidence of muscle weakness elsewhere
- Class II: Eye muscle weakness of any severity; mild weakness of other muscles
- Class IIa: Predominantly affecting limb or axial muscles
- Class IIb: Predominantly affecting bulbar and/ or respiratory muscles
- Class III: Eye muscle weakness of any severity; moderate weakness of other muscles
- Class IIIa: Predominantly affecting limb or axial muscles
- Class IIIb: Predominantly affecting bulbar and/or respiratory muscles
- Class IV: Eye muscle weakness of any severity; severe weakness of other muscles
- Class IVa: Predominantly affecting limb or axial muscles
- Class IVb: Predominantly affecting bulbar and/or respiratory muscles (can also include feeding tube without intubation)
- Class V: Intubation needed to maintain airway

Clinical presentation of myasthenia gravis

Patients with MG classically present with fatigability of voluntary muscles that worsens with repetitive activities and improves with rest. The weakness is usually noticed at the specific skeletal muscle groups, such as the extraocular muscles, bulbar, proximal extremities, and neck muscles. Involvement of the facial muscle gives rise to *expressionless* face. When the neck muscles are affected, they lose the ability to hold the weight of the head leading to *dropped head syndrome*.

Extraocular muscle involvement with pupillary sparing is one of the most important clinical features. Ptosis and diplopia are the initial presentation in most of the patients. Medial rectus is most commonly affected. When the patient is asked to look laterally for more than 20–30 s, extraocular muscle fatigability leads to diplopia. This is one of the simple maneuvers to elicit diplopia in patients with MG.

Bulbar myasthenia is seen in 85% of patients with MG presenting with generalized weakness in the form of dysphagia, dysphonia, dysarthria, dyspnea, or respiratory failure. Patients may also present with difficulty in handling secretions due to weakness in the pharyngeal and laryngeal muscles, leading to pulmonary aspiration.[6] The patient's ability to generate adequate ventilation and to clear bronchial secretions are of utmost concern with severe exacerbations of MG, which is termed as *myasthenic crisis*.[7] Thymic abnormality is seen in 85%–95% of patients with MG.

Precipitating factors of myasthenia gravis

Common precipitating factors for myasthenic crisis include respiratory infections, aspiration, sepsis, surgical procedures, rapid tapering of immune modulation, beginning treatment with corticosteroids, exposure to drugs that may increase myasthenic weakness, and pregnancy. Some drugs that exacerbate myasthenic crisis are macrolides, fluoroquinolones, aminoglycosides, tetracycline and chloroquine, beta-blockers, calcium channel blockers, diphenylhydantoin, lithium, chlorpromazine, muscle relaxants, levothyroxine, adrenocorticotropic hormone (ACTH), and, paradoxically, corticosteroids.

Diagnosis of myasthenia gravis

1. *Tensilon (edrophonium) test*: This is useful in diagnosing MG and in distinguishing myasthenic crisis from cholinergic crisis.

A positive response is not completely specific for MG because several other conditions (e.g., amyotrophic lateral sclerosis, brain tumors, and motor neuron disease) may also respond to edrophonium with increased strength.[8,9]

Edrophonium chloride has rapid onset (within 30 s) and short duration (5 min) of action which is administered intravenously. It increases the concentration of acetylcholine by inhibiting acetylcholinesterase at the NMJ, thus improving muscle weakness. If the muscle strength improves, the test results are considered positive. Development of increased weakness suggests abnormal neuromuscular transmission. Hence, resuscitation equipment and drugs should be kept ready. A total of up to 10 mg edrophonium is administered with a small dose to begin with. This is especially to avoid the muscarinic side effects of edrophonium at larger bolus doses. Side effects of edrophonium include bradycardia, increased salivation, sweating, nausea, stomach cramps, and muscle fasciculations. The sensitivity of edrophonium test is 85% for ocular MG and 96% for generalized MG.[10]

2. *Ice pack test*: Cooling may improve neuromuscular transmission. A positive test is clear resolution of the ptosis when ice is placed lightly over an eyelid. The test is thought to be positive in about 80% patients with ocular MG.
3. *Electrophysiological testing*: Repetitive nerve stimulation (RNS) and single-fiber electromyography (SFEMG) are the two principal tests performed in patients with MG.

RNS testing: This reduces the amount of acetylcholine available at the NMJ, leading to decremental response to RNS. A 10% decrease in the first and fourth evoked muscle action potential is diagnostic of MG.

SFEMG: This is the most sensitive test for detecting abnormal neuromuscular transmission. A fine-needle electrode is used for generating and recording evoked action potentials from the motor axon. Neuromuscular jitter refers to the abnormality of neuromuscular transmission noticed between the second and first action potentials. In MG, increased neuromuscular jitter is seen in 95%–99% patients.[11]

4. *Serologic testing*: Anti-AChR antibodies are the most specific pathognomonic for the diagnosis of MG.[12] They are 80%–85% sensitive to generalized MG and 50% for ocular MG.[13] Patients who are negative for anti-AChR antibodies should be screened for the presence of anti-MuSK antibodies.
5. *Radiologic testing*: A chest X-ray is indicated to determine the presence of aspiration or other pneumonias. A CT scan or MRI is highly accurate to detect thymoma.
6. *Arterial blood gas (ABG) test*: In severe disease state, an elevated $PaCO_2$ suggests progressive respiratory failure and may indicate the need for mechanical ventilator support.

Management of myasthenia gravis

Management of MG is based on the following two approaches:

- Increase in the number and duration of acetylcholine available to bind with the postsynaptic AChRs.
- Immunosuppressive therapy to reduce binding of antibodies to postsynaptic AChRs.

Acetylcholinesterase inhibitors

Acetylcholinesterase inhibitors are used as the first-line symptomatic treatment for MG. These drugs do not alter the disease progression or outcome. They inhibit acetylcholinesterases and increase the availability of acetylcholine to bind to postsynaptic AChR. Oral pyridostigmine is the most commonly used drug. The onset of action of the drug is within 15–30 min and the action lasts up to 4–6 h. It is started with an initial dose of 15–30 mg every 4–6 h and the dosage is increased until the desired effect is achieved. Neostigmine is the other commonly used drug that can be used for the treatment of MG. It can be administered by oral, IV, and IM route.

Adverse effects are due to their muscarinic properties that include bradycardia, nausea, vomiting, abdominal cramps, diarrhea, diaphoresis, and increased salivation, bronchial secretions, and lacrimation. Glycopyrrolate may be used for the management of these side effects.

Excessive dosing of anti-acetylcholinesterases may lead to cholinergic crisis. The symptoms include severe muscular fatigue with increased oropharyngeal and tracheobronchial secretions, with increased risk of aspiration pneumonia. The muscular weakness of cholinergic crisis is similar to that of myasthenic crisis but the former can be distinguished by the presence of muscle fasciculations, increased secretions, and bradycardia.

Long-term immune-modulating therapy

Corticosteroids

These are the most commonly used immune-modulating therapy in MG. Steroids are usually used in MG patients with unsatisfactory response to acetylcholinesterase inhibitors. The addition of corticosteroids may rapidly improve the symptoms, but these agents are associated with dose-dependent side effects and may exacerbate the symptoms in the initial 2 weeks of therapy. This initial dosing regimen of prednisone 1.5–2 mg/kg/day can be maintained for 2–4 weeks and then gradually tapered to a low dose or an alternative dosage regimen. Rapid tapering of corticosteroids may actually precipitate exacerbations or crises.

Nonsteroidal immunosuppressive agents

Azathioprine

This inhibits nucleotide synthesis, thereby interfering with T- and B-cell proliferation. It is usually effective after a long-term therapy of 6–8 months in 70%–90% patients with MG. The initial dose is 50 mg/day and is increased by 50 mg/day every week up to a total dose of 2–3 mg/kg/day. Side effects include dose-dependent myelosuppression and hepatotoxicity.

Cyclosporine

This is another immunomodulating agent that is used as a steroid sparing agent in the treatment of MG.[14] Clinical improvement is usually seen after 2 months of treatment. The typical dose in MG is 2.5 mg/kg every 12 h.

Mycophenolate mofetil

This is another steroid sparing agent that inhibits T- and B-cell proliferation. Improved strength is generally seen in patients after 2 months of mycophenolate mofetil (MMF) therapy. The dose is 1–1.5 g twice daily. Myelosuppression is seen at higher doses.

Cyclophosphamide

More than 50% patients on cyclophosphamide therapy become asymptomatic within 1 year of therapy for MG. Side effects include hair loss, nausea and vomiting, and skin discoloration.

Other agents

Rituximab and etanercept have also been shown to have steroid sparing effect in patients with MG.[15]

Short-term immune-modulating therapy

Plasma exchange/plasmapheresis

Plasma exchange (PEX) removes the AChR antibodies from plasma of patients with MG. It is done with either albumin or fresh frozen plasma. A large bore vein–like antecubital vein or central vein is preferred. In general, five to six PEXs are carried out on alternate days. The total exchange for each setting is around 200–250 mL/kg. The improvement is seen after the second or third PEX and the effect lasts for a short time unless the other forms of therapy are used. PEX is done to bring rapid improvement in myasthenic crises or during the preoperative period for thymectomy.

Intravenous immunoglobulin therapy

Intravenous immunoglobulin (IVIg) may provide a short-term improvement in patients with MG. The total dose of IVIg is 2 g/kg/day administered in equal doses for 5 days. Studies have shown comparable efficacy in patients who received either PEX or IVIg therapy.[16] Side effects of IVIg therapy include volume overload, renal failure, and idiosyncratic reactions such as fever, chills, nausea, vomiting, and headaches.

Surgical therapy

Thymectomy

Thymectomy is strongly recommended in MG patients with thymoma. However, the evidence is not very clear for nonthymomatous patients. Thymectomy is associated with drug-free remissions in patients with MG. Surgery is usually recommended in patients below 50 years of age.

Anesthetic implications

For neurosurgery, general anesthesia is preferred in 98% of cases. The main concern in myasthenic patients who come for surgery under anesthesia is the use of muscle relaxants. It is difficult to predict the response of the patient to muscle relaxants. Patients show marked resistance to succinylcholine due to decreased postsynaptic receptors at NMJ.[17] The ED95 dose of succinylcholine is 2.6 times that of normal patients. The anticholinesterases and plasmapheresis used to treat myasthenia decreases the plasma cholinesterase and pseudocholinesterase responsible for degradation of succinylcholine. So prolonged duration and chances of phase 2 block are increased with higher dose of succinylcholine in MG. These patients show marked sensitivity and ED95 is reduced to 50% in non-depolarizing muscle relaxants.[18] However short-acting non depolarizing muscle relaxants can be used with careful neuromuscular monitoring, which may avoid the requirement of reversal with anticholinesterase. The use of anticholinesterase may trigger cholinergic crisis.[19]

Preoperative assessment and preparation

The preoperative assessment should include assessment of severity of disease and the treatment regimen of the patient. It is better to optimize anti-cholinesterase and corticosteroid therapy preoperatively. Plasmapheresis is recommended in patients with severe respiratory failure.[3] Studies suggest that the usual morning dose of anticholinesterase be skipped or halved to decrease the dose of muscle relaxant needed during intraoperative period. Patients have to be assessed for predictors for the postoperative requirement of ventilation in the preoperative period itself. These are duration of disease (> 6 years), coexisting chronic respiratory disease, dose requirement of pyridostigmine (>750 mg/day), and vital capacity (<2.9 L).[20] The anesthetic plan has to be individualized depending on the condition of the patient and the type of surgery. Adequate hours of nil-per-oral (NPO) status have to be advised (usually 8 h).

Intraoperative managements

The monitoring during intraoperative period includes electrocardiogram (ECG), blood pressure, pulse oximetry, and temperature. In addition, a train of four (TOF) monitor is strongly recommended for perioperative monitoring. Preoperative TOF < 0.9 suggests decreased requirement of intraoperative muscle relaxants. Arterial cannulation is done to sample for $PaCO_2$ to monitor ventilator management and beat-to-beat variability of hemodynamic status. For surgeries, IV or inhalational anesthetics are used for induction, intubation, and maintenance of anesthesia in these patients. To facilitate endotracheal intubation, intermediate-acting muscle relaxants can be used in smaller doses (10%–25% of ED95). The deeper plane of anesthesia with these agents may help eliminate the requirement of muscle relaxants[21] and allow neuromuscular transmission to recover at the end of the surgery.

Postoperative management

Ventilatory function must be monitored carefully after surgery. Patients with severity grades III and IV have a higher incidence of postoperative respiratory failure.[22] Patients have to be assessed for extubation criteria; both clinical parameters (head-lift, tongue protrusion, adequate tidal volume generation) and TOF monitoring would be useful. The different response of peripheral versus bulbar muscles may be more evident in patients with MG, particularly those having bulbar and/or respiratory muscle weakness. In patients with MG, giving reversal at the end of surgery is controversial. However, if preoperative symptom control has been good, a standard dose of reversal inj. neostigmine 50 µg/kg and glycopyrrolate 10 µg /kg can be given. But case reports have shown that sugammadex (relaxant-binding agent) has been safely used to reverse vecuronium in patients with MG.[23] It is essential that sustained respiratory muscle strength be confirmed before extubation of the trachea and resumption of spontaneous ventilation.

Clinicians are well aware of the risk of postoperative respiratory failure that may result from stress-induced exacerbation of MG (myasthenic crisis), an overdose of anticholinesterases (cholinergic crisis), the residual effects of myorelaxants, or other adverse drug interactions (with antibiotics or antiarrhythmics). Therefore, routine postoperative ventilatory support and planned extubation in the intensive care unit (ICU) have been recommended in high-risk patients.[24]

Myasthenic crisis

This is an acute exacerbation of the myasthenic symptoms, a life-threatening medical emergency resulting from acute respiratory failure. It may manifest as either hypoxemic or hypercapnic acute respiratory failure due to worsening of weakness, necessitating admission to the ICU. The central drive for ventilation usually remains intact during myasthenic crisis. But the ventilator response to carbon dioxide accumulation is lost.[25] Use of concomitant drugs may precipitate crisis in patients with MG. Other precipitating factors include emotional stress, hot environment, and elevation of body temperature.

Clinical picture

The respiratory muscle weakness in myasthenic crisis is characterized by reduction in forced vital capacity less than 1 L, a negative inspiratory force of $\leq 20\,cmH_2O$, and decreased or inability to cough, thus necessitating mechanical respiratory support.

Diagnosis

Edrophonium (Tensilon) test is performed to support the diagnosis in previously unknown MG patients. The test can also be used to distinguish myasthenic crisis from cholinergic crisis. The test should be carried out with caution as it can increase the weakness further leading to ventilator failure.

Management

The most important aspect of management is providing adequate pulmonary support. Most of the patients in crisis require intubation and mechanical ventilation. To provide rest to the respiratory muscles is the most important aspect of the management of patients in crisis. Once the patients are started on mechanical ventilation, anticholinesterase medications should be temporarily stopped. These medications worsen the crisis by further increasing secretions. These medications should be restarted just before extubation after the crisis period weans off and the patient shows definite improvement in muscle strength with PEX or IVIg therapy.

References

1. Hirsch NP. Neuromuscular junction in health and disease. *Br J Anaesth* 2007;99(1):132–138.
2. Robertson N. Enumerating neurology. *Brain* 2000;123:663–664.
3. Drachman DB. Myasthenia gravis. *N Engl J Med* 1994;330:1797–1810.
4. Jaretzki A 3rd, Barohn RJ, Ernstoff RM et al. Myasthenia gravis: Recommendations for clinical research standards. Task Force of the Medical Scientific Advisory Board of the Myasthenia Gravis Foundation of America. *Ann Thorac Surg* 2000;70:327–334.
5. Osserman KE, Genkins G. Studies in myasthenia gravis: Review of a twenty-year experience in over 1200 patients. *Mt Sinai J Med* 1971;38:497–537.
6. Stoelting RK, Dierdorf SP. *Anesthesia and Coexisting Disease*, 3rd ed. New York, NY: Churchill Livingstone; 1993, pp. 439–444.
7. Keesey JC. Clinical evaluation and management of myasthenia gravis. *Muscle Nerve* 2004;29:484–505.
8. Dirr LY, Donofrio PD, Patton JF, Troost BT. A false-positive Edrophonium test in a patient with a brainstem glioma. *Neurology* 1989;39:865–867.
9. Moorthy G, Behrens MM, Drachman DB et al. Ocular pseudomyasthenia or ocular myasthenia "plus": A warning to clinicians. *Neurology* 1989;39:1150–1154.
10. Phillips LH 2nd, Melnick PA. Diagnosis of myasthenia gravis in the 1990s. *Semin Neurol* 1990;10:62–69.
11. Oh SJ, Kim DE, Kuruoglu R, Bradley RJ, Dwyer D. Diagnostic sensitivity of the laboratory tests in myasthenia gravis. *Muscle Nerve* 1992;15:720–724.
12. Lindstrom JM, Seybold ME, Lennon VA, Whittingham S, Duane DD. Antibody to acetylcholine receptor in myasthenia gravis. Prevalence, clinical correlates, and diagnostic value. *Neurology* 1976;26:1054–1059.

13. Lennon VA. Serologic profile of myasthenia gravis and distinction from the Lambert–Eaton myasthenic syndrome. *Neurology* 1997;48:S23–S27.

14. Tindall RS, Phillips JT, Rollins JA, Wells L, Hall K. A clinical therapeutic trial of cyclosporine in myasthenia gravis. *Ann N Y Acad Sci* 1993;681:539–551.

15. Tüzün E, Meriggioli MN, Rowin J, Yang H, Christadoss P. Myasthenia gravis patients with low plasma IL-6 and IFN-gamma benefit from etanercept treatment. *J Autoimmun* 2005;24:261–268.

16. Gajdos P, Chevret S, Clair B, Tranchant C, Chastang C. Clinical trial of plasma exchange and high-dose intravenous immunoglobulin in myasthenia gravis. Myasthenia Gravis Clinical Study Group. *Ann Neurol* 1997;41:789–796.

17. Eisenkraft JB, Book WJ, Mann SM, Papatestas AE, Hubbard M. Resistance to succinylcholine in myasthenia gravis: A dose response study. *Anesthesiology* 188;69:760–763.

18. Nilsson E, Meretoja OA. Vecuronium dose-response and maintenance requirements in patients with myasthenia gravis. *Anesthesiology* 1990;73:28–32.

19. Ceremuga TE, Yao XL, McCabe JT. Etiology, mechanisms, and anesthesia implications of autoimmune myasthenia gravis. *AANA J* 2002;70(4):301–309.

20. Leventhal R, Orkin FK, Hirsch RA. Prediction of the need for postoperative ventilation in Myasthenia gravis. *Anesthesiology* 1980;53:26–30.

21. Gissen AJ, Karis JH, Nastuk WL. Effect of halothane on neuromuscular transmission. *JAMA* 1966;197:770–774.

22. Gracey DR, Divertie MB, Howard FM Jr. Mechanical ventilation for respiratory failure in myasthenia gravis: Two year experience with 22 patients. *Mayo Clin Proc* 1983;58:597–602.

23. Rudzka-Nowak A, Piechota M. Anaesthetic management of a patient with myasthenia gravis for abdominal surgery using sugammadex. *Arch Med Sci* 2011;7(2):361–364.

24. Sahin S, Çolak A, Inal M, Arar C. Total intravenous anesthesia management of a patient with myasthenia gravis. *Internet J Anesthesiol* 2008;16(1):14.

25. Chaudhuri A, Behan PO. Myasthenic crisis. *QJM* 2009;102:97–107.

40

Guillain–Barré syndrome

PRASANNA U. BIDKAR

Introduction

Guillain–Barré (GB) syndrome is a peripheral nervous system disorder characterized by acute onset, ascending motor weakness. The term is also considered to be synonymous with acute inflammatory demyelinating polyradiculopathy (AIDP). Worldwide, the reported incidence rate is 1–2 per 100,000 persons.[1–3] No clear data are available regarding the incidence of GB syndrome in the Indian population. The features of GB syndrome were first described by Landry in 1877.[4] In 1916, Guillain and Barré described the typical cerebrospinal fluid (CSF) findings of two French soldiers who spontaneously recovered from acute flaccid paralysis.[5]

Clinical features

GB syndrome can occur at any age and men are more affected (1.5 times) than women. The clinical presentation usually begins with onset of sensory symptoms in the lower limbs followed by a rapid onset flaccid paralysis. The weakness spreads from distal to proximal and then ascends to involve abdominal, thoracic, upper limb, and pharyngeal muscles. Lumbar pain is common and may represent the inflammation in nerve roots and breach of the nerve CSF barrier.

Approximately 60%–70% of cases of GB syndrome are preceded by either respiratory tract or gastrointestinal infections in the previous 10–14 days,[1,6] suggesting an autoimmune mechanism behind its occurrence. Many infectious pathogens have been identified. These include *Campylobacter jejuni*, cytomegalovirus, influenza virus, Epstein–Barr virus, and *Mycoplasma pneumoniae*.[7,8] Even surgery and immunizations are also associated with GB syndrome.

Onset of weakness

GB syndrome begins with acute onset of paresthesia, which is symmetrical, followed by progressive lower-limb weakness. Progression is generally rapid with nearly half of patients achieving peak weakness by 2 weeks and more than 90% of patients by the end of 4 weeks.[9] The deep tendon reflexes are either weak or absent. The weakness is more in distal muscles compared to proximal muscles. More than two-thirds of patients are nonambulatory during weakness[10]; patients also complain of moderate-to-severe muscular pain. Neurological examination reveals widespread hyporeflexia or areflexia with prominent distal weakness compared to proximal muscles. Sensory examination may often be normal with only loss of vibration and proprioception senses.

Respiratory involvement

Facial and laryngeal muscles reflect the involvement of cranial nerves. Phrenic nerve involvement causes diaphragmatic palsy. These together eventually can lead to acute respiratory failure and the need for mechanical ventilation in one-third of patients with GB syndrome.[11–15] Approximately 60% of mechanically ventilated patients with GB syndrome experience major complications such as pneumonia, sepsis, gastrointestinal bleeding, and pulmonary embolism.

In approximately 50% of patients, autonomic disturbance is observed and is a significant cause of death. Cardiac and hemodynamic disturbances are frequently encountered. Occasionally, bowel and bladder dysfunction is observed. Sympathetic overactivity is the common pattern of autonomic imbalance. These include acute onset of tachycardia and hypertension, but serious life-threatening arrhythmia can also occur during the course of illness.[16–21]

Investigations

1. *CSF analysis*: A lumbar puncture is done to rule out infectious etiology. The CSF analysis may be normal in the early phases of disease.

The characteristic albuminocytological dissociation is observed in 50% of patients in the first week of illness, which increases to 75% by the end of the third week.[22] Hence, it is important for clinicians to have a high index of suspicion of GB syndrome and they should not rely on CSF findings alone.

2. *Electrodiagnostic testing*: Electrodiagnostic testing is performed to support the diagnosis of flaccid paralysis due to peripheral neuropathy. The features of demyelination include slow conduction velocities, temporal dispersion, and increased latencies.[23] Another characteristic of electrodiagnostic testing in patients with GB syndrome is "sural nerve sparing." The sensory response pattern to the sural nerve is normal, but there is impaired sensory conduction in the upper limb. This pattern is observed within 1 week of illness in half of the patients with GB syndrome.[23,24]

3. *Antoganglioside antibodies*: The patient should be screened for the presence of anti-GM1, anti-GD1a, and anti-GQ1b antibodies in different variants of GB syndrome.

4. *Magnetic resonance imaging (MRI)*: MRI of spine and brain may be carried out to rule out other causes of paralysis such as myelopathy and polyradiculopathy. Enhancement of the involved nerve roots can be observed in MRI.[25–27]

Variants of GB syndrome

GB syndrome has been classified into different subtypes based on the neurological injury (Table 40.1). The injury can be demyelinating, axonar degeneration with or without sensory involvement.

Table 40.1 Variants of GB syndrome

Variant	Clinical features	Pathophysiology
Acute inflammatory demyelinating polyradiculopathy (AIDP)	Demyelination of motor neurons. Most common variant. Secondary axonal damage can be present	Destruction of myelin sheath by leukocyte infiltration
Acute motor axonal neuropathy (AMAN)	Primarily children. Primarily axonal degeneration. No sensory involvement. Early respiratory involvement. Positive for C. Jejuni infection	Positive for anti-GM1 and anti-GD1a antibodies

Variant	Clinical features	Pathophysiology
Acute motor-sensory axonal neuropathy (AMSAN)	Usually adults. Motor and sensory involvement. Severe respiratory involvement seen. Poor outcome	Both dorsal (sensory) and ventral (motor) roots are affected
Miller–Fisher syndrome	Characterized by a triad of sensory ataxia, areflexia, and ophthalmoplegia. Good outcome	Anti-GQ1b positive in most of the cases

Differential diagnosis

Various other conditions causing acute flaccid paralysis can mimic GB syndrome (Table 40.2). Acute onset of illness, symmetry of neurological weakness, and ascending type of symptoms in the absence of other infectious causes should point toward the diagnosis of GB syndrome. Table 40.3 depicts the commonly practiced diagnostic criteria for GB syndrome.[9]

Management

General supportive care

The patients with suspected/proven GB syndrome should be admitted to a neurointensive care unit (NICU) or a high-dependency unit where the patient can be closely monitored for the development of respiratory failure. Approximately 30% of patients develop respiratory failure and require mechanical ventilation. Routine monitoring should include heart rate, respiratory rate, effort of breathing, use of accessory muscles of respiration, and signs and symptoms of autonomic dysfunction.[13] Forced vital capacity and negative inspiratory force should be monitored to detect respiratory dysfunction early. A vital capacity of <20 mL/kg or a negative inspiratory force of <30 cmH$_2$O or a maximal expiratory pressure <40 cmH2$_O$ indicates an imminent respiratory failure and is an indication for endotracheal intubation and mechanical ventilation.[28,29] Endotracheal intubation should also be considered in patients

Table 40.2 Conditions Mimicking GB Syndrome

Causes	Examples
1. Neurological/ Neuromuscular	Myasthenia gravis, Eaton–Lambert syndrome, transverse myelitis, multiple sclerosis
2. Infectious	Poliomyelitis, botulism, tick paralysis
3. Metabolic	Hypokalemic periodic paralysis, hypermagnesemia, hypophosphatemia Acute intermittent porphyria
4. Drugs and toxins	Lead poisoning, biological toxins (snake and scorpion toxins), drugs (nitrofurantoin, aminoglycosides)

Table 40.3 Diagnostic Criteria for GB Syndrome

Required for diagnosis	Symmetrical progressive weakness in lower/upper limbs Acute onset Progression of disease <4 weeks
Supporting features	Mild sensory symptoms Cranial nerve involvement, especially the facial nerve Autonomic dysfunction Albuminocytological dissociation in CSF analysis Typical electrodiagnostic features Pain
Exclusionary criteria	Other causes mimicking GB syndrome are excluded

Source: Adapted from Asbury AK, Cornblath DR. *Ann Neurol* 27(Suppl.), S21–S24, 1990.

with excessive secretions, a weak cough, inability to lift the head, and with signs of atelectasis in chest radiograph.[30-32] The duration of mechanical ventilation is around 2–4 weeks. If the patient fails to show significant improvement in 2 weeks, then tracheostomy can be performed.

Immunotherapy

Both plasma exchange (PEX) and intravenous immunoglobulin (IVIG) therapies are effective in treating the early weeks of illness.

Plasma exchange therapy

Plasma exchange therapy still remains the mainstay treatment of GB syndrome. In the PEX, patient's plasma is exchanged with either albumin or fresh-frozen plasma from allogenic donors. This process removes humoral antibodies, immune complexes, cytokines, complement, and other inflammatory mediators. The earlier two studies from American and French groups, which included patients with plasmapheresis within 2 weeks of onset of symptoms, showed a faster motor recovery, time to walk, and rapid weaning from mechanical ventilation.[33] The usual dose of plasma exchange is 200–250 mL/kg divided equally over five occasions in a span of 1–2 weeks.[34-36] A meta-analysis, which included six available studies comparing plasma exchange with standard treatment alone, showed fewer patients on ventilator at the end of 4 weeks in patients who received PEX therapy.[37] Another meta-analysis showed significant motor recovery at the end of 1 year in patients who received PEX therapy.[34] PEX therapy is shown to be cost-effective as it significantly reduces the ventilator days and hospital stay.[38,39] The American Academy of Neurology Subcommittee recommended that PEX can be used up to 4 weeks of onset of symptoms.[34]

Intravenous immunoglobulins

The exact mechanism of action of IVIG is not clearly known. Several mechanisms have been proposed. These include the following:[40]
1. Interference in antigen presentation
2. Modulation of autoantibodies, cytokines, and adhesion molecules
3. Prevention of complement activation and membrane attack complex formation
    The dose of IVIG is 2 g/kg, administered over 5 days. The infusion should be started slowly at the rate of 25–50 mL/h and the patient observed for any adverse reactions. Then, it is gradually increased to 150–200 cc/h. Side effects are usually mild and can be limited to headache, nausea, and back pain.

PEX versus IVIG therapy

In 1992, a Dutch study group compared PEX with IVIG therapy in patients with GB syndrome. They demonstrated that IVIG therapy is equally or more effective than PEX therapy.[41] A subsequent larger study showed that there is no difference in outcome with either PEX or IVIG therapy.[42] Because of the ease of administration and the risk complications due to plasma exchange, many centers prefer to use IVIG therapy as the first line of treatment. There is no significant improvement when one therapy is followed by another (PEX followed by IVIG).[43] Hence, the decision to use PEX or IVIG should be based on cost, availability, and risk of harmful side effects.

Corticosteroids

The role of corticosteroids has been studied in patients with GB syndrome. They have been found to be ineffective in multiple trials, hence they are not recommended in the treatment of GB syndrome.[44-46]

Autonomic dysfunction

Autonomic dysfunction is frequently observed in patients with GB syndrome. The patients should be monitored in the NICU with electrocardiography and blood pressure monitoring. Severe bradycardia may occur during endotracheal intubation or suctioning. One hundred percent oxygen before suctioning reduces the incidence of bradyarrhythmias. The fluctuations in blood pressures are frequent. Sustained increases in blood pressure necessitate treatment. Antihypertensive agents with short half-life are preferred.

Deep vein thrombosis and pain management

A nonambulatory patient is at risk for developing deep vein thrombosis and subsequent pulmonary embolism. Low molecular weight heparins are the preferred drugs for the prevention of deep vein thrombosis in these patients. A majority of patients complain of back and lower extremity pain and should be treated aggressively. Nonsteroidal anti-inflammatory agents are generally ineffective. Opioids are effective in the management of musculoskeletal pain. Other drugs that have been used are gabapentin and carbamazepine.

Prognosis

Several researchers have studied the prognosis in patients with GB syndrome. Generally, the recovery begins in 28 days in the majority of the patients. Mean time to complete recovery is 200 days in 70%–80% of patients. Two-thirds of patients may experience minor residual weakness.[22] The most common cause of death in patients with GB syndrome is acquired infections such as pneumonia secondary to mechanical ventilation. Relapse can be seen in 5% of patients in the first 8 weeks.

References

1. Chiò A, Cocito D, Leone M et al. Guillain–Barré syndrome: A prospective, population-based incidence and outcome survey. Neurology 2003;60:1146–1150.
2. Hughes RA, Rees JH. Clinical and epidemiologic features of Guillain–Barré syndrome. J Infect Dis 1997;176(S2):S92–S98.
3. Alter M. The epidemiology of Guillain–Barré syndrome. Ann Neurol 1990;27(Suppl.):S7–S12.
4. Prineas JW. Pathology of the Guillain–Barré syndrome. Ann Neurol 1981;9(Suppl.):6–19.
5. Guillain G, Barré J, Strohl A. Sur un syndrome de radiculo-nevrite avec hyperalbuminose du liquidecephalorachidien sans reaction cellulaire. Remarques sur les caracterescliniquesetgraphiques des reflexes tendineux. Bull Soc Med Hop Paris 1916;28:1462–1470.
6. Willison HJ. The immunobiology of Guillain–Barré syndromes. J Peripher Nerv Syst 2005;10:94–112.
7. Jacobs BC, Rothbarth PH, van der Meché FG et al. The spectrum of antecedent infections in Guillain–Barré syndrome: A case-control study. Neurology 1998;51:1110–1115.
8. Visser LH, van der Meché FG, Meulstee J et al. Cytomegalovirus infection and Guillain–Barré syndrome: The clinical, electrophysiologic, and prognostic features. Dutch Guillain–Barré Study Group. Neurology 1996;47:668–673.
9. Asbury AK, Cornblath DR. Assessment of current diagnostic criteria for Guillain–Barré syndrome. Ann Neurol 1990;27(Suppl.):S21–S24.
10. Efficiency of plasma exchange in Guillain–Barré syndrome: Role of replacement fluids. French Cooperative Group on Plasma Exchange in Guillain–Barré syndrome. Ann Neurol 1987;22:753–761.
11. Chevrolet JC, Deleamont P. Repeated vital capacity measurements as predictive parameters for mechanical ventilation need and weaning success in the Guillain–Barré syndrome. Am Rev Respir Dis 1991;144:814–818.
12. Lawn ND, Fletcher DD, Henderson RD, Wolter TD, Wijdicks EF. Anticipating mechanical ventilation in Guillain–Barré syndrome. Arch Neurol 2001;58:893–898.
13. Hughes RA, Wijdicks EF, Benson E et al. Supportive care for patients with Guillain–Barré syndrome. Arch Neurol 2005;62:1194–1198.
14. Ropper AH, Kehne SM. Guillain–Barré syndrome: Management of respiratory failure. Neurology 1985;35:1662–1665.
15. Massam M, Jones RS. Ventilatory failure in the Guillain–Barré syndrome. Thorax 1980;35:557–558.
16. Burns TM, Lawn ND, Low PA, Camilleri M, Wijdicks EF. Adynamic ileus in severe Guillain–Barré syndrome. Muscle Nerve 2001;24:963–965.
17. Truax BT. Autonomic disturbances in the Guillain–Barré syndrome. Semin Neurol 1984;4:462–468.
18. Lichtenfeld P. Autonomic dysfunction in the Guillain–Barre syndrome. Am J Med 1971;50:772–780.
19. Flachenecker P, Wermuth P, Hartung HP, Reiners K. Quantitative assessment of cardiovascular autonomic function in Guillain–Barré syndrome. Ann Neurol 1997;42:171–179.

20. Zochodne DW. Autonomic involvement in Guillain–Barré syndrome: A review. *Muscle Nerve* 1994;17:1145–1155.

21. Tuck RR, McLeod JG. Autonomic dysfunction in Guillain–Barré syndrome. *J Neurol Neurosurg Psychiatry* 1981;44:983–990.

22. Ropper AH. The Guillain–Barré syndrome. *N Engl J Med* 1992;326:1130–1136.

23. Albers JW, Kelly JJ Jr. Acquired inflammatory demyelinating polyneuropathies: Clinical and electrodiagnostic features. *Muscle Nerve* 1989;12:435–451.

24. Gordon PH, Wilbourn AJ. Early electrodiagnostic findings in Guillain–Barré syndrome. *Arch Neurol* 2001;58:913–917.

25. Gorson KC, Ropper AH, Muriello MA, Blair R. Prospective evaluation of MRI lumbosacral nerve root enhancement in acute Guillain–Barré syndrome. *Neurology* 1996;47:813–817.

26. Crino PB, Zimmerman R, Laskowitz D, Raps EC, Rostami AM. Magnetic resonance imaging of the cauda equina in Guillain–Barré syndrome. *Neurology* 1994;44:1334–1336.

27. Weiss MD. Root enhancement in GBS. *Neurology* 1997;48:1477.

28. Sunderrajan EV, Davenport J.The Guillain–Barré syndrome: Pulmonary–neurologic correlations. *Medicine* (Baltimore) 1985;64:333–341.

29. Pontoppidan H, Geffin B, Lowenstein E. Acute respiratory failure in the adult. 2. *N Engl J Med* 1972;287:743–752.

30. Lawn ND, Wijdicks EF. Post-intubation pulmonary function test in Guillain–Barré syndrome. *Muscle Nerve* 2000;23:613–616.

31. Durand MC, Porcher R, Orlikowski D et al. Clinical and electrophysiological predictors of respiratory failure in Guillain–Barré syndrome: A prospective study. *Lancet Neurol* 2006;5:1021–1028.

32. Sharshar T, Chevret S, Bourdain F, Raphael JC, French Cooperative Group on Plasma Exchange in Guillain–Barré Syndrome. Early predictors of mechanical ventilation in Guillain–Barré syndrome. *Crit Care Med* 2003;31:278–283.

33. Plasmapheresis and acute Guillain–Barré syndrome. The Guillain–Barré syndrome Study Group. *Neurology* 1985;35(8):1096–1104.

34. Hughes RA, Wijdicks EF, Barohn R et al. Practice parameter: Immunotherapy for Guillain–Barré syndrome: Report of the Quality Standards Subcommittee of the American Academy of Neurology. *Neurology* 2003;23(61):736–740.

35. Plasma exchange in Guillain–Barré syndrome: One-year follow-up. French Cooperative Group on Plasma Exchange in Guillain–Barré Syndrome. *Ann Neurol* 1992;32:94–97.

36. Jansen PW, Perkin RM, Ashwal S. Guillain–Barré syndrome in childhood: Natural course and efficacy of plasmapheresis. *Pediatr Neurol* 1993;9:16–20.

37. Raphael JC, Chevret S, Hughes RA, Annane D. Plasma exchange for Guillain–Barré syndrome. *Cochrane Database Syst Rev* 2001;(2):CD001798.

38. Esperou H, Jars-Guincestre MC, Bolgert F, Raphael JC, Durand-Zaleski I. Cost analysis of plasma-exchange therapy for the treatment of Guillain–Barré syndrome. French Cooperative Group on Plasma Exchange in Guillain–Barré Syndrome. *Intensive Care Med* 2000;26:1094–1100.

39. Osterman PO, Fagius J, Lundemo G et al. Beneficial effects of plasma exchange in acute inflammatory polyradiculoneuropathy. *Lancet* 1984;2:1296–1299.

40. Dalakas MC. Intravenous immunoglobulin in autoimmune neuromuscular diseases. *JAMA* 2004;291(19):2367–2375.

41. van der Meché FG, Schmitz PI. The Dutch Guillain–Barré Study Group. A randomized trial comparing intravenous immune globulin and plasma exchange in Guillain–Barré syndrome. *N Engl J Med* 1992;326:1123–1129.

42. Plasma Exchange Sandoglobulin Guillain–Barré Syndrome Trial Group. Randomized trial of plasma exchange, intravenous immunoglobulin and combined treatments in Guillain–Barré syndrome. *Lancet* 1997;349:225–230.

43. Hughes RA. Plasma exchange versus intravenous immunoglobulin for Guillain–Barré syndrome. *Ther Apher* 1997;1:129–130.

44. Hughes RA, Swan AV, van Doorn PA. Corticosteroids for Guillain–Barré syndrome. *Cochrane Database Syst Rev* 2010;2:CD001446.

45. Double-blind trial of intravenous methylprednisolone in Guillain–Barré syndrome. Guillain–Barré Syndrome Steroid Trial Group. Lancet 1993;341(8845):586–590.

46. Treatment of Guillain–Barré syndrome with high-dose immune globulins combined with methylprednisolone: A pilot study. The Dutch Guillain–Barré Study Group. *Ann Neurol* 1994;35:749–752.

41

Status epilepticus

SALLY H. VITALI

Definitions

- *Seizure*: A transient occurrence of signs and/or symptoms due to abnormal excessive or synchronous neuronal activity in the brain.
- *Status epilepticus (SE)*: A neurological emergency that occurs when a seizure continues for longer than 5 min or two or more discrete seizures occur over 5 min without a return to baseline level of consciousness.[1]
- *Refractory status epilepticus (RSE)*: An episode of SE that does not stop after appropriate doses of first-line (benzodiazepine) and one second-line (e.g., fosphenytoin, levetiracetam, or phenobarbital) medication.
- *Super-refractory status epilepticus (SRSE)*: RSE that continues or recurs 24 h or more after initiation of treatment with third-line, anesthetic, antiepileptic drug (AED) therapy (e.g., high-dose midazolam or pentobarbital).
- *Nonconvulsive status epilepticus (NCSE)*: SE with altered state of consciousness and electroencephalogram (EEG) evidence of seizure but without clinically evident seizures. NCSE should be considered on the differential for any patient with altered mental status or coma of unknown etiology.

Mechanisms of status epilepticus

- Seizures occur because of an *imbalance between excitatory and inhibitory neurotransmission* that favors excitation.
  - *Glutamate* is the most common *excitatory* neurotransmitter and acts predominately through the *N*-methyl-D-aspartate (NMDA) receptor.
  - *Gamma-aminobutyric acid (GABA)* is the most common *inhibitory* neurotransmitter and works through the GABA receptor.
- *The majority of seizures are self-limited*, lasting less than 30–60 s.[2] Excitatory signaling dominates for a short time and then the balance is regained as excitation diminishes and inhibitory mechanisms help to successfully halt the seizure. In SE, excitatory signaling persists, GABA inhibition fails, and *excitation continues unabated*.
- A seizure that has continued for 2–3 min is rare, becomes increasingly less likely to stop spontaneously, and should be treated. This *self-perpetuating nature of SE* is caused in part by changes in trafficking of postsynaptic neuronal receptors during a seizure. As SE progresses, the number of excitatory (e.g., NMDA)

receptors increases and the number of GABA receptors decreases.[3,4] This leads to increased excitatory action from glutamate and greater challenges to GABA inhibition.

- The diminishing number of GABA receptors also contributes to *increasing refractoriness to the AEDs that work through the GABA receptor* (e.g., benzodiazepines, barbiturates, and valproates) as the SE progresses. This phenomenon drives modern SE treatment protocols that emphasize early treatment with appropriate doses of AEDs with the goal of halting seizures before they become refractory.

Consequences of status epilepticus

- Most seizures are accompanied by a systemic catecholamine surge that leads to tachycardia, hypertension, elevated cerebral blood flow, and elevated cerebral perfusion pressure. This mechanism usually serves to deliver a plentiful supply of oxygen and glucose to the brain during the event. *Although careful monitoring and support of respiratory and cardiovascular function during a seizure is important, these steps alone will not prevent brain injury* from an episode of prolonged SE.

- Despite the supply of substrate, prolonged SE causes neuronal loss and gliosis (scarring) in the neocortex, the amygdala and hippocampus, the dorsomedial thalamic nuclei, and the cerebellar Purkinje cell layer. This pattern of injury is seen in humans who die from SE and in animal models of the disease. These areas of the brain are known to have excessive presynaptic glutamate levels. Humans with RSE have elevated serum levels of neuron-specific enolase, a biomarker for neuronal injury.[5]

- Excess glutamate release by excitatory neurons and binding to NMDA receptors leads to *glutamate-mediated excitotoxicity*. The toxicity is related to increased calcium influx into the neuron, leading to cell injury and death by many different mechanisms. Achieving pharmacological control of SE reduces the excitotoxicity and curtails the ongoing potential for neuronal injury.

- SE that continues unrecognized and untreated (e.g., in the prehospital setting) may lead to *secondary brain injury from hypoxic–ischemic injury and/or intracranial hypertension*.

Systemically, prolonged, untreated seizures can cause aspiration pneumonia, dysrhythmias, rhabdomyolysis, hypotension, acidosis, and multiorgan system failure that complicate clinical management and outcome.

- The patient with SRSE that requires prolonged, continuous sedation with or without coma and accompanying mechanical ventilation and hemodynamic support is at risk of *multiple complications of critical illness*, including infection, aspiration pneumonia, thrombosis, hemorrhage, malnutrition, myopathy, and decubitus ulcers. Aggressive prevention protocols for these conditions are crucial to improve outcome.

- Morbidity and mortality of SE are associated with the following:
  - *Underlying cause of SE*: Generally, SE caused by a chronic condition (e.g., epilepsy) has less morbidity and mortality than SE caused by an acute pathophysiology.[6] When an acute neurological process leading to SE carries a high morbidity and mortality, the association between SE and mortality is confounded.
  - *Increasing duration of the SE episode*: Seizures lasting longer than 30 min are associated with greater morbidity and mortality than those lasting less than 30 min. Mortality of SE lasting 30 min or more in adults is widely reported to be around 20%. Longer episodes of RSE and SRSE that are more refractory to therapy have higher morbidity and mortality.[7] Mortality from RSE is about three times higher than that from non-RSE.
  - *Increasing patient age*.
  - *Impaired consciousness at SE presentation*.
  - *Medical comorbidities*.

Treatment

- Many hospitals and medical organizations have guidelines for the management of SE. An example is shown in Figure 41.1 and the medications are described in Table 41.1. The objective of these guidelines is to *deliver effective doses of appropriate AEDs to patients with SE and, when a medication fails to halt SE, to progress immediately to trialing the*

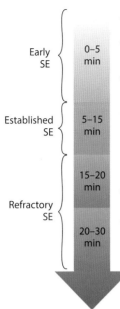

- Monitor and assist with airway, breathing (provide O$_2$), and circulation as needed
- Work to establish IV access and obtain serum glucose, chemistries, and AED levels if applicable, treat hypoglycemia or hyponatremia if present
- Give benzodiazepine (e.g., lorazepam 0.1 mg/kg IV slow push/IM (max/adult 4 mg), midazolam 0.1 mg/kg IM/IN/buccal (max/adult 10 mg), diazepam 0.5 mg/kg PR (max/adult 20 mg))
- Repeat benzodiazepine dose above AND simultaneously
- Load fosphenytoin 20 mg/kg PE IV (150 mg PE/min) or IM (max/adult 1g) or another second-line AED*
- Give levetiracetam 20–60 mg/kg IV/IO (100 mg/min) or another second-line AED* not given above
- Consider transfer to ICU for cEEG and potential need for life support during third-line AED therapy
- Consider another dose of fosphenytoin 10 mg/kg PE IV (150 mg/min) or IM (high phenytoin levels may provoke seizure activity)
- If not successful give phenobarbital 20–30 mg/kg IV/IO (50–75 mg/min) or another second-line AED* not already given
- Start third-line AED (continuous infusion) and cEEG monitoring. Consider intubation/mechanical ventilation if not already done

Early SE: 0–5 min; Established SE: 5–15 min; Refractory SE: 15–20 min, 20–30 min

Figure 41.1 Example guideline for the management of status epilepticus. *Second-line AEDs: fosphenytoin or phenytoin (20 mg/kg at 50 mg/min), levetiracetam, phenobarbital, valproate (20–40 mg/kg IV/IO at 6 mg/kg/min), and lacosamide (for adults 400 mg IV over 5 min). (SE, status epilepticus; IV, intravenous; IM, intramuscular; IN, intranasal; PR, per rectum; max, maximum recommended dose; PE, phenytoin equivalents; IO, intraosseous; AED, antiepileptic drug; cEEG, continuous electroencephalography.)

Table 41.1 First-, Second-, and Third-Line Medications for the Management of Status Epilepticus

	Drug/class	Mechanism	Advantages	Disadvantages
First line	Benzodiazepine (lorazepam, midazolam, diazepam)	GABA agonist	Rapid onset, multiple routes	Can cause respiratory depression, particularly if repeated dosing required
Second line	Fosphenytoin	Na channel blockade, slows Na channel recovery rate	May be loaded rapidly with little cardiovascular toxicity (compared with phenytoin), may be given IM, little respiratory depression, can target serum levels	High levels provoke seizure activity, use with caution in patients already taking phenytoin unless levels are known or likely to be low
	Phenytoin	Na channel blockade, slows Na channel recovery rate	Little respiratory depression, can target serum levels	Potential for arrhythmia and hypotension, requires slow loading, high levels provoke seizure activity (see above)
	Levetiracetam	Unknown, works via binding to SV2A, affects intracellular Ca^{2+} levels	May be loaded rapidly, large therapeutic window, minimal respiratory depression, no hepatic metabolism	Renal excretion, doses must be adjusted in renal failure

(continued)

Table 41.1 First-, Second-, and Third-Line Medications for the Management of Status Epilepticus (*continued*)

	Drug/class	Mechanism	Advantages	Disadvantages
	Phenobarbital	GABA agonist	Can target serum levels	Requires slower loading because of cardiovascular toxicity (hypotension), causes sedation, respiratory depression
	Valproate	GABA agonist, modulates Na and Ca channels	May be loaded rapidly, little respiratory depression, can target serum levels	Larger potential side effect profile (e.g., hepatic dysfunction, pancreatitis, pancytopenia, hypersensitivity reactions)
	Lacosamide	Inactivates Na channels	May be loaded rapidly, little respiratory depression	Can prolong P-R interval, obtain ECG, no pediatric dosing guidelines in SE
Third line	High-dose midazolam infusion	GABA agonist, slows Na channel recovery rate	Rapid onset, can be titrated quickly to control clinical or electrographic seizures, little hypotension or ileus, may avoid need for pressors and parenteral nutrition	Not universally successful in controlling RSE, some patients will require pentobarbital coma to control seizures
	Pentobarbital	GABA agonist	Rapid onset, can be titrated quickly to burst-suppression pattern on cEEG	Causes significant hypotension, ileus, long half-life
	Propofol	GABA agonist, decreases neuronal calcium influx, antioxidant	Rapidly effective to stop seizures, very short half-life, titrated to burst-suppression pattern on cEEG	Hypotension, likely pressor requirement, ileus, propofol-related infusion syndrome limits usefulness
	Isoflurane	GABA agonist	Rapidly effective to stop seizures, very short half-life	Difficult to deliver, SRSE often requires very high MAC for long periods, toxicities unknown

GABA, gamma aminobutyric acid; Na, sodium; IM, intramuscular; Ca²⁺, calcium; SV2A, synaptic vesicle protein 2A; ECG, electrocardiogram; cEEG, continuous electroencephalogram; MAC, mean alveolar concentration; SRSE, super-refractory status epilepticus; SE, status epilepticus; RSE, refractory status epilepticus.

next agent. By continuing through agents one after the other and without delay in between, patients with severe RSE who need to be treated with anesthetics by continuous infusion can be identified within 30–60 min and started on appropriate therapy, reducing the chances of neuronal injury, morbidity, and mortality.

- In contrast to maintenance AED treatment of patients with epilepsy that is targeted toward preventing seizures from starting (prophylaxis), the treatment of SE is focused on stopping an ongoing seizure. *Halting a seizure generally requires higher doses of medications than are required for seizure prophylaxis.* In addition, oral medications cannot be used in SE treatment and many maintenance AEDs do not have an IV formulation and therefore are not useful early in SE management.

- While initiating management of acute SE according to a guideline, the *potential underlying etiologies of prolonged seizure must be considered and treated if possible* (Table 41.2). Malignant hypertension, hypoglycemia, and hyponatremia are important treatable etiologies. AEDs may temporarily halt seizures caused by these metabolic disturbances, but recurrence is likely until the underlying cause is treated. When alcohol intoxication may be a cause of hypoglycemia, if thiamine is readily available during the emergency it should be given simultaneously with dextrose to avoid precipitating the Wernicke–Korsakoff syndrome. For hyponatremia, hypertonic saline (3%) is infused intravenously but stopped as soon as the seizure terminates. The remainder of the sodium correction can be more prolonged to avoid osmotic demyelination. Hypocalcemia and hypomagnesemia are more

Table 41.2 Etiologies of Status Epilepticus

Patients with prior seizures	• Recent medication change or missing medications (low AED levels) • Intercurrent illness ± fever • Metabolic abnormalities (e.g., hyponatremia, hypoglycemia) • Sleep deprivation

Patients with new-onset seizure	• Metabolic abnormalities (e.g., hypo/hyperglycemia, hyponatremia, hypocalcemia, hypomagnesemia, uremia)
	• Drug-related
	  • Medication-induced/intoxication/overdose (e.g., local anesthetic toxicity, penicillin, metronidazole, isoniazid, tricyclic antidepressants, theophylline, clozapine, cyclosporine, flumazenil, organophosphates, alcohol, cocaine, sympathomimetics)
	    • Drug withdrawal (e.g., alcohol, benzodiazepines, barbiturates, opioids, baclofen)
	  • Fever-induced (e.g., febrile SE)
	  • Hypertensive encephalopathy/PRES
	  • Cerebrovascular disorders
	  • Intracranial hemorrhage
	  • Brain trauma
	  • Brain tumor
	  • Meningitis/encephalitis/brain abscess/parasitic infections
	  • Inflammatory, autoimmune, and paraneoplastic syndromes
	  • Inborn errors of metabolism
	  • Genetic causes of epilepsy

Patients with intraoperative seizure	• Consider above etiologies • Intraoperative cortical stimulation

AED, antiepileptic drug; SE, status epilepticus; PRES, posterior reversible leukoencephalopathy.

Table 41.3 Adjunctive Therapy for Empiric Management of SRSE

Vitamins (empiric treatment for metabolic epilepsies)	• Pyridoxine • Pyridoxyl-5-phosphate • Folinic acid • Biotin
Medications	• Any of the medications listed in Table 41.1 or Figure 41.1 that have not been attempted previously • Topiramate and other new AEDs • Ketamine
Other therapies	• Immunomodulatory therapy (steroids, IVIG, plasma exchange) • Ketogenic diet • Therapeutic hypothermia • Epilepsy surgery • Vagal nerve stimulator • Electric or magnetic stimulation therapy

Note: When attempts to wean third-line agents fail, these therapies are often attempted individually, using potential toxicities and likely etiologies of SE to guide the order.
AED, antiepileptic drug; IVIG, intravenous immunoglobulin.

rare causes of seizures but are important to correct if present.

- Once seizures have stopped, the patient should be monitored closely for return to baseline mental status. Although there may be a postictal phase, *continued encephalopathy should prompt EEG evaluation for NCSE* since convulsive status epilepticus (CSE) may evolve into NCSE in some cases. If prolonged seizures are likely to recur, maintenance AED therapy should be started, continued, or modified.

- After several second-line agents have failed, the patient should be started on high-dose midazolam or pentobarbital infusion. Intensive care unit (ICU) transfer, continuous electro-encephalogram (cEEG) monitoring, central venous access, and arterial access are indicated. If the patient has not already required intubation for respiratory failure or airway protection (from either seizures or medications), consider endotracheal intubation. Both anesthetic agents require bolus dosing prior to starting the infusion, and then a subsequent bolus each time the infusion rate is increased. Midazolam is titrated to halting clinical and EEG seizures, while pentobarbital is titrated to an EEG burst-suppression pattern. Propofol infusion and isoflurane are alternative options but have higher risks of complication.

- After 24–48 h of seizure control and/or burst suppression with a third-line agent, an attempt is usually made to wean the sedative infusion. *If seizures recur on weaning, the patient has SRSE.* Generally, the patient's anesthetic infusion is then uptitrated to regain seizure control and adjunctive medications or therapies (Table 41.3) are added to increase the likelihood of success during subsequent weaning attempts. The aggressive pursuit of an etiology for SE should continue during this time, including repeat magnetic resonance imaging (MRI) or lumbar puncture (LP) at reasonable, regular intervals as the findings may evolve over time and eventually elucidate a diagnosis.

Summary

SE is a neurological emergency. The best possible outcome from this condition is achieved with early recognition of seizure and close adherence to a guideline to provide appropriate doses of recommended AEDs in an expedient manner. Although respiratory and cardiac functions must be supported, prevention of neuronal damage from SE requires the seizure to be stopped as soon as possible. A minority of patients will require continuous sedative infusion to halt their seizures. In patients without preexisting epilepsy, imaging and LP results will help narrow the list of possible etiologies and guide therapeutic trials to achieve seizure control.

References

1. Brophy GM, Bell R, Claassen J et al. Guidelines for the evaluation and management of status epilepticus. *Neurocrit care* 2012;17(1):3–23.
2. Theodore WH, Porter RJ, Albert P et al. The secondarily generalized tonic-clonic seizure: A videotape analysis. *Neurology* 1994;44(8):1403–1407.
3. Naylor DE, Liu H, Niquet J, Wasterlain CG. Rapid surface accumulation of NMDA receptors increases glutamatergic excitation during status epilepticus. *Neurobiol Dis* 2013;54:225–238.
4. Naylor DE, Liu H, Wasterlain CG. Trafficking of GABA(A) receptors, loss of inhibition, and a mechanism for pharmacoresistance in status epilepticus. *J Neurosci* 2005;25(34):7724–7733.
5. DeGiorgio CM, Heck CN, Rabinowicz AL, Gott PS, Smith T, Correale J. Serum neuron-specific enolase in the major subtypes of status epilepticus. *Neurology* 1999;52(4):746–749.
6. Claassen J, Lokin JK, Fitzsimmons BF, Mendelsohn FA, Mayer SA. Predictors of functional disability and mortality after status epilepticus. *Neurology* 2002;58(1):139–142.
7. Madzar D, Geyer A, Knappe RU et al. Association of seizure duration and outcome in refractory status epilepticus. *J Neurol* 2016;263(3):485–491.

42

Stroke

SHAHEEN SHAIKH

Introduction

Stroke is the leading cause of disability worldwide and the fourth leading cause of death in the United States.[1] Stroke may be hemorrhagic or ischemic in etiology, although a majority of them (85%) are ischemic in origin. According to the World Health Organization (WHO), stroke is defined as, "rapidly developing signs of focal (or global) disturbance of cerebral function, with symptoms lasting 24 hours or longer, or leading to death, with no apparent cause other than of vascular origin."

Anesthesiologists are involved in the care of the patients with acute ischemic stroke (AIS) at several levels. This may include airway management in the emergency department, neurointerventional procedures under anesthesia, and operating room including hemicraniectomy and the neurocritical care unit. They present as acute emergencies, requiring rapid assessment and treatment, with the same urgency as a trauma patient. It is very important for anesthesiologists to understand the concept of "Time Is Brain." Urgent treatment may prevent severe disability in patients who meet eligibility criteria to receive intravenous (IV) tissue plasminogen activator (tPa), intra-arterial tPa, or interventional thrombectomy.

Pathophysiology

The causes of AIS may be embolic, for example, atrial fibrillation or thromboembolic including carotid artery disease.[2] Sudden occlusion of a large vessel, often the middle cerebral artery (MCA), causes vascular occlusion and interruption of flow. This creates a penumbra, characterized by an ischemic core, with gradients of hypo perfusion and oligemia. The ischemic core represents irreversible cell death whereas the penumbra represents a potentially salvageable tissue. If the patient does not receive treatment in a timely manner, the entire tissue supplied by the occluded vessel will suffer infarction and even death (Figure 42.1).

The penumbra is targeted with the aim of restoring perfusion to the occluded vessel within the time frame of 3 h from symptoms of onset. Current treatment of AIS includes treatment with IV recombinant tissue plasminogen activator (rtPa), clot lysis with intra-arterial tPa, or mechanical clot extraction (thrombectomy).

Initial assessment

In the emergency department, medical stabilization includes airway and ventilatory support,

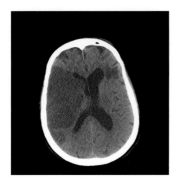

Figure 42.1 CT scan of the brain showing a right hemispheric infarction.

hemodynamic management, a quick neurologic assessment, followed by brain imaging and determining the eligibility for treatment with IV tPa. Recent surgery, head trauma, gastrointestinal bleeding, coagulopathy, and hypoglycemia are some of the contraindications to IV tPa therapy.

Airway management

Patients may be at risk for aspiration if they develop facial or bulbar weakness or altered mental status.

Neurogenic pulmonary edema may occur with severe cerebral ischemia and lead to hypoxemia.

Since hypoxemia is extremely deleterious, the oxygen saturation must be maintained at 94% or higher.

Patients may develop respiratory failure and require urgent intubation. Every effort must be made for a quick neurologic assessment prior to intubation, to determine baseline status. Short-acting agents must be used and hemodynamic stability should be maintained. Medications such as propofol may cause hypotension, which can compromise cerebral perfusion pressure. Hypercarbia worsens intracranial blood volume by cerebral vasodilation. Extreme hyperventilation must be avoided to prevent cerebral vasoconstriction and cerebral ischemia.

Hemodynamic management

Blood pressure (BP) ≥185/110 mmHg must be lowered before IV tPa is administered, if the patient meets eligibility criteria. BP ≥185/110 mmHg increases the risk of intracranial bleeding. Once tPa is initiated, BP must be maintained ≤180/105 mmHg. IV agents such as labetalol, nicardipine, and clevidipine (if available) that do not cause profound cerebral vasodilation are preferred. Hypotension must be avoided. Both hypotension and hypertension are associated with worse outcomes.

Preprocedure assessment

History may be obtained from the patient or next of kin if the patient has aphasia. It is important to perform preprocedure anesthetic evaluation as quickly as possible, with understanding of the risk of limited preanesthetic evaluation versus delayed clot lysis and worse neurological outcome.

Relevant history must include the following:

- Time of onset of symptoms[3] or last seen normal.
- History of comorbidities including hypertension, diabetes, ischemic heart disease, which also cause AIS.
- History of alcohol abuse, liver disease. Anticoagulant use and atrial fibrillation must be sought, which predispose the patient to hemorrhagic stroke.
- NIHSS (National Institutes of Health Stroke Scale), which focuses on the level of consciousness, focal neurologic deficits, and speech abnormalities. Higher NIHSS scores have been shown to be associated with a worse outcome.
- Computed tomography (CT)/magnetic resonance imaging (MRI) findings, particularly arterial territory involved.
- 12-lead ECG (arrhythmias especially atrial fibrillation).
- Neurological status including NIHSS score.
- Sex, ethnicity.
- Serum glucose.
- Complete blood count, platelet count
- International normalized ratio (INR), prothrombin time, partial thromboplastin time.
- Baseline serum electrolytes and creatinine to assess renal function.
- Weight.
- Age.
- Allergies to iodinated contrast medium.
- Contraindications to MRI.
- Administration of IV tPA and total dose given.
- Patient's medication list, if available.

History of preexisting hypertension is significant. It is a major risk factor for stroke.

The autoregulation curve is shifted to the right and sudden lowering of the BP may predispose the patient to cerebral ischemia. Autoregulation is impaired in the ischemic areas of the brain. Presence of atrial fibrillation may be a risk factor for embolic stroke. If the patient is on warfarin, an urgent INR must be requested. An INR ≥1.7 is a contraindication for IV tPa therapy.[4] A platelet count ≤100,000 is also a contraindication for thrombolytic therapy. Baseline creatinine must be documented. Hypoglycemia may mimic stroke symptoms and must be ruled out. Hyperglycemia has been associated with worse outcomes and must be treated. Diabetes is a risk factor for renal impairment. Contrast-induced nephropathy may occur post procedure. If time of onset of symptoms is between 3 and 4.5 h, some institutions might administer IV tPa. This may also be an indication for intra-arterial tPa for clot lysis, since the total dose of tPa is much lower. Beyond 6 h, interventional therapy includes thrombectomy and clot extraction.

Physical examination

The patient's vital signs and neurological status must be noted. Hypotension (systolic BP ≤140 mmHg) is associated with worse outcomes. Hypertension can lead to intracranial hemorrhage, especially after administration of tPa. Arterial BP must be monitored when possible provided no delay occurs to recanalization therapy. Examination of the patient's mental status, ability to lie flat, and airway must be conducted to assess the suitability of general anesthesia (GA) versus monitored anesthesia care. Catecholamine release secondary to cerebral ischemia predisposes patients with AIS to cardiac arrhythmias, myocardial ischemia, and neurogenic pulmonary edema.

Diagnostic tests

Blood tests that must be conducted include complete blood count with platelet count, coagulation profile, blood glucose, serum electrolytes, and blood glucose. Unnecessary tests must be avoided. A 12-lead electrocardiogram (ECG) must be performed to exclude cardiac arrhythmias and myocardial ischemia. A chest X-ray is no longer routinely recommended unless there is evidence of aspiration or neurogenic pulmonary edema.

A noncontrast CT scan is conducted to rule out intracranial hemorrhage or mass lesion within 25 min of arrival in the emergency department. Intracranial hemorrhage or infarction involving one-third of the cerebral hemisphere is a contraindication to tPa therapy. CT angiography will indicate large vessel occlusion in the presence of an MCA hyperdense sign. MRI has a better resolution of the brain parenchyma and evaluates the brain stem and cerebellum with higher resolution. Diffusion-weighted MRI shows an abnormal signal within minutes of ischemia onset and detects early cytotoxic edema whereas CT may take several hours for an infarction to become apparent. If the time of onset of symptoms is not known, an MRI will guide the physician better. A mismatch between the diffusion-weighted imaging (DWI) and perfusion-weighted imaging (PWI) indicates the presence of salvageable tissue, and tPa therapy may be given provided there are no contraindications. MRI is not practical due to time constraints.[5]

Management of acute ischemic stroke

- *Airway and breathing*: Hypoxia may cause secondary neurological injury and must be avoided. Oxygen saturation must be maintained ≥94%. However, hyperoxia must also be avoided since it causes cerebral vasoconstriction. Hypercarbia causes cerebral vasodilation. Severe hypocarbia causes cerebral vasoconstriction and cerebral ischemia. Recommended arterial pCO_2 range is between 30 and 45 mmHg. Patients with AIS must be monitored continuously since they may develop altered central regulation of respiration, sleep apnea, or aspiration.[6,7]
- *Hemodynamic management*: Hypotension is associated with worse outcomes. BP ≥185/110 mmHg is also associated with poor outcomes. The recommended systolic BP range is 160–180 mmHg.[8,9]
- *Temperature management*: There is no evidence to suggest routine use of hypothermia for cerebral protection in patients with AIS. Increased body temperature in the setting of AIS is associated with a poor neurological outcome. Febrile patients must be treated with antipyretic medications and cooling devices.[10,11]

- *Fluid management*: Glucose-containing solutions must be avoided unless blood glucose is ≤50 mg/dL. Hyperglycemia, which is associated with worse outcomes in the setting of cerebral ischemia, must be avoided. Hypovolemia and hypotension are detrimental. Hence euvolemia is recommended.
- *Blood sugar management*: Hyperglycemia is common in patients with AIS. In patients with cortical infarction, it predicts higher mortality and larger infarct size. There is an increased risk of intracranial hemorrhage with hyperglycemia after treatment with tPA. It is unclear if hyperglycemia is itself detrimental or is a marker of stroke severity. The Society for Neuroscience in Anesthesiology and Critical Care (SNACC) guidelines recommend a protocol-driven IV treatment of blood sugar ≥140 mg/dL and maintaining levels within a range of 70–140 mg/dL.
- *Management of anticoagulation*: The goals are to prevent catheter-, stent-, and thrombus-related embolic and thrombotic events and to avoid hemorrhagic events. IV heparin is used during the procedure, guided by activated clotting time (ACT) measurements. Aspirin and/or clopidogrel may be used if an endovascular stent was used.
- *General versus local anesthesia*: Several retrospective studies indicate patients who were intubated or received heavy sedation or pharmacological paralysis had higher mortality. Patients who were not intubated had a lower infarct volume on imaging studies and shorter length of stay in the intensive care unit (ICU). In one study, patients who received little sedation or no sedation had better angiographic reperfusion rates. However, none of these studies were randomized and the choice of general versus local plus sedation was driven by institutional preferences. It is likely that patients with the best preprocedure neurological status were more likely to have the procedure performed awake. Since a selection bias is present, the quality of the existing data is insufficient to influence clinical practice. Local anesthesia with sedation allows neurological monitoring in an awake patient and does not delay the procedure. However, it does expose the patient to the risk of aspiration, respiratory depression, and undesirable movement. GA provides a secure airway and immobility and protects against aspiration, but requires qualified anesthesia personnel and may delay the procedure. GA is also associated with significant hypotension, restricts neurological monitoring, and exposes the patient to intubation hazards including sepsis and pneumonia.[12–15]
- *Thrombolysis*: If the patient presents within 3 h of symptom onset and has no contraindications, he or she must receive IV rtPA to dissolve the clot.[16–18] If the patient's symptoms occur between 3 and 4.5 h, and the patient is aged ≤80 years and is not a diabetic, he or she may still be eligible to receive IV tPA, depending on institutional practice, although this is not approved by the US Food and Drug Administration (FDA). If the patient has a large-vessel occlusion, for example, MCA, intracranial internal carotid artery sign, and basilar or vertebral artery, and symptoms have occurred within 6 h, intra-arterial thrombolysis is an option in the neurointerventional suite. If the patient presented within 8 h of symptom onset, mechanical clot extraction may be considered. If the hyperdense sign is seen on noncontrast CT scan, the patient will undergo thrombectomy. If the patient has received tPa therapy, intracranial bleeding is a potential complication. If the patient showed initial improvement followed by mental status deterioration, an urgent CT scan must be conducted to rule out an intracranial bleed. The tPa infusion must be stopped and the patient must be treated with fresh-frozen plasma and cryoprecipitate, and neurosurgery must be consulted for possible evacuation of hematoma (Figure 42.2).

Complications

Complications related to acute ischemic stroke are the following:

Procedure-related complications:

- Hemorrhagic transformation of infarct
- Intracranial bleeding—direct vessel trauma, which may be procedure related, anticoagulation, or increased BP (Figure 42.3)
- Blood vessel dissection
- Vasospasm
- Groin hematoma
- Limb ischemia

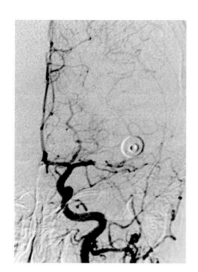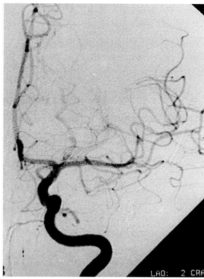

Figure 42.2 Left MCA stroke before and after thrombolysis.

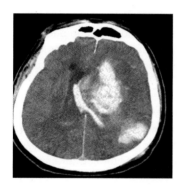

Figure 42.3 CT scan of an intraparenchymal bleed after thrombolysis.

- Retroperitoneal hematoma
- Pseudoaneurysm formation

Anesthesia-related complications:

- Aspiration
- Seizures
- Airway obstruction
- Excessive patient movement
- Conversion of local anesthesia to GA
- Hemodynamic instability

Post-procedure complications:

- Increased intracranial pressure from cerebral edema[19]
- Cerebral infarction needing hemicraniectmy[20]

Post-procedure management

Observation in a dedicated neurointensive ICU
Decision to extubate after communication with a neurointerventional team
Continued hemodynamic and neurological monitoring
Use of short-acting sedatives/hypnotics to allow neurological examination
Continued monitoring of airway and breathing

References

1. Jauch EC, Saver JL, Adams HP Jr et al. Guideline for the early management of patients with acute ischemic stroke. *Stroke* 2013;44:870–947.
2. Caulfield AF, Wijman CA. Management of acute ischemic stroke. *Neurol Clin* 2008;26:345–371.
3. Talke PO, Sharma D, Heyer EJ, Bergese SD, Blackham KA, Stevens RD. Society for Neuroscience in Anesthesiology and Critical Care Expert consensus statement: Anesthetic management of endovascular treatment for acute ischemic stroke. *J Neurosurg Anesthesiol* 2014;26(2):95–108.
4. The National Institute of Neurological Disorders and Stroke rt-PA Stroke Study Group. Tissue plasminogen activator

for acute ischemic stroke. *N Engl J Med* 1995;333(24):1581–1587.

5. Kelley RE, Martin-Schild S. Ischemic stroke: Emergencies and management. *Neurol Clin* 2012;30:187–210.

6. Flexman AM, Donovan AL, Gelb AW et al. Anesthetic management of patients with acute stroke. *Anesthesiol Clin* 2012;30:175–190.

7. Adams HP Jr, del Zoppo G, Alberts MJ et al. Guidelines for the early management of adults with ischemic stroke. *Stroke* 2007;38(5):1655–1711.

8. Leonardi-Bee J, Bath PM, Phillips SJ et al. Blood pressure and clinical outcomes in the International Stroke Trial. *Stroke* 2002;33(5):1315–1320.

9. Castillo J, Leira R, Garcia MM et al. Blood pressure decrease during the acute phase of ischemic stroke is associated with brain injury and poor stroke outcome. *Stroke* 2004;35(2):520–526.

10. Kollmar R, Schwab S. Hypothermia in focal ischemia: Implications of experiments and experience. *J Neurotrauma* 2009;26(3):377–386.

11. Hajat C, Hajat S, Sharma P. Effects of poststroke pyrexia on stroke outcome: A meta-analysis of studies in patients. *Stroke* 2000;31(2):410–414.

12. Abou-Chebl A, Lin R, Hussain MS et al. Conscious sedation versus general anesthesia during endovascular therapy for acute anterior circulation stroke: Preliminary results from a retrospective, multicenter study. *Stroke* 2010;41(6):1175–1179.

13. Nichols C, Carrozzella J, Yeatts S et al. Is periprocedural sedation during acute stroke therapy associated with poorer functional outcomes? *J Neurointerv Surg* 2010;2(1):67–70.

14. McDonagh DL, Olson DM, Kalia JS et al. Anesthesia and sedation practices among neurointerventionalists during acute ischemic stroke endovascular therapy. *Front Neurol* 2010;1:118.

15. Jumaa MA, Zhang F, Ruiz-Ares G et al. Comparison of safety and clinical and radiographic outcomes in endovascular acute stroke therapy for proximal middle cerebral artery occlusion with intubation and general anesthesia versus the non-intubated state. *Stroke* 2010;41(6):1180–1184.

16. Cohen JE, Leker RR, Rabinstein A. New strategies for endovascular recanalization of acute ischemic stroke. *Neurol Clin* 2013;31:705–719.

17. Meyers PM, Schumacher HC, Higashida RT et al. Indications for the performance of intracranial endovascular neurointerventional procedures. *Circulation* 2009;119(16):2235–2249.

18. Lee M, Hong KS, Saver JL. Efficacy of intra-arterial fibrinolysis for acute ischemic stroke: Meta-analysis of randomized controlled trials. *Stroke* 2010;41(5):932–937.

19. Ropper AH, Shafran B. Brain edema after stroke. Clinical syndrome and intracranial pressure. *Arch Neurol* 1984;41(1):26–29.

20. Vahedi K, Hofmeijer J, Juettler E et al. Early decompressive surgery in malignant infarction of the middle cerebral artery: A pooled analysis of three randomised controlled trials. *Lancet Neurol* 2007;6(3):215–222.

43

Cerebral venous sinus thrombosis

MARC-ALAIN BABI and MICHAEL L. JAMES

Introduction

Cerebral venous thrombosis (CVT) is an important etiology of stroke. Cerebral and dural vein thromboses are less common than other stroke subtypes and manifest with myriad neurological symptoms, making CVT a challenging diagnosis. Owing to increased use and advancement of neuroimaging, as well as increased awareness of its signs and symptoms, CVT may become more easily recognizable. In this chapter, epidemiology, pathogenesis, diagnosis, therapeutic approaches, complications, and prognosis of CVT are reviewed.

Epidemiology

Overall, CVT is less common than most other stroke subtypes, but is increasingly recognized as an important cause of stroke, especially in young adults (aged 20–55).[1,2] In fact, CVT may occur at a young age. In hospital-based series, it is found that CVT is more common in neonates and children than in adults.[1,3] For example, in one multicenter Canadian registry of infants and children (newborn until age of 18 years), the incidence of CVT was reported as 0.67 per 100,000 children per year.[2] For adults, one large epidemiological study from Portugal reported an incidence of 0.22 per 100,000 persons per year (95% CI 0–0.47).[4] Another large hospital-based population study from the Netherlands identified 94 CVT cases among adults over a 3-year period, corresponding to an overall incidence of 1.32 per 100,000 persons (95% CI 1.06–1.6). The same study reported a higher annual incidence of CVT among women compared to men (1.86 versus 0.75 per 100,000 persons).[5] In fact, CVT appears to be more common in women than men, with an overall reported female/male ratio of 3:1.[1,6] This may be explained by associations between CVT and oral contraceptive use and higher incidence during pregnancy and puerperium.[1,6,7] One large US registry database reported the incidence of CVT during pregnancy as 11.6 per 100,000 deliveries.[8] In another large epidemiological study (International Study on Cerebral Vein and Dural Sinus Thrombosis, ISCVT),[1] women comprised 75% of all cases and were significantly younger (mean age 34 compared to 42 for men). This difference may be explained by the finding that gender-specific risk factors were identified in 65% of women.

Pathogenesis

The exact etiology and pathophysiologic mechanisms of CVT remain incompletely understood due to variability of the venous anatomy and mechanisms of thrombosis. However, mechanisms that may lead to CVT include the following:

- Thrombosis of the cerebral veins or dural sinuses leading to venous outflow obstruction, cerebral congestion, and elevated intracranial pressure (ICP)
- Parenchymal dysfunction and occlusion of dural sinuses resulting in decreased cerebrospinal fluid (CSF) absorption and elevated ICP

Obstruction of cerebral veins and dural sinuses outflow leads to increased cerebral blood volume, increased venous pressure, and decreased capillary perfusion. In turn, the increase in venous and capillary pressure leads to disruption of the blood–brain barrier, with extravasation of plasma into the interstitial space (i.e., vasogenic edema). As intravenous pressure continues to increase, further parenchymal changes occur, leading to venous or capillary rupture into brain parenchyma. Thus, CVT leads to an overall picture of vascular congestion, breakdown of the blood–brain barrier, diffuse vasogenic edema, small vessel rupture, and parenchymal blood extravasation. The increased intravenous pressure, coupled with space-occupying hematoma, results in overall increased ICP, which then further lowers cerebral perfusion pressure and cerebral blood flow. Ultimately, energy failure occurs with Na^+/K^+ ATPase pump failure and leads to cellular death. Consequently, cytotoxic edema adds to vasogenic edema with resultant irreversible end-stage sequelae of CVT.[9,10] In fact, advances in neuroimaging and understanding of the pathogenesis of CVT have demonstrated the coexistence of both vasogenic and cytotoxic cerebral edema in patients with CVT.[11,12]

A separate sequela of cerebral veins and dural sinuses outflow obstruction resulting from CVT is impaired CSF absorption. Normal absorption of CSF occurs through the arachnoid granulations, which drain into the superior sagittal sinus. As the superior sagittal sinus thrombose, CSF drainage can no longer happen. In addition, thrombosis of other dural sinuses leads to increased venous pressure throughout the sinus network, which impairs CSF absorption and consequently elevates ICP.

Etiology

The most frequently reported conditions associated with CVT are shown in Box 43.1:[1,4,5,8,13]

However, risk factors for development of CVT vary by age. In the Canadian pediatric registry, risk factors for CVT were identified in approximately 98% of the children.[2] In that study cohort, acute systemic illness occurred in 84% of neonates. A prothrombotic state was found in 41% of infants older than 4 weeks. In infants older than 4 weeks, infections and other chronic systemic illnesses of the head and neck disorders were responsible. In older adults, the proportion of cases without associated risk factors were higher (37%) than those in adults younger than 65. The most common risk factors for older adults (>65) were genetic or acquired thrombophilia, malignancy, and hematological disorders.[19] Gender-specific etiologies also exist. The most common risk factor for CVT in women is the use of oral contraception. Two case–control studies have shown increased risk of CVT with the use of oral contraceptive.[18,20] This risk is further increased in the setting of prothrombotic states.[20]

BOX 43.1

- Prothrombotic conditions: either acquired or inherited[14–17]
- Antithrombin deficiency
- Protein C or protein S deficiency
- Factor V Leiden mutation
- G20210A prothrombin gene mutation
- Hyperhomocysteinemia
- Lupus anticoagulant
  - Anticardiolipin and anti-beta 2 glycoprotein-I antibodies
- Systemic illness
- Oral contraceptive[18]
- Malignancy
- Infection
- Head injury and mechanical precipitant
- Spontaneous/cryptogenic
- Dehydration

Clinical manifestations

CVT has highly variable manifestations and clinical presentations. Onset of symptoms can be acute, subacute, or chronic. CVT may also masquerade as other neurological diseases. Overall, signs of CVT can be grouped into the following:[1,4,7,21]

- Isolated symptoms reflective of intracranial hypertension (headache, blurry vision, vomiting, or nausea)
- Focal findings (focal neurological findings, seizures, or both)
- Encephalopathy (fluctuating levels of consciousness, stupor, or coma)

Other but less common manifestations include isolated cranial nerve palsies (single or multiple), subarachnoid hemorrhage, and cavernous sinus syndrome.

Development of CVT signs and symptoms depends on several factors: site and burden of occluded veins or dural sinuses, presence of parenchymal brain lesions (cerebral edema, cerebral infarction, or intraparenchymal hemorrhage), gender, and interval from CVT onset to presentation.

The single most common symptom of CVT is headache, reported in over 89% of patients in the ISCVT cohort.[1] Headache associated with CVT is more frequently observed in women than men. Headache may also be the only symptom of CVT[22] and may be variable in nature, that is, diffuse or localized, abrupt, or subacute onset. There is often no clear relationship between the localization of headache and the location of the occluded sinus or the parenchymal lesion.[22-24] Migraine-like phenomena with aura has also been reported.[25]

Disturbance in the level of consciousness, delirium, cognitive dysfunction, and frontal lobe syndrome has also been reported in the setting of CVT. Overall, coma associated with CVT portends a worse prognosis.[1]

Focal or generalized seizures in the setting of CVT are more common than those in other subtypes of stroke.[1,4,26] In the ISCVT cohort,[1] seizures at presentation occurred in 39% of patients, and seizures after the diagnosis occurred in 7% of patients.[26] In another retrospective cohort of children, seizures at presentation occurred in 44% of patients.[27] Risk factors associated with seizures include supratentorial lesions, sagittal sinus, and cortical veins thrombosis as well as focal motor deficits.[28]

Diagnosis

Appropriate imaging remains the gold standard for diagnosis. In patients with suspected venous thrombosis, the demonstration of absence of venous flow by magnetic resonance or computed tomography (CT) venography confirms the diagnosis of CVT.[13] However, these findings are not always conclusive and clinicians should be aware of the potential diagnostic pitfalls. In fact, normal anatomical variations, such as arachnoid granulations, sinus atresia, sinus hypoplasia, and asymmetric sinus drainage, may mimic CVT.[28,29] Unfortunately, early brain CT is most often normal in patients with CVT. Signs on noncontrast CT that may indicate CVT include an "empty delta sign," reflective of thrombosis of the convergence of sinuses. Intraparenchymal lesions may also be apparent. When the diagnosis of CVT is uncertain, cerebral intra-arterial angiography (digital subtraction angiography) is recommended. Angiography may be helpful for ascertaining this diagnosis by revealing abrupt termination of a cortical vein or tortuous collaterals, or a filling defect.[13]

There is no single confirmatory laboratory test for the diagnosis of CVT. Current guidelines for suspected CVT from the American Heart Association/American Stroke Association (AHA/ASA) recommend obtaining routine blood studies with a complete blood count, chemistry panel, and coagulation panel.[13] The utility of D-dimer in the diagnosis of CVT is uncertain, as an elevated D-dimer may further support the diagnosis of CVT whereas a normal value does not exclude this diagnosis when symptoms are suggestive of CVT. In one study of 233 patients with suspected CVT of symptom onset less than 7 days, D-dimer demonstrated a specificity and sensitivity of 98% and 94%, respectively, for predicting CVT.[30] A 2012 meta-analysis that included 14 studies of patients with suspected or confirmed CVT (a total of 1134 patients) found similar sensitivity and specificity in seven studies of patients with suspected CVT. However, the D-dimer performed less well in the remaining seven studies of subjects with confirmed CVT with a sensitivity of 89% and a specificity of 83%. This sensitivity was similar for patients with isolated headache as the presenting symptom (82%), subacute or chronic clinical presentations of CVT (83%), and single affected venous sinus (84%).[31]

Finally, lumbar puncture may be helpful in excluding other masquerading conditions (e.g., meningitis, and subarachnoid hemorrhage); however, CSF analysis is unlikely to be diagnostic of CVT. If abnormal, CSF findings in patients with CVT may be nonspecific, including elevated levels of protein, elevated levels of red blood cell (RBC), or a lymphocytic pleocytosis. These findings have been reported in 30%–50% of patients with CVT.[21,32]

Treatment

The immediate goals of treatment of patients with CVT should always include hemodynamic and neurological stabilization, including assessment of airway patency. Prevention of thrombus propagation to adjacent sinuses/veins through anticoagulation should follow. The mainstay of CVT treatment is systemic anticoagulation with either unfractionated heparin or low molecular weight heparin (LMWH).[33,34] Antiplatelet drugs are an option when systemic anticoagulation is contraindicated, but there is no evidence regarding their effectiveness and safety in CVT. Evaluation and treatment of underlying prothrombotic states should be undertaken to prevent further recurrence of CVT. Finally, mechanical recanalization of occluded veins should be considered in refractory cases or as life-saving therapy. Endovascular therapies remain investigational and often reserved for cases of patients with otherwise poor prognoses who have not responded to anticoagulation therapy.[7,13] Hematoma or localized focal mass evacuation may also be a necessary life-saving procedure in select cases.

The general consensus and current recommended AHA/ASA guidelines suggest primary treatment of CVT should consist of anticoagulation through administration of unfractionated heparin or LMWH.[1,13,35] In fact, anticoagulation appears to be safe in patient, especially in adult patients with intracranial hemorrhage related to CVT. In two trials,[34,36] no new intracranial hemorrhages were detected in patients randomly assigned to heparin, and only one case of major extracranial bleeding was reported. These findings are in concordance with the pathogenesis of hemorrhage in CVT that is probably caused by

venous outflow blockade or the very high intradural and intravenous pressures leading to rupture of the venules or hemorrhagic transformation of venous infarct.[1,37] Similarly, observational studies suggest that anticoagulant therapy appears to be safe in children with CVT.[38–42] The European Federation of Neurological Societies (EFNS) guidelines on the treatment of CVT, published in 2010, recommended that patients with CVT and no contraindications for anticoagulation should be treated with either weight-adjusted LMWH or dose-adjusted unfractionated heparin, with a goal of two times the mean of the control activated partial thromboplastin time (aPTT) value or the upper limit of the normal aPTT range.[34] The 2014 AHA/ASA guidelines for the prevention of stroke in patients with stroke or transient ischemic attack state that anticoagulation is reasonable for patients with acute CVT, even in selected patients with intracranial hemorrhage, and that it is reasonable to administer anticoagulation for at least 3 months, followed by antiplatelet therapy. Long-term anticoagulation might be reasonable for those with CVT and an inherited thrombophilia.[43] Guidelines from the American Academy of Chest Physicians (ACCP) issued in 2012 suggest anticoagulation over no anticoagulation during the acute and chronic phases of CVT.[44] Either dose-adjusted unfractionated or LMWH can be used as initial treatment, even in the presence of hemorrhage within a venous infarction. Patients who have stabilized can be switched to oral anticoagulation, which is generally continued for a period of 3–6 months.[44]

Some patients continue to clinically decline despite anticoagulation therapy. In select cases, direct endovascular or open craniotomy approaches may be used in adjunct to anticoagulation.[45–52] The aim of these approaches is to directly remove the venous thrombosis and to restore intravenous or dural flow. There are no randomized controlled trials that have evaluated endovascular or open interventions for the treatment of CVT. The published literature consists of case reports and uncontrolled case series. A systemic review published in 2015 included 185 patients with CVT treated with mechanical thrombectomy. In this study, many of these patients were severely ill with stupor or coma present in 47%. A variety of devices were used, including the AngioJet Rheolytic catheter, balloon angioplasty, stents and microsnares, and concurrent local thrombolysis was used in 71% patients. Overall, favorable outcome was reported for 84% of patients and mortality was reported as 12%. New or worsened intracerebral hemorrhage affected 10%.[53] The EFNS guidelines also concluded that there is insufficient evidence to support the routine use of local or systemic thrombolysis for CVT, but state that endovascular thrombolysis may be performed as a therapeutic option in centers with expertise in interventional radiology for patients with a poor prognosis, such as those who worsen despite best medical treatment and anticoagulation, provided that other causes of worsening are excluded and treated.

Management of other complications

General recommendations for the management of elevated ICP should be followed. This may include elevation of the head of bed, admission to a specialist neurocritical care unit or other high-volume center, sedation, hyperosmotic therapy with mannitol or hypertonic saline, modest hyperventilation, and/or ICP monitoring.[13,37] Benefits of glucocorticosteroid administration have not been established; therefore, their routine use cannot be recommended.[54]

In patients who develop seizures during the acute phase of CVT, symptomatic management with antiepileptic medications is recommended. The optimal dose and duration of treatment are not yet established. Patients with CVT are more likely to develop seizures if they demonstrate a supratentorial lesion, cerebral edema, infarction, or hemorrhage. Seizure prophylaxis in the setting of CVT remains controversial, as there is no consensus among experts. Some advocate prophylaxis for all patients with CVT because of the moderately high incidence of seizures during the acute phase of the disease (reported as 5%–11% in the literature) while others prescribe antiepileptic treatment only for patients with symptomatic seizures.[1,13,26,36,55] The optimal duration of antiepileptic treatment in the setting of CVT is unknown. The risk of epilepsy after CVT ranges from 5% to 11%.[1,4,26,56] The 2010 EFNS guidelines for CVT state that it may be reasonable to continue antiepileptic drug treatment for 1 year in patients with early seizures and hemorrhagic lesions on admission brain scan.[35]

Prognosis

Overall CVT has a more favorable prognosis compared to the other subtypes of strokes. However, CVT may also result in severe disability and death. Overall, the reported mortality in CVT is approximately 3%–6%.[1,4,13,37,57,58]

Predictors of mortality at 30 days include the following:[57,58]

- Depressed consciousness and coma state on presentation
- Thrombosis of the deep venous system
- Right hemisphere hemorrhage
- Posterior fossa lesion

The main cause of early mortality in CVT is transtentorial herniation secondary to a large hemorrhagic lesion.[57,58] Other causes of early death include herniation due to diffuse cerebral edema, status epilepticus, pulmonary embolism, and other systemic complications.

Long-term mortality after CVT is related to underlying thrombotic conditions and other secondary complications after the acute injury. In the ISCVT study, at the end of follow-up (median of 16 months), death was reported in 8.3% patients.[1] The following predictors of poor long-term prognosis are reported in the ISCVT databases:

- Central nervous system infection
- Malignancy
- Thrombosis of the deep venous system
- Hemorrhage on head CT or magnetic resonance imaging (MRI)
- Altered mental status
- Male gender
- Age older than 37 years

The rate of recurrence of CVT is low. The overall reported risk of recurrent CVT is 1%–4%, depending on the epidemiological study.[1,4,59–61]

Management of chronic symptoms

Despite the overall good prognosis of CVT, several chronic symptoms may persist long after acute CVT has resolved. For example, nearly half of survivors report depression and other minor cognitive or language changes.[1,13,27,43,62–64] Chronic headache and recurrent severe headaches may also occur after CVT.[1,4] In fact, up to 14% of patients develop severe headaches requiring bed rest or hospital admission. Different options of headache management may warrant referral to headache specialists. A detailed discussion of headache management is beyond the scope of this chapter.

Severe visual loss is a rare but devastating sequela of CVT.[19,65] If visual acuity decreases during follow-up and is otherwise not explained by a prior intracranial or intraocular cause related to CVT, elevated ICP as a cause of vision decline must be ruled out. Fenestration of the optic nerve sheath, repeat lumbar puncture, and use of carbonic anhydrase inhibitors may be considered. Because of the potential for visual loss caused by elevated ICP, serial assessment of visual fields and acuity is recommended for children with CVT. It is reasonable to do the same for adults with visual complaints, chronic headaches, or papilledema.[1,13,27,35,43,62]

As pregnancy and puerperium are known risk factors for CVT, all women should be counselled regarding the risk of CVT in subsequent pregnancies. However, prior CVT is not a contraindication for future pregnancy. However, the rate of spontaneous abortion and recurrence is higher in women with a history of CVT have a higher rate of spontaneous abortion than women without a history of CVT.[1,4,66–70] The role of antithrombotic prophylaxis in the prevention of CVT in subsequent pregnancies is unproven in women. There is no expert consensus on the optimal regimen regarding this issue. However, oral contraceptive should be stopped in women with a history of CVT.[62,67,69]

Conclusion

Cerebral venous thrombosis is uncommon, with an estimated incidence of 0.5–1.5 per 100,000 people annually. This disorder is more common in neonates and children than adults, and is more common in females than males. The clinical presentation of CVT is highly variable, with symptoms that may be acute, subacute, or chronic. The range of symptoms may vary from headache, focal neurological deficits, change in vision, focal or generalized seizure, or encephalopathy and coma. Parenchymal brain lesion including cerebral edema, hemorrhage, and stroke may occur secondary to venous occlusion as well. Noncontrast head CT may be normal in up to 30% of patients and most of the findings on noncontrast

CT may be nonspecific. MR or CT venography may be obtained for diagnosis of CVT. Treatment of CVT involves anticoagulation. The duration of treatment is tailored according to the risk factors of recurrent thrombosis. Overall, CVT is associated with good outcome; however, up to 5% of patients may also die in the acute setting, and longer-term mortality may reach up to 10%.

References

1. Ferro JM, Canhão P, Stam J et al. Prognosis of cerebral vein and dural sinus thrombosis: Results of the International Study on Cerebral Vein and Dural Sinus Thrombosis (ISCVT). *Stroke* 2004;35:664.
2. deVeber G, Andrew M, Adams C et al. Cerebral sinovenous thrombosis in children. *N Engl J Med* 2001;345:417.
3. Lancon JA, Killough KR, Tibbs RE et al. Spontaneous dural sinus thrombosis in children. *PediatrNeurosurg* 1999;30:23.
4. Ferro JM, Correia M, Pontes C et al. Cerebral vein and dural sinus thrombosis in Portugal: 1980–1998. *Cerebrovasc Dis* 2001;11:177.
5. Coutinho JM, Zuurbier SM, Aramideh M, Stam J. The incidence of cerebral venous thrombosis: A cross-sectional study. *Stroke* 2012;43:3375.
6. Coutinho JM, Ferro JM, Canhão P et al. Cerebral venous and sinus thrombosis in women. *Stroke* 2009;40:2356.
7. Stam J. Thrombosis of the cerebral veins and sinuses. *N Engl J Med* 2005;352:1791.
8. Lanska DJ, Kryscio RJ. Risk factors for peripartum and postpartum stroke and intracranial venous thrombosis. *Stroke* 2000;31:1274.
9. Schaller B, Graf R. Cerebral venous infarction: The pathophysiological concept. *Cerebrovasc Dis* 2004;18:179.
10. Gotoh M, Ohmoto T, Kuyama H. Experimental study of venous circulatory disturbance by dural sinus occlusion. *Acta Neurochir* (Wien) 1993;124:120.
11. Röther J, Waggie K, van Bruggen N et al. Experimental cerebral venous thrombosis: Evaluation using magnetic resonance imaging. *J Cereb Blood Flow Metab* 1996;16:1353.

12. Chu K, Kang DW, Yoon BW, Roh JK. Diffusion-weighted magnetic resonance in cerebral venous thrombosis. *Arch Neurol* 2001;58:1569.

13. Saposnik G, Barinagarrementeria F, Brown RD Jr et al. Diagnosis and management of cerebral venous thrombosis: A statement for healthcare professionals from the American Heart Association/American Stroke Association. *Stroke* 2011;42:1158.

14. Lauw MN, Barco S, Coutinho JM, Middeldorp S. Cerebral venous thrombosis and thrombophilia: A systematic review and meta-analysis. *Semin Thromb Hemost* 2013;39:913.

15. Weih M, Junge-Hülsing J, Mehraein S et al. [Hereditary thrombophilia with ischemic stroke and sinus thrombosis. Diagnosis, therapy and meta-analysis]. *Nervenarzt* 2000;71:936.

16. Lüdemann P, Nabavi DG, Junker R et al. Factor V Leiden mutation is a risk factor for cerebral venous thrombosis: A case–control study of 55 patients. *Stroke* 1998;29:2507.

17. Enevoldson TP, Russell RW. Cerebral venous thrombosis: New causes for an old syndrome? *Q J Med* 1990;77:1255.

18. Martinelli I, Sacchi E, Landi G et al. High risk of cerebral-vein thrombosis in carriers of a prothrombin-gene mutation and in users of oral contraceptives. *N Engl J Med* 1998;338:1793.

19. Ferro JM, Canhão P, Bousser MG et al. Cerebral vein and dural sinus thrombosis in elderly patients. *Stroke* 2005;36:1927.

20. De Bruijn SF, Stam J, Koopman MM, Vandenbroucke JP. Case–control study of risk of cerebral sinus thrombosis in oral contraceptive users and in [correction of who are] carriers of hereditary prothrombotic conditions. The Cerebral Venous Sinus Thrombosis Study Group. *BMJ* 1998;316:589.

21. Biousse V, Ameri A, Bousser MG. Isolated intracranial hypertension as the only sign of cerebral venous thrombosis. *Neurology* 1999;53:1537.

22. Cumurciuc R, Crassard I, Sarov M et al. Headache as the only neurological sign of cerebral venous thrombosis: A series of 17 cases. *J Neurol Neurosurg Psychiatry* 2005;76:1084.

23. Ameri A, Bousser MG. Headache in cerebral venous thrombosis: A study of 110 cases. *Cephalalgia* 1993;13(Suppl. 13):110.

24. Lopes MG, Ferro J, Pontes C et al. Headache and cerebral venous thrombosis. *Cephalalgia* 2000;20:292.

25. Newman DS, Levine SR, Curtis VL, Welch KM. Migraine-like visual phenomena associated with cerebral venous thrombosis. *Headache* 1989;29:82.

26. Ferro JM, Canhão P, Bousser MG et al. Early seizures in cerebral vein and dural sinus thrombosis: Risk factors and role of antiepileptics. *Stroke* 2008;39:1152.

27. Wasay M, Dai AI, Ansari M et al. Cerebral venous sinus thrombosis in children: A multicenter cohort from the United States. *J Child Neurol* 2008;23:26.

28. Ayanzen RH, Bird CR, Keller PJ et al. Cerebral MR venography: Normal anatomy and potential diagnostic pitfalls. *AJNR Am J Neuroradiol* 2000;21:74.

29. Zouaoui A, Hidden G. Cerebral venous sinuses: Anatomical variants or thrombosis? *Acta Anat* (Basel) 1988;133:318.

30. Meng R, Wang X, Hussain M et al. Evaluation of plasma D-dimer plus fibrinogen in predicting acute CVST. *Int J Stroke* 2014;9:166.

31. Dentali F, Squizzato A, Marchesi C et al. D-dimer testing in the diagnosis of cerebral vein thrombosis: A systematic review and a meta-analysis of the literature. *J Thromb Haemost* 2012;10:582.

32. Bousser MG, Chiras J, Bories J, Castaigne P. Cerebral venous thrombosis—A review of 38 cases. *Stroke* 1985;16:199.

33. Bousser MG. Cerebral venous thrombosis: Nothing, heparin, or local thrombolysis? *Stroke* 1999;30:481.

34. de Bruijn SF, Stam J. Randomized, placebo-controlled trial of anticoagulant treatment with low-molecular-weight heparin for cerebral sinus thrombosis. *Stroke* 1999;30:484.

35. Einhäupl KM, Villringer A, Meister W et al. Heparin treatment in sinus venous thrombosis. *Lancet* 1991;338:597.

36. Einhäupl K, Stam J, Bousser MG et al. EFNS guideline on the treatment of cerebral venous and sinus thrombosis in adult patients. *Eur J Neurol* 2010;17:1229.

37. deVeber G, Chan A, Monagle P et al. Anticoagulation therapy in pediatric patients with sinovenous thrombosis: A cohort study. *Arch Neurol* 1998;55:1533.
38. Johnson MC, Parkerson N, Ward S, de Alarcon PA. Pediatric sinovenous thrombosis. *J Pediatr Hematol Oncol* 2003;25:312.
39. Sébire G, Tabarki B, Saunders DE et al. Cerebral venous sinus thrombosis in children: Risk factors, presentation, diagnosis and outcome. *Brain* 2005;128:477.
40. Schobess R, Düring C, Bidlingmaier C et al. Long-term safety and efficacy data on childhood venous thrombosis treated with a low molecular weight heparin: An open-label pilot study of once-daily versus twice-daily enoxaparin administration. *Haematologica* 2006;91:1701.
41. Golomb MR. The risk of recurrent venous thromboembolism after paediatric cerebral sinovenous thrombosis. *Lancet Neurol* 2007;6:573.
42. Moharir MD, Shroff M, Stephens D et al. Anticoagulants in pediatric cerebral sinovenous thrombosis: A safety and outcome study. *Ann Neurol* 2010;67:590.
43. Kernan WN, Ovbiagele B, Black HR et al. Guidelines for the prevention of stroke in patients with stroke and transient ischemic attack: A guideline for healthcare professionals from the American Heart Association/American Stroke Association. *Stroke* 2014;45:2160.
44. Lansberg MG, O'Donnell MJ, Khatri P et al. Antithrombotic and thrombolytic therapy for ischemic stroke: Antithrombotic therapy and prevention of thrombosis, 9th ed: American College of Chest Physicians Evidence-based Clinical Practice Guidelines. *Chest* 2012;141:e601S.
45. Bagley LJ, Hurst RW, Galetta S et al. Use of a microsnare to aid direct thrombolytic therapy of dural sinus thrombosis. *AJR Am J Roentgenol* 1998;170:784.
46. Scarrow AM, Williams RL, Jungreis CA et al. Removal of a thrombus from the sigmoid and transverse sinuses with a rheolytic thrombectomy catheter. *AJNR Am J Neuroradiol* 1999;20:1467.

47. Mortimer AM, Bradley MD, O'Leary S, Renowden SA. Endovascular treatment of children with cerebral venous sinus thrombosis: A case series. *Pediatr Neurol* 2013;49:305.
48. Horowitz M, Purdy P, Unwin H et al. Treatment of dural sinus thrombosis using selective catheterization and urokinase. *Ann Neurol* 1995;38:58.
49. Frey JL, Muro GJ, McDougall CG et al. Cerebral venous thrombosis: Combined intrathrombus rtPA and intravenous heparin. *Stroke* 1999;30:489.
50. Kim SY, Suh JH. Direct endovascular thrombolytic therapy for dural sinus thrombosis: Infusion of alteplase. *AJNR Am J Neuroradiol* 1997;18:639.
51. Wasay M, Bakshi R, Kojan S et al. Nonrandomized comparison of local urokinase thrombolysis versus systemic heparin anticoagulation for superior sagittal sinus thrombosis. *Stroke* 2001;32:2310.
52. Stam J, Majoie CB, van Delden OM et al. Endovascular thrombectomy and thrombolysis for severe cerebral sinus thrombosis: A prospective study. *Stroke* 2008;39:1487.
53. Siddiqui FM, Dandapat S, Banerjee C et al. Mechanical thrombectomy in cerebral venous thrombosis: Systematic review of 185 cases. *Stroke* 2015;46:1263.
54. Canhão P, Cortesão A, Cabral M et al. Are steroids useful to treat cerebral venous thrombosis? *Stroke* 2008;39:105.
55. Ameri A, Bousser MG. Cerebral venous thrombosis. *Neurol Clin* 1992;10:87.
56. Ferro JM, Correia M, Rosas MJ et al. Seizures in cerebral vein and dural sinus thrombosis. *Cerebrovasc Dis* 2003;15:78.
57. Canhão P, Ferro JM, Lindgren AG et al. Causes and predictors of death in cerebral venous thrombosis. *Stroke* 2005;36:1720.
58. Borhani Haghighi A, Edgell RC, Cruz-Flores S et al. Mortality of cerebral venous-sinus thrombosis in a large national sample. *Stroke* 2012;43:262.
59. Martinelli I, Bucciarelli P, Passamonti SM et al. Long-term evaluation of the risk of recurrence after cerebral sinus-venous thrombosis. *Circulation* 2010;121:2740.

60. Miranda B, Ferro JM, Canhão P et al. Venous thromboembolic events after cerebral vein thrombosis. *Stroke* 2010;41:1901.

61. Dentali F, Poli D, Scoditti U et al. Long-term outcomes of patients with cerebral vein thrombosis: A multicenter study. *J Thromb Haemost* 2012;10:1297.

62. Roach ES, Golomb MR, Adams R et al. Management of stroke in infants and children: A scientific statement from a Special Writing Group of the American Heart Association Stroke Council and the Council on Cardiovascular Disease in the Young. *Stroke* 2008;39:2644.

63. Madureira S, Canhão P, Ferro JM. Cognitive and behavioural outcome of patients with cerebral venous thrombosis. *Cerebrovasc Dis* 2001;11(Suppl. 4):108.

64. de Bruijn SF, Budde M, Teunisse S et al. Long-term outcome of cognition and functional health after cerebral venous sinus thrombosis. *Neurology* 2000;54:1687.

65. Purvin VA, Trobe JD, Kosmorsky G. Neuro-ophthalmic features of cerebral venous obstruction. *Arch Neurol* 1995;52:880.

66. Rondepierre P, Hamon M, Leys D et al. [Cerebral venous thromboses: Study of the course]. *Rev Neurol* (Paris) 1995;151:100.

67. Lamy C, Hamon JB, Coste J, Mas JL. Ischemic stroke in young women: Risk of recurrence during subsequent pregnancies. French study group on stroke in pregnancy. *Neurology* 2000;55:269.

68. Srinivasan K. Cerebral venous and arterial thrombosis in pregnancy and puerperium. A study of 135 patients. *Angiology* 1983;34:731.

69. Bushnell C, McCullough LD, Awad IA et al. Guidelines for the prevention of stroke in women: A statement for healthcare professionals from the American Heart Association/American Stroke Association. *Stroke* 2014;45:1545.

70. Jilma B, Kamath S, Lip GY. Antithrombotic therapy in special circumstances. I—Pregnancy and cancer. *BMJ* 2003;326:37.

44

Brain stem death

JOHN ANDRZEJOWSKI and ANDREW DAVIDSON

Hypothetical scenario

A 25-year-old previously fit and healthy man presents to the emergency department after a severe, sudden onset headache yesterday while driving. After self-presentation at hospital, he suddenly deteriorates from Glasgow Coma Scale (GCS) 15 without neurological deficits to GCS 3, apnea, with one fixed dilated pupil and the other 3 mm and reactive. Blood pressure is 170/100 mmHg, pulse 40/min.

He is sedated, he has tracheal intubation and ventilation, and urgent head CT scan shows widespread subarachnoid hemorrhage without hydrocephalus. He rapidly proceeds to have bilateral fixed dilated pupils despite adequate sedation, ventilation, and cardiovascular support.

The neurosurgical and intensive care multidisciplinary team (MDT) opinion is that no further life-sustaining treatment is possible, so sedation is stopped. Normal physiological homeostasis is maintained, brain stem death tests are performed, which show no response on two occasions, and the patient is declared dead. Next of kin are approached and consent to organ donation is obtained.

As an occasional neuroanesthetist, it is unlikely that you will ever be involved in diagnosing brain stem death (BSD); however, neuropatients (e.g., with head injuries or those undergoing decompressive craniotomy following ischemic stroke) are some of the most likely to deteriorate and become ventilator dependent with a subsequent diagnosis of brain death. Likewise, you may be asked to "anesthetize" for organ retrieval in heart-beating donors, so an understanding of the criteria used in brain stem death testing (BSDT) is desirable.

In most circumstances outside critical care, death follows cardiorespiratory arrest and its confirmation involves observation of the patient for up to 5 min for signs of life.

According to the UK Code of Practice for the Neurological Determination of Death from the Academy of Medical Royal Colleges (AoMRC), BSD "entails the irreversible loss of those essential characteristics which are necessary to the existence of a living human person. Thus the definition of death should be regarded as the irreversible loss of capacity for consciousness, combined with the irreversible loss of the capacity to breath."[1]

In North America and Australia the term "brain death" is used.

In other words, because of continued artificial ventilation, a patient can be clinically and legally dead while having a cardiac output. This condition was first described in 1959 as "coma dépassé" by Mollaret and Goulon in the increasing number of patients receiving artificial respiration while in a coma.[2] It was first defined by Harvard Medical School in 1968 and the 1976 UK code of practice by the AoMRC was revised to its current version in 2008. One major change since this revised version of the Royal College of Paediatrics and Child Health (RCPCH) guidelines is that they now allow a diagnosis of BSD in infants less than 2 months.[3]

For the purposes of this chapter, we will consider patients in a coma and ventilated in a critical care unit. These patients may have been in a coma for a varying duration, and since dying is a process rather than an event, subtle changes or deterioration in neurology or new pathology may raise the possibility of the onset of "BSD." The neural control of cardiac, respiratory, and endocrine functions is damaged in these patients; however, the onset of cardiac arrest varies considerably. Thus, a patient's cardiac output can continue for some time, so it should be remembered that failure to recognize this can lead to undue distress for relatives who may be at the patients' bedside, as well as unnecessary and expensive ongoing care.

By having well laid out and clear criteria for diagnosing BSD, the process of organ donation is also facilitated. This is discussed in the latter half of the chapter.

Diagnosing brain stem death

Step 1: Ascertain cause of coma

Most causes will be fairly obvious from the patient's admission history, for example, trauma, stroke (cerebrovascular accident [CVA]), and poisoning. Other etiology may involve careful diagnostics and review by appropriate neurologists and/or neurosurgeons. Tests such as computed tomography (CT), magnetic resonance imaging (MRI), and electroencephalography (EEG) as well as blood tests or drug levels may be needed. If there is doubt about the potential reversibility (particularly if the cause is unknown), then BSDT should not be undertaken.

Step 2: Exclude depressant drugs

Review the patient's drug card. Exclude the administration of long-acting drugs known to cumulate such as morphine and benzodiazepines. If present, they must be given ample time to wear off with extra time needed in patients with liver or kidney dysfunction, which can affect drug metabolism and excretion. Thiopentone may need several days to wear off. Drug-level testing is not mandatory but is recommended if any doubt exists as to the ongoing effects of thiopentone or benzodiazepines. Thiopentone levels less than 5 mg/L and midazolam levels less than 10 µg/L are needed prior to BSDT. Reversal agents such as naloxone and flumazenil can also be administered. A peripheral nerve stimulator can be used if muscle relaxants have been discontinued recently, to confirm full reversal.

Step 3: Exclude primary hypothermia

Patients can be obtunded with temperatures of <34°C and brain stem reflexes are affected at <28°C. It is recommended that hypothermia is treated and BS testing should be undertaken only if temperature is >34°C.

Step 4: Exclude other causes of unconsciousness

Many endocrine and metabolic disturbances can result in a state of unconsciousness. Thyroid dysfunction and addisonian crisis can affect muscle function or result in coma. They should be excluded by hormonal assay, if suspected, when ascertaining the primary cause of coma.

Electrolyte disturbance can lead to muscle weakness that might interfere with BSDT. Mildly abnormal levels need not preclude testing. Rapid correction of deranged glucose and sodium levels can be damaging, so it should be undertaken cautiously. Ideally BSDT should take place with levels as follows:

- Sodium: 115–160 mmol/L
- Glucose: 3–20 mmol/L
- Magnesium and phosphate: 0.5–3 mmol/L
- Potassium: 1–2 mmol/L
- Oxygen: >10 kPa

- Carbon dioxide: < 6 kPa
- Mean arterial pressure: > 60 mmHg

Step 5: Exclude reversible causes of apnea

Narcotics and hypnotics should again be excluded as a cause of respiratory depression. Muscle function can be confirmed by demonstrating the presence of deep tendon reflexes or use of a nerve stimulator. High cervical spine injury would invalidate apnea testing and must be excluded following traumatic head injury using radiological imaging, as indicated by the history and examination. Ancillary tests (such as CT angiography) to show no cerebral blood flow can be used in these cases if required.

Brain stem death: Testing cranial nerve function

Since the cranial nerve (CN) nuclei are found in the brain stem, to make a diagnosis of BSD, the clinicians must demonstrate absence of CN function. We describe the way tests are carried out in the United Kingdom and which CNs are tested at each point.

In the United Kingdom, BSDT is performed by two doctors who must have been registered for at least 5 years. At least one doctor must be of consultant (specialist) status. Neither should have any conflict of interest (e.g., be a member of the transplant team). The tests are carried out by both doctors simultaneously:

1. *Fixed pupils:* Tests CNs II and III. Pupils may be an irregular shape or asymmetrical; however, the only criterion to be assessed is that there is no change to size or shape of the pupils when a bright light is shone into each eye. Take care to look at ipsilateral and contralateral pupils when shining the light into each pupil in turn.
2. *No corneal reflexes:* Tests CNs V and VII. Hold open the eye gently. There is no eye movement or eyelash reflex (e.g., eyes closing) when the cornea is stimulated. This can be done very carefully with sterile gauze.
3. *Absence of oculovestibular reflexes:* Test CNs III, VI, and VIII. Turn the head away from the side to be tested and use an auroscope to

inspect the ear canal and confirm that there is no debris or ear wax in the outer ear. This test relies on stimulating both tympanic membranes with 50 mL of ice-cold saline injected over a minute into the external auditory meatus. This stimulus would normally result in the eye movement of nystagmus. No movement of the eyes should be seen if brain stem death is present.

4. *No motor responses:* No motor responses are seen in the CN V and VII or somatic when applying pressure in the supraorbital notch on both sides. It is possible that limb or trunk movements will be seen before or during testing.[4] They can be related to spinal reflexes and do not preclude a diagnosis of BSD being made.
5. *No cough or gag response:* No cough or gag response is elicited. Test CNs IX and X. Pass a suction catheter down the endotracheal tube (ETT) to the carina. Use a laryngoscope to visualize the posterior pharynx, then stimulate using a spatula; there should also be no gag response.
6. *No respiration seen on apnea testing:* It is important to avoid hypoxia during the test while simultaneously allowing the $PaCO_2$ to climb to a level high enough to allow the clinician to be certain that respiration would be triggered in a patient with some remaining brain stem function. The FiO_2 is increased to 1.0. Decrease the respiratory rate to allow the $ETCO_2$ to climb. Once the $ETCO_2$ is >6kPa, a confirmatory arterial blood gas is sent to make sure the $PaCO_2$ is >6 kPa (or >6.5 kPa in patients with chronic CO_2 retention) and the pH is less than 7.4. The patient is then disconnected from the ventilator and observed for respiratory effort for a 5 min period. If there is a risk of hypoxia, then a catheter with oxygen flow can be passed down the ETT or continuous positive airway pressure (CPAP) can be applied. Cardiovascular stability should be maintained during this period. At the end of 5 min, a second blood gas should confirm that $PaCO_2$ has risen by >0.5 kPa.

These tests are repeated a second time in full, after the CO_2 has been allowed to return to its pre-test level. Time of death is recorded as the time of absent brain stem reflexes at the end of the first set of tests. In the United Kingdom, a form for the recording of BSDT has been endorsed by the Faculty of Intensive Care Medicine (FICM) and the Intensive Care Society (ICS).

Brain stem death: Ancillary or confirmatory tests

BSDT protocols may vary throughout the world. Studies show heterogeneity in testing between different states and also different institutions in the USA.[5,6] In some countries additional neurophysiological or imaging tests are used to confirm BSD.[7] These can also be used if any uncertainty exists as to the nature of any metabolic or endocrine derangement or if routine testing as outlined in the previous section is not possible (e.g., extensive maxillofacial injury). The tests rely on showing either loss of electrical activity or lack of blood flow in the brain. The most common ancillary tests include the following:

* EEG
* Four-vessel angiography
* Positron emission tomography
* Transcranial Doppler

Managing the potential organ donor in critical care

Sometimes, a variety of profound physiological instabilities accompany BSD and must be recognized and managed. The changes that occur are the consequence of either the loss of the neurological and humoral functions of the brain stem or the treatment of the cause of BSD.

Hypotension occurs due to hypovolemia, loss of sympathetic tone, and temporary myocardial dysfunction after the "catecholamine storm" of the coning period. Hypoxia may occur due to neurogenic pulmonary edema, systemic inflammatory response to BSD, sepsis, or atelectasis from the presence of retained tracheal secretions.

Appropriate support at this time will optimize the chances of successful transplantation following subsequent organ retrieval. Guidance for the unstable potential BSD patient is available from the UK organ donation and transplantation website.[8] The main summary points of this chapter are the following:

* Correct hypovolemia
* Maintain cardiac output and vascular tone

* Continue strategies to optimize lung function
* Treat diabetes insipidus
* Avoid hypernatremia
* Avoid hypothermia

Managing the potential organ donor in the operating theater

Caring for a patient in theater undergoing multi-organ retrieval is a major undertaking involving multiple theater and surgical personnel. Extensive laparotomy and sternotomy are performed to allow inspection and retrieval of thoracic and abdominal organs, resulting in large fluid losses. The procedure may take several hours and timing needs to be coordinated with the potential recipients' surgical preparation elsewhere. Standard WHO (World Health Organization) safer surgical checks are mandatory. A secure wide-bore venous access, intra-arterial monitoring, and central venous pressure (CVP) monitoring are needed.

Following are the suggested targets with initial cardiovascular goal:

* Sinus rhythm: 60–100 beats per minute
* CVP: 4–10 mmHg
* Pulmonary arterial pressure: < 12mmHg
* Mean arterial pressure: 60–80 mmHg
* Cardiac index: >2.1 L/min/m²

Cardiovascular instability at the time of transfer to theater and during retrieval will be minimized by close attention to $PaCO_2$ control as BSD donors lack vasomotor control and are susceptible to vasodilatation. Cardiac output is best maintained with the lowest level of combined fluid loading and inotrope (or vasoconstrictor) possible. This avoids further lung injury from fluid and myocardial or splanchnic injury from inotropes or vasoconstrictors. Cardiac output monitoring may help guide this balance although these parameters may be relaxed if not all organs are being considered for retrieval. A vasopressin infusion at 1–4 IU/h may be used to help maintain a stable blood pressure.

Anesthesia is not required as the patient is dead; however, if the anesthetist personally wishes to administer volatile anesthesia, this is not contraindicated and may benefit liver transplant outcome. Full neuromuscular blockade is needed throughout the retrieval process, to allow surgical access to body cavities. A fall in blood pressure due to fluid shifts and surgical manipulation of organs is best minimized by limited fluid loading and cautious inotrope use. Rarely, rises in blood pressure may require opiates or direct antihypertensive drugs.

Steroids, if lung donation is possible, antibiotics, and the need for full heparinization will be guided by attending retrieval teams.

Privacy and respect for the patient's body must be maintained at all times and last offices should be performed by the attending nursing teams at the conclusion of the retrieval. Support for all staff members through a potentially challenging and stressful situation must be offered during the process and afterward.

Organ retrieval after circulatory death

This process allows organ donation when BSD has not occurred. After appropriate consent, withdrawal of life-sustaining treatment, such as extubation, occurs. Treatment withdrawal near the operating theater increases the potential for a successful retrieval and transplantation, honoring the wishes of the donor and family. Normal end-of-life care of the patient and family should continue. If the patient dies within a timeframe (normally up to 3 h) that avoids undue warm ischemia to potential donor organs, confirmation of death and the rapid transfer of the body to theater for retrieval can occur. In the United Kingdom, death is declared after 5 min of asystole. If lungs are considered for retrieval, the trachea is then intubated to avoid soiling; however, a further 5 min must be allowed to elapse before giving a single vital capacity breath of oxygen-enriched air. A variety of ante mortem interventions such as heparinization, bronchoscopy, femoral vessel cannulation,

and administration of vasodilators are practiced worldwide.

References

1. Academy of the Medical Royal Colleges, London. A code of practice for the diagnosis and confirmation of death, 2008. Available at: http://www.aomrc.org.uk/publications/reports-guidance/ukdec-reports-and-guidance/code-practice-diagnosis-confirmation-death/
2. Mollaret P, Goulon M. Le coma dépassé. *Rev Neurol* 1959;101:3–15.
3. Royal College of Paediatrics and Child Health. The diagnosis of death by neurological criteria (DNC) in infants less than two months old. Available at: http://www.rcpch.ac.uk/system/files/protected/page/DNC%20Guide%20FINAL.pdf
4. Saposnik G, Bueri JA, Mauriño J, Saizar R, Garretto NS. Spontaneous and reflex movements in brain death. *Neurology* 2000;54:221–223.
5. Greer DM, Varelas PN, Haque S, Wijdicks EF. Variability of brain death determination guidelines in leading US neurologic institutions. *Neurology* 2008;70:284.
6. Gardiner D, Shemie S, Manara A, Opdam H. International perspective on the diagnosis of death. *Br J Anaesth* 2012;108(Suppl. 1):i14–28.
7. Escudero D, Valentro MO, Escalante, JL. Intensive care practices in brain death diagnosis and organ donation. *Anaesthesia* 2015;70:1130–1139.
8. Organ Donation and Transplantation Website. Available at: http://www.odt.nhs.uk/pdf/donor_optimisation_guideline.pdf

Appendix: Scales and scores

Score/Scale	Reference	Web address
Glasgow Coma Scale (GCS)	Teasdale G, Maas A, Lecky F, Manley G, Stocchetti N, Murray G. The Glasgow Coma Scale at 40 years: Standing the test of time. *Lancet Neurol* 2014;13(8):844–854.	http://www.sciencedirect.com/science/article/pii/S1474442214701206
FOUR score	Widjicks EFM, Bamlet WR, Maramattorn BV, Manno EM, McLelland FL. Validation of a new coma scale: The FOUR score. *Ann Neurol* 2005;58:585–593.	http://onlinelibrary.wiley.com/doi/10.1002/ana.20611/abstract
Modified Hunt and Hess Scale	Hunt WE, Hess RM. Surgical risk as related to time of intervention in the repair of intracranial aneurysms. *J Neurosurg* 1968;28:14–20.	http://thejns.org/doi/abs/10.3171/jns.1968.28.1.0014
Fisher Grade	Fisher CM, Kistler JP, Davis JM. Relation of cerebral vasospasm to subarachnoid hemorrhage visualized by computerized tomographic scanning. *Neurosurgery* 1980;6:1–9.	http://journals.lww.com/neurosurgery/Abstract/1980/01000/Relation_of_Cerebral_Vasospasm_to_Subarachnoid.1.aspx
Modified Fisher Grade	Frontera JA, Claassen J, Schmidt JM et al. Prediction of symptomatic vasospasm after subarachnoid hemorrhage: The modified Fisher scale. *Neurosurgery* 2006;59:21–27.	http://journals.lww.com/neurosurgery/Abstract/2006/07000/PREDICTION_OF_SYMPTOMATIC_VASOSPASMAFTER.3.aspx
Botterell's Clinical Grades	Botterell EH, Lougheed WM, Scott JW, Vandewater SL. Hypothermia, and interruption of carotid, or carotid and vertebral circulation, in the surgical management of intracranial aneurysms. *J Neurosurg* 1956;13:1–42.	http://thejns.org/doi/abs/10.3171/jns.1956.13.1.0001?url_ver=Z39.88-2003&rfr_id=ori:rid:crossref.org&rfr_dat=cr_pub%3dpubmed
Spetzler–Martin Scale	Spetzler RF, Martin NA. A proposed grading system for arteriovenous malformations. *J Neurosurg* 1986;65:476–483.	http://thejns.org/doi/abs/10.3171/jns.1986.65.4.0476
Modified Spetzler-Martin scale	Spetzler RF, Ponce FA. A 3-tier classification of cerebral arteriovenous malformations. *J Neurosurg* 2011;114:842–849.	http://thejns.org/doi/abs/10.3171/2010.8.JNS10663?url_ver=Z39.88-2003&rfr_id=ori:rid:crossref.org&rfr_dat=cr_pub%3dpubmed
National Institute of Health Stroke Scale (NIHSS) scoring system	Adams HP Jr, Davis PH, Leira EC et al. Baseline NIH Stroke Scale score strongly predicts outcome after stroke: A report of the Trial of Org 10172 in Acute Stroke Treatment (TOAST). *Neurology* 1999;53:126–131.	http://www.neurology.org/content/53/1/126.long

(Continued)

(*Continued*)

Score/Scale	Reference	Web address
Modified Mallampati Scale	Mallampati SR, Gatt SP, Gugino LD, Waraksa B, Freiburger D, Liu PL. A clinical sign to predict difficult intubation: A prospective study. *Can Anaesth Soc J* 1985;32:429–434. Samsoon GLT, Young JRB. Difficult tracheal intubation: A retrospective study. *Anaesthesia* 1987;42:487–490.	http://link.springer.com/article/10.1007%2FBF03011357 http://onlinelibrary.wiley.com/doi/10.1111/j.1365-2044.1987.tb04039.x/abstract
Cormack–Lehane grading	Cormack RS, Lehane J. Difficult tracheal intubation in obstetrics. *Anaesthesia* 1984;39:1105–1111.	http://onlinelibrary.wiley.com/doi/10.1111/j.1365-2044.1984.tb08932.x/abstract
Richmond Agitation–Sedation Scale	Sessler CN, Gosnell MS, Grap MJ et al. The Richmond Agitation—Sedation Scale: Validity and reliability in adult intensive care unit patients. *Am J Respir Crit Care Med* 2002;166:1338–1344.	http://www.atsjournals.org/doi/abs/10.1164/rccm.2107138#.V02YC_l97IU
Ramsay Sedation Scale	Ramsay MA, Savege TM, Simpson BR et al. Controlled sedation with alphaxalone-alphadolone. *Br Med J* 1974;2(5920):656–659.	http://www.bmj.com/content/2/5920/656
Riker Sedation–Agitation Scale	Riker RR, Fraser G, Cox PM. Continuous infusion haloperidol controls agitation in critically ill patients. *Crit Care Med* 1994;22:433–440.	http://journals.lww.com/ccmjournal/Abstract/1994/03000/Continuous_infusion_of_haloperidol_controls.13.aspx
Wong–Baker FACES Scale	Wong D, Baker C. Pain in children: Comparison of assessment scales. *Pediatr Nurs* 1988;14(1):9–17.	http://www.wongbakerfaces.org/wp-content/uploads/2010/08/pain-in-children.pdf
FLACC Scale	Merkel SI, Voepel-Lewis T, Shayevitz JR, Malviya S. The FLACC: A behavioral scale for scoring postoperative pain in young children. *Pediatr Nurs* 1997;23:293–297.	https://www.ncbi.nlm.nih.gov/pubmed/?term=Pediatr+Nurs.+1997%3B+23%3A293-7
Wilson–Hardy classification	Hardy J, Vezina JL. Transsphenoidal neurosurgery of intracranial neoplasm. *Adv Neurol* 1976;15:261–273. Wilson CB. Neurosurgical management of large and invasive pituitary tumors. In: Tinadall GT, Collins WF, editors. *Clinical Management of Pituitary Disorders.* New York: Raven Press; 1979, p. 335–342.	https://www.ncbi.nlm.nih.gov/pubmed/945663
Simpson's classification	Simpson D. The recurrence of intracranial meningiomas after surgical treatment. *J Neurol Neurosurg Psychiatry* 1957;20:22–39.	http://jnnp.bmj.com/content/20/1/22
Glasgow Outcome Scale	Jennett B, Bond M. Assessment of outcome after severe brain damage. *Lancet* 1975;1:480–484.	http://www.thelancet.com/journals/lancet/article/PIIS0140-6736(75)92830-5/abstract

Score/Scale	Reference	Web address
Glasgow Outcome Scale extended	Wilson JTL, Pettigrew LEL, Teasdale GM. Structured interviews for the Glasgow Outcome Scale and the extended Glasgow Outcome Scale: Guidelines for their use. *J Neurotrauma* 1997;15:573–585.	http://online.liebertpub.com/doi/abs/10.1089/neu.1998.15.573
Modified Rankin Scale	Rankin J. Cerebral vascular accidents in patients over the age of 60. *Scott Med J* 1957;2:200–215. Bonita R, Beaglehole R. Recovery of motor function after stroke. *Stroke* 1988;19:1497–1500.	http://scm.sagepub.com/content/2/5/200.full.pdf+html http://stroke.ahajournals.org/content/19/12/1497

Index